T0074074

Procurement, Preservation and Allocation of Vascularized Organs

Procurement, Preservation and Allocation of Vascularized Organs

Edited by

G.M. Collins
California Pacific Medical Center, Department of Transplantation, San Francisco, California, USA

J.M. Dubernard
Transplantation Pavillon V, Hôpital Edouard Herriot, Lyon, France

W. Land
Division of Transplant Surgery, Department of Surgery, Klinikum Grosshadern, University of Munich, Munich, Germany

G.G. Persijn
Eurotransplant Foundation, Leiden, The Netherlands

Springer-Science+Business Media, B.V.

Library of Congress Cataloging-in-Publication Data
Procurement, preservation, and allocation of vascularized organs /
    edited by G.M. Collins ... [et al.].
        p.   cm.
    Includes bibliographical references and index.
    ISBN 978-94-010-6280-0   ISBN 978-94-011-5422-2 (eBook)
    DOI 10.1007/978-94-011-5422-2
    1. Donation of organs, tissues, etc.   2. Preservation of organs,
tissues, etc.   I. Collins, G.M.
    [DNLM: 1. Organ Procurement.   2. Organ Preservation.   3. Tissue
Donors.   WO 660 P964 997]
RD129.5.P754   1997
617.9′5 – dc21
DNLM/DLC
for Library of Congress   96–38863

ISBN 978-94-010-6280-0

Printed on acid-free paper

Contents

SECTION II: ORGAN PRESERVATION

SECTION III: ALLOCATION AND LOGISTICS

SECTION IV: ETHICS AND LEGISLATION IN ORGAN DONATION

Preface

At the brink of the third millennium organ transplantation will become routine and the results will be so excellent that every patient in need of a transplant deserves to be transplanted. How to provide every patient with his or her organ and how to guarantee that the organ is in a superb condition? That is the challenge for all of us privileged to work in this magnificent field of medicine.

In this book, an international team of experts has laid down their intellectual knowledge on the process that precedes successful transplantation: Procurement, Preservation and Allocation. In four sections important aspects of this preamble of the actual transplantation are dealt with.

Section 1 concerns donor conditioning and surgery, Section 2 the organ preservation, Section 3 allocation and logistics, while in Section 4 the important aspects of ethics and legislation in organ donation are covered. Experts from all over the world have contributed to this book, which therefore gives a unique overview of the topics from different angles. In particular, the section on allocation provides the reader with information how, in the case of shortage, a fair allocation of the scarce organs can be achieved. This is a very timely subject that continues to be discussed between doctors and between laymen.

This book serves the needs of several groups of specialists working with transplant patients. Firstly, the doctors who are directly involved in the care of the multi-organ donor, and who have to collaborate to do the best for their recipients. Heart surgeons might like to learn from liver surgeons and vice versa. Secondly, the paramedical specialist who is involved in the treatment of transplant patients and their families will find in this book many answers to questions. Students can also use it as a source for general information.

This book will be of great help in defining the material to be studied in educational courses and I hope it will find its way to the library shelf of every transplant program.

G. Kootstra
Maastricht, March 20, 1997

List of Contributors

Dr. D. Anaise
1001 West San Martin
TUCSON, AZ 85704
USA

Dr. H. Angstwurm
Neurologer Klinik
Universität München
Ziemssentrasse 1
D-80336 MUNCHEN
Germany

Dr. Nancy L. Ascher
Department of Transplantation
University of California San Francisco
505 Parnasus Avenue n. 886
SAN FRANCISCO, CA 94143-0780
USA

Dr. G. Bagou
Service d'Anesthésie Réanimation VII
Hôpital Edouard Herriot
69437 LYON Cedex 03
France

Dr. C. Baude
Service d'Anesthésie Réanimation
Hôpital Edouard Herriot
Pavillon V
69437 LYON Cedex 03
France

Dr. Dieter Birnbacher
Universität Dortmund
Fachbereich 14
D-44221 DORTMUND
Germany

Dr. O. Boillot
Unité de Transplantation Hépatique
Fédération des Spécialités Digestives
Hôpital Edouard Herriot
F-69437 LYON Cedex 03
France

Dr. G.E. Chatrian
Professor Emeritus
Division of Electroencephalography and Clinical
Neurophysiology
Department of Neurology,
University of Washington School of
Medicine
Seattle, WA.
USA

Dr. P. Cloix
Service d'Urologie et Chirurgie de
Transplantation
Hôpital Edouard Herriot
Place d'Arsonval
69437 LYON Cedex 03
France

Dr B. Cohen
Eurotransplant Foundation
P.O. Box 2304
2301 CH LEIDEN
The Netherlands

Dr. G.M. Collins
Chairman, Department of Transplantation
California Pacific Medical Center
2340 Clay Street, Suite 251
SAN FRANCISCO, CA 94115
USA

Dr. J.J. Colpart
Coordination Center
Regionale et hospitalier
Hôpital Edouard Herriot
F-69437 LYON CEDEX 03
France

Dr. A.S. Daar
Department of Surgery
P.O. Box 35
Al-Khod
123-MUSCAT
Sultanate of Oman

Dr. M. Dawahra
Service d'Urologie et Chirurgie de Transplantation
Hôpital Edouard Herriot
Place d'Arsonval
69437 LYON Cedex 03
France

Dr. F. Th. De Charro
Eurotransplant Foundation
P.O. Box 2304
2301 CH LEIDEN
The Netherlands

Dr. B. Delafosse
Service d'Anesthésie Réanimation V
Hôpital Edouard Herriot
69437 LYON Cedex 03
France

Dr. Ronald M. Ferguson
Department of Surgery
Ohio State University
327 Means Hall
1654 Upham Drive
COLUMBUS, OH 43210
USA

Ms Patricia Franklin
44 Axtell Road
Kidlington
OXFORD
UK

Dr. D. Gille
Unité de Transplantation Hépatique
Fédération des Spécialités Digestives
Hôpital Edouard Herriot
69437 LYON Cedex 03
France

Dr. M.C. Graber
Pavillon H.
Hôpital Edouard Herriot
69437 LYON Cedex 03
France

Dr. Thomas Gutmann
Leopold Wenger-Institut für Rechtsgeschichte
(Abt.B) Universität München
Prof-Huber-Platz 2
D-80539 MUNCHEN
Germany

Drs B. Haase-Kromwijk
St. Eurotransplant Nederland
Postbus 2304
2301 CH LEIDEN
The Netherlands

Professor Axel Haverich
Medizinische Hochschule Hannover
Klinik fur Thorax-, Herz – und
Gefasschirurgie
Konstanty Gutschowstrasse 8
D-30625 HANNOVER
Germany

Dr. E. Heineman
Afdeling Chirurgie
Academisch Ziekenhuis Maastricht
P.O. Box 5800
6202 AZ MAASTRICHT
The Netherlands

Dr. M.L. Henry
Ohio State University
Department of Surgery
Division of Tansplantation
259 Means Hall, 1654 Upham Drive
COLUMBUS, OH 43210-1228
USA

Dr. N.V. Jamieson
Department of Surgery
Addenbrooke's Hospital
Hills Road
CAMBRIDGE CB2 2QQ
UK

Dr. Uwe Jost
Universität Leipzig
Bereich Medizin
Transplantationsburo
Liebigstrasse 20a
D-04103 LEIPZIG
Germany

Dr. G. Kootstra
Department of Surgery
Academisch Ziekenhuis Maastricht
Heelkunde
P.O. Box 5800
6202 AZ MAASTRICHT
The Netherlands

Dr. C. Kopp
Service d'Anesthésie Réanimation IV
Hôpital Edouard Herriot
69437 LYON Cedex 03
France

Dr M.M. Koerner
Herz-& Diabeteszentr. Nordhein-Westfalen
Univ. Klin d. Universität Bochum
Klinik für Thorax und Kardiovaskularchirurgie
Georgstrasse 11
D-32545 BAD OEYNHAUSEN
Germany

Professor W. Land
Head of Division Transplantation Surgery
Klinikum Grosshadern
University of Munich
Marchioninistrasse 15
D-81366 MUNCHEN
Germany

Dr N. Lenfrancois
Service de Medicine de La Transplantation
Hôspital E. Herriot
Place d'Arsonval
F-69437 LYON
France

Dr. J.J. LeMasters
Laboratory of Cell Biology
Department of Cell Biology and Anatomy
The University of North Carolina
Campus Box 7090, 236 Taylor Hall
CHAPEL HILL, NC 27599-7090
USA

Dr. D. Long
Service d'Anesthésie Réanimation IV
Hôspital E. Herriot
Place d'Arsonval
F-694377 LYON
France

Dr K. McNeil
Transplant Unit
Papworth Hospital
Papworth Everard
CAMBRIDGE CB3 8RE
UK

Dr. M.J. Lindop
Department of Anaesthesia
Addenbrookes Hospital
CAMBRIDGE CB2 2QA
UK

Dr. R. Margreiter
Department of Transplant Surgery
University Hospital
Anichstrasse 35
A-6020 INNSBRUCK
Austria

Dr. V. Marshall
Department of Surgery
Monash University
Prince Henry's Hospital
St. Kilda
MELBOURNE, VICTORIA 3004
Australia

Dr. X. Martin
Service d'Urologie et de Chirurgie de Transplantation
Pavillon V
Hôpital Edouard Herriot
Place d'Arsonval
69437 LYON Cedex 03
France

Dr. J.M.J. De Meester
St. Eurotransplant Nederland
Postbus 2304
2301 CH LEIDEN
The Netherlands

Dr. A. Mercatello
Centre d'acceuil de la mort cérébrale
Service d'anesthésie et réanimation
Pavillon P
Hôpital Edouard Heriot
69437 LYON Cedex 03
France

Dr. J. Ninet
Hôpital Louis Pradel
F-69500 BRON
France

Dr. D. Novitzky
The University of South Florida
College of Medicine, Dept. of Surgery
Harbourside Medical Tower, Suite 730
4 Columbia Drive
TAMPA, FL 33606
USA

Dr. G.G. Persijn
Eurotransplant Foundation
P. O. Box 2304
2301 CH LEIDEN
The Netherlands

Dr. Rutger J. Ploeg
Department of Surgery
University Hospital Groningen
P.O Box 30 001
9700 RB GRONINGEN
The Netherlands

Dr. Leo Roels
CPTC
The Leuven Colloborative
Group for Transplantation
Heerestraat 49
B-3000 LEUVEN
Belgium

Dr. X. Rogiers
Universität Hamburg
Chirurgische Klinik
Martinistrasse 52
D-20246 HAMBURG
Germany

Dr. P. Sagnard
Pavillon D
Hôpital Edouard Herriot
F-69437 LYON Cedex 03
France

Professor Klaus A. Schneewind
Institut für Psychologie
Universität München
Leopoldstrasse 13
D-80802 MUNCHEN
Germany

Dr. Robert A. Sells
Director Renal Transplant Unit
Royal Liverpool University Hospital
Prescot Street
LIVERPOOL, L7 8XP
UK

Dr. J.M.A. Smits
St. Eurotransplant Nederland
Postbus 2304
2301 CH LEIDEN
The Netherlands

Dr. J.H. Southard
Department of Surgery
University of Wisconsin
H4/332 Clinical Science Center
600 Highland Avenue
MADISON, WI 53792-3236
USA

Professor D.E.R. Sutherland
Department of Surgery
Box 280 UMHC
University of Minnesota
420 Delaware Street S.E.
Minneapolis, MN 55455
USA

Professor G. Thiel
Abteilung für Nephrologie
Universitätskliniken
Kantonspital Basel
Petersgraben 4
CH-4031 Basel
Switzerland

Dr. Luis H. Toledo-Pereyra
The Michigan Transplant Institute
at Borgess Medical Center
1521 Gull Road
KALAMAZOO, MI 49001
USA

Dr. M.E. Wachs
Department of Transplantation
University of California San Francisco
505 Parnasus Avenue, n 886
SAN FRANCISCO, CA 94143-0780
USA

Dr.J. Wallwork
Cambridge
Transplant Unit
Papworth Hospital
Papworth Everard
CAMBRIDGE CB3 8RE
UK

Dr. A. de Wit
Stichting Renine
p/a Erasmus Universiteit
Faculteit Rechtsgeleerdheid
Postbus 1738
3000 DR ROTTERDAM
The Netherlands

Dr. W.N. Wicomb
Department of Transplantation
California Pacific Medical Center
2340 Clay Street, Suite 251
SAN FRANCISCO, CA 94115
USA

Celia Wight
Donor Action Secretariat
The White House
67 London Road
Harston
CAMBRIDGE CB2 5QJ
UK

Dr. R.M.H. Wijnen
Catharina Ziekenhuis Eindhoven
Michel Angeloolaan 2
5623 EJ EINDHOVEN
The Netherlands

Section I
Donor Conditioning and Surgery

1 | Living kidney donation: preoperative evaluation and preparation for surgery

N. Lefrancois and J.L. Touraine

1. Introduction – justification

Patients developing end stage renal disease can be treated by haemodialysis, peritoneal dialysis or transplantation. Kidney transplantation is now generally accepted as the primary therapy for chronic renal failure in most patients, with the exception of those who cannot tolerate immunosuppressive treatment or transplant surgery [1]. Many reasons justify the use of kidneys from living donors. Although the overall short and long term results for all donor categories have increased in recent years, transplants from living related donors have a higher success rate than those from cadaver donors [2]. In our experience with living donor transplantation since 1966, survival of kidney grafts from living donors is 20% higher at 10 years than for those from cadaver donors. The introduction of cyclosporin was responsible for increased survival of all categories of transplants. In our series this increase was 15% for cadaveric donors and 20% for living donors. The benefit was more pronounced in patients receiving kidneys from parents (+35%) and, in this category, no effect of age was observed in the long term analysis.

The use of kidneys from living donors is also justified by the increasing shortage of cadaver kidneys, which are far from fulfilling the needs of recipients awaiting transplantation. As results of kidney trans-plantation have improved during recent years, high-risk patients can be safely transplanted, increasing the numbers on waiting lists. In France, more than 4000 patients are awaiting transplantation, and less than 2000 are transplanted every year. Some high-risk patients, such as those highly sensitized or awaiting retransplantation, may wait for more than 10 years for an adequate cadaver kidney [3].

An additional argument for the use of living donor is that transplantation can be planned for a specific date, reducing waiting time on dialysis or even being performed before the beginning of chronic dialysis. This is important for economic reasons. Furthermore a planned operation can be performed at a time that does not interfere with the patient's employment or education. Another advantage of shortening the period of dialysis is the avoidance of the risk of necessary blood transfusions and consequent limitation of anti-HLA immunization.

Living related donors potentially reduce immuno-suppressive treatment and, therefore, the risk of complications such as viral infections in the short term or malignancies in the long term. Finally, kidneys from living donors do not suffer from cold ischaemia and they may be less susceptible to cyclosporin nephro-toxicity [4].

Despite these reasons favouring the use of living donors, the removal of a normal kidney for transplanta-

G.M. Collins, J.M. Dubernard, W. Land and G.G. Persijn (eds). Procurement, Preservation and Allocation of Vascularized Organs 3–10
© 1997 Kluwer Academic Publishers.

tion should not be associated with significant morbidity or mortality for the donor. Donation must be carefully evaluated in order to minimize the risks of nephrectomy in the healthy donor. Our policy is to inform systematically the recipient and the family considering living related donation. The donor must be perfectly and objectively informed and there must be adequate indications regarding the recipient's prognosis. To minimize risks for the potential living donor, a detailed and extensive pretransplantation evaluation is necessary. This should consider the donor's emotional health, the strength of his motivation to donation and the possible consequences on the donor and his family. Evaluation of donor's physical health and renal function is mandatory in order to select a donor without disease and with no predictable adverse consequences of nephrectomy.

2. Preoperative evaluation

Preoperative evaluation is carefully performed in several stages. We carry out the analyses shown in Table 1, to evaluate kidney donors.

2.1. The search for an ABO-compatible family donor

ABO blood compatibility between donor and recipient is considered an absolute requirement for transplantation. Several groups have reported successful results following ABO-incompatible transplants after removal of ABO isoagglutinins by plasmaphoresis and splenectomy of the recipient [5,6]. However, extensive preoperative preparation of the recipient and higher rates of morbidity suggest that these procedures can be performed only under certain circumstances. The prospective donor is first screened for motivation and emotional stability. On ethical grounds, to exclude paid donors, and for genetic reasons (compatibility being comparable with that of cadaver donors), non-family volunteers and remote family members are presently excluded as organ living donors in most developed countries.

2.2. Clinical evaluation

The second stage is clinical analysis to confirm the general good health of the potential donor. Many of the

---

Table 1. Evaluation of potential intrafamilial donors.

Clinical approach
   History, physical and psychological evaluation
   ABO blood group
   Repeated blood pressure determinations
   Electrocardiogram, chest X-ray, abdominal echography
   Pelvic examination for women

Biological and immunological tests
   Laboratory studies: Na, K, Cl, CO_2, BUN, creatinine, Ca, phos, uric acid, AST, ALT, LDM, Alk phos, T. bili, chol, trigly, Apo A, Apo B, FBS, OGTT, HbAlc, urine culture, proteinuria, urine cytology
   HbS, HIV, HTLV, EBV, VHC, CMV serologies
   Tissue typing

Renal function tests

Polyfructosan and PAH clearance
Morphological evaluation
   Intravenous pyelogram
   Renal arteriogram

Over 50 years
   Pulmonary evaluation
   Cardiac evaluation

studies aim to detect unsuspected extrarenal pathology in the donor. This step includes medical history and physical examination with blood pressure measurement, electrocardiogram, chest X-ray, abdominal echography and pelvic examination in women.

2.3. Biological and immunological evaluation

Biological and immunological evaluation includes blood and urinary tests to evaluate kidney, liver, pancreas and haemopoietic function. Parasitic, mycotic, viral and bacteria screening is also performed. Tissue typing and leucocyte cross-matching identify the most compatible donor–recipient pair. The cross-match is a laboratory test in which recipient serum is added to donor lymphocytes in the presence of complement. If the cross-match is positive the donor's lymphocytes are lysed by preformed antibodies directed against donor cells. Identical twins and HLA identical siblings are very good donors but they are comparatively rare. If several potential donors are equally compatible (e.g. parent or haplo-identical sibling) mixed lymphocyte culture (MLC) can identify the potential donor showing the least stimulation of host cells.

In overweight patients, measurement of haemoglobin A_{1C} and an oral glucose tolerance test (OGTT) using 50 g of glucose are performed to identify subclinical diabetes.

2.4. Renal function evaluation

The fourth stage includes physiological tests to confirm excellent bilateral function of the kidneys: lack of proteinuria, urine cytology, renal function study and kidney scintigraphy. In our unit, renal function study is performed as follows: after overnight fasting, polyfructosan (Inutest®, Laevoson, Linz, Austria) and sodium paraminohippurate (PAH, Nephrotest®, BA GmBH, Lich, Germany) are administered by an i.v. infusion of 30 mg/kg polyfructosan and 15 mg/kg PAH (made up to 120 ml with mannitol 10%) and given at a rate of 10 ml for 12 minutes. This is followed by an infusion of 40 mg/kg polyfructosan and 30 mg/kg PAH in mannitol 10% at 1 ml/min. After a 30 minute equilibration period, the urine is discarded and 30 minute control periods are considered. For each period of urine collection, the following measurements are made in plasma and urine: concentrations of sodium and potassium, chloride, creatinine, urea, osmolality, polyfructosan and PAH. GFR is calculated as polyfructosan clearance and renal plasma flow as PAH clearance. Creatinine clearance, excretion rate of

sodium, potassium, chloride and urea and fractional tubular reabsorption of sodium, chloride and potassium are also determined [8].

2.5. Morphological evaluation

The final step is a morphological approach, including intravenous pyelography and kidney arteriography by the classic Seldinger femoral route. Angiography is required to determine the exact status of the renal arteries and to eliminate unsuspected intrarenal lesions.

3. Criteria for exclusion

In most countries, the use of living volunteer donors less than 18 years of age is not usually allowed. Kidney donation from elderly living donors can be considered in rare circumstances.

Our transplant unit analysed criteria for exclusion in 248 ABO compatible potential volunteers investigated for potential kidney donation between August 1975 and February 1984. Ninety (36%) of these 248 volunteers were not accepted for various reasons [9]. Thirty-five per cent of volunteers were refused on the basis of their medical history or clinical examination. The reasons for refusal at this stage were: 14 donors (mean age 54 years) had high blood pressure (mean systolic blood pressure 170.5 mmHg; mean diastolic blood pressure 100.5 mmHg). Patients with systolic pressure above 140 mmHg and diastolic pressure above 90 mmHg, measured by 24 h blood pressure monitoring or patients requiring antihypertensive drugs to normalize blood pressure were excluded as kidney donors.

Eighteen other potential donors presented other clinical manifestations or biological abnormalities: six patients had a past history of proteinuria. Potential kidney donors must have no evidence of abnormal proteinuria in a 24 h collection of urine. Any nephrological or urological abnormality that might present a future risk to either donor or recipient is an exclusion criterion. A history of duodenal ulcer (2), Down's syndrome (1), glomerulonephritis (1), tuberculosis (1), congenital hip subluxation (1), non-insulin dependent diabetes (2) and psychosis (1) were additional reasons for refusal as kidney donors. We have a routine policy of obtaining psychiatric evaluation for all donors to detect psychiatric disorders. A stable emotional relationship between donor and recipient should exist and the donor's motivation must be altruistic, donation for profit being considered as condemnable. Three other patients were eliminated on the basis of cardiovascular disease (myocardial infarction), chronic bronchitis and asthma, and obesity with varicose vein in the lower limbs (which may be an increased risk for pulmonary embolism after surgery).

Specific caution was taken when renal failure in the recipient had resulted from an hereditary disease. The risk of the potential donor developing diabetes in the future is very high when both parents are diabetic [10]. In the case of adult polycystic kidney disease, selection is generally limited to individuals over 30 years of age and with no abnormality on intravenous pyelography, ultrasonography of the kidneys and the liver, and arteriography [11] when there is a family history of hereditary nephritis, it is considered that progressive disease is associated with proteinuria or with haematuria at a relatively early age. In such families, the use of a 25-year-old donor with no evidence of renal disease is possible [12].

At the third stage, 36 patients (40% of these rejected) were refused for biological abnormalities or immunological incompatibilities. Eight potential donors had abnormal proteinuria or microscopic haematuria, probably related to glomerulonephritis. Eleven potential donors presented liver abnormalities (cytolysis or HbsAg positive). At present, patients positive for hepatitis C virus are not considered for kidney donation because of the risk of viral transmission to the recipient. If the HIV antibody test is positive, the donor is rejected. In all cases, information is given to the individuals for their future care. Two donors had suspected systemic lupus erythematosus (SLE). Relatives of patients with SLE have an increased frequency of autoimmune disease [13]. Two further patients were excluded as a result of a serological evidence of syphilis.

If glucose tolerance detected by fasting blood glucose, OGTT and haemoglobin A_{1C} measurement is normal, the donor is considered to be non-diabetic. In patients with obesity, impaired glucose tolerance (IGT) and hyperlipidaemia were often found. Twenty potential donors (22%) were obese, 27 (30%) had IGT and 31 (34%) had hyperlipidaemia type II, abnormalities mostly found after 40 years; among our potential donors presenting a normal OGTT 85% were normal weight and 15% were obese. Among the potential donors presenting with disturbed OGTT, 52% had normal weight and 48% were obese. Patients with a disturbed OGTT and obesity must be carefully studied before any decision is made since the risk of developing diabetes after donation of the kidney is important. Weight must always be reduced to normal range before nephrectomy.

Seventeen patients were refused for immunological incompatibilities: seven had a positive cross-match with recipients, six potential donors had major HLA incompatibilities, one had Lewis incompatibility and three had high stimulation indices in MLC. A negative cross-match is an absolute requirement for transplantation. An HLA-identical sibling is the ideal donor, but if serological testing identifies several equally compatible potential donors (either haplo-identical sibling or parent), selection of the best intrafamilial donor may be determined on the basis of age and results of MLC. In a previous study we found a strong association between a weak allogenic proliferative response and graft survival: in 65 haplo-identical recipients, graft survival rate was better in patients with a stabilized relative response (SRR) < 30%: 100% at 5 years vs. 69% in patients with an SRR > 30%. There was also a strong association between the number of patients with rejection and SRR > 30% [14].

At the fourth stage, 18 (20%) patients were refused for abnormal renal glomerular filtration rate or renal blood flow. In our laboratory, normal glomerular filtration measured as inulin clearance per 1.73 m^2 is 2.1 ± 0.5 ml/s and normal plasma renal flow measured by PAH clearance is 10.8 ± 2.8 ml/s. In our patients, there was a statistically significant difference in age ($p < 0.001$) in the group of patients with normal clearance (40.4 ± 10.6 years) and those with abnormal clearance (50.2 ± 9.4). Precise evaluation of renal function is therefore mandatory and pre-existing renal disease excludes a potential donor because of the future likelihood of decreased renal function and increased incidence of hypertension with nephrectomy.

Finally 4 donors were excluded for morphological abnormalities: three donors presented renal fibromuscular dysplasia and one had a pelvic kidney with multiple arteries. Most transplant teams avoid transplanting abnormal kidneys. It is preferable to transplant a kidney with a single artery, although it is possible to transplant a kidney with multiple arteries. The left kidney is usually chosen because the longer renal vein contributes to easier nephrectomy and transplantation. Others have, however, reported long term rates using anatomically abnormal kidneys. The types of abnormalities present in these transplanted kidneys were: hypoplasia [15], fibromuscular or mild atherosclerotic disease of the renal artery, presence of multiple arteries, microaneurysms or hydronephrosis [16,17].

To summarize our experience in selecting potential living donors, 36% of potential living donors were excluded from donation. Of these 75% were refused as a result of simple tests and not following invasive tests. However, refused donors were further investigated to determine the causes of their abnormalities and

Table 2. Criteria for exclusion of potential donors.

Age < 18 years

Medical history of HTA, diabetes, malignancy, generalized bacterial or viral infection (HBS, HIV, VHC), deep vein thrombophlebitis

Evidence of primary renal disease: history of kidney stone, proteinuria, abnormal glomerular filtration rate or plasmatic renal flow, microscopic haematuria, urological abnormalities

Psychiatric disorders

---

invasive tests had to be performed to document three renal arterial stenoses, five renal tumour syndromes, one ureteropelvic function abnormality, two renal artery aneurysms and two cases of renal tuberculosis.

Table 2 reviews the reasons for exclusion of potential donors.

4. Short and long term risks for the donor

4.1. Short term complications and mortality

The short and long term risks to the donor are minimal in any evaluation. Mortality as a result of nephrectomy was rare in a survey of the literature [18–21]. One series reported two deaths in a total of 5698 living donor transplants [12]. A more recent assessment of perioperative mortality of donors was achieved by a survey of all members of the American Society of Transplant Surgeons. Between January 1980 and January 1991, the estimated perioperative mortality in the USA was 0.03% among 19 368 living related donor nephrectomies [18]. The most common cause is pulmonary embolism.

Major but reversible complications occur in the immediate postoperative period in 1.8–3% of donors. These include deep wound infections, local haemorrhages, thrombophlebitis with or without pulmonary emboli, and myocardial infarction [18,21]. Minor complications are observed with an incidence of 10–20% superficial wound infection, atelectasis and pneumothorax, urinary infection, reversible renal failure, acute retention or prolonged ileus [22,23].

4.2. Long term risks

Late complications related to nephrectomy can be seen after the operation: incisional pain, incisional hernia,

keloid or lumbar pain. Beekman reported six long term complications related to the incision and one incisional hernia required surgical correction in 47 donors [24].

4.2.1. Renal function

Unilateral nephrectomy was long considered to be without adverse consequences because survival of subjects following nephrectomy was no different from that of the general population [25]. Indeed, uninephrectomy in a patient with two normally functioning kidneys results in early functional adaptation, with compensatory hypertrophy and hyperfiltration in the remaining kidney.

However, this compensatory hyperfiltration may be detrimental to renal function: rats show progressive glomerulosclerosis after severe reduction in renal mass [26]. The increase in renal blood flow and glomerular filtration rate per nephron in the remaining kidney after unilateral nephrectomy may be relevant to the kidney donor. However, many long term clinical arguments indicate that patients with a single normal kidney are not at increased risk for progressive renal failure. After a mean follow up of 23 years (range 17–33) in 27 patients who had undergone unilateral nephrectomy in childhood, creatinine clearance was 83.9 ± 6.5 ml/min/1.73 m² or 74.3% of that in healthy controls with two kidneys [27], a value similar to that reported 3–6 months post-nephrectomy in kidney donors. None of these patients had clinically important hypertension or proteinuria.

Long term follow-up also indicates that kidney donors are not at increased risk for progressive renal failure, and glomerular filtration rate is independent of mean post-operative follow up, ranging between 66 ml/min/1.73 m² and 87 ml/min/1.73 m² [24,28–33]. In the longest mean follow up of kidney donors (23.7 years, range 21–29 years), Najarian et al. [18] found no significant difference in serum creatinine, BUN or creatinine clearance in donors and sibling controls. Furthermore, 53% of donors whose creatinine clearance was below normal had one or more sibling with an abnormal value, in contrast to the donors whose clearance was normal [20]. We studied 99 living donors before and after nephrectomy from 1967 to 1994 [32–34]. The mean follow up was 4.25 years (range 1.4 months to 19 years). Mean inulin clearance decreased from 115 ± 15 ml/min before donation to 80 ± 12 ml/min after donation, corresponding to an increase of 40%. Comparison between two groups age < 37 years and > 37 years confirmed a significant adaptation in young donors at nephrectomy. No significant sex-related changes were seen in our patients. However, Anderson et al. reported a significantly greater degree of compensatory hypertrophy in male patients (46.9% at 1 week) than in female patients (26.7%) [35]. Secondary and prolonged increase in glomerular filtration may be observed according to time post nephrectomy. In our patients, longitudinal studies showed no deterioration with time up to 22 years; inulin and PAH clearances showed some tendency to increase progressively until 20 years post-nephrectomy, results also observed by Higashihara et al., who showed a progressive increase in creatinine clearance from 70 ml/min less than 5 years after nephrectomy to 78 ml/min more than 21 years after nephrectomy [36].

4.2.2. *Proteinuria*

Proteinuria is reported in relatively few donors and is generally mild; it appears to be non-progressive and not associated with renal dysfunction. About one-third of donors develops microalbuminuria or proteinuria with long time follow up, with a maximum of 94% in the study of Higashihara et al. [36]. In our study 21% of donors had microalbuminuria [33]. Only one study shows a group of 21 donors with no microalbuminuria 12 years after nephrectomy [37].

Higashihara et al. found a significant correlation between proteinuria and post-operative follow up in patients who underwent nephrectomy for various reasons [36]. In our patients and in other studies, no correlation was found between proteinuria and the length of follow up [33].

4.2.3. *Hypertension*

In our kidney donors, no hypertension was observed 1.4 month to 22 years after nephrectomy. Williams et al. and Najarian et al. found no increase in frequency of hypertension in donors when siblings were used as controls and hypertensive patients show no significant modification of renal function compared with patients with no hypertension [18,28]. Anderson et al. found that the prevalence of hypertension in kidney donors was similar to that in the general population, with the exception of male donors aged 50–69 years who had a higher frequency of hypertension than matched controls [38]. Talseth et al. re-examined 92% of living donors 9–15 years after donation and found 15% to be hypertensive, with an age range of 53–84 years. Of these, only 5% could be considered completely normotensive preoperatively [39].

4.2.4. *Psychosocial consequences of kidney donation*

Morris et al. [40], in a retrospective study of 15 living related donors over the period 1980–1985, showed that in one-third of subjects the post-donation period was complicated by significant reductions in quality of life. They conclude that factors likely to predict psychosocial complications for living related kidney donors include older donors, rejection of the graft, lower level of educational attainment and absence of stable personal relationships.

The donation of a kidney is a loss to the individual concerned but it may also have a great impact on the family of the donor. It is advisable to perform pre-transplant evaluation of psychosocial status of all potential kidney donors and, if possible, of other members of the family in order to detect patients at high risk for psychological post-donation sequelae.

Renal transplantation with an intrafamilial donor may avoid problems due to anonymity, especially those related to the donor identity. The amputation for one and the transplantation for the other relates to the idea of 'giving' and 'losing' for some and 'taking' and 'receiving' for others [41]. Long term follow up indicates that some donors tend to view donation more as a moral decision; with time they continue to feel that they made the best decision and would do it again if the opportunity were again available [1].

Many donors report increased self-esteem after donation, whatever the transplant kidney outcome was in the recipient [7]. Bonomini and Gozzetti showed minimal negative psychological reactions in donors even in the long term and when the transplantation is unsuccessful, but among their 54 donors, 9.2% had increased feelings of depression, though 100% of them found their efficiency at work unchanged [21].

5. Preparation for surgery

The donor is generally admitted in hospital 2 days before nephrectomy. General biological status and co-agulation are again studied and the negativity of the cross-match is confirmed. The mean hospital stay for donors is approximately 2 weeks after nephrectomy. Beekman et al. [24] reported the same mean hospital stay in those with and without complications: 10.8 ± 1.8 days (range 8–14 days) and 11.2 ± 2.2 days (range 8–17 days), respectively. Donors usually resume their employment 1–2 months after nephrectomy.

6. Conclusion

We can suggest some guidelines for prospective living donors elaborated on the basis of selection, evaluation and long term evolution. First, the donor's motives must be altruistic and donation for profit is condemnable. The donation must be voluntary and it should not be a response to family pressures. The donation must be based on full awareness after significant information. Furthermore, stringent medical evaluation and selection has to be performed to exclude any evidence of disease and any increased risk for the nephrectomy.

HLA compatibilities between donor and recipient should be optimal, the ideal donor being an HLA-identical sibling. A negative cross-match between donor and recipient is mandatory.

Regular postoperative evaluation of the donor is recommended, including psychological and clinical examinations (blood pressure, biological analysis with 24 h microalbuminuria and proteinuria, serum creatinine level and creatinine clearance).

In such conditions, short and long term morbidity related to donor nephrectomy appears to be low. Long term studies, 20 years after nephrectomy, have shown that glomerular changes observed after nephrectomy remain stable. Although about 20–30% of donors develop proteinuria or hypertension, there is no evidence that removal of a kidney represents a long term risk for deterioration of function in the remaining kidney.

References

1. Briggs JD. The recipient of a renal transplant. In: Morris PJ (ed.) Kidney Transplantation. WB Saunders Co., Philadelphia 1988, pp. 71–92.
2. Najarian JS, Matas AJ. The present and future of kidney transplantation. Transplant Proc 1991; 23: 2075–82.
3. France Transplant. Rapport annuel, 1993.
4. Canadian Transplant Study Group. Examination of parameters influencing the benefit detriment ratio of ciclosporine in renal transplantation. Am J Kidney Dis 1985; 5: 328–32.
5. Breimer ME, Samuelsson BE. The specific distribution of glycolipid-based blood group A antigens in human kidney related to A1/A2, Lewis and secretor status of single individuals. Transplantation 1986; 42: 88–91.
6. Alexandre GP, Squifflet JP, Debruyere M et al. Present experience in a series of 26 ABO incompatible living donor renal allografts. Transplant Proc 1987; 19: 4538–42.
7. Kamstra-Hennen L, Beebe J, Stumm S et al. Ethical evaluation of related donation: the donor after five years. Transplant Proc 1981; 13: 60–1.
8. Hadj-Aissa A, Bankir L, Eraysse M et al. Influence of the level of hydration on the renal response to a protein seal. Kidney Int 1992; 42: 1207–16.
9. Cantarovich D, Alcazar-Flores R, Piatti PM et al. Selection of living kidney donors: 90 of 248 compatible volunteers were not accepted. In: Touraine JL et al. (eds). Transplantation and Clinical Immunology. Elsevier Science Publishers, Amsterdam 1985; 24: 241–43.
10. Goto Y, Kakizaki M, Toyota T. Heredity of diabetes mellitus. In: Melish JS, Hanna J, Baba S (eds). Genetic Environmental Interaction of Diabetes Mellitus. Excerpta Medica, Amsterdam 1982; pp. 18–29.
11. Milutinovic J, Fialkow PJ, Phillips LA et al. Autosomal dominant polycystic kidney disease: early diagnosis and data for genetic counselling. Lancet 1980; 1: 1203–6.
12. Bay WH, Hebert LA. The living donor in kidney transplantation. Ann Intern Med 1987; 106: 719–27.
13. Lahita RG, Chiorazzi N, Gibotesky A, Winchester RJ, Kunkel HG. Family systemic lupus erythematosus in males. Arthritis Rheum 1983; 26: 39–44.
14. Pouteil Noble C, Betuel H, Freidel AC, Dubernard JM, Touraine JL. Correlation between the allogenic proliferative response and the outcome of renal transplantation. Transplant Proc 1987; 19: 3637–9.
15. Dandavino R, Beaudry C. Girard R, Bastiene E, Pison C, Houde M. Growth response of an adult hypoplastic kidney transplanted in a living related recipient. Transplantation 1985; 40: 723–4.
16. Waltzer WC, Engen DE. Stanson AW et al. Use of radiographically abnormal kidneys in living related donor renal transplantation. Nephron 1985; 39: 302–5.
17. Brandina L, Fraga AMA, Bergonse MRR et al. Kidney transplantation: the use of abnormal kidneys. Nephron 1983; 35: 78–81.
18. Najarian S, Chavers BM. McHugh LE, Matas AJ. 20 years or more of follow-up of living kidney donors. N Engl J Med 1992; 340: 807–10.
19. Bennett AM. Harrison JM. Experience with living familial related donors. Surg Gynecol Obstet 1974; 139: 894–8.
20. Starzl TE. Living donors. Transplant Proc 1987; 19: 174–6.
21. Bonomini V. Gozzetti G. Is living donation still justifiable? Nephrol Dial Transplant 1990; 5: 407–9.
22. Levey AS, Hou S, Bush HL. Kidney transplantation from unrelated living donors. N Engl J Med 1986; 314: 914–16.
23. Weiland D, Sutherland DER, Chavers B et al. Information on 628 living-related kidney donors at a single institution, with long term follow-up in 472 cases. Transplant Proc 1984; 16: 5–7.
24. Beekman GM, Van Dorp WT, Van Es LA et al. Analysis of donor selection procedure in 139 living-related kidney donors and follow-up results of donors and recipients. Nephrol Dial Transplant 1994; 9: 163–8.
25. Andersen B. Hansen JB, Jorgensen SJ. Survival after nephrectomy. Scand J Urol Nephrol 1968; 2: 91–4.
26. Brenner BM. Hemodynamically mediated glomerular injury and the progressive nature of kidney disease. Kidney Int 1983; 23: 647–55.
27. Robitaille P, Mongeau JG, Lortie L et al. Long term follow-up of patients who underwent unilateral nephrectomy in childhood. Lancet 1985; x: 1297–9.
28. Williams S. Oler J, Jorkasky DK. Long term renal function in kidney donors: a comparison of donors and their siblings. Ann Intern Med 1986; 105: 1–8.
29. Watnick TJ, Jenkins RR, Rackoff P et al. Microalbuminuria and hypertension in long term renal donors. Transplantation 1988; 45: 59–65.
30. Vicentini F, Amen WJC, Keysen G et al. Long term renal function in kidney donors: sustained compensatory hyperfiltration with no adverse effects. Transplantation 1983; 36: 626–9.
31. Ogden DA. Consequences of renal donation in man. Am J Kidney Dis 1983; 105: 1–8.
32. Hadj-Aissa A, Cochat P. Pozet N et al. Renal function studies before and after nephrectomy in renal donors. Transplant Clin Immunol 1985; 16: 249–52.
33. Fourcade J. Evolution à long de la fonction rénale chez 99 donneurs vivants. Thèse Lyon 1994.
34. Hadj-Aissa A. Pozet N. Facteurs d'adaptation fonctionnelle du rein restant après néphrectomie chez les donneurs vivants. Pédiatrie 1993; 48: 102–4.
35. Anderson RG, Bueschen AJ, Lloyd K et al. Short term and long term changes in renal function after donor nephrectomy. J Urol 1991; 145: 11–13.
36. Higashihara E, Horie S, Takeuchi T et al. Long term consequences of nephrectomy. J Urol 1990; 143: 239–43.
37. Schmitz A, Christensen CK, Christensen T et al. No microalbuminuria or other adverse effects of long standing hyper-

filtration in humans with one kidney. Am J Kidney Dis 1989; 13: 131–6.

38. Anderson C, Velosa JA, Frohnert PP *et al.* The risks of unilateral nephrectomy: status of kidney donors 10 to 20 years postoperatively. Mayo Clin Proc 1985; 60: 367–74.

39. Talseth T, Fauchald P, Skrede S *et al.* Long term blood pressure and renal function in kidney donors. Kidney Int 1986; 29: 1072–6.

40. Morris P, St George B, Waring T *et al.* Psychosocial complications in living related kidney donors: an Australian experience. Transplant Proc. 1982; 19: 2840–4.

41. Boisriveaud C. Les problèmes psychologiques des donneurs vivants dans la transplantation renale. Psychol Méd 1994; 26: 159–61.

42. Bonomini V. Ethical aspects of living donation. Transplant Proc 1991; 23: 2497–9.

2 | Kidney recovery from living related donors

X. Martin, P. Cloix, M. Dawahra and J.M. Dubernard

1. Introduction

The superiority of short and long term results obtained with transplants from living related donors was particularly notable in the era before cyclosporin. Since the availability of cyclosporin and improved immunosuppression protocols, the difference between the results obtained with cadaveric and living related donors are less extreme; however, transplants from living related donors continue to produce better long term results [1]. An additional reason for the use of living related donors for transplantation is the increasing shortage of cadaver donors. It would, however, not be possible to justify the use of living related donors if the procedure had significant morbidity or mortality. A study of the experience at the Cleveland Clinic Hospital in over 100 transplants from living related donors performed using a flank approach reported an overall donor complication rate of 12.2%. The most frequent complication was pneumothorax. None of the patients who had postoperative complications suffered any long term sequelae [2]. Experimental studies and clinical data have suggested that glomerulosclerosis and impaired renal function can occur in individuals with decreased nephron mass, possibly due to glomerular hyperfiltration [3]. Long term follow up of living related donors has not confirmed this assessment [4].

The number of complications related to surgery in the recipient of a living donor kidney seems to be very low, though some authors have suggested a higher incidence of renal artery stenosis due to the performance of end-to-end anastomosis versus end-to-side when a cadaver kidney is used [5,6].

2. Surgical techniques

The two most common surgical approaches for donor nephrectomy are the flank approach and the transperitoneal approach (Fig. 1). There are advocates for both techniques and both have valid reasons for favouring one over the other. It must be remembered that regardless of the approach chosen, the primary goal of donor nephrectomy is to deliver an intact, well-functioning graft for transplantation with minimal morbidity to the donor.

The principles of the operation are to dissect the main renal vessels, avoiding excessive dissection in the true renal hilum to prevent vascular damage leading to ureteral or parenchymal ischaemia. Kidney vessels should be taken long enough to make an easy vascular anastomosis in the recipient. It is important that the ureter is dissected with a large amount of periureteral tissue to decrease the risk of ureteral ischaemia or necrosis, leading to stenosis or fistula. The renal artery must not be stretched to prevent intimal damage or vasospasm. During dissection, careful and adequate mobilization of the kidney and surrounding tissues is important: blood flow in the kidney is very dependent upon mobilization during dissection. Adequate exposure is crucial, and the incision should be lengthened if greater exposure is necessary. When there is no

G.M. Collins, J.M. Dubernard, W. Land and G.G. Persijn (eds). Procurement, Preservation and Allocation of Vascularized Organs 11–14
© 1997 Kluwer Academic Publishers.

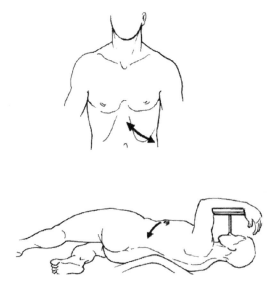

Figure 1. Living donor nephrectomy. Flank incision or transperitoneal incision.

anatomical or physiological reason to favour the use of either kidney, the left kidney is chosen since it has a longer renal vein, which can improve the technical ease of the transplant.

2.1. Flank approach technique

2.1.1. *Left kidney procurement* (Fig. 2)
The patient is rolled into the lateral position with the tip of the twelfth rib directly overlying the kidney-rest on the operating table. After the patient is secured with tape, the table is flexed and the kidney rest raised so that there is the greatest possible separation between iliac crest and lower costal margin. The position of the incision depends on patient morphology. An incision in the tenth intercostal space gives usually a good exposure to the renal pedicle. Care must be taken not to open the pleura when extending the incision upward. If the pleura is opened it is repaired at the time of wound closure and a thoracic drain is placed. The peritoneum is reflected medially and the kidney identified within Gerota's fascia. The peritoneal content is retracted with a large retractor to gain adequate exposure.

The ureter and gonadal vessels are identified as they course in the retroperitoneum. The ureter is blunt dissected as far as possible in the pelvis in order to obtain maximal length. The anterior aspect of the renal vein is exposed and its tributaries are ligated and divided (Fig. 3). The gonadal vein is usually easy to identify as it is close to the ureter. Its identification helps identification

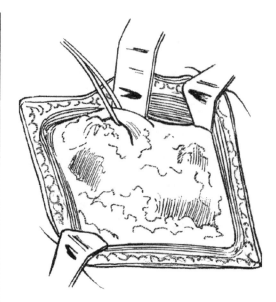

Figure 2. Dissection of the retroperitoneal space. Identification of the ureter.

of the left renal vein. The gonadal vein is ligated. Another tributary of the renal vein can be identified as it joins the renal vein posteriorly: the posterior lumbar branch. Its identification is very important as damage can result in significant bleeding and damage to the renal vein. The third tributary to be identified is the

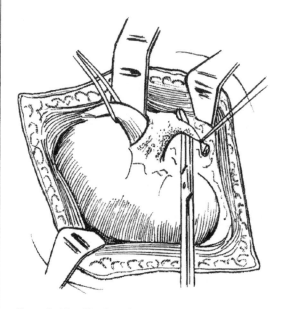

Figure 3. Identification of renal vein.

adrenal vein. This can be recognized when dissecting the superior border of the left renal vein. Its ligation and division gives access to the renal artery just below the superior border of the vein. The renal vein is then cleaned of adjacent adventitial tissue, at least up to the point where it crosses the aorta. This allows enough room for vascular clamp placement and an adequate cuff for ligation. The lymphatics of the kidney are divided between ligatures or vascular clips to avoid the development of lymphocoele in the donor or recipient. Once the artery is recognized, it is dissected. The kidney is then mobilized outside of Gerota's fascia and rotated medially, taking care not to put any tension on its pedicle. The injection of periadventitial papaverin or 4% lidocaine may be helpful in reducing spasm. The renal artery is dissected from its origin on the aorta to its division (Fig. 4). Adrenal branches are divided. Excessive traction on the renal artery can lead to intimal disruption; this can be recognized by softness in the kidney with a periadventitial haematoma around the renal artery. The medial and superior aspects of the kidney are then mobilized. Along the superior aspect of the kidney the adrenal gland is dissected bluntly within its own compartment of Gerota's fascia leaving the kidney within its Gerota's fascia. The posterior aspect of Gerota's fascia is opened and the surface of the kidney is identified in an attempt to inspect most of the renal surface. The ureter and its surrounding tissue are mobilized at the level of the iliac vessels up to the

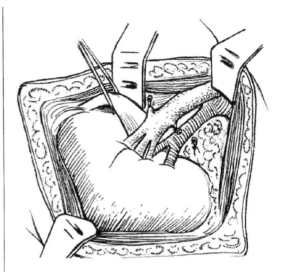

Figure 5. Liberation of the posterior attachment completed.

lower pole of the kidney (Fig. 5). The ureter is then divided distally and observed for urine flow. Prior to vascular cross-clamping, the donor is given a bolus of mannitol and the renal artery is inspected to ensure there is no evidence of vascular spasm. Systemic heparinization (1 mg/kg) can be used a few minutes before the renal artery is ligated. Vascular clamps are then applied and the vessels are transected; the kidney is given to an assistant for flushing with preservative solution. It is then transferred to an adjacent operating room for transplantation. It is important when applying the vascular clamps that an adequate cuff be maintained to allow easy repair of the donor vessels. Fine vascular sutures may be used for repair. Another option is simple ligation combined with suture ligation. After the kidney has been flushed, the excess of perinephric tissue is dissected away, allowing visual inspection of the renal surface.

The wound is then irrigated with antibiotic solution and haemostasis is ensured. The fascial layers are closed in the usual fashion with absorbable monofilament suture. Wound drains can be used. If there has been any injury to the pleura, it is closed at this time.

2.1.2. *Right donor nephrectomy in the flank approach technique*

For a right nephrectomy a similar incision is made. Because of the difference in venous anatomy on the right side, the gonadal vein is not routinely divided; however, many small venous tributaries course between the gonadal vein and periureteral tissue and

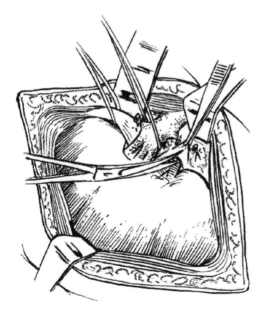

Figure 4. Identification of renal artery.

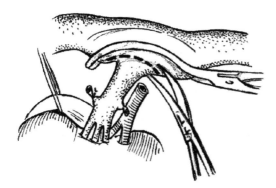

Figure 6. Division of the right renal pedicle. Division of the right renal vein with a patch of vena cava.

must be spot fulgurated as close to the gonadal vein as possible. The vena cava and the right renal vein are dissected anteriorly. They should also be dissected posteriorly to allow for placement of a Satinsky clamp on the origin of the renal vein. It is sometimes necessary to ligate and divide posterior lumbar branches of the vena cava. This allows a patch of vena cava to be taken with the renal vein (Fig. 6). This dissection also provides exposure to the medial aspect of the aorta so that the renal artery can be taken at its origin from the aorta. Once the kidney has been removed a running suture is performed on the lateral aspect of vena cava to close the cavotomy. The renal artery is usually ligated posterior to the vena cava.

2.2. Transperitoneal approach technique (left kidney removal)

This can be performed through a midline incision or a subcostal abdominal incision. A transverse incision is preferable for the patient with a wide subcostal angle. After the abdomen is opened the left colon is retracted medially after incision of the Told ligament and the anterior aspect of Gerota's fascia is dissected (on the right side the colon and duodenum are reflected medially to expose the renal pedicle). The ureter is individualized and vessels are dissected as with a lumbar approach. Ruiz has reported a 2.3% incidence of splenectomy in 171 donors operated on through an anterior approach [7]. The most serious long term complication of transperitoneal donor nephrectomy is small bowel obstruction, 2% in the series of Dunn *et al.* [8].

References

1. Fryd DS, Canafax DM, Atatas AD. A comparison of two cyclosporine protocols at the University of Minnesota. In: PI Tarasaki (ed). Clinical Transplants. UCLA, Los Angeles 1988; pp 79–89.
2. Streem S, Novick AC, Steinmuller DR. Flank donor nephrectomy: efficacy in the donor and recipient. J Urol 1989; 141: 1099.
3. Hayes JM, Steinmuller DR, Streem S, Novick AC. The development of proteinuria and focal-segmented glomerulosclerosis in recipients of pediatric donor kidneys. Transplantation 1991; 52: 813.
4. Anderson RG, Bueschen AJ, Lloyd LK, Dubovsky EV, Burns JR. Short-term and long-term changes in renal function after donor nephrectomy. J Urol 1991; 145: 11.
5. Lacombe MA. Arterial stenosis complicating renal transplantation in man: a study of 38 cases. Ann Surg 1975; 181: 283.
6. Sutherland RS, Spees EK, Jones JW, Fink DW. Renal artery stenosis after renal transplantation: the impact of the hypogastric artery anastomosis. J Urol 1993; 149: 980.
7. Ruiz R, Novick AC, Braun WE, Montague DK, Stewart BH. Transperitoneal live donor nephrectomy. J Urol 1979; 123: 819.
8. Dunn JF, Richie RE, MacDonell RC Jr, Nylander WA Jr, Johnson HK, Sawyers JL. Living related kidney conors: a 14-year experience. Ann Surg 1986; 203: 637.

3 | Anaesthesia and resuscitation of the genetically related living donor in liver transplantation

D. Gille, O. Boillot, M.C. Graber, P. Sagnard, C. Beaude, B. Chabrol, C. Kopp, D.Long, B. Delafosse and G. Bagou

1. Introduction

Liver transplantation has become a method used in the treatment of an increasing number of adults and children suffering from end stage liver disease. As a consequence, there is a discrepancy between the availability of grafts from cadaver donors and the number of waiting recipients at high risk of impending death, especially children.

In spite of the development of various technical solutions designed to increase the number of grafts available for children, such as size reduction or bipartitioning of adult cadaver livers, the still relatively high shortage of available organs led, as early as 1989 in Brazil and Australia, to the use of livers from genetically related living donors. Owing to the very low surgical risk during hepatectomy performed on non-cirrhotic livers, the concept of procurement of partial liver grafts from living donors gained approval from several medical ethics committees and this procedure has been performed in our transplantation unit, 1992. We describe our anaesthetic procedure and the pre-, intra- and postoperative management which offers optimal physical and psychological safety during and after surgery, as well as in the longer term.

2. Methodology

2.1. Selection of genetically related donors

When the transplant team is considering transplanting a liver from a living donor to a child, the feasibility of the procedure should be established after a thorough medical and psychological evaluation of the donor. Preanaesthetic donor assessment should include all the criteria required prior to any hepatic surgery: personal history, clinical examination, non-invasive exploration of hepatic, renal, cardiac and pulmonary function, and biological parameters. Some additional data may be taken into account in order to preserve the donor from predictable operative and postoperative complications. A donor should be free of any physical and psychological problems, i.e. rated ASA 1 according to the classification of the American Society of Anesthesiologists. We consider obesity and heavy smoking as high risk factors since they are a source of known postoperative complications such as infections, respiratory and thromboembolic complications. Female donors must not be pregnant and must discontinue the use of oestrogen–progestogen drugs if these are being taken.

G.M. Collins, J.M. Dubernard, W. Land and G.G. Persijn (eds). Procurement, Preservation and Allocation of Vascularized Organs 15–17
© 1997 Kluwer Academic Publishers.

2.2 Donor management

Donor management and the anaesthetic technique chosen is dermined by the need for optimal safety and depends on the nature of the surgery performed: lobectomy or left hepatectomy, carried out without clamping the hepatic pedicle is a procedure with a limited though not negligible risk of bleeding.

The risk of viral disease transmission associated with exogenous transfusion can be avoided by the use of methods combining normal blood volume haemodilution with two methods of autologous transfusion: autotransfusion planned 3–4 weeks before surgery, including collection of packed RBCs, fresh frozen plasma and platelet concentrates, and intraoperative autotransfusion using a 'cell saver' system. Prevention of thromboembolism begins 12 h before surgery with the administration of a suitable minimum dose of low molecular weight heparin; this treatment is continued for 1 month. Screening tests for venous thromboses based on the levels of d-dimers, biological markers of coagulation, make it possible to control the degree of anticoagulation and alert the clinician to the need for specific investigations for incipient thromboses.

Short term prophylactic antibiotic therapy is included in the protocol, and vaccination against bepatitis B is performed if this is considered necessary.

Anxiolytic and amnestic premedication with a benzodiazepine and hydroxyzine is administered orally in the evening of the day before surgery and 2 h before the patient is taken to the operating suite.

2.3. Anaesthetic technique

The usual general anaesthesia used for any liver surgery is also the method of choice where organ removal is limited either to one lobe (segments II and III) or to left hepatectomy (trisegmentectomy: II, III and IV). This anaesthesia is both deep and easy to control, and offers the patient maximum comfort. Hepatic surgery requires the use of powerful analgesics, capable of both suppressing pain and the main nociceptive reactions caused by the manipulation of the liver and abdominal viscera and ensuring relaxation of abdominal muscles, diaphragm and viscera. Quality of surgery, patient safety and postoperative outlook will depend on these two prerequisites. The technique of general anaesthesia we use is called 'balanced anaesthesia', for it combines various hypnotics, curare and analgesic agents to meet the requirements of this type of surgery.

2.3.1. *The choice of anaesthetic agents is subject to certain conditions*

In order to preserve the donor's hepatic function and the quality of the graft, the choice of volatile or intravenous anaesthetics must show an absence of hepatotoxicity, low hepatic metabolism and maintenance of blood flow rate in the arterial and portal system, with respect to reciprocal arterial and portal flow rates. Narcosis is usually induced with a rapidly acting hypnotic such as penthotal or etomidate and maintained by isoflurane, a volatile halogenated agent which does not alter hepatic blood flow, respects the regulation of arterial and portal hepatic flow rates and has very little hepatotoxicity owing to its low hepatic metabolism.

Analgesia is obtained with the use of a potent, highly lipid-soluble morphinic drug such as fentanyl or sulfentanyl, the kinetics of which is controlled by redistribution phenomena. The latter must be taken into account during recovery from anaesthesia. Atracurarium is the muscle relaxant of choice since it is not metabolized in the liver and is eliminated rapidly.

2.3.2. *Monitoring*

Intraoperative monitoring methods meet the mandatory safety standards adopted by the Société Française d'Anesthésie Réanimation and the World Federation of Societies of Anesthesiologists. Protection of airways by orotracheal tubing and peroperative assisted ventilation are essential. Invasive cardiovascular monitoring methods are limited to continuous monitoring of blood pressure by catheterization of the radial artery and of central venous pressure by internal jugular catheterization. The haemodynamic impact of lobectomy or left hepatectomy is negligible since this type of surgery does not require exclusion of the liver vasculature. Haemodynamic stability must be obtained by adequate vascular filling, guided by continuous arterial blood pressure and measurement of central venous pressure, maintained between 6 and 7 cm/H_2O, in order to preserve the liver from any congestive episode, which would be deleterious to the liver function and a source of haemorrhage.

During hepatic arterial dissection (left hepatic artery), we administer prostaglandin E_1 at a dose of 500 μg per 24 h in order to protect hepatic arterial vascularization from spasmodic vasomotor disorders and protect hepatic arterial circulation from any thrombogenic element.

Vascular filling and blood volume expansion are obtained on the basis of water and electrolyte requirements using Ringer's lactate and artificial solutes (starch) which are free from any allergenic effect. Haematocrit monitoring is essential and maintained at levels of 30–35%. Blood returning from the cell saver is transfused together with the harvested RBCs. Fresh frozen plasma and platelet concentrates are transfused at the time of haemostasis.

3. Postoperative period

Patients are monitored in the intensive care unit for the first 24 h after surgery. Invasive monitoring systems are removed as early as possible and their maintenance is limited to the postanaesthetic recovery phase. Postoperative assisted ventilation is not indicated and may be a source of complications. Postoperative analgesia is required: the patient receives morphine-type drugs through a programmed delivery system. Short term parenteral feeding and water–electrolyte delivery are maintained until resumption of complete oral nutrition. Clinical, paraclinical and biological monitoring, in particular for liver function, are performed as usual during hepatic surgery follow-up, and any treatment required is prescribed.

4. Conclusion

Donor safety is the essential goal. With thorough pre- and intraoperative methodology, liver transplantation from a genetically related living donor to a child should be a reliable technical choice, performed by a team of highly qualified and experienced operators in the field of liver surgery and liver transplantation in order to secure optimal donor safety.

References

1. Sann L et al. Ethical considerations on hepatic transplantation from living related donors. J Pediatrie 1993; 48: 435–45.
2. Lery N Droit éthique de la santé: l'expérience d'une consultation. Med Hyg 1990; 48: 2161–6.
3. Singer PA et al. Ethics of liver transplantation with living donor. N Engl J Med 1989; 321: 620–2.
4. Boillot O et al. Transplantation hépatique pédiatrique et donneur vivant apparenté. Pédiatrie 1993; 48: 435–45.
5. Boillot O et al. Controlled hepatic bipartition for transplantation in two recipients: surgical technique, results and perspectives. Br J Surg 1993; 80: 75–80.
6. Liehn et al. Risk of living related donors for liver transplantation. Liver intensive care group of Europe. 7th meeting. April 15–16, 1994.
7. Delva et al. Vascular occlusions for liver resections. Operative management and tolerance to hepatic ischemia: 142 cases. Ann Surg 1989; x; x–x.
8. Gavelli A et al. Risk factors associated with hepatectomy: results of a multivariate analysis of 113 cases. Ann Chir 1993; 47: 586–91.
9. Goldfarb G Influence of anaesthetic drug on hepatic blood flow. Ann Fr Anesth Réan 1987; 6: 498–506.
10. Russel E et al. Effects of anesthetic agents and abdominal surgery on liver blood flow. Hepatology 1991; 14: 1161–6.
11. Gilman S Anesthesia and the liver. In Barash PG, Cullen BF and Stoelung RK (eds) Clinical Anesthesia Lippincott, Philadelphia; pp. 1133–62.
12. Goldfarb G et al. Comparative effects of halothane and isoflurane anesthesia on the ultrastructure of human hepatic cells. Analgesia, 1989; 69: 491–5.

4 | Living related liver transplantation (LRLT)

N. Habib, X. Rogiers and C.E. Broelsch

1. Preoperative evaluation and preparation

1.1. The donor

Most adult donors reaching a centre for living related liver transplantation have some idea about living related liver transplantation (LRLT) and about the possibility that they themselves might become a donor. From the outset there is, therefore, some form of consent to the concept or principle of donating part of the liver to their child. However, selection and preparation of the donor is of the utmost importance.

Preparation should include complete explanation of the potential operative mortality and morbidity of the donor as well as the risk of graft failure in the recipient. This should be weighed against the potential morbidity and mortality for the recipient remaining on a waiting list.

The transplanting team should make sure that there is as little coercion and psychological pressure as possible involved in the decision of a parent to donate to his or her child. Whenever possible the consent is obtained twice at separate times, to ensure the donor has enough time to reflect and possibly to change his or her mind. It is important to exclude any psychological disorder in the donor and to ensure that love rather than guilt, marriage difficulties or emotional instability is the motive for organ donation.

A thorough standard medical history and examination is performed in order to exclude major risk factors for surgery and, more specifically, for liver resection. Viral screening is performed to prevent transmission of diseases from donor to recipient. In addition, the donor's liver is assessed by CT scan (with volume measurement of the left lateral lobe) to confirm the presence of an anatomical left lobe and to ensure that its size is compatible with the size of the recipient.

Duplex doppler ultrasound scan and visceral angiography are important to delineate any anatomical anomalies, such as a left hepatic artery originating from a left gastric artery or the presence of two arteries to the left liver. Indirect phase portography will exclude the presence of portal vein thrombosis. It will also display abnormal anatomy such as the right anterior-median or the right posterior lateral portal vein branch originating from the main left portal vein rather than from the main right portal vein.

It has not been our custom to perform routine endoscopic retrograde cholangiography (ERC) to detect biliary anomalies. ERC should, however, be performed when the recipient has a familial cholestatic disorder, since problems with abnormally small bile ducts in the donor liver have been reported.

Table 1 illustrates our standard donor investigation programme. In summary, following the consent of a suitable parent, clinicians need to make sure that there is a healthy liver of adequate volume, with conventional arterial and portal supply in a donor with a low surgical risk. In the weeks prior to surgery up to three units of autologous blood should be obtained from the donor for intraoperative transfusion. Mini-dose low molecular weight heparin is administered routinely, starting 12 h before surgery.

G.M. Collins, J.M. Dubernard, W. Land and G.G. Persijn (eds). Procurement, Preservation and Allocation of Vascularized Organs 19–22
© 1997 Kluwer Academic Publishers.

Table 1. Preoperative investigations in potential living related donors.

Full history and clinical examination
Psychological examination
Chest X-ray
Lung function tests
ECG, stress ECG
Abdominal US
CT liver with size measurements
Coeliac angiography
ERC (only on specific indication)
Laboratory investigations:
    CBC, differential count, electrolytes, BUN, creatinine, blood group, HLA typing, thyroid function tests, coagulation
    tests, alfa 1 antitrypsin, transferrin, coeruloplasmin, CEA, α-fetoprotein, ferritin, CRP
Serology:
    hepatitis A, B, C, CMV, EBV, HSV, HIV
Urine sediment
Blood self donation

1.2. The recipient

The preparation and investigation of the recipient undergoing LRLT are the same as in cadaveric liver transplantation with the difference that one can plan the operation for a time which is optimal for the recipient. Many centres have shown the importance of performing elective paediatric liver transplantation. This major advantage of living related liver transplantation over cadaveric transplantation should be used at best.

Normally blood group compatibility between donor and recipient is required. However, in young infants liver transplantation across ABO barriers can be performed safely in certain specific circumstances.

2. Operative procedures

Donor and recipient operations can be performed either simultaneously or consecutively.

2.1. The donor procedure

Anaesthetic preparation of the patient includes arterial, CVP, pulse and core temperature monitoring. A nasogastric tube and urinary catheter are routinely placed. The patient is placed in a supine position. The abdomen, and right and left groins are prepared. A cell saver is used. The abdominal incision is a limited mercedes incision. The transverse limb of the incision allows incision of the recti muscle. The vertical limb is a median incision that joins the transverse limb to the

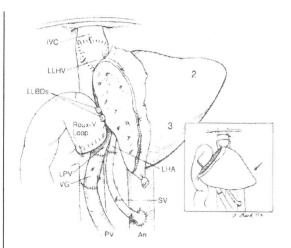

Figure 1. Living related left lateral segment after implantation. From Broelsch C.E., Whitington P.F., Emond J.C., Heffron T.G., Thistlethwaite J.R., Stevens L., Piper J., Whitington S.H., Lichtor J.L., Liver transplantation in children from living related donors. Surgical techniques and results. Ann Surg 1991; 214: 428–439.

xiphoid process. Once the abdomen is opened a routine exploration is performed and a retractor (f. ex. Rochard retractor) is placed to retract the costal margins in a cephalad direction.

The left lateral lobe of the liver is mobilized by incising the falciform ligament and the left triangular ligament. The gastrohepatic ligament is opened while confirming the absence of a *left hepatic artery originating from the left hepatic artery*. The ligamentum teres is cut across and the hepatic end of the ligament is used as a retractor to dissect the structures running at its base.

The first structure to be dissected is the left hepatic artery, which is freed throughout its length to its origin from the hepatic artery. It is important to exclude the presence of two left hepatic arteries: preoperative angiography is always helpful in this respect. When a major branch or a separate artery to segment 4 is present it should be conserved if possible. No adverse effects of arterial devascularization of segment 4 have been reported thus far. There is usually a bridge of parenchyma underneath the ligamentum teres that joins segments III and IV. This can be cut across with the diathermy. One or two suture(s) might be needed to ensure haemostasis.

The left portal vein is the next structure to be dissected, up to its branching from the common portal vein. The round ligament is pulled upwards and all the branches to segment 4 at its base are carefully dissected, suture ligated and transected. The same procedure is performed with the portal vein branches to the caudate lobe. In this way the left portal vein is completely mobilised, and now services only the left lateral liver lobe.

Once the left branch of the portal vein has been mobilized, the hilar plate in which the bile duct(s) to segments 2 and 3 run(s) can be seen on the medial-caudal side. It is important to cut this structure sharply and to avoid electrocoagulation in its vicinity: impaired vascularization of the bile duct is a major cause of bile leakage in the recipient. For the same reason, and for reasons of safety, the transection should be performed closely to the parenchyma of the left lateral lobe. Doing so will provide a separate bile duct to segments 2 and 3 in one-third of cases. All the structures entering the left liver have now been dissected without the need for mobilization of the right liver, removal of the gall bladder or dissection of the hilus.

An attempt should be made to encircle the left hepatic vein with a tape. Although this is usually possible it is not essential to perform this manoeuvre when it is difficult.

During the parenchymatous phase the remaining bridge of liver tissue is progressively transected using one of the classical techniques in liver surgery. This part of the operation is performed very patiently, performing haemostasis of both section surfaces as necessary. Importantly, no vascular exclusion is used. Parenchymatous transection continues until the left hepatic vein is completely freed, and two livers, each with its own vascular supply, have been created in the donor. Explantation can now be performed easily by clamping and transecting the left hepatic artery, left portal vein and left hepatic vein.

On the back-table the graft is flushed with UW solution via the artery and portal vein and the bile duct(s) are rinsed. Vascular reconstructions may be needed to lengthen artery and/or portal vein. For this purpose one can use saphenous vein, procured from the donor, or cryopreserved veins.

The vascular stumps are oversewn with running prolene sutures. The bile duct stump is oversewn with a 5/0 PDS suture. The abdomen is closed and one drain is left adjacent to the hepatotomy surface.

2.2. The recipient procedure (Fig. 1)

The patient is placed supine and a Mercedes or bilateral subcostal incision is performed. The hilar structures are identified following dissection of adhesions. Early ligation of the hepatic artery will diminish bleeding from the liver capsule and facilitate liver mobilization. The common bile duct, when present, is then identified and cut across with the distal end oversewn. The portal vein is then dissected free up to the splenomesenteric bifurcation and the retro-portal lymphatics are tied. The liver is now fully mobilized by cutting across the falciform, right and left triangular ligaments. Finally the portal vein is clamped and transected.

Next the hepatectomy is performed, with preservation of the recipient vena cava. A long curved vascular clamp (Satinski's clamp) is applied to the vena cava in such a way that its keel clamps the infrahepatic inferior vena cava (IVC), its jaws the retrohepatic IVC and its distal part the suprahepatic IVC. This technique saves time and prevents the bleeding associated with IVC mobilization in the presence of portal hypertension. The liver is now excised by cutting across the caudate and hepatic veins. All these vena cava tributaries are now sutured carefully, including the hepatic vein orifices. Once all these tributaries are tied, the Satinski clamp is removed. Alternatively one can progressively dissect the branches on the anterior surface of the IVC until the whole liver is detached from it.

The diaphragm can be dissected upwards for 1 or 2 cm in order to lengthen the IVC above the hepatic vein sutures. A smaller clamp is applied, if possible only partially occluding the IVC, and a large triangular venotomy is performed. This is important to minimize the risk of outflow obstruction to the graft. The hepatic vein anastomosis is made with continuous 5/0 PDS. Once completed the IVC clamp is removed and substituted with a smaller vascular clamp which is applied to the hepatic vein anastomosis, so as to permit free blood flow through the vena cava. All anastomoses are performed using magnifying lenses. Following this, the portal vein anastomosis is completed. After arterioportal flushing of the graft with 200 cm³ of 5% albumin, the hepatic vein and portal vein clamps are removed. This will allow partial vascularization of the graft. Usually only minimal additional haemostasis is needed.

Arterial flow is established by anastomosis of the saphenous vein to the graft hepatic artery. If the recipient hepatic artery is large (3 mm or more) the saphenous vein segment can be shortened and anastomosed directly to the recipient hepatic artery with 7/0 PDS. If the recipient hepatic artery is smaller it is safer to anastomose the saphenous vein segment to the infrarenal aorta directly. The saphenous vein can be placed in a retro-pancreatic precaval position. A final check should ensure haemostasis at the resection margin, IVC and all vascular anastomoses, as once the hepatico–jejunostomy anastomosis has been performed liver mobilization should be avoided in order not to disturb the biliary anastomoses.

The next step is to ensure a long (50 cm) Roux-en-Y-jejunal loop for the hepatico–jejunostomy. In one-third of patients two bile duct anastomoses will have to be performed. Good vascularization of the bile duct(s), a tensionless anastomosis and the use of magnification are essential for this delicate part of the operation.

The abdomen is closed with the placement of two drains against the cut surface of the graft. During closure the liver will be pushed by the abdominal organs in such a way that the cut surface of the graft will face the right diaphragm. The abdomen should be closed without tension, otherwise a generous Goretex 1 mm patch should be placed temporarily and removed 48 h later.

3. Postoperative care

The postoperative care and complications of the donor are no different to those of other liver resection patients. The postoperative management of the recipient is identical to that of recipients of cadaver reduced size livers.

4. Conclusion

Living related liver transplantation provides a unique opportunity for children with end-stage liver disease and their parents to avoid the mortality and morbidity associated with remaining on a waiting list for a cadaver organ. We have given an overview of the perioperative and intraoperative course of such a procedure. It should be stressed, however, that, in order to guarantee maximal safety for the donor and potential benefit for the recipient, these procedures should only be performed in experienced paediatric liver transplant centres with additional expertise in adult liver resections.

Bibliography

1. Broelsch CE, Emond JC, Whitington PF, Thistlethwaite JR, Baker AL, Lichtor JL. Application of reduced-size liver transplants as split grafts, auxiliary orthotopic grafts and living related segmental transplants. Ann Surg 1990; 214: 368–77.
2. Broelsch CE, Whitington PF, Emond JC, Heffron TG, Thistlethwaite JR, Stevens L, Piper J, Whitington SH, Lichtor JL. Liver transplantation in children from living related donors. Surgical techniques and results. Ann Surg 1991; 214: 428–39.
3. Broelsch CE, Lloyd DM. Living related donors for liver transplants. Adv Surg 1993; 26: 209–31.
4. Emond JC, Heffron TG, Kortz EO, Gonzales-Vallina R, Contis JC, Black DD, Whitington PF. Improved results of living related liver transplantation with routine application in a pediatric program. Transplantation 1993; in press.
5. Emond JC, Heffron TG, Whitington PF, Broelsch CE. Reconstruction of the hepatic vein in reduced size hepatic transplantation. Surg Gynecol Obstet 1993; 176: 11–17.
6. Makuuchi M, Kawarazaki H, Iwanaka T, Kamada N, Takayama T, Kumon M. Living related liver transplantation. Surg Today 1992; 22: 297–300.
7. Ozawa K, Uemoto T, Tanaka K, Kumada L, Yamaoka Y, Kobayashi N, Inamoto T, Shimahara Y, Mori K, Honda K et al. An apprasial of pediatric liver transplantation from living relatives. Ann Surg 1992; 216: 547–53.
8. Singer PA, Siegler M, Whitington PF, Lantos JD Emond JC, Thistlethwaite JR, Broelsch CE. Ethics of liver transplantation with living donors. N Engl J Med 1989; 321: 620–22.
9. Tanaka K, Uemoto S, Tkunaga Y, Fujita S, Sano K, Nishizawa T, Sawada H, Shirahase I, Kim HJ, Yamaoka Y et al. Surgical techniques and innovations in living related liver transplantation. Ann Surg 1993; 217: 82–91.

5 | Diagnosis of brain death

GIAN-EMILIO CHATRIAN

(Received: 16 September 1994)

1. Death of the brain as death of the person

Traditionally, death has been defined in medicine as the permanent cessation of heart beat and respiration. Whenever the loss of these functions is not promptly reversed by appropriate resuscitative measures, profound and irreversible pathological alterations occur in the brain within minutes under normothermic conditions. During the last three decades, the increasing effectiveness of resuscitative techniques and life-support systems made it possible to restore and artificially maintain cardiovascular and respiratory functions in countless individuals. However, it soon became apparent that the extreme vulnerability of the brain to anoxia, which exceeded that of other systems of the body, was a major limiting factor in assuring a favourable outcome of resuscitation. In patients who had suffered sufficiently prolonged cardiorespiratory arrest, the restoration and maintenance of pulmonary, cardiac and other functions was not accompanied by recovery of conscious adaptive behaviour and those higher faculties that represent the very essence of human life.

In France, Mollaret and Goulon [1] and Mollaret *et al.* [2] coined the term 'coma dépassé' (a state beyond coma) to describe conditions in which even autonomic control was lost and that were believed to be associated with destruction of the brain. In the USA, Adams and Jequier [3] proposed the term 'brain death syndrome' to designate these states.

Because, in the face of complete and permanent abolition of brain functions, preservation of other organs was inconsequential, brain death was soon equated with death of the person by medical, legal and religious authorities. Moreover, it was recognized that the futile use of extraordinary measures to support certain body functions in individuals with dead brains demanded unreasonable expenditure of human and financial resources, unnecessarily prolonged the sorrow and grief of relatives and friends, and was contrary to the individual's right to die with dignity. The advent of transplant surgery provided further impetus to redefining death of the individual as death of the brain, since its success depended on the use of viable organs removed from patients with permanently abolished brain function before their circulation failed. Identification of death of the brain with death itself was felt to permit removal of organs either simultaneously

G.M. Collins, J.M. Dubernard, W. Land and G.G. Persijn (eds). Procurement, Preservation and Allocation of Vascularized Organs 23–46
© 1997 Kluwer Academic Publishers.

with or shortly before cessation of artificial supporting measures.

2. Concept and neuropathology of brain death

In 1968, a circular of the Ministry of Social Affairs of the French Republic stated that 'irreversibility of lesions incompatible with life' was characterized by the *'destructive and irreparable nature of the alterations of the central nervous system in its totality'* (italics added) [4]. In contrast to this holistic concept, the Conference of Medical Royal Colleges and their Faculties in the United Kingdom, embracing earlier formulations of Mohandas and Chou [5], identified brain death with *'permanent functional death of the brain stem'* (italics added [6]). This notion was reiterated in subsequent UK documents on this subject, including a report by a Working Party of the British Paediatric Association [7] and a review by a Working Group of the Royal College of Physicians [8]. In turn, in the USA, a Report of the Medical Consultants on the Diagnosis of Death defined brain death as *'irreversible cessation of all functions of the entire brain, including the brain stem ... that are clinically ascertainable.'* [9].

That permanent cessation of brain functions which characterizes the death of the brain involves the diencephalon and the cerebral hemispheres in addition to the brain stem is irrefutably demonstrated by electroencephalogram (EEG) and brain perfusion studies, and by pathological findings. However, in this author's opinion, the concept that brain death is characterized by irreversible cessation of all functions of the entire brain, including the brain stem [9], is by no means irreconcilable with the notion that irreversible loss of brain stem functions [8] is central to the pathophysiological mechanisms, the clinical manifestations, and the ultimate cardiac outcome of brain death [10,11].

As the concept of brain death evolved, so did the knowledge of the neuropathological changes characterizing this condition [12]. Early work had suggested that marked oedema, extensive softening and necrosis, particularly in the grey matter, and severe neuronal alterations without inflammatory reaction or vascular thrombosis characterized the brains of individuals who had been in 'coma dépassé' and had been artificially ventilated [1,2,13]. Adams and Jequier [3] noted a similar pathological picture. However, subsequent publications revealed a greater diversity of findings in individuals with brain death who had been maintained on a respirator for variable periods of time. Most commonly, swelling and softening as well as transtentorial

herniations, haemorrhages, infarcts and necroses were found in the cerebrum, cerebellum, and brain stem of individuals with brain death. These alterations varied considerably in extent, severity and distribution [12,14–23]. Moreover, the brains of some patients who died less than 12–36 h, but usually about 24 h after the onset of coma and apnoea displayed minimal or no pathological alterations, indicating that some time must elapse after the onset of coma and apnoea for the changes of the 'respirator brain' to develop [12,16,17,22–26].

3. Operational criteria for determining brain death in the adult

Acceptance of the notion of brain death and identification of this condition with death of the individual made it necessary to formulate operational criteria for diagnosing this state in persons with artificially sustained cardiac and respiratory functions. The definition of these standards was intended to help physicians to identify the circumstances under which continuation of extraordinary supportive measures was both unnecessary and inadvisable, as well as to protect patients against premature termination of these efforts. A complete survey of the criteria of brain death throughout the world is beyond the scope of this chapter. Thus, almost exclusive consideration will be given to regulations legislated in France and guidelines suggested in the USA and the UK, each of which is representative of a fundamentally different approach to the determination of death of the brain. Additional information is provided by books [12,22,23,27], a serial monograph [28], an atlas [29], and review articles [10,30–36].

In April 1968, a circular of the Ministry of Social Affairs of the French Republic [4] (Table 1) mandated that the determination of death in patients who were maintained on a respirator after an event requiring prolonged resuscitative efforts be based on the following criteria: (1) systematic analysis of the circumstances of the accident, (2) lack of spontaneous respiration, (3) abolition of all reflexes, complete loss of muscle tones, and mydriasis, and (4) absence of all spontaneous and stimulus-evoked activities in the EEG over a sufficient period of time, in the absence of effects of hypothermia and sedative drugs. This document specified that the determination and certification of death was to be made by two concurring physicians having certain specified qualifications, with the support of a specialist in EEG when needed. The determination of death authorized the discontinuation of all measures of artificial support of cardiac and respiratory functions. When the removal of organs for transplantation was considered, continuation of the supporting measures was authorized to avoid premature interruption of perfusion of the organ to be removed. Moreover, when organ transplantation was envisaged, no physician or surgeon belonging to the transplantation team could participate in the determination and certification of death (Table 1).

A few months later, similar criteria of 'irreversible coma', a term used at the time as a synonym of brain death, were formulated in the USA by an Ad Hoc Committee of the Harvard Medical School [37]. The Harvard standards required that the following conditions be met: (1) unreceptivity and unresponsivity, (2) absent movements and breathing, (3) absent reflexes, (4) a 'flat' EEG of at least 10 minutes' duration, and possibly twice as long, and (5) confirmation of findings at least 24 h later. The validity of these criteria as indicators of brain death depended on the exclusion of effects of hypothermia and central nervous system depressants such as barbiturates. Since these original formulations, criteria for determining irreversible extinction of brain functions have evolved under the influence of clinical experience and technological developments. In the UK, standards for the diagnosis of brain death were first promulgated by an initial statement of the Conference of Medical Royal Colleges and their Faculties in the United Kingdom (Table 2). These criteria emphasized the role of clinical observation and ordinary laboratory tests, and denied the need for using ancillary methods, including EEG, evoked potential, and brain perfusion studies [6,8]. The American views found official expression in a Report of the Medical Consultants on the Diagnosis of Death to the President's Commission for the Study of Ethical Problems in Medicine and Biomedical and Behavioral Research [9] (Table 3). Recently, the French regulations were reasserted and expanded by a circular of the Ministry of Social Affairs and of Solidarity [38] (Table 1). This document established the need to repeat an EEG demonstrating electrocerebral inactivity (ECI) after an adequate period of observation, generally about 6 h, and to ensure that 'blood and urine assays do not detect any drug depressing the nervous system and the subject is not hypothermic, or that hypothermia has been corrected'.

Comparison of the French, UK, and American standards (Tables 1–3) reveals substantial agreement on the preconditions to be met and the conditions to be excluded for establishing brain death as well as the

neurological criteria to be fulfilled to ascertain this state. Deep coma ('cerebral unresponsivity') [9], apnoea, and absent cephalic reflexes emerge as the clinical criteria attesting to global loss of brain functions. However, certain complicating conditions may reversibly cause the manifestation of this clinical triad. These conditions, reviewed in detail elsewhere [11,22] include: the effects of CNS depressant drugs, neuromuscular blocking agents, hypothermia (core temperature below 32.2°C), profound hypotension (systolic blood pressure ≤ 80 mmHg), and severe metabolic derangements, such as those associated with hepatic encephalopathy, hyperosmolar coma, and preterminal uraemia. Total paralysis due to exposure to neuromuscular blocking agents and diseases such as myasthenia gravis could also mimic loss of brain functions. In order to demonstrate that the loss of these functions determined by an initial examination was irreversible, a period of observation was required, long enough to allow the performance of tests aimed at determining the primary cause of coma, exclude complicating and remediable conditions, stabilize the patient's cardiovascular status, normalize body temperature, take other essential therapeutic measures, and determine whether or not the clinical signs of extinguished brain functions persisted. When, at the end of this period an irreversible condition was established, drug intoxication was excluded, the patient's body temperature and blood pressure were normal, and deep coma, apnoea and absent cephalic reflexes were confirmed, it could be assumed that the loss of brain functions was irreversible, i.e., that the brain was dead. The duration of observation was a matter of medical judgment. However, the US guidelines [9] suggested that, in the circumstances specified, brain death could be established within approximately 6 h if the clinical diagnosis was confirmed by ancillary methods, such as studies of cerebral blood flow or the EEG. In the absence of this corroborative evidence, the observation period should be extended to at least 12 h, and as much as 24 h in cases of anoxic encephalopathy.

Observations by Jørgensen [39] confirmed that, provided certain preconditions were met and certain confounding factors were excluded, the clinical triad of deep coma, loss of cephalic reflexes, and apnoea persisting for an appropriate time reliably indicated that the brain was dead. He studied retrospectively individuals who met these criteria after suffering primary intracranial lesions, circulatory arrest complicating extracranial disorders, or severe drug intoxication requiring resuscitation. Although all patients received full life support, they developed final asystole within days. Jørgensen's findings [39] prompted the

Table 1. French Government regulations on procedures and criteria for ascertaining and certifying death and measures authorized by the determination of death.

Conceptual framework

'the destructive and irreparable nature of the alterations of the central nervous system in its totality' 'is incompatible with life'.

Procedure and criteria for ascertaining and certifying death[a]

.....'the ascertainment of death of a subject who underwent prolonged resuscitation will be established after consultation of two physicians, one of whom must be the head of a hospital service or his duly authorized substitute assisted, whenever deemed desirable, by a specialist in [electro]encephalography (text in brackets added). This ascertainment will be based on the existence of concurring proofs of irreversibility of lesions incompatible with life. This judgement will be prompted by the destructive and irreparable nature of the alterations of the central nervous system in its totality'.

'This determination will be primarily based on:
– a systematic analysis of the circumstances in which the accidents occurred;
– the entirely artificial character of the respiration maintained only by the use of respirators;
– the total abolition of all reflexes, complete hypotonia, and mydriasis;
– the disappearance of all [electro]encephalographic signals (a "null" trace without any evidence of reactivity) either spontaneous or elicited by any artificial stimulation, demonstrated over a time regarded as sufficient, in a patient in whom hypothermia has not been induced and who has not received any sedative medication' (text in brackets added).

'The irreversibility of the functional loss can be established only by the concurrence of these clinical and electroencephalographic criteria; lack of fulfillment of just one of these criteria does not permit declaring the subject dead'.

'The certificate of death of a subject who underwent prolonged resuscitation is written following consultation of these two practitioners'.

Measures authorized by the determination of death and special requirements for the removal of organs for therapeutic purposes[a]

'The determination of death of a subject whose survival is maintained artificially authorizes the cessation of cardio-respiratory support.

'No removal of organ or tissue can be considered before death has been duly determined as defined above. In the event that, following determination of death, removal of organs is considered for therapeutic purposes, the pursuit of maneuvers of resuscitation can be authorized to avoid the premature interruption of circulation in the organ to be removed.

'It is clarified that, in this event, the physicians or surgeons belonging to the team involved in the transplant of the organ removed cannot be under any circumstance one of the two physicians who jointly signed the determination and the certificate of death'.

Current regulations on the criteria for the determination of cerebral death[b]

'Criteria of cerebral death include a "null", non-reactive electroencephalogram, demonstrated by two recordings repeated during an observation period after a sufficient interval (in general of the order of six hours) – after having insured that blood and urine do not detect any drug with depressant effects on the nervous system, and that the subject is not hypothermic, or that hypothermia has been corrected.'

[a] Excerpts from the Circular No. 76 issued on April 24, 1968 by the Ministère des Affaires Sociales [4]. (Translated by G.-E. Chatrian).
[b] Excerpts from the Circular No. 03, Part II – Current rules on the criteria for the determination of cerebral death, issued on January 21, 1991 by the Ministère des Affaires Sociales et de la Solidarité, Ministère de la Santé [38]. (Translated by G.-E. Chatrian).

Table 2. UK criteria for the diagnosis of brain death[a,b].

Conceptual framework
'Permanent functional death of the brain stem constitutes brain death'

Conditions for considering diagnosis of brain death

Condition	Action recommended or special comments
Patient is deeply comatose and the following conditions causing or contributing to coma are excluded:	
a. Depressant drugs	Review carefully drug history and allow adequate time to elapse
b. Primary hypothermia	
c. Metabolic and endocrine disturbances	Exclude profound abnormality of serum electrolytes, acid base balance, or blood glucose concentration
Patient is on ventilator because of previous inadequacy or cessation of respiration	Exclude effects of (a) neuromuscular blocking agents by eliciting spinal reflexes or by using conventional nerve stimulator and (b) hypnotics and narcotics
Patient's condition is due to irremediable structural brain damage. Diagnosis of causal disorder should have been fully established. Most common eventualities include:	
a. Primary intracranial event such as severe head injury, spontaneous intracranial haemorrhage, or neurosurgery.	Irremediable nature of condition may be obvious within hours
b. Patient has suffered primarily from cardiac arrest, hypoxia, or severe circulatory insufficiency with an indefinite period of cerebral anoxia or is suspected of having cerebral air or fat embolism.	To establish diagnosis and be confident of prognosis may take much longer
c. Primary condition is a matter of doubt.	Confident diagnosis may be reached only by continuous observation and investigation

Tests for confirming brain death
All brain stem reflexes should be absent including:
1. Pupillary
2. Corneal
3. Vestibulo-ocular to cold water stimulation of each external auditory meatus
4. Motor responses within the cranial nerve distribution to stimulation of any somatic area
5. Gag reflex or reflex response to bronchial stimulation by suction catheter passed down the trachea
6. Respiratory movement when the patient is disconnected from the mechanical ventilator for long enough to ensure that the arterial CO_2 tension rises above the threshold for stimulating respiration. This is best achieved by measuring blood gases. Because patients in intensive care units tend to be over ventilated, first 5% CO_2 in O_2 should be administered through the ventilator until the $PaCO_2$ reaches 5.3–6.0 kPa (40–45 mmHg), then the patient should be disconnected from the ventilator until the $PaCO_2$ attains at least 6.7 kPa (50 mmHg). During disconnection, delivery of O_2 at 6 l/min through a tracheal catheter is essential to establish diffusion oxygenation and prevent hypoxia during apnoea. When blood gas analysis is not available, an alternate procedure is to supply the ventilator with O_2 then with 5% CO_2 in O_2 for 5 minutes followed by disconnection of the ventilator for 10 minutes while delivering O_2 at 6 l/min by catheter into the trachea. Patients with preexisting chronic respiratory insufficiency who may be unresponsive to raised levels of CO_2 and who depend on hypoxic drive for respiration should be expertly investigated with careful blood gas monitoring.

Other considerations
Repetition of testing is required in conditions in which the outcome is unclear. The interval between tests is a matter for medical judgement and may be as long as 24 hours.

Integrity of spinal reflexes may be observed in brain dead patients.

Table 2. (*Continued.*)

Other considerations

Confirmatory investigations. 'It is now widely accepted that electroencephalography is not necessary for diagnosing brain death.' 'When electroencephalography is used, the strict criteria recommended by the Federation of EEG Societies … must be followed.' 'Other investigations such as cerebral angiography or cerebral blood flow measurements are not required for diagnosing brain death.'

Body temperature should not be less than 35°C before the diagnostic tests are carried out.

Specialist opinion and status of doctors concerned. 'Experienced clinicians in intensive care units, acute medical wards, and accident and emergency departments should not normally require specialist advice. Only when the primary diagnosis is in doubt is it necessary to consult with a neurologist or neurosurgeon. The decision to withdraw artificial support should be made after all the criteria presented above have been fulfilled and can be made by any one of the following combinations of doctors: (a) a consultant who is in charge of the care and one other doctor; (b) in the absence of a consultant, his deputy, who should have been registered for five years or more and who should have had adequate experience in the care of such cases, and one other doctor.'

---

[a] Excerpts from: Diagnosis of Brain Death. Statement issued by the honorary secretary of the Conference of Royal Colleges and Faculties of the United Kingdom on 11 October 1976 [6].
[b] Reviewed by a Working Group convened by the Royal College of Physicians and endorsed by the Conference of Medical Royal Colleges and their Faculties in the United Kingdom[8].

Table 3. US guidelines for determining brain death[a].

Conceptual Framework
'An individual with irreversible cessation of all functions of the entire brain, including the brain stem, is dead.'

Neurologic Criteria for Determining Death
1. Cessation of all functions of the entire brain (that are clinically ascertainable) is recognized when evaluation discloses that both cerebral and brain stem functions are absent.
    a. Cerebral functions are absent when the examination reveals 'deep coma, that is, cerebral unreceptivity and unresponsivity. Medical circumstances may require the use of confirmatory study such as an EEG or blood-flow study.'
    b. Brain stem functions are absent when the examination reveals absence of 'Pupillary light, corneal, oculocephalic, oculovestibular, oropharyngeal, and respiratory (apnoea) reflexes.' 'When these reflexes cannot be adequately assessed, confirmatory tests are recommended.' An accepted method for demonstrating apnoea is 'ventilation with pure oxygen or an oxygen and carbon dioxide mixture for 10 minutes before withdrawal of the ventilator, followed by passive flow of oxygen. A 10-minute period of apnoea is usually sufficient to allow $PaCO_2$ to rise above 60 mmHg.' 'Testing of arterial blood gases can be used to confirm this level …Spontaneous breathing efforts indicate that part of the brain stem is functioning … True decerebrate or decorticate posturing or seizures are inconsistent with the diagnosis of death … Peripheral nervous system activity and spinal cord reflexes may persist after death.'
2. Irreversibility of cessation of function of the entire brain is recognized when evaluation discloses the following:
    a. 'The cause of coma is established and is sufficient to account for the loss of brain function … In addition to a careful clinical examination and investigation of history, relevant knowledge of causation may be acquired by computed tomographic scan, measurement of core temperature, drug screening, EEG, angiography, or other procedures.'
    b. 'The possibility of recovery of any brain function is excluded… The most important reversible conditions are sedation, hypothermia, neuromuscular blockade, and shock. In the unusual circumstances where sufficient cause cannot be established, irreversibility can be reliably inferred only after extensive evaluation for drug intoxication, extended observation, and other testing. A determination that blood flow to the brain is absent can be used to demonstrate a sufficient and irreversible condition.'
    c. 'The cessation of all brain functions persist for an appropriate period of observation and/or trial of therapy.' The duration of this period 'is a matter of clinical judgment.' However, when an irreversible condition is well established, cessation of brain function over a period of about 6 hours, 'documented by clinical examination and confirmatory EEG or a period of observation of at least 12 hours' in the absence of confirmatory tests is recommended. An exception is anoxic brain damage in which a period of observation of 24 hours 'is generally desirable.' This 'may be reduced if a test shows cessation of cerebral blood flow or if an EEG shows electrocerebral silence in an adult patient with drug intoxication, hypothermia, or shock.'

Table 3. *(Continued.)*

Complicating Conditions

Condition	Action recommended or special comments
Drug and metabolic intoxication Effects of sedative and anaesthetic drugs especially when multiple drugs are used.	When suspected, 'Toxicology screen for all likely drugs is required. If exogenous intoxication is found, death may not be declared until the intoxicant is metabolized or intracranial circulation is tested and found to have ceased.'
Total paralysis causing unresponsiveness, areflexia, and apnoea due to: Exposure to drugs such as neuromuscular blocking agent and aminoglycoside antibiotics, and diseases like myasthenia gravis.	Careful review of history, evaluation for pseudocholinestherase deficiency after use of succinylcholine chloride. In case of doubt, low-dose atropine stimulation, EMG, peripheral nerve stimulation, EEG, tests of intracranial circulation, short-latency auditory or somatosensory evoked potentials, or extended observation, as indicated.
Some severe illness (e.g. hepatic encephalopathy, hyperosmolar coma, and preterminal uremia)	Metabolic abnormalities should be considered and, if possible, corrected. Confirmatory tests of intracranial circulation or EEG 'may be necessary'.
Hypothermia (core temperature below 32.2°C)	Criteria for reliable recognition of death in the presence of hypothermia are not available. In case of doubt, 'restore normothermia'.
Children 'younger than 5 years'	'Physicians should be particularly cautious.'
Shock	'Physicians should be particularly cautious.'

[a] Excerpts from the Guidelines for the Determination of Death: Report of the Medical Consultants on the Diagnosis of Death to the President's Commission for the Study of Ethical Problems in Medicine and Behavioral Research [9].

affirmation that 'apnoeic coma with absent brain stem reflexes, in a patient with a primary intracranial lesion or after resuscitation from cardiac arrest reliably indicates that brain stem functions will never return. These signs also reliably predict both total brain death and asystole, i.e., 'whole body' death'. Jørgensen's observations [39] were complemented by a prospective study by Jennett and co-workers [40] of 1003 patients still alive 3 months after severe head injury followed by coma of at least 6 h duration. None of these individuals had demonstrated at any time the combination of deep coma, absent eye movements, and unreactive pupils, or had received artificial ventilation not required as a result of chest or trunk injuries or pulmonary complications.

It should be noted that both the UK Code and the US guidelines require that before the final determination of brain death, absence of spontaneous respiration be confirmed by an apnoea challenge test during which artificial ventilation is interrupted long enough to allow the pCO_2 to rise to levels sufficient to stimulate respiration while adequate oxygenation is provided [5,9]. Three problems deserve additional comment: the pupillary diameter, the status of cephalic reflexes and the drug levels of CNS depressants in brain-dead patients. The size of the pupils is not a con-

sistent and reliable indicator of brain death. Allen *et al.* [41] investigated 63 patients with coma, apnoea and ECI for 24 h or more who were not drug-intoxicated and did not survive. In their series, pupils of normal diameter were observed in 25% of cases shortly after onset of apnoeic coma was and in at most 40% of cases in subsequent examinations. Myotic pupils were also noted, although less frequently. Only in those patients who had suffered cardiac arrest was pupillary dilatation consistently observed. In this study, one or more cephalic reflexes were present at some time during the 24 h observation period in seven of 63 patients (11%). Light pupillary, vestibular, oculocephalic, and corneal reflexes were the most useful in that they were most consistently associated with brain death. Walker [22] pointed out that in the American Collaborative study, cephalic reflexes could not always be tested adequately. The presence of an intratracheal tube compromises cough and pharyngeal reflexes, and other cranial nerve reflexes are sometimes impaired by local oedema and drying of tissues. Injuries to the head and face may hinder the study of cranial nerve reflexes. In the same multicentre study, individuals demonstrating the clinical signs of absent brain functions, with the possible exception of pupillary dilatation, frequently had barbiturate blood levels no higher than those regarded as therapeutic for epilepsy. Potentiation of the effects of barbiturates by other drugs and local or systemic conditions that alter the blood–brain barrier were regarded as possibly responsible for the poor correlation between clinical states and blood concentrations of barbiturates. Because of this observation, the presence of even small amounts of barbiturates or other CNS depressants in the blood of brain-dead suspects was thought to be a sign of possible drug toxicity requiring prompt treatment and special caution in interpreting the significance of clinical findings [42].

In this author's opinion [11], brain death can be determined in ordinary circumstances by good history, competent clinical examination, and ordinary laboratory tests alone, as advocated by the UK Code [5]. However, in some instances, doubt exists regarding the cause of coma or the role of certain complicating factors. In other cases the clinical criteria are ambiguously or incompletely fulfilled, such as when brain stem reflexes cannot be tested adequately. In patients intoxicated with CNS depressants or receiving high-dose barbiturate treatment to control intracranial pressure, sometimes combined with the administration of neuromuscular blocking agents and hypothermia, the clinical examination is likely to be uninformative. In these, and other circumstances, prolongation of observation, sometimes over a period of days, may be necessary to establish by purely clinical means that failure of brain function is irreversible [6,8]. Such extended clinical assessment has major disadvantages in that it prolongs the agony of relatives and friends, increases the burden on hospital facilities and personnel, augments already heavy expenditures, deprives the patients of dignity in death, and delays the removal of organs for life-saving transplantation. This approach appears to be justified only when the instrumentation and human skills required for these ancillary studies are not available. This author feels strongly that, whenever brain death is suspected, no effort should be spared to decrease the chances of error, expedite the diagnosis, and provide objective proof of irreversible extinction of brain functions by using appropriate confirmatory procedures [9] (Table 3). Acceptance of this notion invites a critical assessment of the studies proposed to corroborate the clinical diagnosis of brain death.

In principle, ancillary procedures designed to confirm the clinical determination of brain death, should be non-invasive and safe, readily performed at the patient's bedside in the intensive care unit, executed rapidly and reasonably inexpensively, interpretable by intensive care physicians without the assistance of skilled specialists, highly sensitive, highly specific, and independent of aetiology – particularly with regard to those conditions that may reversibly cause the clinical manifestations of brain death. These methods presently include: electrophysiological examinations designed to demonstrate lack of spontaneous and stimulus-elicited electrical activity of the brain, brain perfusion studies intended to establish cessation of intracranial circulation, and tests of brain metabolism devised to demonstrate cessation of vital metabolic processes. A brief review should help determine to what extent each technique fulfils these requirements, if at all.

3.1. Electrophysiologic studies

Corroboration of loss of brain viability by electrophysiologic testing in the adult relies mostly on monitoring of the EEG and evoked potentials.

3.1.1. The EEG

To the extent that the EEG was an indicator of brain and, more specifically, cerebral cortical, function, it seemed natural that it be called upon to provide objective proof of failure of this capacity when the notion of 'coma dépassé' was first developed. Thus, as early as 1959 Fischgold and Mathis [43] reported that scalp records of patients in this condition showed absence of demonstrable EEG potentials, a finding they termed 'silence cérébral' (cerebral silence). Subsequent studies confirmed that brain death was characterized by an enduring state of electrocortical inactivity [44–51]. This electrocerebral silence (ECS) or, more properly, electrocerebral inactivity (ECI) is characterized by 'absence over all regions of the head of identifiable electrical activity of cerebral origin, whether spontaneous or induced by physiological stimuli and pharmacological agents' [52].

Evidence reviewed elsewhere [10,11,32,35] reveals that, in the absence of certain complicating conditions, the demonstration of stringently recorded and properly interpreted ECI [53] indicates that cerebral cortical function has ceased. In the face of persisting clinical evidence of cessation of brain stem functions, the additional demonstration of absent electrocerebral activity attests to a global loss of brain viability that characterizes death of the brain. Complicating conditions that may reversibly cause ECI include overdoses of CNS depressants [22,29,54], hypothermia [9,55], profound hypotension [9,22,55], severe metabolic and endocrine disorders [9], and very young age [9,56]. It should be noted that those same conditions that may reversibly cause ECI may also reversibly produce the clinical manifestations of deep coma, apnoea, and loss of cephalic reflexes. This is a major limitation for a test designed to confirm objectively the clinical diagnosis of permanent loss of brain viability [10,11,35]. Medically sound and cost-effective management of brain death suspects would require that, whenever these complicating conditions are suspected or known, a confirmatory test other than the EEG be used.

It has long been assumed that allowing about 6 h to elapse between the onset of apnoeic coma and the application of EEG criteria of brain death would give adequate protection against 'false positive' determinations of ECI [22]. However, this notion was not supported by careful, detailed studies of Jørgensen and Malchow-Møller [57]. They reported that in individuals who demonstrated ECI immediately after resuscitation from circulatory arrest but subsequently regained consciousness, electrocerebral activity reappeared within 10 min to as long as 8 h after restoration of circulation. Hence, it would seem prudent to let at least 8 h elapse between resuscitation and EEG recording to ensure valid ECI determination [10,11,32]. Fulfilling this widely ignored requirement would add a delay of at least 2 h to the application of EEG criteria of brain death in the adult.

Preparing for and performing EEG recordings on brain death suspects in the intensive care unit that satisfy current stringent technical requirements [53,58] frequently takes as long as 2 h and sometimes longer [59]. These procedures must be performed by highly trained technologists, and interpreted by experienced clinical neurophysiologists [53,58], both of whom are in short supply throughout the world. The EEGs so obtained frequently contain artefacts, including electrical potentials generated by instruments close to or connected to the patient, such as ECG monitors, cardiac pacemakers and dialysis units, and potentials generated by the patient, such as those of muscular, respiratory and cardiovascular origin [29]. Identifying and eliminating or reducing, and monitoring these extracerebral potentials, is a difficult and sometimes unsuccessful task. Hence, in some instances, ambiguity exists as to whether electrocerebral activity is present or absent in the EEGs of patients whose brain viability is in question. Disagreements may arise even among qualified interpreters [10,11,22].

Instances of recovery of EEG activity following ECI have been described in individuals suffering from conditions other than those known to produce reversible depression of electrocerebral potentials and who survived for a long time. Most of these occurrences were not adequately demonstrated. A few more credible reports of recovery of at least some electrocerebral activity in children will be discussed later. In contrast, it has been unambiguously established that electro-

cerebral activity may persist in the EEGs of individuals who satisfy all preconditions and criteria for brain death, have no evidence of blood flow to their brains, and succumbed. In the American Collaborative Study, the presence of at least some EEG activity in patients with apnoeic coma who succumbed characterized those individuals whose brains showed only patchy swelling, oedema, infarction, and necrosis classified as 'partial respirator brain' [19,20,26]. Hence, it was felt that persistence of some EEG activity in clinically brain-dead individuals did not predict prolonged survival or restoration of any form of sentience [60] and that it did not justify the continuation of life-supporting measures [10]. Grigg et al. [61] further reported that 11 of 56 consecutive patients (19.6%) who met the clinical criteria of brain death and did not survive, demonstrated unequivocal EEG activity 3–168 h after this condition was diagnosed. These authors hypothesized that: 'Brain death is present when a critical number of neurones has been irreversibly damaged, such that all the integrative neuronal capacities of the brain are lost' and affirmed that the demonstration of residual EEG activity, 'possibly derived from patchy islands of electrophysiologically active cortical or subcortical tissue' did not change 'the final mortal outcome'. Unfortunately, how much EEG activity is compatible with this judgment and justifies cessation of life-supporting measures is a highly subjective matter.

In some countries, including France and the USA, the EEG has long enjoyed the status of test of choice for confirming the clinical diagnosis of death of the brain in adults. Other corroborative methods have been used, if at all, as adjuncts to, or substitutes for, the EEG. Growing recognition of the limitations and pitfalls of the EEG suggests that at present other techniques are better suited to fill this role. Levy-Alcover and Goulon [62] reported confirming brain death by EEG by performing a first 30-minute recording demonstrating ECI ('tracé nul') at the time brain death was clinically diagnosed. This test was followed by a second 15-minute recording of ECI obtained 6–8 h after the first. Assuming that the clinical diagnosis was established about 6 h after the brain insult, and taking into consideration preparation time, total time required for EEG confirmation would have been in excess of 13–15 h and probably substantially longer. In the event of complicating clinical conditions, repeating clinical and EEG observations after at least 24 h [63] would have required substantially more than 30 h and 45 min, probably 33–34 h if not longer. At variance with the conclusions of Levy-Alcover and Goulon [62], it appears that EEG recording is a slow and cumbersome process of sometimes uncertain results that does not guarantee the expeditious determination of brain death in the adult.

3.1.2. *Evoked potentials*

The determination of ECI in patients fulfilling the clinical criteria of brain death requires special efforts visually to resolve minute electrical potentials of cerebral origin from spurious potentials of instrumental or biological origin. In contrast to the spontaneous EEG, the detection of neural responses to stimuli benefits from the use of computer averaging techniques capable of extracting small stimulus-locked signals from unrelated noise. Moreover, unlike the EEG, which primarily reflects cerebral cortical activity, these evoked potentials provide objective measures of both brain stem and cortical capacities. Standards for their performance and interpretation have been published by the American Electroencephalographic Society [53].

In studies of patients suspected of having non-viable brains, evoked potentials have been obtained in response to sensory stimuli, generally visual, auditory, and somatosensory excitations and, more recently, by transcranial magnetic stimulation of the motor cortex.

Visual evoked potentials [64], generally elicited by light flashes in visual and related cortices and recorded from the intact scalp, were shown to be abolished in individuals fulfilling all clinical criteria of brain death [27,65,66] or with incompletely specified clinical criteria but with complete arrest of intracranial circulation demonstrated by contrast angiography [67]. Because the retina is more resistant than the brain to anoxia, electroretinograms may be detected over the anterior head regions in the absence of cerebral visual evoked potentials. Preservation of these retinal responses is irrelevant to the outcome of clinically brain-dead patients [10,11,32,35]. A limitation of visual evoked potentials in the study of brain death is that they are highly vulnerable to hypothermia [68,69] and CNS depressant drugs.

Brainstem auditory evoked potentials [70] are generated by the auditory nerve and brain stem auditory pathways in response to click stimuli and are detected from the surface of the head. These potentials were found to be abolished in brain death, with the possible exception of waves I (from the auditory nerve), I and II (the latter presumably also generated, at least in part, by the auditory nerve) [67,71–77] or, in a few cases, I–III [67]. Obliteration of these responses probably results from anoxic–ischaemic changes secondary to arrest of the intracranial circulation [73]. However, other pathological circumstances summarized elsewhere [11,35] may cause loss of brain stem auditory

evoked potentials. These include peripheral deafness or profound hearing loss, whether pre-existing or caused by conditions such as trauma, meningitis, or anoxia. In head-injured patients in particular, cochlear or auditory nerve damage secondary to fracture of the temporal bone, blood in the external auditory canal and injury to the tympanic membrane and the middle ear may cause, or contribute to, loss of brain stem auditory evoked potentials.

Brief electrical excitations of peripheral nerves, most commonly the median nerve at the wrist, were used to elicit early (short-latency) somatosensory evoked potentials [78]. In brain-dead patients, responses to stimulation of this nerve showed obliteration of their cortical components (the N20 and subsequent waves) [66,67,73], loss of a low medullar (P14) and of spinal (N13) components, and frequent persistence of brachial plexus potentials (P9-N10) [11,35]. Reports of variable preservation of the low medullar P14 wave in brain death [79,80] have not been confirmed. Injuries to peripheral nerves may preclude the performance or confound the interpretation of somatosensory evoked potentials. Moreover, on occasion, myogenic contamination may complicate them [81].

In a recent study of brain perfusion by radioisotope scintigraphy, Schlake *et al.* [77] alluded to lack of all central potentials to both clicks and median nerve stimuli in patients with brain death, and similarly absent or delayed responses in persistently vegetative and deeply comatose individuals.

Magnetic transcutaneous stimulation of the motor cortex or the spinal cord elicits motor potentials, i.e. compound motor action potentials in appropriate muscles [82]. In patients with irreversibly extinguished brain functions, these responses were absent to transcranial stimulation, but those to cervical stimulation were preserved [83].

Available evidence suggests that demonstration of abolished brain stem and cortical potentials in response to auditory, somatosensory and visual stimulation, and inability to elicit motor responses to transcranial magnetic stimulation, indicates widespread failure of cerebral functions. This finding adds substance to the clinical evidence of brain death. An especially interesting feature of short-latency auditory and somatosensory evoked potentials is that, unlike the spontaneous EEG, they are not significantly altered by CNS depressants even in large doses [72,84], at least in the absence of hypothermia [72,85]. However, because each evoked potential modality study suffers from limitations and only explores topographically limited pathways, a minimum of two modalities, generally somatosensory and auditory, should be assessed in patients whose brain viability is in question. Multimodality evoked potential studies performed at the bedside on patients receiving intensive care are time consuming and require superior technical expertise and interpretive skills. They are, therefore, ill-suited for the routine and rapid confirmation of the clinical diagnosis of brain death in the adult. Different opinions have been expressed by Guérit [76].

3.2. Brain perfusion studies

Wertheimer *et al.* [86] first made the observation that blood flow to the brain had ceased in patients in coma dépassé. Subsequently, the notion that the mechanisms responsible for brain death, however complex, ultimately led to arrest of intracranial circulation won general acceptance [23]. Thus, techniques designed to assess brain perfusion were extensively used to confirm the clinical diagnosis of irreversible failure of brain functions. Methods designed to demonstrate absence or critical deficits of brain perfusion include contrast angiography, radioisotope scintigraphy, Doppler ultrasonography and tests of brain metabolism.

3.2.1. *Contrast angiography*
Early studies demonstrated that the clinical and EEG manifestations of irreversible loss of brain function were consistently associated with the demonstration of non-filling of brain vessels by contrast angiography [87–93]. In Scandinavian countries, the demonstration of arrest of intracranial circulation by transfemoral four-vessel brain angiography was included among the cardinal criteria of brain death [94]. This method encountered little favour in the USA for routine use in brain-dead suspects primarily because of its invasive nature, its relative complexity and cost, the danger that intra-arterial administration of contrast material may produce further critical diminution of brain perfusion [22], and the risks involved in the transportation of respirator-dependent patients to the angiography suite. Yet, it remained the gold standard for determining the arrest of intracranial circulation in brain death suspects. Some of the problems of contrast angiography were obviated by the advent of intravenous digital subtraction angiography [95,96], a technique that also distinguished intracranial from extracranial vessels. Rapid contrast-enhanced computed tomography [97] had the advantage of providing information on intracranial pathology while establishing the absence of blood flow to the brain.

3.2.2. *Radioisotope scintigraphy*
The advent of intravenous radioisotope scintigraphy [98] provided safe alternatives to contrast angiography,

although the latter remained the gold standard for assessing blood flow to the brain. Initially, radionuclide cerebral scintigraphy was limited to detecting the passage through the intracranial circulation of an intravenously injected radioisotopic bolus displayed as a characteristic curve. Lack of this cranial bolus tracing attested to absence or critical decrease of cerebral blood flow to less than 24% of normal [99], a finding believed to be incompatible with preservation of cerebral functions. The results of this technique were confirmed by contrast angiography [100] and were associated with clinical, EEG, and pathological evidence of brain death [101–103]. Subsequently, visualization of radioactive uptake within the anterior and middle cerebral arteries provided a more direct method for assessing cerebral blood flow. Lack of uptake in early dynamic images, even when associated with faint visualization of the sagittal sinus in static images [104], attested to a critical deficit of cerebral perfusion. This finding was associated with clinical signs of brain death [98,105–110], confirmation of cessation of blood flow to the brain by four-vessel contrast angiography [104,111], lack of electrocerebral activity in EEG recordings, with some exceptions [105,108,112], and severe autolytic changes in the brain at autopsy [98,108]. In more than 25 000 radionuclide angiograms performed in one centre, no condition other than brain death was associated with the absence of cerebral perfusion [106]. An advantage of radionuclide cerebral scintigraphy was that it could be readily performed at the patient's bedside in the intensive care unit using a portable gamma camera [106]. The results of this technique, unlike those of the EEG, were not appreciably confounded by barbiturate intoxication or treatment [106,108,113,114] and hypothermia [108].

Objections to cerebral radionuclide scintigraphy as a confirmatory test of brain death were that it did not adequately distinguish between severely diminished and absent cerebral blood flow and provided no assessment of brain stem perfusion [114]. In recent years, these problems have been alleviated by the introduction of technetium-99m hexamethyl-propylene amine oxide (^{99m}Tc-HMPAO). This lipophilic agent crosses the intact blood–brain barrier and is extracted by brain tissue in proportion to regional perfusion [115,116]. ^{99m}Tc-HMPAO brain scintigraphy provides adequate imaging of brain stem perfusion and differentiates between severely decreased and absent brain perfusion with greater accuracy than conventional radionuclide scintigraphy [77,114,117]. Hypothermia and toxic/metabolic factors do not appreciably alter the brain uptake of this compound [118,119]. ^{99m}Tc-HMPAO tomographic brain scintigraphy can also be performed at the bedside with a single photon emission computed tomography (SPECT) system [120]. Unfortunately, ^{99m}Tc-HMPAO is a labile compound the preparation of which requires special care and the cost of brain scintigraphy with this isotope substantially exceeds that of conventional radionuclide scintigraphy.

This review suggests that both conventional radionuclide and ^{99m}Tc-HMPAO brain scintigraphy are non-invasive, safe, rapid, easily and quickly interpretable, and reliable methods for confirming at the bedside the clinical diagnosis of brain death in the adult.

3.2.3. Doppler ultrasonography and xenon-enhanced computed tomography

In recent years, several investigators have used Doppler ultrasonography to corroborate the clinical diagnosis of brain death in adults. Early studies demonstrated a close association between absence of midline pulsatile echoes in normotensive patients and cessation of cerebral blood flow [121]. Subsequent investigations focused on the analysis of blood flow velocity wave form in the common carotid [122] and the middle cerebral and basilar arteries. Wave form alterations most commonly consisted of brief, sharp systolic peaks followed by reverse or absent flow during diastole [59,123–127]. However, preserved forward flow throughout diastole was observed in some patients with skull defects or ventricular drains [59] and Doppler signals were unobtainable, or the studies were incomplete, in up to 10% of cases [59,127]. Moreover, the incidence of false-negative and false-positive results of transcranial Doppler has not been definitely established. Powers et al. [126] reported that identification of flow velocity reversal alone was inadequate to demonstrate brain death. Net flow velocity measurements more sensitively indicated this condition and closely paralleled neurological status. In keeping with this belief, Payen et al. [128] used Doppler common carotid flow velocity measurements as indices of mean hemispheric perfusion and established quantitative criteria which discriminated between brain-dead and deeply comatose patients. Due to potential confounding effects of carotid artery disease, they recommended that their method should be used primarily for assessing cerebral circulation in patients younger than 35 years. These more quantitative approaches deserve special attention in future research which is needed to determine the validity of Doppler ultrasonography as a confirmatory test of death of the brain.

Only limited information is available on the use in adults of xenon-enhanced computer tomography,

which is capable of measuring cerebral blood flow in multiple brain regions in brain death suspects [129]. Further study is needed to establish the validity of this method in determining loss of brain viability

3.3. Metabolic studies

Tests have been devised to demonstrate the cessation of vital metabolic processes in patients with dead brains. Cerebral metabolic rates of oxygen ($CMRO_2$) below 1 ml/g/min and arteriovenous oxygen differences ($AVDO_2$) of less than 2 vol % were believed to indicate extinction of brain functions [22,130]. Assaying cerebrospinal fluid lactic acid content [22] and enzymes [131] was also felt to be useful. Recently, Kato et al. [132] reported preliminary results of P-31 magnetic resonance (MR) spectroscopy. In brain death, this technique showed high monopeak and absence of adenosine triphosphate (ATP) and phosphocreatine (PCr) detectable in healthy brains. Whether these findings will prove useful in substantiating the diagnosis of brain death remains to be determined.

4. Diagnosis of brain death in neonates and infants

4.1. US guidelines and a review of the available literature

Since the earliest formulations of criteria of brain death, doubts were expressed whether standards derived from observations on adults are applicable to newborns, infants and young children. In keeping with these uncertainties, the US guidelines [9] cautioned that the recommended clinical and ancillary criteria of brain death may not be valid under the age of 5 years (Table 3). However, Solomon et al. [33] found no evidence in the literature that any patient between the ages of 3 months and 6 years who had fulfilled all clinical criteria of brain death formulated for adults had survived. Guidelines for establishing brain death in neonates and infants, subsequently issued by a Special Task Force for the Determination of Brain Death in Children [133] stated that establishing cessation of cerebral and brain stem functions and determining its irreversibility was possible no earlier than 7 days after severe insults to the brains of newborns at term. Clinical criteria of brain death applicable after this time (Table 4) did not differ from those recommended for adults. However, between the ages of 7 days and 1 year, the validity of these criteria

Table 4. Physical examination and laboratory criteria for determining brain death in newborns and infants.

Physical examination[a]	EEG[b]	Cerebral angiography[a,c]
Coma and apnoea Absence of brain stem function Lack of significant hypothermia or hypotension for age 'Flaccid tone and absence of spontaneous or induced movements, excluding spinal cord events such as reflex withdrawal or spinal myoclonus'. The above findings should remain constant throughout the observation period.	Electrocerebral inactivity (ECI) as defined by the AEEGS guidelines [9]. For neonates and young infants up to the age of 2 months, effective recording time should be no less than 1 hour and numbers and locations of electrodes, and montages should meet the AEEGS guidelines for paediatric EEG [132] Extreme caution should be used in the presence of even small blood concentrations of CNS depressants.	Lack of visualization of intracranial arterial circulation in radionuclide cerebral angiogram, or lack of effect on blood flow to brain in contrast angiography.

[a] Based on: Guidelines for the determination of brain death in children. Report of Special Task Force for the Determination of Brain Death in Children [133].
[b] Modified from the recommendations included in: Guidelines for the determination of brain death in children. Report of Special Task Force for the Determination of Brain Death in Children [133].
[c] Value of EEG and radionuclide cerebral angiogram in infants under 2 months is under investigation.

Table 5. Types of studies and observation periods for determining brain death in newborns and infants[a].

Patient's age	Types of studies and observation periods
7 days–2 months	Two physical examinations and two EEGs demonstrating ECI at least 24 h apart
> 2 months–1 year	Two physical examinations and two EEGs showing ECI at least 24 h apart; or a physical examination, an EEG demonstrating ECI, and a radionuclide cerebral angiogram showing no visualization of cerebral arteries
> 1 year	Assuming demonstration of irreversible cause of coma, there should be two physical examinations fulfilling criteria of brain death 24 h apart without laboratory testing. Period of observation should be prolonged by at least 24 h if the extent and irreversibility of brain damage are uncertain (especially in hypoxic–ischaemic encephalopathy), or it may be reduced if the EEG demonstrates ECI or if the radionuclide cerebral angiogram does not visualize cerebral arteries

[a] Based on: Guidelines for the determination of brain death in children. Report of Special Task Force for the Determination of Brain Death in Children [133].

depended on their persistence during specified periods of clinical observation as well as on their confirmation by EEG, visualization of intracranial circulation, or both (Table 5). No such constraints were advocated after the age of 1 year (Table 5).

The recommendations of the Special Task Force [133] drew sharp criticism from Freeman and Ferry [134] and Shewmon [135] who felt that the proposed standards were premature and based on combined clinical and auxiliary criteria, none of which had been validated. To inquire into the bases for these guidelines, the author of this chapter reviewed the available literature on brain death in young patients ranging in age from premature to 5 years old. Because of paucity and limitations of published data, this inquiry identified only 97 patients whose ages had been specified and in whom current clinical criteria, of brain death [133] appeared to have been met. This number is substantially smaller than in previous reviews based on less stringent criteria, wider age ranges, or both [110,136]. The individuals included in this review consisted of (1) 19 clinically brain-dead newborns, of whom nine were premature infants of 28–38 weeks gestation, examined, when specified, within a few hours to 10 days after birth, and 10 of whom were term newborns up to 7 days old [137–140], (2) 12 term newborns and young infants over 7 days old to 2 months [137,139,141], (3) 28 infants over 2 months to 1 year of age [108,137, 140–147] and (4) 38 children 1–5 years old [104,108,137,140,141,143–146]. Of these 97 clinically brain-dead patients, 86 were studied with methods designed to corroborate the clinical determination, consisting of single or multiple EEGs in 65 patients and individual or repeated brain perfusion tests in 82. The latter techniques included intravenous radionuclide cerebral scintigraphy [104,108,137,139,140,142, 144,145], sometimes complemented by transfemoral four-vessel brain angiography [104,142] or xenon-enhanced computed tomography [140,145], transcutaneous [138,148] and transcranial [146] Doppler ultrasonography and real-time cranial ultrasonography

[143]. Extreme scarcity of data made it essential to combine the results of these heterogeneous methods.

Both EEG and brain perfusion studies were used in 68 individuals. Results of final tests (Tables 6–8) are limited in number. However, it is noteworthy that only half (7 of 14) premature and term newborns up to the age of 7 days demonstrated ECI in their last EEGs (Table 6) whereas nearly three-quarters (5 of 14) showed no detectable cerebral blood flow in their final brain perfusion studies (Table 7). Remarkably, when both EEGs and brain perfusion tests were performed (Table 8), the joint demonstration of ECI and absent cerebral blood flow confirmed the clinical diagnosis in only four of 14 neonates up to 7 days of age and the combined finding of persistent electrocerebral activity and blood flow contradicted the clinical assessment in

Table 6. Results of final EEGs in 65 young patients with clinically determined brain death.

Results	Age groups							
	0–7 days[a]		> 7 days–2 months[b]		> 2 months–1 year[c]		> 1–5 years[d]	
	n	%	n	%	n	%	n	%
ECI[e]	7	50	12	100	14	78	16	76
ECA[f]	7	50	0	0	4	22	5	24
Total	14		12		18		21	

[a] From references 137, 139, 142.
[b] From references 137, 138, 139, 140, 145.
[c] From references 108, 137, 140, 142, 143, 145, 146.
[d] From references 108, 137, 140, 143, 145, 146.
[e] ECI: Electrocerebral inactivity.
[f] ECA: Electrocerebral activity.

Table 7. Results of final brain perfusion studies in 82 young patients with clinically determined brain death.

Results	Age groups							
	0–7 days[a]		> 7 days–2 months[b]		> 2 months–1 year[c]		> 1–5 years[d]	
	n	%	n	%	n	%	n	%
No CBF[e]	9	64	11	92	19	83	28	85
CBF	5	36	1	8	4	17	5	15
Total	14		12		23		33	

[a] From references 137, 139, 142.
[b] From references 137, 138, 139, 140, 145.
[c] From references 108, 137, 140, 142, 143, 145, 146.
[d] From references 108, 137, 143, 145, 146.
[e] CBF: cerebral blood flow.

two. In over half of cases (8 of 14) the two methods gave conflicting results in that electrocerebral activity persisted in the absence of detectable blood flow in five patients and ECI was demonstrated in the presence of flow in three. This discordance was complete in five premature infants studied by Ashwal and Schneider [139], three of whom had ECI despite cerebral blood flow whereas two showed preserved electrocerebral activity but no flow. However small, these numbers suggest that the frequency of preserved electrocerebral activity (Table 6) and of discordant EEG and brain perfusion findings (Table 8) is lower in young patients between the ages of 7 days and 5 years than in newborns up to 7 days old, whereas the frequency of preserved cerebral blood flow showed no substantial changes (Table 7). These impressions were validated by χ^2 analysis, which demonstrated statistically significant differences between the age group of 0–7 days and the combined totals of the three remaining groups with respect to the frequency of EEG findings (Table 6, χ^2, 1 df = 4.56, $p < 0.05$) and of combined EEG and brain perfusion results (Table 6, χ^2, 3 df = 12.51, $p < 0.01$), but not with respect to the results of cerebral blood flow studies alone. These data cast serious doubt on the validity of EEG and combined EEG and brain perfusion studies, but not of brain perfusion studies alone, as confirmatory tests of clinically determined brain death in the immediate neonatal period. All prematures and term neonates up to 7 days succumbed 2–15 days after brain death was recognized, either due to somatic death or following with-

drawal of respiratory support. It appears that, in the face of discordant results of auxiliary methods, persistent clinical evidence of absent brain functions ultimately guided the physicians' decision to discontinue life-supporting measures in those neonates in whom death did not occur spontaneously. However limited, these data add substance to the contention of the Special Task Force [133] that establishing cessation of brain functions and determining its irreversibility cannot be made less than 7 days after the initial brain insult in newborns at term. The results of this review also invite the suspicion that combining tests subject to different and mutable influences may on occasion hinder rather than facilitate the determination of brain death, especially in the immediate neonatal period.

The notion is widely accepted that unique problems are met in attempting to determine by clinical observation and ancillary methods that brain functions have ceased in newborns and young infants and in establishing that this functional failure is irreversible. In a thoughtful introductory commentary to the guidelines of the Special Task Force [133], Volpe [149] emphasized that 'many of the critical functions to be assessed are either still in the process of developing or have only recently developed' and that 'developing systems or recently acquired developmental functions are exquisitely vulnerable to injury by exogenous insults'. Rapid changes occur during the last 12–15 weeks of gestation in such functions as level of alertness, pupillary size and reaction to light, and the control of venti-

Table 8. Results of final combined EEG and brain perfusion studies in 68 young patients with clinically determined brain death[a].

Results	Age groups							
	0–7 days[a]		> 7 days–2 months[b]		> 2 months–1 year[c]		> 1–5 years[d]	
	n	%	n	%	n	%	n	%
ECI,[e] no CBF[f]	4	29	11	92	12	60	17	77
ECA,[g] CBF	2	14	0	0	3	15	3	14
ECI, CBF	3	21	1	8	1	5	2	9
ECA, no CBF	5	36	0	0	4	20	0	0
Total	14		12		20		22	

[a] From references 137, 139, 142.
[b] From references 137, 138, 139, 140, 145.
[c] From references 108, 137, 140, 142, 143, 145, 146.
[d] From references 108, 137, 143, 145, 146.
[e] ECI: electrocerebral inactivity.
[f] CBF: cerebral blood flow.
[g] ECA: electrocerebral activity.

lation, eye movements and bulbar reflexes [149]. Some brain stem reflexes, such as pupillary and oculocephalic reflexes, are not fully developed before 32 weeks of gestation, and caloric stimulation is difficult to perform and assess in neonates [150]. Clinical experience suggests that recovery from prolonged unresponsive coma is not uncommon among neonates, infants and children [150], although no data are available to indicate that this outcome is more frequent than in adults. Even the reliability of apnoea tests in this age group has been questioned [150]. In addition to developmental factors, other conditions may confound the clinical assessment of brain viability in the early developmental period. Profound systemic hypotension, frequent among newborns and young infants suspected of having dead brains, may so reduce cerebral perfusion as to cause potentially reversible clinical manifestations of loss of brain functions. A major complicating factor is that a substantial number of neonates and infants suspected of having dead brains are treated with high-dose intravenous pentobarbital to control intracranial pressure or have received high-dose intravenous phenobarbital because of proven or suspected seizures. Barbiturates have profound depressing effects on the CNS of severely brain damaged neonates [110]. However, the blood concentrations of barbiturate drugs associated with these effects have not been established with certainty and may be far lower than it is commonly assumed, as reported in adults [42]. The inclusion in the therapeutic protocol of neutomuscular blocking agents and hypothermia may further complicate the clinical assessment of these young patients. Volpe [149] also pointed out that a large proportion of newborns with suspected irreversible loss of brain functions suffer from hypoxic–ischaemic encephalopathies secondary to perinatal asphyxia of unclear duration and severity. In this age group, the extent and gravity of hypoxic–ischaemic injury is thought to be inadequately assessed by the clinical examination. These factors limit the validity of the clinical criteria of deep coma, apnoea and abseat brain stem reflexes as indicators of global loss of brain functions in neonates and young infants, and periods of observation longer than in older patients are felt to be essential to determine their irreversibility [149,150]. Unfortunately, how long these periods should be is difficult to establish on the basis of the available literature. Because of uncertain reliability of the clinical examination, confirmation of the diagnosis by auxiliary methods would strengthen and expedite the determination of brain death. Regrettably, a number of factors conspire to limit the validity of these methods in neonates and young infants.

4.2. Technical and interpretive requirements of the EEG

The EEGs of neonates and small infants have features which evolve particularly rapidly between prematurity and 2 months after term. Neonatal EEGs are characteristically discontinuous, displaying bursts of activity separated by periods of apparent inactivity [151]. The duration of these featureless intervals may increase under the influence of a variety of physiological and pathological factors, including those conditions that may reversibly cause clinical signs of loss of brain functions, such as hypotension, hypothermia, and toxic/metabolic disorders. Hence, to determine whether electrocerebral activity is present or absent in the EEGs of neonates and young infants suspected of having dead brains, the effective duration of EEG recording must be at least 1 h. Unfortunately, published EEG studies of brain death suspects of these ages consisted of recordings lasting 30 minutes, in keeping with the standards recommended for older patients [152] recently endorsed by the Special Task Force for the Determination of Brain Death in Children [133], conceptional, as distinct from gestational, ages were frequently not specified. The small heads of these patients require the use of a smaller number of scalp electrodes in standardized locations (as opposed to smaller interelectrode distances) [133]. It should also be noted that, despite some preliminary data [139] the blood concentrations of CNS depressant drugs insufficient to suppress EEG activity have not been determined [133], and that even low concentrations may influence the EEGs of young patients suspected of having dead brains, as is the case in adults [42]. Because the EEGs of neonates and infants are extremely sensitive to a variety of endogenous and exogenous factors, recordings demonstrating ECI in patients of these ages should be repeated after an appropriate interval to ensure that electrocerebral activity is still absent. To this end, an interval of 24 h [133] may be appropriate, but this is not based on adequate published data. A matter of additional concern is the lack of expressed recognition [133] that because of their peculiarities the EEGs of neonates and young infants must be interpreted by clinical neurophysiologists with special experience in this age group. There are few individuals with adequate training in this field among adult and paediatric neurologists as well as neonatologists. How many published reports of ECI, and perhaps also of preserved EEG activity in this age group, were influenced by these technical and interpretive factors cannot be determined.

Although the exclusion of complicating conditions that may reversibly suppress the EEG remains a pre-requisite for the validity of ECI in older infants and children, the interpretation of this finding generally is viewed with greater confidence by most authors after the age of 2–3 months. Alvarez *et al.* [153] studied retrospectively 52 patients aged 7 days to 5 years (mean: 2.25 years) who had ECI in at least one EEG (presumably the last one) and met for at least 6 h prior to the recording the clinical criteria of brain death used for adults. All patients in this series succumbed, either spontaneously (31) or following withdrawal of respiratory support (21). When examined, their brains showed pathological changes characteristic of brain death. The authors concluded that even a single EEG demonstrating ECI in the absence of toxic/metabolic disorders, hypotension, and hypothermia is sufficient to confirm permanent loss of brain viability in patients above the age of 3 months. Indeed, most cases of recovery of EEG activity following ECI, whether temporary or long lasting, were not documented beyond doubt in the absence of hypothermia, hypotension, and CNS depressants [33,154]. It is difficult to exclude that diminishing effects of phenobarbital may also have played a role in the restoration of EEG activity associated with partial, transient neurological recovery in a 5-year-old child [108] (case 18) and in a 3-month-old infant [147]. However, in a term newborn reported by Ashwal and Schneider [139] (patient 6) and in a 3-month old infant not receiving barbiturates examined by Ashwal *et al.* [140] (patient 11) restoration of at least minimal EEG activity ('near ECS') was described. Of these patients, only the last survived, in a vegetative state. Hence, with rare and somewhat questionable exceptions, ECI, once established, generally persists in successive EEGs obtained in young clinically brain-dead patients free of hypotension, toxic/metabolic factors, and hypothermia [110].

Even in the absence of complicating and potentially reversible conditions, ECI may occur in clinically brain-dead neonates and young infants in whom cerebral blood flow is present [137,139,155]. Conversely, electrocerebral activity can be detected in the absence of cerebral blood flow [108,110,137,139,140,142,145], although in several instances repeated recordings often ultimately demonstrate ECI [110,137,139,142].

Half of the brain-dead neonates up to 7 days after term displayed some degree of EEG activity 3–10 days (mean: 7 days) after admission (Table 8). Islands of electrophysiologically active brain tissue in otherwise non-functional brains are likely to generate this residual activity. However, on occasion, loss of brain stem functions with relative preservation of cerebral functions may account for this finding [129]. Whatever its origin, it is generally agreed that preserved EEG activity in the face of persisting clinical evidence of loss of brain functions does not rule out brain death and does not warrant continuation of life-supporting measures in neonates, infants and children [108,110,142, 149,157], as in adults [11,19,20,26,61]. This belief is further strengthened when additional brain perfusion studies show absence or critical reduction of cerebral blood flow. It is of interest that in the cases reviewed in this chapter, the frequency of persistent EEG activity in brain-dead infants and young children approached that reported in adults [61].

The limitations of the EEG and considerations of cost-effectiveness require that this method be used with special restraint and caution to assess brain viability in neonates and young infants, especially before the age of 2 months, and only when the appropriate technical and interpretative skills are available.

4.3. Evoked potentials

Limited and primarily anecdotal data have also been reported on evoked potentials obtained on very young brain death suspects. In a few individuals with this diagnosis, Setzer *et al.* [158] demonstrated obliteration of brain stem auditory and cortical somatosensory evoked potentials, a combination of findings apparently not observed in children suffering from other conditions. However, Steinhart and Weiss [159], Dear and Godfrey [160], Taylor *et al.* [161] and Drake *et al.* [110] reported that following hypoxic episodes, brain stem auditory evoked potentials disappeared transiently in a few newborns, infants and small children who did not fulfil criteria of brain death and survived, although mostly with neurological sequelae. Of additional interest is the case of a 3-year-old child who met incompletely current clinical criteria of brain death and demonstrated ECI, preserved cerebral blood flow, absent visual evoked potentials, prolonged I–III intervals of brain stem auditory evoked potentials, and succumbed after 26 days [155]. These data suggest that, until sufficiently extensive information is obtained evoked potentials should not be routinely relied upon to confirm irreversible loss of brain viability in neonates, infants, and small children [11,35].

4.4. Brain perfusion and other studies

Single or repeated brain perfusion tests ultimately demonstrated cessation or critical deficit of cerebral blood flow in 67 of 82 newborns, infants and children included in Table 7. All 53 patients without detectable cerebral blood flow in whom EEGs were additionally performed (Table 8) died within 2–30 days , irrespective of whether electrocerebral activity was absent or present. However limited, these findings suggest that failure to detect cerebral blood flow in young patients with persisting clinical signs of brain death reliably establishes lack of potential for recovery of brain functions [110,139]. However, Volpe [149] cautioned that cerebral blood flow values below which cerebral radionuclide scintigrams detect no flow may be close to values compatible with preservation of brain functions and may in fact be relatively frequent in newborns without clinical or pathological evidence of brain death. The legitimacy of this concern is confirmed by the case briefly alluded to by Coulter [162] of a brain-dead newborn in whom cerebral blood flow was not detected by radionuclide scintigrams but was demonstrated by high pressure contrast angiography. However, this finding is at variance with the experience of other authors who found no disagreements between the two methods in their young patients [104,142]. Hence, careful consideration should be given to the patient's systemic blood pressure before interpreting lack of cerebral blood flow in brain perfusion tests as confirmatory of brain death in newborns and small infants. It has been suggested that in spite of shortcomings, transfemoral four-vessel contrast angiography, still the gold standard for visualizing the intracranial circulation, may be resorted to in particular cases in which brain death viability remains in question and must be demonstrated beyond doubt, such as when donation of vascularized organs is considered [104,135,142]. A remarkable advantage of radioisotope scintigraphy and other brain perfusion methods is that their results, unlike those of the EEG, are not demonstrably altered by hypothermia and CNS depressants [77,108,114].

That cerebral blood flow may persist in some clinically brain-dead neonates in the presence or in the absence of electrocerebral activity [108,137,139] has been explained by postulating that, due to the presence of open fontanelles and sutures, the skull of the newborn behaves as an expandable chamber. Because of this peculiarity, the oedema associated with brain death may be insufficient to raise the intracranial pressure above the mean arterial pressure, thus allowing continued cerebral blood flow [153]. However likely, this explanation does not account for the demonstration of the same phenomenon in older patients, including young children [108]. Moreover, lack of scintigraphic evidence of cerebral perfusion in some young brain-dead suspects with mean arterial pressure

higher than intracranial pressure, suggests that intracranial pressure exceeding mean arterial pressure is not the sole explanation for the absence of cerebral perfusion [108,136].

All young patients included in this review died, whether spontaneously or following withdrawal of respiratory support, except for three: a 3-month old [145] and a 4-year-old with near drowning [108] both of whom survived in a vegetative state, and a 3-month old with Reye's syndrome who had full neurologic recovery [108]. Three additional patients, aged 3 months [147], 20 months and 5 years [108], had transient neurologic recovery but subsequently died spontaneously. In all these cases, both cerebral blood flow and EEG activity were preserved, except for the first [145] in whom slow cerebral blood flow was associated with ECI. Hence, the possibility of survival in a vegetative state or even of neurologic recovery should be considered in young patients up to the age of 5 years who demonstrate preserved cerebral blood flow, especially if associated with persistent EEG. In these instances, more prolonged clinical observation and repeated brain perfusion and, eventually, EEG testing are indicated. Additional information on the clinical course and outcome of brain dead patients was given by Rowland et al. [141], Drake et al. [110] and Alvarez et al. [153]

P-31 MR spectroscopy failed to detect adenosine triphosphate (ATP) and phosphocreatinine (PCr) in 5 brain-dead patients aged 2–19 months [132]. The potential of this method as a confirmatory test of irreversible loss of brain viability remains to be established.

4.5. UK recommendations

Recently, the problems posed by the diagnosis of brain death in children received consideration by a Working Party of the British Paediatric Association [7]. This group concluded that for infants below 37 weeks gestation 'the concept of brain stem death is inappropriate...' and that in this age group, 'Decisions on whether to continue intensive care should be based on an assessment of the likely outcome of the condition, after close discussion with the family.' The Working Party also concluded that 'given the current state of knowledge it is rarely possible confidently to diagnose brain stem death...' between the ages of 37 weeks gestation and 2 months. For children older than 2 months, it was recommended that the formal assessment of brain stem death be 'approached in an unhurried manner' to ensure that all preconditions are satisfied and all excluding conditions are ruled out. 'The assessment of children in this age group' should be carried out separately by two experienced clinicians of consultant or senior registrar status; at least one should be a paediatrician, one should be a consultant, and one should not be primarily involved in the child's care.' This Working Party did not feel confident, given the current state of knowledge, that the EEG and evoked potential recordings would be helpful additions in the diagnosis of brain stem death. It also concluded that angiographic, radio-isotope, and Doppler techniques were complex to carry out and that 'low or absent cerebral blood flow does not necessarily equate with brain stem death'.

5. Summary and conclusions

In formulating criteria for determining brain death, the notion is often overlooked that substantial numbers of small hospitals in developed countries and most hospitals in the developing world lack the instrumentation and skills required to perform and interpret ancillary studies designed to corroborate the clinical diagnosis of irreversible loss of brain viability. In these circumstances, unless the patient can be safely transported to a properly equipped medical centre, there are no alternatives but to establish the diagnosis of brain death by prolonged clinical observation. To this end, the guidelines of the UK criteria may prove especially helpful [8]. However, in this author's opinion, whenever appropriate instrumentation and human skills are available, ancillary tests confirming the clinical diagnosis should be conducted to decrease the chances of error and expedite the determination of brain death. This is viewed as essential to ensure dignity in death, diminish the human and monetary costs of unnecessarily prolonging artificial supportive measures, provide objective proof of irreversible loss of brain viability, and increase the opportunities for removal of viable organs for life-saving transplantation [10,11]. Performance of these auxiliary procedures is recommended by the U.S. Guidelines [9] and mandated by French governmental regulations [4,38].

Confirmatory methods critically analysed in this chapter include EEG, evoked potentials, brain perfusion, and metabolic studies. In many countries, including France and the USA, the EEG has long been used as the method of choice for corroborating the clinical diagnosis of brain death. Unfortunately, this technique is time-consuming, requires specialized technical and professional expertise, is subject to failures and misinterpretations, and has inadequate sensitivity and specificity in the context of brain death.

Persistence of some form of EEG activity does not exclude brain death, and electrocerebral inactivity (ECI) may be reversibly caused by complicating factors, including large doses of CNS depressants, other severe toxic/metabolic disorders, profound hypotension, and hypothermia, all of which are common among brain death suspects. These same conditions may also transiently cause clinical manifestations of global loss of brain functions, the irreversibility of which the EEG is called to confirm. Because of these limitations and pitfalls, French laws require the finding of electrocerebral inactivity (ECI) to be confirmed by repeating the EEG after an interval of at least 6 h, a requirement that further delays the determination of brain death. Data analysed in this chapter strongly suggest that, at present, intravenous radionuclide cerebral scintigraphy performed at the patient's bedside with a portable gamma camera is the method of choice for corroborating the clinical diagnosis of brain death in the adult. Advantages of this non-invasive and safe method over the EEG include rapidity and ease of performance and interpretation, lack of demonstrable effects of those conditions that may reversibly cause both ECI and clinical signs of loss of brain functions, with the exception of profound hypotension. Given the limited tolerance of the human brain for anoxia, absence of blood flow for the duration of radionuclide cerebral angiography in adult patients who have been in deep coma with apnoea and absent cephalic reflexes for 6 h or longer attests to irreversible loss of brain functions, regardless of aetiology. Thus, this method generally makes it possible to establish irreversible loss of brain viability even when the primary aetiology is unknown or uncertain and when the criteria of brain death are not fully met, such as when brain stem reflexes cannot be adequately tested, the pupils are small, the results of a toxicology screen are not available, or the EEG is not or is ambiguously interpretable or demonstrates residual electrocerebral activity. Whenever two neurological examinations no less than 6 h apart demonstrate loss of brain functions, the subsequent finding of lack of detectable cerebral blood flow allows accurate and expeditious determination of brain death in the adult. The use of other tests of brain perfusion, Doppler ultrasonography, real time cranial ultrasonography, and xenon-enhanced computed tomography requires further investigation. In cases of special complexity in which doubts persist on the viability of the brain, transfemoral four-vessel contrast angiography may be called upon to define definitely the status of the intracranial circulation, if safe transportation of the patient to the angiography suite can be arranged. Tests of brain metabolism may also be helpful but have not found widespread application as tests of choice for confirming brain death.

The performance of multimodality evoked potential studies at the bedside of patients receiving intensive care is a time-consuming task that requires superior technical expertise and interpretive skills. Thus, this technique is less suitable than brain perfusion tests for routinely assessing brain viability.

The methods chosen to confirm irreversible extinction of brain functions may vary according to the instrumentation and the technical and professional skills available in each institution, and may be dictated in some countries by governmental regulations. Moreover, it is highly likely that the nature of the auxiliary tests of brain death will change with the advent of new technologies. Hence, the validity of current methods should be periodically reassessed and new corroborative tests should undergo stringent scrutiny before they are included in institutional protocols or governmental directives.

Special problems are posed by the diagnosis of brain death in neonates and infants. A review of the published cases in which the patient's age was specified and the clinical diagnosis of brain death appeared to be established by current criteria revealed extraordinary paucity of data. However limited, the available information appeared to confirm the contention of the US Special Task Force [133] that brain death cannot be established by clinical examination and auxiliary methods before the age of 7 days in neonates at term whereas this determination becomes increasingly less difficult in older newborns and infants up to the age of year. This Special Task Force [133] recommended that between the ages of 7 days and 1 year loss of brain viability be established by combined clinical assessments, and evaluations by EEG, radionuclide cerebral angiography, or both, repeated at specified time intervals. Presumably, the guidelines issued by this prestigious body stemmed in part from the extensive personal experience of its members and their sincere desire to provide cautious, yet specific advice in a previously uncharted area. However, the lack of prospective studies and the paucity of retrospective reports supporting their recommendations are so striking as to justify some of the reservations expressed by concerned physicians in the USA as well as the scepticism pervading the report of the UK Working Party [7,134,135]. Not included among the criticisms published so far is the inadequacy of the techniques proposed for the EEG evaluation of these young patients. Some remedies to this deficiency are suggested in this chapter. It is hoped that the sensible but somewhat tentative nature of the guidelines of the Special Task Force [133] will be recognized by the physicians responsible for assessing the viability of the brains of neonates and infants and that this realization will inspire due caution and stimulate prospective studies designed to establish or refute their legitimacy.

I wish to thank Mrs. Silvana Brevik for editorial assistance.

References

1. Mollaret P, Goulon M. Le coma dépassé (mémoire préliminaire). Rev Neurol 1959; 101: 3–15.
2. Mollaret P, Bertrand I, Mollaret H. Coma dépassé et nécroses nerveuses centrales massives. Rev Neurol 1959; 101: 116–39
3. Adams RD, Jequier M. The brain death syndrome: hypoxemic panencephalopathy. Schweiz Med Wochenschr 1969; 99: 65–73.
4. Ministère des Affaires Sociales. Circulaire No. 67 du 24 avril 1968 relative à l'application du décret n° 47–2057 du 20 octobre1947 relatif aux autopsies et prélèvements. Journal Officiel de la République Française 1968; S.P./18, 12.262: 1–3.
5. Mohandas A, Chou SN. Brain death: a clinical and pathological study. J Neurosurg 1971; 35: 211–18.
6. Diagnosis of brain death. Statement issued by the honorary secretary of the Conference of Royal Colleges and Faculties of the United Kingdom on 11 October 1976. Br Med J 1976; 2: 1187–8.
7. Working Party Report on the Diagnosis of Brain Stem Death in Children. British Paediatric Association, London 1991; 6 p.
8. Working Group Convened by the Royal College of Physicians and endorsed by the Conference of Medical Royal Colleges and their Faculties in the United Kingdom. Criteria for the diagnosis of brain stem death. J R Coll Physicians Lond 1995; 29: 381–2.
9. Guidelines for the Determination of Death: Report of the Medical Consultants on the Diagnosis of Death to the President's Commission for the Study of Ethical Problems in Medicine and Behavioral Research. JAMA 1981; 246: 2184–6.
10. Chatrian G-E. Electrophysiologic evaluation of brain death: a critical appraisal. In: Aminoff MJ (ed.), Electrodiagnosis in Clinical Neurology. 2nd edn. Churchill Livingstone, New York 1986; pp. 669–736.
11. Chatrian G-E. Electrophysiological examination of brain death: a critical appraisal. In: Aminoff MJ (ed.) 3rd edn. Churchill Livingstone, New York 1992; pp. 737–93.
12. Walker AE. Cerebral Death. 3rd edn. Urban and Schwarzenberg Baltimore, 1985; 206 p.
13. Bertrand I, Lhermitte F, Antoine B, Ducrot T. Nécroses massives du système nerveux central dans une survie artificielle. Rev Neurol 1959; 101: 101–15.
14. Kramer W. Progressive posttraumatic encephalopathy during reanimation. Acta Neurol Scand 1964; 40: 249–58.
15. Kimura J, Gerber HW, McCormick WF. The isoelectric electroencephalogram. Significance in establishing death in patients maintained on mechanical respirators. Arch Intern Med 1968; 121: 511–17.
16. Schneider H, Masshoff W, Neuhaus GA. Klinische und morphologische Aspeckte des Hirntodes. Klin Wschr 1969; 47: 844–59.
17. Lindenberg R. Systemic oxygen deficiencies: the respirator brain. In: Minckler J (ed.), Pathology of the Nervous System, vol 2. McGraw-Hill, New York 1972; pp. 1583–1617.

18. Fujimoto T. "Brain death" and vital phenomena; autopsy findings in cases maintained on a respirator for a prolonged period. Jap J Clin Med 1973; 31: 700–6.

19. Walker AE, Diamond EL, Moseley JI. The neuropathological findings in irreversible coma: a critique of the 'respirator brain'. J Neuropathol Exp Neurol 1975; 34: 295–323.

20. Moseley JI, Molinari GF, Walker AE. Respirator brain: report of a survey and review of current concepts. Arch Pathol Lab Med 1976; 100: 61–4.

21. Collaborative Study. An appraisal of the criteria of cerebral death: a summary statement. JAMA 1977; 237: 982–6.

22. Walker AE. Cerebral Death. Professional Information Library Dallas, 1977; 241 p.

23. Walker AE. Cerebral Death. 2nd edn. Urban and Schwarzenberg Baltimore, 1981; 212 p.

24. Nedey R, Brian S, Jedynak P, Arfel G. Neuropathologie du coma dépassé. Ann Anesth Fr 1974; 15: 3–11.

25. Hughes JR, Boshes B, Leestma J. Electro-clinical and pathological correlations in comatose patients. Clin Electroencephalogr 1976; 7: 13–30.

26. Leestma JE, Hughes JR, Diamond ER. Temporal correlates in brain death: EEG and clinical relationships to the respirator brain. Arch Neurol 1984; 41: 147–52.

27. Arfel G. Problèmes électroencéphalographiques de la mort. Mason, Paris 1970; 140 p.

28. Korein J (ed.) Brain Death: Interrelated Medical and Social Issues. New York: 1978: 454. (Ann NY Acad Sci; vol 315).

29. Bennett DR, Hughes JR, Korein J et al. Atlas of Electroencephalography in Coma and Cerebral Death. EEG at the Bedside or in the Intensive Care Unit. Raven Press New York, 1976; 244 p.

30. Black PM. Brain death (first of two parts). N Engl J Med 1978; 299: 338–44.

31. Black PM. Brain death (second of two parts). N Engl J Med 1978; 299: 393–401.

32. Chatrian G-E. Electrophysiological evaluation of brain death: A critical appraisal. In: Aminoff MJ (ed.), Electrodiagnosis in Clinical Neurology. Churchill Livingstone, New York 1980: pp. 525–588.

33. Solomon L, Moshé SL, Alvarez LA. Diagnosis of brain death in children. J Clin Neurophysiol 1986; 3: 234–49.

34. Vernon DD, Holzman BH. Brain death: considerations for pediatrics. J Clin Neurophysiol 1986; 3: 251–65.

35. Chatrian G-E. Coma, other states of altered responsiveness, and brain death. In: Daly DD, Pedley TA (eds), Current Practice of Clinical Electroencephalography. 2nd edn. Raven Press, New York 1990; 425–87.

36. Vecchierini-Blineau MF, Moussalli-Salefranque F. Diagnostic de la mort cérébrale chez le nouveau-né et l'enfant. Neurophysiol Clin 1992; 22: 179–90.

37. A definition of irreversible coma. Report of the Ad Hoc Committee of the Harvard Medical School to examine the definition of brain death. JAMA 1968; 205: 337–40.

38. Ministère des Affaires Sociales et de la Solidarité, Ministère de la Santé. Circulaire N° 03 du 21 janvier 1991 relative à l'application du décret n° 90–844 du 24 septembre 1990 modifiant le décret n° 78–501 du 31 mars 1978 pour l'application de la loi n° 76–1181 du 22 décembre 1976 relative aux prélèvements d'organes. II- La réglementation en vigueur sur les critères du constat de la mort cérébrale. 1991: 3–4.

39. Jørgensen EO. Brain death: retrospective surveys. Lancet 1981; 1: 378–9.

40. Jennett B, Gleave J, Wilson P. Brain death in three neurosurgical units. Br Med J 1981; 282: 533–9.

41. Allen N, Burkholder J, Comiscioni J. Clinical criteria of brain death. Ann NY Acad Sci 1978; 315: 70–96.

42. Walker AE, Molinari GF. Sedative drug surveys in coma: how reliable are they? Postgrad Med J 1977; 61: 105–9.

43. Fischgold H, Mathis P. Obnubilations, comas et stupeurs. Etudes électroencéphalographiques. Electroencephalogr Clin Neurophysiol Suppl 11 1959; 125 p.

44. Jouvet M. Diagnostic électroencéphalographique de la mort du système nerveux central au cours de certains comas. Electroencephalogr Clin Neurophysiol 1959; 11: 805–8.

45. Arfel G, Fischgold H, Weiss J. Le silence cérébral. In: Fischgold H. Dreyfus-Brisac C. Pruvot P (eds), Problèmes de base en électroencéphalographie. Masson, Paris 1963; pp. 118–52.

46. Hockaday JM, Potts F, Epstein E, Bonazzi A, Schwab RS. Electroencephalographic changes in acute cerebral anoxia from cardiac or respiratory arrest. Electroencephalogr Clin Neurophysiol 1965; 18: 575–86.

47. Müller HR. Zur Problematik der flaschen Hirnstromkurve und der Diagnose 'Hirntod' nach akuter zerebraler Anoxie. Med Klin 1966; 61: 1955–9.

48. Scharfetter C, Schmoigl S. Zum isoelektrischen Enzephalogramm. Aussagewert nach Aussetzen der Spontanatmung. Dtsch Med Wochenschr 1967; 92: 472–5.

49. Spann W, Kugler J. Liebhardt E. Tod und elektrische Stille im EEG. Munch Med Wschr 1967; 109: 2161–7.

50. Pampiglione G. Harden A. Resuscitation after cardiocirculatory arrest: prognostic evaluation of early electroencephalographic findings. Lancet 1968; 1: 1261–4.

51. Rosoff SD. Schwab RS. The EEG in establishing brain death. A 10-year report with criteria and legal safeguards in the 50 states. Electroencephalogr Clin Neurophysiol 1968; 24: 283–4.

52. International Federation of Societies for Electroencephalography and Clinical Neurophysiology. Recommendations for the Practice of Clinical Neurophysiology. A Glossary of Terms Most Commonly Used by Clinical Electroencephalographers. Elsevier, Amsterdam 1983; pp. 11–26.

53. American Electroencephalographic Society. Guideline nine: Guidelines on evoked potentials. J Clin Neurophysiol 1994; 11: 40–73.

54. Silverman D, Saunders MG. Schwab RS, Masland RL. Cerebral death and the electroencephalogram. Report of the Ad Hoc Committee of the American Electroencephalographic Society on EEG Criteria for Determination of Cerebral Death. JAMA 1969; 209: 1505–10.

55. Arfel G, Weiss J. Electroencéphalogramme et hypothermie profonde. Ann Chir Thorac Cardiovasc 1962; 16: 666–74.

56. Masland RL. Report of the Inter-Agency Committee on Irreversible Coma and Brain Death. Trans Am Neurol Assoc 1975; 100: 280–2.

57. Jørgensen EO, Malchow-Møller A. Natural history of global and critical brain ischaemia. I. EEG and neurological signs during the first year after cardiopulmonary resuscitation in patients subsequently regaining consciousness. Resuscitation 1981; 9: 133–53.

58. International Federation of Societies for Electroencephalography and Clinical Neurophysiology. Recommendations for the Practice of Clinical Neurophysiology. Appendix 1 E: Standards of Clinical Practice of EEG in Cases of Suspected 'Cerebral death'. Elsevier, Amsterdam 1983; pp. 66–8.

59. Petty GW, Mohr JP, Pedley TA, et al. The role of transcranial Doppler in confirming brain death: sensitivity, specificity, and suggestions for performance and interpretation. Neurology 1990; 40: 300–3.

60. Hughes JR. Limitations of the EEG in coma and brain death. Ann NY Acad Sci 1978; 315: 121–36.

61. Grigg MM. Kelly MA, Celesia GG, Ghobrial MW, Ross ER. Electroencephalographic activity after brain death. Arch Neurol 1987; 44: 948–54.

62. Levy-Alcover MA. Goulon M. Evolution des conditions d'enregistrement de l'EEG pour le diagnostic de la mort cérébrale. Neurophysiol Clin 1989; 19: 271–8.

63. Bureau de la Société de Neurophysiologie Clinique de Langue Française. Recommandations quant aux conditions de réalisation d'un enregistrement électroencéphalographique exigibles

pour le constat d'une mort cérébrale. Neurophysiol Clin 1989; 19: 339–41.

64. Epstein CM. Visual evoked potentials. In: Daly DD, Pedley TA (eds), Current Practice of Clinical Electro-encephalography. 2nd edn. Raven Press, New York 1990; pp. 593–623.

65. Walter ST, Arfel G. Réponses aux stimulations visuelles dans les états de coma aigu et de coma chronique. Electro-encephalogr Clin Neurophysiol 1972; 32: 27–41.

66. Trojaborg W, Jørgensen EO. Evoked cortical potentials in patients with 'isoelectric' EEGs. Electroencephalogr Clin Neurophysiol 1973; 35: 301–9.

67. Ganes T, Lundar T. EEG and evoked potentials in comatose patients with severe brain damage. Electroencephalogr Clin Neurophysiol 1988: 69: 6–13.

68. Reilly EL, Kondo C, Brunberg JA, Doty DB. Visual evoked potentials during hypothermia and prolonged circulatory arrest. Electroencephalogr Clin Neurophysiol 1978; 45: 100–6.

69. Russ W, Kling D, Loesevitz A, Hempelmann G. Effect of hypothermia on visual evoked potentials (VEP) in humans. Anesthesiology 1984; 61: 207–10.

70. Picton TW. Auditory evoked potentials. In: Daly DD, Pedley TA (eds), Current Practice of Clinical Electro-encephalography. 2nd edn. Raven Press New York, 1990; pp. 625–78.

71. Starr A. Auditory brain stem responses in brain death. Brain 1976; 99: 543–54.

72. Stockard JJ, Stockard JE, Sharbrough FW. Brainstem auditory evoked potentials in neurology: methodology, interpretation, clinical application. In: Aminoff J (ed.), Electrodiagnosis in Clinical Neurology. Churchill Livingstone, New York 1980; pp. 370–413.

73. Goldie WD, Chiappa KH, Young RR, Brooks EG. Brainstem auditory and short-latency somatosensory evoked responses in brain death. Neurology 1981; 31: 248–56.

74. Lutschg J, Pfenninger J, Lundin HP, Vassella F. Brainstem auditory and early somatosensory evoked potentials in neurointensively treated comatose children. Am J Dis Child 1983; 137: 421–6.

75. Desbordes JM, Krémer C, Mesz M, et al. Potentiels évoqués auditifs du tronc cérébral dans la mort cérébrale. Ann Fr Anesth Réanim 1988; 7: 13–16.

76. Guérit JM. Evoked potentials: a safe brain-death confirmatory tool? Eur J Med 1992; 1: 233–43.

77. Schlake H-P, Böttge IG, Grotemeyer K-H, et al. Determination of cerebral perfusion by means of planar brain scintigraphy and ^{99m}Tc-HMPAO in brain death, persistent vegetative state and severe coma. Intensive Care Med 1992; 18: 76–81.

78. Emerson RG, Pedley TA. Somatosensory evoked potentials. In: Daly DD, Pedley TA (eds), Current Practice of Clinical Electroencephalography. 2nd edn. Raven Press New York, 1990; pp. 679–705.

79. Mauguière F, Grand C, Fisher C, Courjon J. Aspects des potentiels évoqués auditifs et somesthésiques précoces dans les comas neurologiques et la mort cérébrale. Rev EEG Neurophysiol Clin 1982; 12: 280–6.

80. Facco E, Casartelli-Liviero M, Munari M, et al. Short-latency evoked potentials: new criteria for brain death? J Neurol Neurosurg Psychiatry 1990; 53: 351–3.

81. Guérit JM. Unexpected myogenic contaminants observed in the somatosensory evoked potentials recorded in one brain-dead patient. Electroencephalogr Clin Neurophysiol 1986; 64: 21–6.

82. Murray NMF. Motor evoked potentials. In: Aminoff MJ (ed.), Electrodiagnosis in Clinical Neurology. 3rd edn. Churchill Livingstone, New York 1992; pp. 605–26.

83. Firsching R, Wilhelms S, Cs'escei G. Pyramidal tract function during onset of brain death. Electroencephalogr Clin Neurophysiol 1992; 84: 321–4.

84. Starr A, Achor LJ. Auditory brainstem responses in neurological disease. Arch Neurol 1975; 32: 761–8.

85. Hall JW III, Mackey-Hargadine J, Allen SJ. Monitoring neurologic status of comatose patients in the intensive care unit. In: Jacobson JT (ed.) The Auditory Brainstem Response. College-Hill Press, San Diego 1985; pp. 253–83.

86. Wertheimer P, Jouvet M, Descotes J. A propos du diagnostic de la mort du système nerveux dans les comas avec arrêt respiratoire traités par respiration artificielle. Presse Méd 1959; 67: 87–8.

87. Heiskanen O. Cerebral circulatory arrest caused by acute increase of intracranial pressure. A clinical and roentgenological study of 25 cases. Acta Neurol Scand 1964; 40 (Suppl. 7): 1–57.

88. Langfitt TW, Kassell NF. Nonfilling of cerebral vessels during angiography. Correlation with intracranial pressure Acta Neurochir 1966; 14: 96–104.

89. Gros C, Vlahovitch B, Frèrebeau P, et al. Critères artériographiques des comas dépassés en neurochirurgie. Neurochirurgie 1969; 15: 477–86.

90. Vlahovitch B, Frèrebeau P, Kuhner A, Billet M, Gros C. Les angiographies sous pression dans la mort du cerveau avec arrêt circulatoire encéphalique. Neurochirurgie 1971; 17: 81–96.

91. Baslev-Jørgensen P, Heilbrun MP, Boysen G, Rosenklint A. Jørgensen, EO. Cerebral perfusion pressure correlated with regional cerebral blood flow, EEG, and aortocervical angiography in patients with severe brain disorders progressing to brain death. Eur Neurol 1972; 8: 207–12.

92. Greitz T, Gordon E, Kolmodin G, Widén L. Aortocranial and carotid angiography in determination of brain death. Neuroradiology 1973; 5: 13–19.

93. Rosenklint A, Jørgensen P. Evaluation of angiographic methods in the diagnosis of brain death: correlation with systemic arterial pressure and intracranial pressure. Neuroradiology 1974; 7: 215–19.

94. Ingvar DH, Widén L. Hjärndöd-Sammanfattning av et Symposium. Läkartidningen 1972; 69: 3804–14.

95. Gomes AS, Hallinan JM. Intravenous digital subtraction angiography in the diagnosis of brain death. AJNR 1983; 4: 21–4.

96. Van Bunnen Y, Delcour C, Wery D, Richoz B, Struyven J Intravenous digital subtraction angiography. A criteria of brain death. Ann Radiol 1989; 32: 279–81.

97. Arnold H, Kühne D, Rohr W, Heller M. Contrast borus technique with rapid CT scanning. A reliable diagnostic tool for the determination of brain death. Neuroradiology 1981; 22: 129–32.

98. Goodman JM, Mishkin FS, Dyken M. Determination of brain death by isotope angiography. JAMA 1969; 209: 1869–72.

99. Braunstein P, Korein J, Kricheff IL, Lieberman A. Evaluation of the critical deficit of cerebral circulation using radioactive tracers (bolus technique). Ann NY Acad Sci 1978; 315: 143–67.

100. Kricheff II, Pinto RS, George AE, Braunstein P, Korein J. Angiographic findings in brain death. Ann NY Acad Sci 1978; 315: 168–83.

101. Braunstein P, Korein J, Kricheff I, Corey K, Chase N. A simple bedside evaluation for cerebral blood flow in the study of cerebral death: a prospective study on 34 deeply comatose patients. Am J Roentgenol Radium Ther Nucl Med 1973; 118: 757–67.

102. Korein J, Braunstein P, Kricheff I, Lieberman A, Chase N. Radioisotopic bolus technique as a test to detect circulatory deficit associated with brain death. Circulation 1975; 51: 924–39.

103. Korein J, Braunstein P, George A, et al. Brain death: 1. Angiographic correlation with the radioisotopic bolus technique for evaluation of critical deficit of cerebral blood flow. Ann Neurol 1977; 2: 195–205.

104. Schwartz JA, Baxter J, Brill DR, Burns JR. Radionuclide cerebral imaging confirming brain death. JAMA 1983; 249: 246–7.
105. Mishkin F. Determination of cerebral death by radio-nuclide angiography. Radiology 1975; 115: 135–7.
106. Goodman JM, Heck LL. Confirmation of brain death at bedside by isotope angiography. JAMA 1977; 238: 966–8.
107. Tsai SH, Cranford RE, Rockswold GL, Koehler S. Cerebral radionuclide angiography: its application in the diagnosis of brain death. JAMA 1982; 248: 591–2.
108. Holzman BH, Curless RG, Sfakianakis GN, Ajmone-Marsan C, Montes JE. Radionuclide cerebral perfusion scintigraphy in determination of brain death in children. Neurology 1983; 33: 1027–31.
109. Goodman JM, Heck LL, Moore BD. Confirmation of brain death with portable isotope angiography: a review of 204 consecutive cases. Neurosurgery 1985; 16: 492–7.
110. Drake B, Ashwal S, Schneider S. Determination of cerebral death in the pediatric intensive care unit. Pediatrics 1986; 78: 107–12.
111. Schwartz JA, Baxter J, Brill DR. Diagnosis of brain death in children by radionuclide cerebral imaging. Pediatrics 1984; 73: 14–18.
112. Arfel G, Akerman M, Hertzog E, Bamberger-Bozo C. Données radiologiques, électro-encéphalographique et isotopiques dans les comas dépassés. Acta Radiol Diagn 1972; 13: 295–300.
113. Nordlander S, Wiklund PE, Asard E. Cerebral angioscintigraphy in brain death and in coma due to drug intoxication. J Nucl Med 1973; 14: 856–67.
114. de la Riva A, González F, Llamas-Elvira J, et al. Diagnosis of brain death: superiority of perfusion studies with 99Tcm-HMPAO over conventional radionuclide cerebral angiography. Br J Radiol 1992; 65: 289–94.
115. Neirinckx RD, Nowotnik DP, Pickett RD, Harrison RC, Ell PJ. Development of a lipophilic Tc99m complex useful for brain perfusion evaluation with conventional SPECT imaging equipment. In: Biersack HJ, Winkler C (eds), Amphetamine and pH-shift Agents for Brain Imaging: Basic Research and Clinical Results. De Gruyter, Berlin 1986; pp. 59–70.
116. Sharp PF, Smith FW, Gemmel HG, et al. Technetium–99m HMPAO stereoisomers as potential agents for imaging regional blood flow: human volunteer study. J Nucl Med 1986; 27: 171–7.
117. Wilson K, Gordon L, Selby JB Sr. The diagnosis of brain death with Tc99m HMPAO. Clin Nucl Med 1993; 18: 428–34.
118. Laurin NR, Driedger AA, Hurwitz GA, et al. Cerebral perfusion imaging with technetium-99m-HM-HMPAO in brain death and severe nervous system injury. J Nucl Med 1989; 30: 1627–35.
119. Reid RH, Gulenchyn KY, Ballinger JR. Clinical use of technetium–99m HM-PAO for determination of brain death. J Nucl Med 1989; 30: 1621–6.
120. Wieler H, Marohl K, Kaiser KP, Klavki P, Frössler H. Tc-99m HMPAO cerebral scintigraphy. A reliable, noninvasive method for determination of brain death. Clin Nucl Med 1993; 18: 104–9.
121. Uematsu S, Smith TD, Walker AE. Pulsatile cerebral echo in diagnosis of brain death. J Neurosurg 1978; 48: 866–73.
122. Kreutzer EW, Rutherford RB, Lehman RAW. Diagnosis of brain death by common carotid artery velocity waveform analysis. Arch Neurol 1982; 39: 136–9.
123. Ropper AH, Kehne SM, Wechsler L. Transcranial Doppler in brain death. Neurology 1987; 37: 1733–5.
124. Hassler W, Steinmetz H, Gawlowski J. Transcranial Doppler ultrasonography in raised intracranial pressure and in intracranial circulatory arrest. J Neurosurg 1988; 68: 745–51.
125. Newell DW, Grady MS, Sirotta P, Winn HR. Evaluation of brain death using transcranial Doppler. Neurosurgery 1989; 24: 509–13.
126. Powers AD, Graeber MC, Smith RR. Transcranial Doppler ultrasonography in the determination of brain death. Neurosurgery 1989; 24: 884–9.
127. Zurynski Y, Dorsch N, Pearson I, Choong R. Transcranial Doppler ultrasound in brain death: experience in 140 patients. Neurol Res 1991; 13: 248–52.
128. Payen DM, Lamer C, Pilorget A, et al. Evaluation of pulsed Doppler common carotid blood flow as a noninvasive method of brain death diagnosis: a prospective study. Anesthesiology 1990; 72: 222–9.
129. Darby JM, Yonas H, Gur D, Latchaw RE. Xenon-enhanced computer tomography in brain death. Arch Neurol 1987; 44: 551–4.
130. Torda TA. Cerebral arterio-venous oxygen difference: a bedside test for cerebral death. Anesth Intensive Care 1976; 41: 148–50.
131. Voisin C, Wattel F, Scherpereel P. Enzymes in the cerebrospinal fluid in diagnosis of brain death. Resuscitation 1975; 4: 61–7.
132. Kato T, Tokumaru A, O'uchi T, et al. Assessment of brain death in children by means of P-31 MR spectroscopy: Preliminary note. Radiology 1991; 179: 95–9.
133. Guidelines for the determination of brain death in children. Report of Special Task Force for the Determination of Brain Death in Children. Pediatrics 1987; 80: 298–9.
134. Freeman JM, Ferry PC. New brain death guidelines in children: further confusion. Pediatrics 1988; 81: 301–3.
135. Shewmon DA. Commentary on guidelines for the determination of brain death in children. Ann Neurol 1988; 24: 789–91.
136. Ashwal S, Schneider S. Brain death in children. Part II. Pediatr Neurol 1987; 3: 69–77.
137. Ashwal S, Smith AJK, Torres F, Loken M, Chou SN. Radionuclide bolus angiography: a technique for verification of brain death in infants and children. J Pediatr 1977; 91: 722–8.
138. McMenamin JB, Volpe JJ. Doppler ultrasonography in the determination of neonatal brain death. Ann Neurol 1983; 14: 302–7.
139. Ashwal S, Schneider S. Brain death in the newborn. Pediatrics 1989; 84: 429–37.
140. Ashwal S, Schneider S, Thompson J. Xenon computed tomography measuring cerebral blood flow in the determination of brain death in children. Ann Neurol 1989; 25: 539–46.
141. Rowland TW, Donnelly JH, Jackson AH, Jamroz SB. Brain death in the pediatric intensive care unit. A clinical definition. Am J Dis Child 1983; 137: 547–50.
142. Ashwal S, Schneider S. Failure of electroencephalography to diagnose brain death in comatose children. Ann Neurol 1979; 6: 512–17.
143. Furgiuele TL, Frank LM, Riegle C, Wirth F, Earley LC. Prediction of cerebral death by cranial sector scan. Crit Care Med 1984; 12: 1–3.
144. Coker SB, Dillehay GL. Radionuclide cerebral imaging for confirmation of brain death in children: the significance of dural sinus activity. Pediatr Neurol 1986; 2: 43–6.
145. Thompson JR, Ashwal S, Schneider S, et al. Comparison of cerebral blood flow measurements by xenon computed tomography and dynamic brain scintigraphy in clinically brain dead children. Acta Radiol 1986, Suppl 369: 675–9.
146. Bode H, Sauer M, Pringsheim W. Diagnosis of brain death by transcranial Doppler sonography. Arch Dis Child 1988; 63: 1474–8.
147. Kohrman MH, Spivack BS. Brain death in infants: sensitivity and specificity of current criteria. Pediatr Neurol 1990; 6: 47–50.

148. Ahmann PA, Carrigan TA, Carlton D, Wyly B, Schwartz JF. Brain death in children: characteristic common carotid arterial velocity patterns measured with Doppler ultrasound. J Pediatr 1987; 110: 723–8.
149. Volpe JJ. Brain death determination in the newborn. Commentary. Pediatrics 1987; 80: 293–7.
150. Ashwal S, Schneider S. Brain death in children: Part I. Pediatr Neurol 1987; 3: 5–11.
151. Stockard-Pope JE, Werner SS, Bickford RG, Curran JS. Atlas of Neonatal Electroencephalography. 2nd edn. Raven Press, New York 1992; 401 p.
152. American Electroencephalographic Society. Guideline three: Minimum technical standards for EEG recording in suspected cerebral death. J Clin Neurophysiol 1986; 3: 139–43.
153. Alvarez LA, Moshé SL, Belman AL, et al. EEG and brain death determination in children. Neurology 1988; 38: 227–30.
154. Moshé SL. Usefulness of EEG in the evaluation of brain death in children: the pros. J Clin Neurophysiol 1989; 73: 272–5.
155. Toffol GJ, Lansky LL, Hughes JR, et al. Pitfalls in diagnosing brain death in infancy. J Child Neurol 1987; 2: 134–8.
156. Determination of brain death. From the Ad Hoc Committee on Brain Death, the Children's Hospital, Boston. J Pediatr 1987; 110: 15–19.
157. Schneider S. Usefulness of EEG in the evaluation of brain death in children: the cons. Electroencephalogr Clin Neurophysiol 1989; 73: 276–8.
158. Setzer NA, McPherson RW, Johnson RM, Gioia F. Evoked potential determinations in children with brain death. Anesthesiology 1983; 59: A130.
159. Steinhart CM, Weiss IP. Use of brainstem audilory evoked potentials in pediatric brain death. Crit Care Med 1985; 13: 560–2.
160. Dear PRF, Godfrey DJ. Neonatal auditory brainstem response cannot reliably diagnose brainstem death. Arch Dis Child 1985; 60: 17–19.
161. Taylor MJ, Houston BD, Lowry NJ. Recovery of auditory brainstem responses after a severe hypoxic ischemic insalt. N Engl J Med 1983; 309: 1169–70.
162. Coulter DL. Neurologic uncertainty in newborn intensive care. N Engl J Med 1987; 316: 840–4.

6 | Selection of multivisceral cadaveric organ donors

MICHAEL E. WACHS AND NANCY L. ASCHER

1. Introduction

The recent improvements in results with solid organ transplantation have led to a relative shortage of donor organs in the USA and Europe [1]. Despite efforts to increase the number of living donors and recent efforts to recover organs from non-heart beating donors, the majority of organs transplanted in the USA are still obtained from brain-dead heart beating cadaver donors [2]. Evans has estimated that 40–60% of potential cadaveric organs are not utilized for transplantation [3]. The cause of this discrepancy between potential and actual cadaver donor utilization in the USA is multifactorial and includes delayed recognition of brain death by non-transplant physicians and, historically, stringent donor selection criteria imposed by transplant surgeons. Attempts are now under way to improve the general understanding of brain death criteria and to liberalize in a safe manner the criteria for organ acceptability [2]. Similar initiatives are under way in Europe, including a policy of presumed consent, which has not been shown to be effective in increasing the donor pool in France and Austria where it has been extensively studied [1].

2. Clinical brain death

Prior to consideration for heart-beating organ donation, a diagnosis of clinical brain death must be established. The definition of clinical brain death used in the USA is based on criteria, outlined in the Uniform Determination of Death Act, which are reliably predictive of irreversible brain injury [4]. These criteria provide the framework in which the physicians caring for a potential donor can make the clinical diagnosis of brain death. They have been refined in the USA over the past 25 years and currently include the absence of reversible causes of coma such as hypothermia, intoxication, shock or neuromuscular blockade; deep coma; the absence of brain stem function; the absence of spontaneous respiration; no spontaneous movement or response to deep painful stimuli (spinal reflexes may be present); and the absence of cranial nerve reflexes [5]. Similar criteria for brain death are used in most European countries [1]. In addition, most hospitals in the USA have their own brain death committees which may require additional confirmatory tests, including EEG, cerebral blood flow scans or angiography. An understanding of these criteria by non-transplant physicians is the first step in the timely selection of potential cadaveric organ donors. It is estimated that up to 50% of potential donors are lost in the first 24 h after head injury due to delayed recognition of clinical brain death [6].

3. Donor evaluation

The essential principles of the cadaveric donor selection process are three-fold: the organs must function adequately, the anatomy of the donor organs must be compatible with transplantation into the proposed recipient and the risk of transmission of donor-derived

G.M. Collins, J.M. Dubernard, W. Land and G.G. Persijn (eds). Procurement, Preservation and Allocation of Vascularized Organs 47–54
© 1997 Kluwer Academic Publishers.

diseases must be reduced to a minimum. The evaluating surgeon uses information from the donor history and physical examination and laboratory and radiological data to assess the organs with regard to these three selection criteria. In addition, inspection of the organs by the donor surgeon and occasional organ biopsy prior to transplantation can provide further information regarding the acceptability of the organs for transplantation.

The selection of a particular donor organ must always be viewed in terms of a risk/benefit analysis which takes into consideration the health status of the potential recipient. While a kidney with multiple arteries, obtained from an older donor, might represent an unacceptable graft for a young, non-sensitized patient, that same kidney may represent a 'chance of a lifetime' for an older, sensitized, six antigen-matched recipient. Similarly, a liver from an unstable donor with slightly elevated serum liver chemistries might be life-saving for a comatose patient in the intensive care unit while it would be suboptimal for a well compensated cirrhotic patient living at home. It is with this risk/benefit analysis in mind that the following selection criteria should be considered. Very few of these parameters represent absolute criteria and exceptions are often made, particularly when considering a recipient who may die without a transplant.

4. Organ function

4.1. Donor history

The most critical part of the donor evaluation is the assessment of donor organ function, which is used to predict the performance of the transplanted organs in the recipient. Primary non-function or poor function in the post-transplant period increases the cost, morbidity and mortality of transplantation. The best predictor of post-transplant organ function is the baseline function of those organs in the donor. The extent to which the circumstances leading to brain death have adversely affected that baseline function is also examined.

After the declaration of brain death a careful review of the donor's past medical and social history is essential as a first step in estimating baseline organ function. Certain pre-existing medical conditions may impair the function of one or all of the transplantable organs. A history of hypertension, stroke or previous myocardial infarction is a sign of generalized atherosclerotic disease which can have deleterious effects on donor organ function. This is particularly true for the heart and kidneys; however, severe disease may also affect

the liver, pancreas and lungs. Due to the variable severity and location of the vascular disease, which can be assessed during back-table inspection, some organs may be transplantable whereas others from the same donor will not be. Within the last 5 years the proportion of donors dying from intracranial haemorrhage secondary to underlying vascular disease has increased in the USA. This change reflects a trend towards accepting older donors and a reduction in deaths due to head injury resulting from motor vehicle accidents [2]. The assessment of the donor organs with regards to cardiovascular disease has therefore taken a more prominent role in our selection process.

A history of other chronic diseases such as chronic obstructive pulmonary disease, chronic renal insufficiency, hepatic cirrhosis and diabetes mellitus may also preclude transplantation of specific organs affected by these diseases. Although the patient may not carry one of these organ-specific diagnoses, a social history of excessive alcohol or tobacco use will alert the selection team to a potentially suboptimal donor. Other aspects of the patient's social history are discussed later in this chapter. Certain diseases may not directly affect the organ being evaluated but are associated with other diseases which do have an adverse effect. For example, patients with a history of ulcerative colitis or Crohn's disease are more likely to have sclerosing cholangitis, which has deleterious effects on liver function. These associated diseases may be subclinical and not apparent from the history or laboratory data: a biopsy may be indicated prior to transplantation. Similarly, patients with multiple sclerosis are more likely to develop diabetes mellitus and do not, therefore represent ideal pancreas donors. Individuals dying from ruptured intracranial aneurysms are more likely to have aneurysms in other vessels, and also have a higher incidence of polycystic liver and kidney disease. This history should heighten the awareness of the donor surgeon during back-table inspection of the organs. The donor's family history also provides clues with regard to underlying organ function: for example, a young non-diabetic donor with a strong family history of type 1 diabetes should probably not be considered for pancreas donation.

A review of the patient's cause of death and hospital course will provide information about any injury which the organs may have sustained during this period. Episodes of cardiopulmonary arrest, their duration and the effectiveness of cardiopulmonary resuscitation, including difficulties in obtaining an airway, can help to predict potential ischaemic injury to the organs. Episodes of hypotension or severe hypertension, their duration and response to therapy are important clues to potential organ injury. Although the majority of donors are maintained on some vasopressor (usually dopamine) during their hospital course, large doses of pressors, the need for multiple pressors, or failure to respond to pressor agents are all suggestive of organ ischaemia. When brain death has occurred secondary to trauma the recipient surgeons must review the management, looking for evidence of injury to other organs. The findings at operative exploration, chest X-rays, abdominal films and CT scans should be reviewed. Occasionally, the most appropriate trauma management is not completed once the severity of head injury has been established. In these cases the selection team must be even more diligent in their evaluation. Patients who remain unstable despite resuscitation, demonstrate falling haematocrits or develop progressive abdominal distension often have undiagnosed abdominal injuries at the time of organ recovery.

The age of the donor is considered in so far as it may effect organ function. Previously, most transplant centres have set arbitrary upper age limits for organ donation. These age limits tended to vary depending on the organ under consideration, and were based on the assumption that organ function deteriorates with age, creating a higher potential for primary non-function as well as limiting the life span of the organ. While it is clear that glomerular filtration rate decreases with age, the effects of ageing on the liver, pancreas, heart and lungs are less clear and difficult to separate from the effects of other diseases commonly seen in the elderly. A recent study by Wall suggests that the function and outcome of livers transplanted from older donors is no different from that of organs obtained from younger donors [7]. Alexander showed similar results in a review of older kidney, liver and heart donors, provided there is no evidence of organ dysfunction on laboratory and radiological assessment (i.e. chest X-ray, echocardiography, coronary angiography) [8]. These studies indicate that the physiological assessment of the donor is more important than a strict chronological assessment, and that older donors can be safely used to increase the donor pool. We tend to rely on donor biopsies, particularly of the kidneys, when evaluating older donors. A kidney which shows 20% or more nephrosclerosis is not transplanted. Transplantation of organs from donors at the lower end of the age spectrum is mostly limited by size and anatomical constraints, which are discussed below.

There is evidence to suggest that the weight of the donor can also adversely affect organ function. Livers from donors over 100 kg in weight have a higher incidence of primary non-function [9]. Studies of back-table liver biopsies have shown that these donors more often have severe steatosis [10]. In addition, obese donors are more likely to have underlying heart disease, nephrosclerosis and diabetes, limiting the utility of their organs for transplantation.

4.2. Donor laboratory and radiological data

Following review of the donor history, laboratory data and radiological studies are used to assess further organ function and corroborate suspicions raised by the donor history. Routine donor screening includes complete blood count, electrolytes, blood urea nitrogen and creatinine (BUN/Cr), serum liver chemistries, serum albumin, amylase, lipase, PT/PTT and platelets. BUN/Cr are used to estimate renal function: they may be elevated due to underlying baseline renal disease or they may reflect a more acute injury sustained during the time surrounding brain death. In these cases the response to fluid resuscitation should be ascertained. A creatinine that remains abnormally elevated or continues to rise despite resuscitation argues against kidney transplantation. Albumin, prothrombin time and bilirubin are used to predict underlying liver function, whereas the serum liver chemistries (AST, ALT) are more reflective of organ injury. Although mild elevations of AST, ALT and bilirubin may be non-specific and transient, worsening function on serial determinations or levels more than two times normal reflects liver damage and a greater chance of primary non-function. These abnormalities must be weighed against the relative urgency of transplantation for the particular recipient. A back-table biopsy of the liver provides valuable information in this situation. Evidence of hepatocyte necrosis or ballooning degeneration are suggestive of severe ischaemic insult. Several investigators have suggested that other tests, including lidocaine metabolism, [11] and arterial ketone body ratios [12] may be more predictive of liver damage and post-transplant dysfunction. These reports are, however, inconclusive and these tests are currently considered experimental.

Elevations of the serum amylase are suggestive of pancreatic injury; however they should be corroborated with serum lipase determinations as elevated amylase can have other causes, particularly in head trauma patients. The serum glucose level is often elevated either secondary to a stress response, or following steroid and glucose administration. Shaffer has shown that an elevated serum glucose is not predictive of poor post-transplant organ function [13]. In the absence of a history of diabetes mellitus and in the face of a normal amylase and lipase, elevated glucose levels should not exclude pancreatic transplantation. Arterial blood gas values are important to identify potential ischaemia in general, but also are essential in determining the potential for pulmonary transplantation. A potential lung donor should have a $pAO_2 > 360$ torr on 100% oxygen [5]. Similarly, myocardial enzymes are useful when reviewing a potential cardiac donor, especially when there has been a cardiac arrest or trauma to the chest wall suggestive of myocardial contusion.

In addition to providing organ-specific information the laboratory values also allow for a general assessment of the adequacy of donor management. Hypernatraemia and acidosis are common findings in a volume-depleted donor and should be corrected quickly to avoid organ ischaemia. These findings, in conjunction with large urinary outputs and hypokalaemia, suggest diabetes insipidus, which is treated aggressively. Progressive hypoxia raises the suspicion of a mechanical ventilatory problem such as inadequate endotracheal tube placement or pneumothorax: treatment can improve the overall donor status. Elevations of the PT/PTT in combination with a drop in platelet count is suggestive of disseminated intravascular coagulation, which can adversely affect renal function. Fibrinogen levels and fibrin split products can aid in the diagnosis. A donor kidney biopsy will occasionally be necessary to evaluate microvascular thrombosis in the renal parenchyma.

Serum toxicology studies should be reviewed when available as certain toxins may have an adverse effect on post-transplant organ function. The use of cocaine has been associated with hepatic necrosis [14] and has been postulated to be the cause of one case of primary non-function of a liver allograft at our institution. Not all positive toxicology results, however, eliminate the donor from consideration. Successful transplantation of the liver and kidneys has been reported from a donor who died from carbon monoxide poisoning [15]. Similarly, the Pittsburgh group has reported no adverse outcome when transplanting livers from trauma patients with elevated blood alcohol levels, provided that they have normal liver function [16].

The ultimate function of the graft is also dependent on donor–recipient immunological compatibility. For this reason the determination of the donor blood type is of utmost importance. Transplantation of ABO-matched organs is considered standard: the use of ABO-incompatible solid organs (particularly kidney and heart) has been associated with hyperacute antibody-mediated rejection, graft loss and even severe haemolytic reactions [17,18]. In an attempt to address the shortage of donor organs and in light of the rarity of hyperacute rejection in liver transplant recipients,

several experimental protocols using ABO-mismatched donor livers are being evaluated. These include the use of plasmaphoresis to remove donor-directed antibodies and transfusion of blood of the donor group to prevent haemolysis in recipients of these mismatched organs. At this point, however, the use of ABO-mismatched organs for transplantation is for the most part investigational. One exception to this policy is the use of ABO-mismatched livers in children less than 1 year old, prior to the initiation of production of anti-ABO antibodies [19]. A second exception is the use of organs from blood type A2 donors in type O and AB recipients. The titre of blood group antigens on tissue from these donors is felt to be low enough to avoid antibody mediated destruction [20]. HLA matching remains an area of controversy in selecting donors for transplantation. For cadaveric organ donors, a prospective cross-match and tissue typing is only used in kidney, pancreas and sensitized heart transplant recipients. There is consensus in the literature of an immunological advantage in transplanting six-antigen-matched kidneys from cadaveric donors [21]. The importance of matching in other organ transplants is less convincing.

Additional studies, such as EKG and chest X-ray are often helpful in identifying patients with underlying cardiopulmonary disease and are most useful n assessing heart and lung function. An echocardiogram or coronary catheterization will occasionally be necessary at the discretion of the thoracic transplant surgeon, especially when considering older donors.

4.3. Evaluation and biopsy by the donor surgeon

The final analysis of organ function rests with the donor surgeon. It is essential for the donor surgeon carefully to review the chart and complete a physical examination in order to ensure that all of the donor information used to assess organ function is accurate. Once in the operating room, a careful exploration should be undertaken to evaluate for organ injury or signs of ischaemia. An unstable patient on high doses of pressors may have a mottled liver or poorly perfused kidneys, which are predictive of poor function. On the back-table the donor surgeon must assess the adequacy of the flush and inspect the organs carefully for injury. The back-table dissection also allows for a biopsy of the organs when there is a question of inadequate function. At our institution these biopsies are carried out selectively: when there is a question of ischaemic insult to the organs, a fatty appearance to the liver (especially in heavy donors) and to exclude significant nephrosclerosis in an older donor. One recent study suggests the routine use of frozen section liver biopsy to help exclude livers which would have resulted in primary non-function [22]. The majority of the livers excluded in this series were those with severe steatosis. The rate of primary non-function in this study was 1.8%. This rate of primary non-function is similar to ours and we feel that the use of selective biopsies based on the donor surgeon assessment is adequate.

A final consideration relates to the predicted ischaemic time prior to transplantation. In an effort to minimize organ ischaemia and post-transplant dysfunction, most transplant networks are organized on a regional basis. There are instances, however, when organs are shipped long distances prior to transplantation, therefore adding to the cold ischaemia time. The tolerance of each individual organ to cold ischaemia must be considered when contemplating accepting organs from outside regions. Jonas has demonstrated that livers shipped in from other centres can be safely transplanted with good results provided that the cold ischaemia time is within standard guidelines and the organs are recovered by experienced surgeons [23].

5. Donor anatomy

The second principle of cadaveric donor organ evaluation is the assessment of the donor anatomy. First, the size of the organs must be compatible with the recipient size. Next, the vascular anatomy is assessed for anomalies, injury and the extent of atherosclerosis. Finally, the organ parenchyma is evaluated for evidence of injury or anomaly. The first consideration, regarding the size of the organ relative to the recipient, is most critical with regard to liver donor selection. While the liver must be large enough to maintain normal function it also must fit into the abdominal cavity. A liver placed in a tight intra-abdominal compartment will not function appropriately and can result in recipient death, particularly in a child. Proper donor size matching can help to avoid this problem. For the paediatric liver recipient several donor options exist, including size-matched paediatric grafts, reduced size adult cadaveric grafts and living related grafts. Reducing the size of an adult liver by removing the entire right lobe on the back-table adds to the technical challenge of paediatric liver transplantation. There is evidence, however, that the risk of hepatic artery thrombosis is lower when reduced size and living related grafts are used rather than size-matched whole organs from paediatric donors [24]. This difference may reflect a historical bias at centres where technical

expertise improved and the use of higher magnification for performing the arterial anastomoses became standardized during the time that these alternative grafts were being developed. Our practice is to utilize all three types of liver grafts for paediatric recipients, depending on availability, in an attempt to limit the time waiting for transplantation. We also use pared down livers for small adult recipients. We feel that the combination of microsurgical technique and experience can lead to comparable results among these donor choices.

The results of kidney allografts transplanted from paediatric donors are less clear cut. There seems to be general agreement that paediatric kidneys transplanted into paediatric recipients show poorer survival [25]. Several hypotheses can be offered for this finding, including greater technical problems related to the size of the artery and ureter, less parenchymal reserve to tolerate rejection, and a higher likelihood of rejection due either to a greater immunogenicity of the paediatric kidneys and/or a heightened immune response in the paediatric recipient [26]. We attempt to place paediatric kidneys into small adult recipients, and paediatric recipients are transplanted via a transperitoneal approach, preferably with an adult living related donor kidney. Kidneys from donors weighing less than 20 kg are usually transplanted using the en-bloc technique.

With regard to cardiac transplantation, the need to place the heart in an orthotopic position and the inability to reduce the size of the graft dictates that younger, smaller donors must be used for younger, smaller recipients, despite the increased technical difficulty associated with these small grafts. Pancreas grafts from paediatric donors have been used successfully for transplantation. Most of these reports, however, state the age and not the weight of the pancreas donor [27]. We believe that pancreas grafts from donors weighing less than 40–50 kg are at a higher risk of thrombosis due to the small size of the iliac conduits and the inherently high resistance in the pancreatic microcirculation. Since we view pancreas transplantation as a relatively elective procedure we prefer not to use allografts from donors below this weight.

Radiological studies are occasionally helpful in elucidating donor anatomy. For example, when assessing an older potential cardiac donor, a pre-recovery coronary catheterization is often obtained to document the absence of significant coronary artery disease. A plain chest X-ray is critical in the assessment of the lungs for transplantation. When the donor has suffered a traumatic death CT scans and other X-rays obtained during the trauma evaluation are used to document organ injury.

Lastly, donor anatomy is most accurately evaluated by the donor surgeon at the time of organ recovery: the size of the organs can be directly visualized as opposed to estimating the size based on donor weight. The organs are inspected carefully for injury either sustained from previous trauma or due to technical error at the time of recovery. In addition, anatomical anomalies are assessed. Multiple arteries and veins and aberrant vessels are more prone to injury at the time of recovery. Such anatomical variations often require complex reconstructions, increasing the technical difficulty and risk of the transplant procedure. Renal and hepatic lacerations due to trauma range from minimal, requiring no intervention, to severe, with associated vascular injury which may be difficult to repair. This anatomical information is used in the risk/benefit equation when determining the suitability of the organs for transplantation into a particular recipient. For example, if the liver is noted to have a lacerated aberrant right hepatic artery arising from the superior mesenteric artery, the recipient surgeon must decide if the recipient is sick enough to warrant an attempt at reconstruction in order to salvage the liver.

6. Donor transmission of disease

The third principle of cadaveric donor assessment is the estimation of the risk of transmission of a donor-derived disease, primarily of infectious or malignant nature. The transmission of underlying medical diseases which affect the function of the organs (i.e. atherosclerosis) has already been discussed. A review of the donor history will establish those donors at high risk for infectious disease transmission. A history of hepatitis (excluding hepatitis A), intravenous drug use, promiscuous sexual activity or a previously positive HIV test are all contraindications to organ donation. Serological testing of prospective donors is routine in order to screen for potentially transmissible infectious diseases and to corroborate the findings from the donor history. A positive test for HIV and hepatitis B surface antigen are generally considered absolute contraindications to organ donation. We have recently shown that there is a variable risk of transmission of hepatitis B from donors who have a positive core antibody in the absence of surface antigen; recipients of hearts and kidneys from these donors are much less likely to seroconvert and develop clinically significant hepatitis than are recipients of the livers [28]. For this reason, we no longer accept livers from hepatitis B core-positive donors and only use the kidneys if the donor liver biopsy is normal. Transmission of cytomegalovirus

from a seropositive donor to a seronegative recipient has also been demonstrated. Although most centers will transplant CMV-positive organs into CMV-negative recipients extended prophylaxis of the recipient with antiviral agents may be needed [29].

The donor is also assessed for the potential to transmit a bacterial or fungal infection. A history of multiple previous urinary tract or pulmonary infections should raise the question of an underlying anatomical abnormality which may preclude transplantation of the affected organ. Urine and sputum microscopy, culture and Gram staining can document the presence of an active urinary tract or pulmonary infection. An elevated white blood cell count is a common finding in the potential organ donor. This can often be attributed to a stress response or the administration of steroids, both of which are common in head-injured patients. When this elevation is associated with a fever or when there is a preponderance of immature forms on the differential, the chance of finding an active infection is increased. Radiological studies, including plain chest X-ray to document pneumonia and abdominal films to document free intra-abdominal air, are also reviewed. Preventative measures are instituted as needed, such as the placement of a functioning nasogastric tube and the changing of intravenous lines and urinary catheters which may have been placed hastily prior to hospital admission or in the emergency room.

The presence of an active infection in one of the potentially transplantable organs is usually a contraindication to transplantation of that particular organ. When transplanted, these infected organs can result in both ongoing parenchymal infection, which is difficult to treat under immunosuppression, as well as infection of the vascular anastomoses, which is potentially life threatening [30]. Infection in one organ, however, does not necessarily exclude transplantation of the other uninfected organs. If the potential donor shows no signs of sepsis, the other organs may be transplanted with appropriate recipient antibiotic coverage based on careful follow-up of donor cultures. The organism responsible for the infection must also be considered in the risk/benefit analysis. For example, none of the organs from a donor with an established fungal infection, particularly *Aspergillus* or *Candida*, would normally be accepted; whereas organs, including the kidneys, from a donor with an easily treatable *Escherichia coli* bladder infection would probably be acceptable. In some cases, a positive donor culture is only obtained after the organs have been transplanted. In these cases the recipient should be treated with antibiotics in accordance with culture sensitivities. Occasionally, a potential donor will have sustained an enterotomy, either as the result of trauma or due to surgical error at the time of recovery. We feel that the risk of transmitting infection in these cases can be correlated with the site of injury (small bowel < large bowel), the degree of contamination and the presence of peritonitis. If organs from these donors are transplanted, peritoneal cultures should be obtained to guide antibiotic coverage in the recipient.

Transmission of malignancies from donors to recipients has been well documented [31]. In a large, retrospective analysis, Penn documented a 45% risk of transmission of malignancy from cadaver donors with a history of previous malignancy, including melanomas, renal cell carcinomas, breast, lung and colon cancers. Transmission occurred despite the fact that all of the allografts were grossly free of tumour by visual inspection at the time of recovery. Furthermore, over half of these malignancies were metastatic at the time of diagnosis in the recipient. Based on these findings, Penn [31] and others [32] suggest that all donors should be carefully screened for a history of previous malignancy, and those with a positive history should be excluded, with the exception of low-grade skin cancers (i.e. basal cell carcinoma) and primary, non-metastatic CNS tumours. Histopathology of these skin and brain lesions should be reviewed prior to transplantation, as they can occasionally be confused with metastatic deposits from other occult primaries. Penn also cautions against the use of organs from patients who have had ventriculo-peritoneal shunts as part of their therapy for primary CNS tumours, as these devices can promote dissemination of malignant cells. Several recent case reports have documented transmission of non-metastatic primary CNS tumours to liver recipients in the absence of a V-P shunt. These reports suggest that post-transplant tumour recurrence is associated with a donor history of previous craniotomy, a long duration of disease and high-grade histopathology (i.e. glioblastoma multiforme) [32].

It is commonly accepted that the risk of malignancy increases with advancing age. As the trend towards using organs from older donors continues the need for a thorough exploration by the donor surgeon assumes an even greater importance. This exploration includes a careful preoperative physical examination, looking for skin lesions, breast masses and lymphadenopathy. In the operating room the organs should be explored in situ and on the back-table, looking for areas suspicious for malignancy. Organs which are not routinely recovered for transplant (i.e. colon, small bowel) should also be inspected. All suspicious lesion should be biopsied by the donor surgeon and the results of these biopsies should be made available to the recipient surgeons.

7. Conclusion

The proper selection of the cadaver organ donor is the first step towards curing the patient with end-stage organ dysfunction. An error in judgment at this stage can be devastating in terms of increased cost, morbidity and mortality. A technically perfect transplant operation, and state of the art postoperative care and immunosuppression cannot make up for a poor donor choice and a non-functioning organ. Kidney recipients with early ATN, requiring dialysis, are more difficult to care for, at an increased cost. In the case of liver or heart transplantation, primary non-function is even more devastating and often lethal. At a time when transplantation is growing in popularity and success around the world it is crucial that efforts to expand the donor pool, to provide organs to those in need, are balanced against the requirement that the results obtained are not compromised.

References

1. Caplan A, Siminoff L, Arnold R. Increasing organ and tissue donation: What are the obstacles? The surgeon general's workshop on increasing organ donation. US Department of Health and Human Services, Washington, 1991.
2. United Network of Organ Sharing Trends in organ transplantation, 1993 annual report of the US scientific registry of transplant recipients and the organ procurement and transplant network. UNOS, Richmond, 1993.
3. Evans RW, Orians GE, Ascher NA. The potential supply of donor organs: An assessment of the efficiency of the organ procurement efforts in the US. JAMA 1992; 267: 239–46.
4. Halevy A, Brody B. Brain death: reconciling definitions, criteria and tests. Ann Intern Med 1993; 119: 519–25.
5. Starzl TE, Shapiro R. Simmons RL. Atlas of Organ Transplantation. New York, Gower Medical Publishing 1992.
6. Stark JL, Reiley P. Osiecki A et al. Attitudes affecting organ donation in the intensive care unit. Heart Lung 1984; 13: 400–4.
7. Wall WJ, Mimeault R. Grant DR et al. The use of older donor livers for hepatic transplantation. Transplantation 1990; 49: 377–81.
8. Alexander JW. Vaughn WK. The use of marginal donors for organ transplantation. The influence of donor age on outcome. Transplantation 1991; 51: 135–41.
9. Mor E, Klintmalm GB. Gonwa TA. The use of marginal donors for liver transplantation. A retrospective study of 365 liver donors. Transplantation 1992; 53: 383–6.
10. D'Alessandro AM. Kalayoglu M. Sollinger HW et al. The predictive value of donor liver biopsies for the development of primary nonfunction after orthotopic liver transplantation. Transplantation 1991; 51: 157–63.
11. Rossi SJ. Schroeder TJ. Vine WH et al. Monoethylglycinexylide formation in assessing pediatric donor liver function. Ther Drug Monit 1992; 14: 452–6.
12. Yamaoka Y. Washida M. Manaka D et al. Arterial ketone body ratio as a predictor of donor liver viability in human liver transplantation. Transplantation 1993; 55: 92–5.
13. Shaffer D, Madras PN. Sahyoun AI et al. Cadaver donor hyperglycemia does not impair long-term pancreas allograft survival or function. Transpl Proc 1994; 26: 439–40.

14. Kanel GC, Cassidy W, Shuster L *et al.* Cocaine induced liver cell injury: comparison of morphological features in man and in experimental models. Hepatology 1990; 11: 646–51.

15. Leikin JB, Heyn-Lamb A, Aks S *et al.* The toxic patient as a potential organ donor. Am J Emerg Med 1994; 12: 151–4.

16. Hassanein TI, Gavaler JS, Fishkin D *et al.* Does the presence of a measurable blood alcohol level in a potential organ donor affect the outcome of liver transplantation? Alcohol Clin Exp Res 1991; 15: 300–3.

17. Triulzi DJ, Shirey RS, Ness PM *et al.* Immunohematologic complications of ABO-unmatched liver transplants. Transfusion 1992; 32: 829–33.

18. Kissmeyer-Nielsen F, Olsen S, Petersen VP *et al.* Hyperacute rejection of kidney allografts associated with pre-existing humoral antibodies against donor cells. Lancet 1966; 2: 662–5.

19. Yandza T, Lambert T, Alvarez F *et al.* Outcome of ABO-incompatible liver transplantation in children with no specific alloantibodies at the time of transplantation. Transplantation 1994; 58: 46–50.

20. Rydberg L, Breimer ME, Brynger H *et al.* ABO-incompatible kidney transplantation (A2 to O). Transplantation 1990; 49: 954–60.

21. Cecka MJ, Terasaki PI. The UNOS scientific renal transplant registry. Clinical Transplants 1993: 1–18.

22. Markin RS, Wisecarver JL, Radio SJ *et al.* Frozen section evaluation of donor livers before transplantation. Transplantation 1993; 56: 1403–9.

23. Jonas S, Bechstein WO, Keck H *et al.* Trarsplantation of shipped donor livers. Transplant Int 1993; 6: 206–8.

24. Stevens LH, Emond JC, Piper JB *et al.* Hepatic artery thrombosis in infants. Transplantation 1992; 53: 396–9.

25. McEnery PT, Stablein DM, Arbus G *et al.* Renal transplantation in children. New Engl J Med 1992; 26: 1727–32.

26. Ilstaad ST, Tollerud DJ, Noseworthy J *et al.* The influence of donor age on graft survival in renal transplantation. J Pediatr Surg 1990; 25: 134–41.

27. Abouna GM, Kumar MSA, Miller JL *et al.* Combined kidney pancreas transplantation from pediatric donors into adult diabetic recipients. Transplant Proc 1994; 26: 441–4.

28. Wachs ME, Melzer JS, Lake JR *et al.* Transmission of HBV infection from HBcAb(+) HBsAg(−) donors. Presented at the American Society of Transplant Surgeons Meeting in Chicago, IL, 18–20 May 1994.

29. Balfour HH, Chace BA, Stapleton JT. A randomized, placebo-controlled trial of oral acyclovir for the prevention of cytomegalovirus disease in recipients of renal allografts. New Engl J Med 1989; 320: 1381–7.

30. Haag BW, Stuart FP. The organ donor: Brain death, seleotion criteria, supply and demand. In: Flye MW (ed.) Principles of Organ Transplantation, WB Saunders, Philadelphia, 1989: 176–93.

31. Penn I. Donor transmitted disease: Cancer. Transplant Proc 1991; 23: 2629–31.

32. Colquhoun SD, Robert ME, Shaked A *et al.* Transmission of CNS malignancy by organ transplantation. Transplantation 1994; 57: 970–3.

7 | Management of the cadaver donor in the intensive care unit

M.J. LINDOP

Intensive care management changes direction at the moment that the patient is declared to be dead. Previously all therapy has been directed to achieving recovery of the patient. Suddenly all therapy is aimed at establishing the best possible function of the various potential donor organs.

1. Management prior to the diagnosis of brain stem death

When a patient whose condition is likely to lead to fulfilment of the criteria for brain stem death is admitted to the intensive care unit it is important to ensure that they do not inadvertently receive unnecessary treatment that would interfere with tests required for the diagnosis of brain stem death. In most instances the application of the usual principles of physiological management will not cause problems, but it is important to limit the use of long acting sedative drugs and long acting muscle relaxants (which will not be required once patients have fulfilled the criteria for brain stem death). At this stage it is useful to ensure that baseline bacteriological samples such as urine and sputum are taken so that culture results will be available later.

2. Management following declaration of death

Once death is declared it is important that organ donation is managed expeditiously for the sake of the rela-

tives and the hospital staff. There is also urgency because 50% of patients who fulfil the criteria for brain stem death will suffer cardiac arrest in the first 24 h despite intensive management [1] and almost all will die in 48–72 h. The transplant co-ordinators must arrange a timetable for surgery to retrieve organs which tolerate only short ischaemia times, such as lungs, and which must link with potential recipient operation timetables. In some hospitals delay can result from competition for theatre space from other emergency surgery.

At times when the intensive care unit is busy it is tempting to reduce the level of care given to patients who are known to be dead. During this waiting period it is essential that maximum therapy is continued. In well instructed units this is no problem, but it is important to emphasize to all unit staff that the success of the recipient operation depends on the quality of donor care during this critical period.

Blood tests, if not already performed, must be completed according to local protocols, but will include ABO grouping, HIV status and HB_sAg status.

2.1. Respiratory management

Patients with raised intracranial pressure will often have been significantly hyperventilated. Brain death lowers metabolic rate and will reduce carbon dioxide production. Hypocapnia reduces peripheral oxygen availability and may disrupt regional blood flow patterns. Ventilation is reduced to bring arterial carbon dioxide up into the normal range (4.5–6 kPa). Inspired

G.M. Collins, J.M. Dubernard, W. Land and G.G. Persijn (eds). Procurement, Preservation and Allocation of Vascularized Organs 55–58
© 1997 Kluwer Academic Publishers.

oxygen is adjusted to ensure arterial oxygen tensions higher than 11 kPa. Minimum oxygen concentrations are used to avoid any risk of oxygen toxicity before lung tranplantation.

Large tidal volumes (12–15 ml/kg) with low rates are used to promote gas exchange and to reduce atelectasis. For the same reasons positive end expiratory pressure (PEEP) is added; this may also reduce the tendency for pulmonary oedema to develop. A modest level of (5 cm water) will be useful and up to 10 cm water is appropriate if the circulation is stable and there are no conditions predisposing to barotrauma. High levels of PEEP will reduce hepatic and renal blood flow. Tracheal toilet using aseptic technique should be continued regularly to prevent accumulation of secretions and risk of segmental collapse. Many patients will have been at risk of aspiration. Where there is a clear history of aspiration prophylactic antibiotic therapy such as cefotaxime and metronidazole is wise. Pneumonia, pulmonary collapse, pneumothorax and pulmonary oedema are all potential complications and management should aim to minimize these risks.

2.2. Cardiovascular management

Hypotension is common and may have various causes (Table 1). Patients will usually have been treated with fluid restriction and diuretic therapy, resulting in hypovolaemia. It is essential that this is quickly corrected with colloid solutions, such as those which are gelatin based (Haemaccel, Gelofusin). If there is not a rapid response to less than a litre of these colloids monitoring must immediately include measurement of cardiac filling pressures. A central venous line will be needed for the donor operation anyway. In the unstable patient a pulmonary artery line must be used to measure pulmonary artery occlusion pressure because this varies more widely with blood volume changes and is more relevant to left ventricular performance.

Loss of vasomotor tone is another cause of persistent hypotension. This loss of tone probably reflects damage to the vasomotor centre. There also seems to be a dependency on antidiuretic hormone (ADH) to maintain vascular tone in the brain stem dead patient. ADH has a synergistic action with adrenaline [2]. The pulmonary artery catheter also allows cardiac output to be measured, and systemic vascular resistance is usually low. From the results of these measurements inotropes and vasoactive drugs may be titrated to restore cardiac output and increase perfusion. Dopamine is useful as it will enhance renal, mesenteric and coronary blood flows: in some protocols it is administered routinely at a dose of 2 μg/kg/min. It depletes noradrenaline stores in the heart which might impair myocardial function after transplantation so it may be better given for only specific indications. Dopamine can be increased to 10 μg/kg/min but higher doses, which carry the risk of vasoconstriction through α-adrenergic stimulation, should be used only when there is an inadequate response to lower doses. Dobutamine starting at 2 μg/kg/min is a useful β-adrenergic agonist to promote cardiac output but can aggravate peripheral vasodilatation. Where there is an excellent cardiac index but very low systemic vascular resistance small doses of α-adrenergic agonists such as noradrenaline (0.02 μg/kg/min) can be used. These should only be administered where specific measurements of cardiac output and systemic vascular resistance have been made. When noradrenaline is given dopamine should be continued at 2 μg/kg/min to defend renal blood flow [3].

Care must be taken not to overload donors, especially of lungs, and it is preferable to accept systolic blood pressures about 80 mmHg in a vasodilated patient rather than aim at a particular filling pressure. The criterion of adequate management is to achieve urine flow of at least 1 ml/kg/h. Note is taken of the minimum arterial and venous pressures at which such urine flows are maintained and these pressures become the target values for that particular patient.

Hypertension can occur. This is managed by reduction of vascular resistance by titration with sodium nitroprusside or nitroglycerine infusion.

2.2.1. Arrhythmias
Atrial and ventricular arrhythmias with a variety of junctional rhythms and conduction blocks are commonly seen and may be resistant to therapy. They may be the result of raised intracranial pressure or of

Table 1. Possible causes of hypotension in organ donors.

1. Hypovolaemia from:
     drug- or hyperglycaemia-induced diuresis
     blood loss
     therapeutic fluid restriction
     diabetes insipidus
2. Loss of vasomotor tone from vasomotor centre damage
3. Myocardial contusion or tamponade
4. Electrolyte and acid base disturbance
5. Hypoxaemia
6. Hormonal imbalance
7. Catecholamine induced cardiomyopathy

myocardial contusion. Tachyarrhythmias are particularly associated with hypovolaemia. Arrhythmias are reduced by avoidance of electrolyte and acid–base imbalance, hypotension, hypothermia and high inotrope doses. Once these factors have been minimized, management is with conventional anti-arrhythmics. Bradycardia may be resistant to atropine. If dopamine or other β-adrenergic agonist does not work, pacing may be required.

It is appropriate to use cardiopulmonary resuscitation to allow the gift of organs to be achieved and the donor procedure to continue. In practice, successful resuscitation may be difficult to accomplish and prolonged efforts are not appropriate.

2.3. Fluid management

Two main patterns are seen. First, prolonged fluid restriction and intense diuretic therapy may have left the patient hypovolaemic, dehydrated and oliguric. This leads to hypotension, the management of which with colloid fluid replacement is described above. Second, patients with brain stem damage will have damage to the pituitary axis, and diabetes insipidus is common. This should be suspected on finding urine flows > 4 ml/kg/h, urine osmolality < 300 mOsm/kg, and < 10 mmols sodium/l urine with rising plasma sodium and osmolality. Diabetes insipidus can lead to major fluid balance problems and arterial and central venous pressure monitoring will certainly be needed. The likely electrolyte derangements shown in Table 2 must be corrected. Colloid plasma expanders all have high sodium contents to match extracellular concentrations. Where diabetes insipidus has developed it will be necessary to limit the sodium load by mixing some of the replacement as 5% dextrose solution. With large fluid volume exchanges potassium will be lost, and monitoring and replacement will be needed, usually by prescribing at least 20 mmol K$^+$/l in the infusion fluids.

Desmopressin (DDAVP) 1–10 μg intramuscularly may be repeated or vasopressin 2 units/h given intravenously to control diabetes insipidus when the urine

flow exceeds 4–5 ml/kg/h. No detriment to organ blood flow has been demonstrated by this management.

The haematocrit may be low as a result of blood losses from trauma and will fall markedly during the early rehydration of the patient. The value should be kept at about 30% and may require packed cell transfusion.

2.4. Hormone therapy

The anterior pituitary axis may also be damaged and this may be the cause of further hormone deficiencies [4]. Cardiovascular stability may be promoted by hormone supplementation. Hydrocortisone 100 mg hourly should be given if the patient is unstable and may have adrenal insufficiency. Over the short period prior to the donor operation there are no adverse effects from generous hydrocortisone supplementation. Insulin may be needed to treat hyperglycaemia and is best given by continuous intravenous infusion at 1–6 units/h. Tri-iodothyronine (5 μg, then 3 μg/h) may help graft function, though donor instability has not been correlated with measurable endocrine deficits [5].

2.5. Temperature

Brain damage leads to loss of hypothalamic control and the patient is virtually poikilothermic. Heat loss to the environment will lead to hypothermia. Inspired gases should be warmed and humidified. Fluids should be warmed. Warm air blankets are the most effective method of restoring core temperature.

Adverse effects of cooling are bradycardias, tachy-arrhythmias and ventricular irritability. Diuresis can be aggravated and platelet function depressed. Oxygen delivery to the tissues will be impaired.

2.6. Blood coagulation

Disseminated intravascular coagulation can be precipitated by release of fibrinolytic substances or plasminogen activators following severe head injury [6]. Characteristic changes include thrombocytopenia with a fall in fibrinogen levels, coupled with the appearance of D dimer fibrin degradation products. Fresh frozen plasma and platelets may be required to improve coagulation integrity before the donor operation. Effective haemostasis is important during the long donor operation to reduce cardiovascular instability and reduce transfusion requirements. Plans for the donor operation should be accelerated where possible before renal impairment supervenes. Anti-

Table 2. Electrolyte changes in diabetes insipidus.

Raised	Lowered
Sodium	Potassium
Osmolality	Calcium
	Magnesium
	Phosphate

fibrinolytics such as ε-aminocaproic acid (EACA) are not used lest they provoke microvascular thrombosis in the donor organs.

2.7. Prevention of infection

Scrupulous asepsis should be maintained to prevent transmission of infection to the recipient. Special care is needed for lung donors. Microscopy and culture of possible sites of infection is routine throughout intensive care stay.

2.8. Preparation for surgery

Blood (four units) should be cross-matched for what will be a 3–4 h operation with possibly a 2 l blood loss. Colloid fluid replacement may suffice but anaemia from blood loss can threaten oxygen delivery if it is allowed to become too severe.

The donor must be transferred to operating theatre at as stable a period as possible. Transfer is a major risk element in the unstable patient and intensive therapy aims to achieve stability particularly for the planned transfer time. Full cardiovascular monitoring must be maintained with portable equipment. A portable ventilator is useful to ensure constancy of ventilation, and the theatre must be warm.

3. Summary

The care of the transplant recipient should be thought of as beginning from the moment that brain stem death

Table 3. Recommended minimum monitoring of the donor.

Intravascular arterial pressure
Central venous pressure
Hourly urine output
Pulse oximetry
Hourly blood gas analysis
Blood electrolyte status, as indicated
Electrocardiogram

has been diagnosed in the donor and consent for organ donation has been given. The aim of management is to support body function in the brain stem dead patient until the organ donation can take place. The continuing perfusion of those organs is the preoccupation of this period. It is achieved by the maintenance of normal values for circulation, maintaining a urine flow > 1 ml/kg/h; arterial pO_2 at > 11 kPa; core temperature at > 35°C, and a normal electrolyte and acid base state. The minimum monitoring requirements are listed in Table 3

All hospital staff must understand that the success of transplantation depends on the quality of organs available as much as the surgical skills of implantation. Once brain stem death has been diagnosed, care must be intensifed at a time when the natural instinct is to limit treatment and divert scarce nursing resources to other intensive care patients who still have hope of recovery. The basic tenet is that the quality of care given to the donor must equal that which will be available to the recipient.

References

1. Mackersie RC, Bronsther OL, Shackford SR. Organ procurement in patients with fatal head injuries. The fate of the potential donor. Ann Surg 1991; 213: 143–50.
2. Yoshioka T, Sugimoto H, Uenishi M, Sakamoto T, Sadamitsu D, Sakano T, Sugimoto T. Prolonged hemodynamic maintenance by the combined administration of vasopressin and epinephrine. Neurosurgery 1986; 18: 565–7.
3. Schaer GL, Fink MP, Parillo JE. Norepinephrine alone versus norepinephrine plus low dose dopamine:enhanced renal blood flow with combination pressor therapy. Crit Care Med 1985; 13: 492–6.
4. Novitsky D, Wicomb WN, Cooper DKC, Rose AG, Fraser RC, Barnard CN. Electrocardiographic, hemodynamic, and endocrine changes during experimental brain death in the Chacma baboon. J Heart Transplant 1984; 4: 63–9.
5. Robertson KM, Hramiak IM, Gelb AW. Endocrine changes and haemodynamic stability after brain death. Transplant Proc 1988; 21: 1197–8.
6. Miner ME, Kaufman HH, Graham SH, Haar FH, Gildenberg PL. Disseminated intravascular coagulation fibrinolytc syndrome following head injury in children. J Pediatrics 1982: 100: 687–91.

8 | Donor conditioning in organ procurement

Dimitri Novitzky

1. Introduction

Achievements in clinical transplantation have created a demand for organs which is currently not being met by the available donor organ pool. It is estimated that approximately 30% of cardiac [1], 30% of liver [2], 30% of heart and lung [3] and 7% of renal patients die [4] or deteriorate further, deeming them unsuitable for transplantation, before a suitable donor becomes available. Furthermore, utilization of suboptimal donors as a desperate, last resort has a major negative impact on the recipient's survival. Following transplantation, the poorest results are observed when an organ is procured from an unstable donor receiving high inotropic support (i.e. dopamine in excess of 20–30 μg/kg/min) and then transplanted to the recipient whose major organs have been progressively deteriorating from low cardiac output. Primary graft failure in this population may be as high as 20% [3]. These critically ill patients frequently require inotropic support, experience hypotensive episodes, are at risk for iatrogenic infections and are nutritionally deficient [5].

To optimize the utilization of this scarce commodity, the transfer of organs from suboptimal donors to marginal recipients should be excluded. Acutely ill patients require rigorous daily assessment to determine whether they continue to meet the criteria required of transplant recipients. A lack of objective clinical parameters may result in a very high risk surgical procedure associated with high morbidity and mortality [6].

Major moral and ethical issues regarding allocation of organs remain unresolved. Furthermore, there is significant risk of incurring exorbitant health care costs in marginal recipients of suboptimal donor organs.

The objectives of this chapter are to analyse the physiological impact of brain death and the events which lead to organ deterioration in the donor, and to review the effect of triiodothyronine (T_3) as a therapeutic modality for the reversal of metabolic graft dysfunction occurring in both the donor and recipient.

Whatever the initiating events resulting in brain death, two major neuro-endocrine responses occur, characterized by an initial autonomic storm (parasympathetic and sympathetic) lasting for minutes to hours (Fig. 1) and the rapid endocrine disintegration of the hypothalamic–hypophyseal axis, which results in a loss of antidiuretic hormone and loss of thyroid releasing hormone, corticotropic releasing hormone and gonadotropic releasing hormone production. This results in diabetes insipidus. There is also a significant alteration of the thyroid hormone profile [7].

2. The autonomic storm

Experimental data obtained during induction of brain death in fully instrumented and ECG monitored baboons revealed significant electrocardiographic, haemodynamic and endocrine changes [7,8]. In the early stages, as a response to intracranial hypertension (Cushing reflex) [9], an initial, marked para-

G.M. Collins, J.M. Dubernard, W. Land and G.G. Persijn (eds). Procurement, Preservation and Allocation of Vascularized Organs 59–68
© 1997 Kluwer Academic Publishers.

EXPERIMENTAL BRAIN DEATH
Plasma Catecholamines

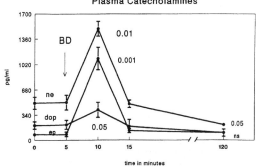

Figure 1. Plasma catecholamine levels before and following induction of brain death in the baboon. The significant peak occurs within 5 minutes and by 15 minute levels returns to control levels. By 3 h these are significantly lower than control values.

EXPERIMENTAL BRAIN DEATH

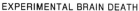
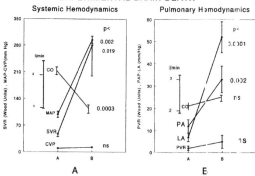

Figure 2. Systemic and pulmonary haemodynamics in the baboon before induction of brain death and at the peak of the systemic vascular resistance. (A) Note the significant increment of the SVR and MAP. There is a simultaneous marked reduction in cardiac output. (B) Note the significantly higher elevation of LAP over PAP, indicating pulmonary blood pooling.

sympathetic activity is observed (Phase I) characterized by sinus bradycardia, sinus standstill, prolonged asystole, junctional escape beats and total atrioventricular dissociation. At the end of Phase I and beginning of Phase II there is an overlapping of initial parasympathetic activity with the release of endogenous and circulating catecholamines leading to a marked sinus tachycardia (without ST segment changes). Phase III is marked by the development of unifocal, multifocal ventricular ectopic beats and runs of ventricular tachycardia. During Phase IV sinus rhythm resumes. Acute ischaemic changes similar to acute myocardial infarction have been observed, with the development of Q waves and significant ST segment changes. Phase V marks the end of the autonomic (adrenergic) storm. The heart remains in sinus rhythm with non-specific ST segment changes, QRS notching, J waves, T wave flattening and biphasic T waves [10].

As result of the adrenergic storm during Phases II, III and IV there is a marked imbalance of oxygen supply and demand, as evidenced by ECG abnormalities. Histological subendocardial necrosis, appearing as scattered patchy areas throughout the heart, is thought to result from the combination of calcium overload, oxygen deficiency and ATP depletion. This is prevalent along the interventricular septum. In some specimens, the observed injury is similar to an acute myocardial infarction [7,10]. Bilateral vagotomy does not prevent myocyte necrosis; however surgical sympathetic denervation of the heart [11] or pretreatment with calcium channel blockers prior to induction of brain death abolishes the catecholamine-induced injury [12]. In addition to affecting the heart, the adrenergic

storm adversely affects other organs: structural changes have been well documented in the lungs, kidneys and liver [13].

In the lung, there is significant alveolar-capillary disruption resulting in a protein-rich transudate producing pulmonary oedema [14]. Pulmonary injury occurs during the peak systemic vascular resistance and arterial hypertension induced by the catecholamine storm (Fig. 2). This produces acute left ventricular geometrical changes inducing sudden mitral valve regurgitation. Significant increases in left atrial pressure up to 90 mm/Hg have been observed on occasion and may well explain the pulmonary oedema seen following head trauma. The left atrial pressure elevation is short-lived, occurring immediately after head injury, and is not seen clinically as it occurs prior to hospital admission.

As a result of the adrenergic storm, pulmonary capillary disruption may be responsible for temporary lung dysfunction immediately post-lung transplant. Preservation solutions and reperfusion injury may also contribute, leading to primary lung failure.

3. Endocrine response to brain death

In the baboon, induction of brain death is followed by rapid endocrine derangement [7] (Figure 3). There is evidence of hypothalamic–hypophyseal axis disruption and lack of stimulation of the peripheral endocrine organs. Peripheral tissue activation of the 5′monodeo-

EXPERIMENTAL BRAIN DEATH
Free T3 and T4

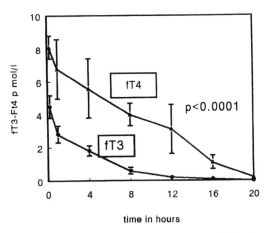

Figure 3. Plasma fT_3 and fT_4 levels before and following induction of brain death in the baboon. Note the rapid reduction within the first 4 h.

dinase (induced by tissue catecholamines) results in thyroxine (T_4) conversion to reverse triodothyronine (rT_3) rather than the triiodothyronine (the active hormone) produced during the healthy state [15]. These changes result in major metabolic dysfunction at the cellular level, affecting mainly mitochondrial function and inhibiting aerobic metabolism. Major cellular fuels can no longer enter the tricarboxylic acid cycle (TCA), efficient ATP production is reduced and lactate accumulation occurs. As a result of brain death, the whole body is globally affected and progressive metabolic deterioration of all organs ensues. Cardiac arrest will occur despite careful donor management [16] and early organ procurement becomes a priority before major metabolic injury can progress contributing to graft dysfunction.

Following the initial catecholamine storm, plasma levels of various hormones are depleted. There is a rapid and significant drop of ACTH, cortisol, ADH, insulin, growth hormone and the thyroid hormones, resulting in the so-called 'euthyroid sick syndrome' (ESS). There is marked reduction of the free T_3 (fT_3) while free T_4(fT_4), total T_3 and T_4 may remain normal or slightly reduced. Reverse T_3 (rT_3) is significantly elevated and thyroid stimulating hormone (TSH) levels remain unchanged [7,17]. ESS is currently considered to be an adaptive, beneficial response to stress in order to save cellular fuels (fats, carbohydrates and proteins) for utilization during the recovery phase, thus thyroid replacement is not indicated [18]. However, our exper-

imental and clinical studies clearly indicate a beneficial effect from T_3 therapy in various conditions, challenging this traditional thinking.

4. The haemodynamic and metabolic impact of brain death and the role of hormonal therapy

The previously described endocrine events indicate the need for further research in this realm. In a study in pigs, T_3, cortisol and insulin were administered with the objective of reversing the effects of brain death on the heart and kidneys. The heart and kidneys were procured from alive anaesthetized animals (Group A), brain-dead animals supported for 4 h with mechanical ventilation, volume replacement and inotropic support (Group B), and brain-dead animals ventilated for 6 h (Group C). During the first 4 h, animals in Group B and C received the same treatment. Animals in Group C were then supported for an additional 2 h and given hormonal therapy as follows: T_3 2 $\mu g/h$, cortisol 100 mg/h and insulin 10 IU/h [20]. The excised hearts underwent haemodynamic testing in an *ex vivo* modified Langendorff model [19] (Fig. 4). Hearts from brain-dead animals in group B had a significant reduction of the dp/dt, peak LV pressure and cardiac output, and elevation of the LVEDP. The *ex vivo* testing of hearts from Group C animals receiving hormonal therapy showed normal haemodynamic parameters. No

EXPERIMENTAL BRAIN DEATH
Ex Vivo Hemodynamics

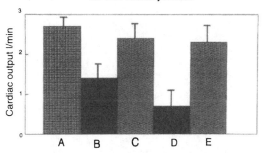

Figure 4. Ex vivo haemodynamic testing of pig hearts procured from alive (Group A), brain-dead (Group B), brain-dead given hormonal therapy (Group C), brain-dead stored hearts (Group D), and brain-dead stored hearts with hormonal therapy administered to donors (Group E) (A vs B, $p < 0.02$; C vs A, ns; D vs A, $p < 0.0002$; E vs A, ns).

difference was observed in those procured from live animals. Hearts procured from similar groups of animals were also evaluated after 24 h of hypothermic perfusion storage [20]. The haemodynamic performance was significantly worse in hearts procured from brain-dead animals (Group B). Hearts procured from animals in Group C showed full functional myocardial recovery and were no different from hearts procured from live animals.

At the completion of the haemodynamic testing, myocardial biopsies were performed. Biochemical assays showed that Group B hearts had significant lactate accumulation, glycogen depletion and reduction of high energy phosphates. Group C hearts were no different from hearts from live animals [19] (Fig. 5).

Intravenous ^{14}C-R (glucose, pyruvate and palmitate) was administered to alive, brain dead and brain dead T_3-treated baboons for 6 h [21]. Brain-dead animals were unable to aerobically metabolize the injected

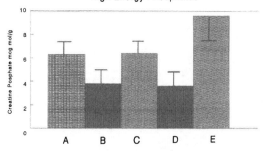

EXPERIMENTAL BRAIN DEATH
High Energy Phosphates

Figure 5. High energy phosphates from myocardial biopsies procured from alive (Group A), brain-dead (Group B), brain-dead given hormonal therapy (Group C), brain-dead stored hearts (Group D), and brain-dead stored hearts with hormonal therapy administered to donors (Group E) (B vs A, $p < 0.02$; C vs A, ns; D vs A, $p < 0.02$; E vs A, $p < 0.02$).

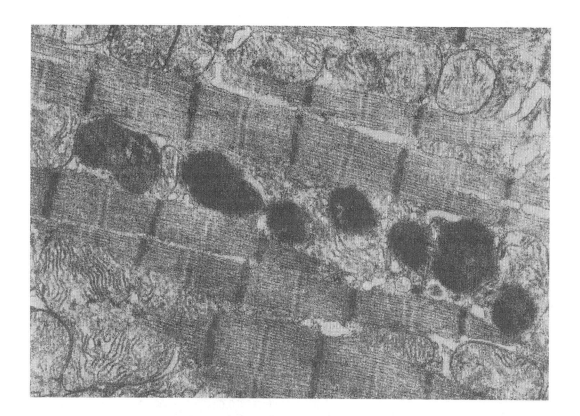

Figure 6. Electron microscopy of a human donor heart prior to implantation. There is a significant disruption of structural integrity, mitochondrial swelling, membrane continuity loss and various degrees of mitochondria degeneration, and loss of cristae integrity. The electron-dense injured mitochondria are no longer functional (×23 500).

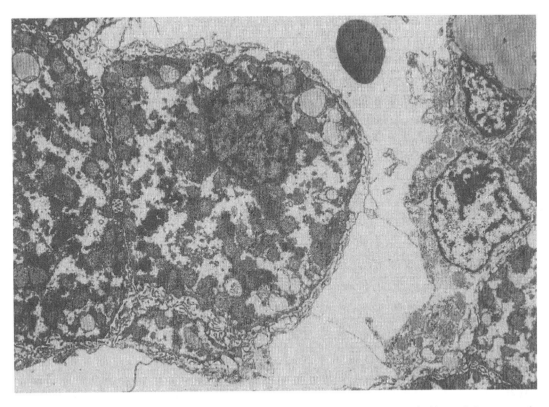

Figure 7. Electron microscopy of a human donor liver prior to implantation. There is marked loss of glycogen, various stages of mitochondrial degeneration, loss of cristae and abundant lipid droplets. The membranous structures are preserved (×7050).

radiolabelled metabolites. Following a single bolus of ^{14}C-R, brain-dead baboons showed a significant reduction in exhaled $^{14}CO_2$ and prolongation of the plasma half-life. The inability to produce $^{14}CO_2$, especially after administration of ^{14}C labelled fatty acids, glucose and pyruvate, indicates inhibition of aerobic metabolism at the mitochondrial level. There is an inability to generate two-carbon compounds, resulting in the depletion of the acetyl CoA pool. Pyruvate can no longer be incorporated in the TCA cycle and is shifted to lactate. This progressive inhibition of aerobic metabolism results in inability of the cells to use fuels aerobically and progressively reduces the cellular energy charge. This affects the whole body and all organs used for transplantation (Figs 6, 7).

Organ injury may occur in the potential donor prior to brain death as events such as trauma, haemorrhage, hypotension, hypoxia and blood transfusion stimulate the catecholamine surge. Release of interleukins, complement activation, and release of free oxygen radicals and endothelial adhesion molecules may further potentiate the tissue injury [22–24].

During the agonal period, while the patient is progressively developing intracranial hypertension, two separate sets of injury take place. The first is the result of a catecholamine storm which affects all organs, and is probably calcium mediated. The second event is the endocrine derangement and loss of aerobic metabolic pathways. The impact on the mitochondria is thought to arise from calcium overload and T_3 deficiency [25,26].

Na/K ratios were measured in renal slices from live or brain-dead pigs and from brain-dead pigs treated with hormones as indicators of organ viability. The ionic gradient is Na^+K^+-ATPase energy dependent. The Na/K ratio was significantly increased in renal slices procured from brain-dead animals. This was not observed following administration of hormonal therapy to brain dead animals [27].

The synergistic negative effects of brain death and catecholamine administration were studied in pigs. Kidneys were harvested from alive, brain-dead and brain-dead dopamine-supported animals, and from brain-dead animals treated with hormonal therapy and transplanted into nephrectomized recipients. Animals receiving kidneys from the brain-dead dopamine-supported group had significantly higher creatinine levels. However, pigs receiving kidneys from brain-dead dopamine-supported and hormone-treated animals had normal creatinine/plasma levels post-transplant. Renal function was no different from animals who received kidneys from living pigs [28].

5. Initial results of hormonal therapy in human brain-dead donors

Initially a T_3 total loading dose of 20 μg (extrapolated from animal weight to humans) combined with cortisol 100 mg and insulin 10 IU was administered to an unstable brain-dead organ donor. Haemodynamic parameters were rapidly normalized, allowing discontinuation of inotropes. This dose precipitated a full thyrotoxic storm evidenced by hyperthermia, hypertension, hypercarbia and respiratory acidosis. Despite body surface cooling, hyperventilation and administration of calcium channel and β-blockers, the heart developed ventricular fibrillation and all organs were lost. A second patient treated with the same regimen had a similar haemodynamic response without the untoward negative metabolic component. All organs were successfully harvested and transplanted, with excellent results in all recipients.

As a result of this early experience we modified the initial T_3 dosage to 2 μ, repeated at hourly intervals until a haemodynamic response was achieved and compared this therapeutic modality with 26 historical brain-dead donors who received standard management. T_3, cortisol and insulin were administered on an hourly basis for 4 h to 21 unstable organ donors who were on high inotropic support, requiring frequent sodium bicarbonate replacement. All had significantly elevated plasma lactate, pyruvate and free fatty acid levels. All donors receiving hormonal therapy became haemodynamically stable with resolution of the lactic acidosis and organs procured were able to be successfully transplanted. In seven donors, the hormonal therapy was continued for several additional hours following haemodynamic stabilization to enable elective cardiac transplantation. In the control group, four donors developed ventricular fibrillation and were excluded from the donor pool [29].

The advantage of hormonal replacement was further confirmed by applying this therapy to human, brain-dead patients. In this study, patients were randomized to placebo and hormonal therapy groups. Vasopressin was introduced and sequential haemodynamic assessments were performed by cardiac catheterization. The control group exhibited similar endocrine changes to those observed in the baboon after brain death. There was progressive haemodynamic deterioration and half of the patients suffered cardiac arrest prior to completion of the study. Conversely, the brain-dead patients who received hormonal replacement demonstrated excellent haemodynamic profiles [30].

Despite optimal volume replacement, ventilatory and inotropic support, neurological patients receiving high-dose steroid therapy for cerebral oedema and insulin for elevated serum glucose levels will experience haemodynamic deterioration following brain death. A total of 72% of patients suffered ventricular fibrillation within 3 days as a terminal event [16]. In this type of patient, the addition of T_3 alone rapidly improves the haemodynamic condition, allowing reduction of inotropic support. Cardiac output improves and lactic acidosis is corrected in these unstable donors, allowing transplantation and subsequent haemodynamic function in the recipient [25,29].

These data are further validated by a prospective randomized trial in which T_3 or a placebo was administered to brain-dead organ donors. Hearts from those receiving T_3 had significantly better post-transplant haemodynamics and a marked reduction in acute rejection episodes [31]. This reduced immunological response could be attributed to the effect of T_3 at the cellular level, resulting in less myocyte necrosis and reduced Class I–II antigen expression. Prior studies have shown up-regulation of antigen expression in injured cells. This study confirmed the relevance and beneficial effects of T_3 therapy upon donor hearts.

6. The euthyroid sick syndrome in the recipient

A profound alteration in thyroid profile has been observed in acute illnesses with profound fT_3 reduction and rT_3 elevation while TSH levels remain unchanged. Lower fT_3 levels correlate with higher patient mortality [32]. This condition lasts several days after an acute event, and in chronic debilitating illnesses, the fT_3 remains low. Hormonal replacement may be of benefit in both acute and chronic illness. The acute physiological changes following brain death and beneficial effects of T_3 have been previously discussed. Acute ESS has also been observed in shock states, acute myocardial infarction, following cardiopulmonary bypass and in sepsis [33–36]. In chronic states ESS has been observed in congestive heart failure, chronic haemodialysis, starvation, diabetes, patients requiring prolonged inotropic support and those awaiting organ transplantation [37–39].

Organs procured from brain-dead donors and transplanted to chronically ill recipients with a low fT_3 level are subjected to another T_3-depleted environment. Functional recovery of organ function may be delayed for hours or days after transplantation. Early adequate graft function may subsequently fail in the low T_3 recipient environment. In heart transplantation, immediate mechanical efficiency is required. Primary graft failure is a major catastrophic event associated with high morbidity and mortality. In the event of pump failure, mechanical support devices and even retransplantation may be required [40]. Triiodothyronine has been administered to five patients with primary graft failure, with remarkable recovery of the transplanted heart to perform work allowing discontinuation of cardiopulmonary bypass support. T_3 is the essential hormone for rapid reversal of graft dysfunction in both the donor and the recipient. We have adopted this approach, administering T_3 to the donor prior to procurement of the heart, and to the recipient.

The haemodynamic and histological appearance of primary graft failure has often been confused with those of severe acute cellular rejection. Differentiation between these entities may be extremely difficult. Myocyte injury occurs at the time of brain death in the donor and triggers an inflammatory response. Mononuclear cells, macrophages and lymphocytes surround necrotic cells [41]. Early biopsies of the heart may confuse the histological interpretation and the recipient may be given unnecessary steroid pulses, for treatment of perceived severe acute rejection. The usual response to steroids will not occur, graft function will remain suboptimal, and further aggressive immunosuppression may result in further deterioration coupled with the possibility of opportunistic infections. Early biopsies of other transplanted organs may demonstrate similar confusing histological patterns.

7. Results of T_3 therapy to both donor and recipient

Extensive data regarding hormonal therapy has been accumulated and therapeutic regimens have been modified. Donors on high inotropic support ($\geq 21/\mu g/kg/min$ of dopamine) require several boluses of T_3 before the dopamine inotropic requirement is reduced to 0–10 $\mu g/kg/min$. It became evident that T_3 requirements in unstable donors are significantly higher than those in stable donors and need to be repeated at more frequent intervals (15–30 minutes) [25]. In unstable donors, the loading dose has been increased to 4–6 μg bolus repeated at 15 minute intervals until the desired effects (haemodynamic stability, reduction of inotropes, normalization of EKG, abolition of arrhythmias, reduction of the heart rate and improvement of cardiac output) are achieved. Stable donors requiring dopamine 2–5 $\mu g/kg/min$ benefit from small (2 μg) boluses repeated hourly.

We have treated 196 consecutive brain-dead organ donors with T_3, improving haemodynamics rapidly and reducing acidosis. The last 154 patients (Table 1), received T_3 until a haemodynamic response was observed. The more unstable donors required a significantly higher dose of T_3 therapy: seven donors in this group were not accepted for cardiac transplantation purposes by other institutions. The dopamine support was reduced to 0–10 $\mu g/kg/min$. Following cardiac transplantation, the 154 recipients received a loading T_3 dose during cardiopulmonary bypass of 0.1–0.2 $\mu g/kg$. T_3 administration was continued for a further 12–72 hours in boluses of 2 $\mu g/kg$ at 1–2 hourly intervals. Cardiac function at the completion of cardiac transplant was poor in one recipient requiring 24 h of support with a biventricular assist device. Twenty-four hours later, cardiac recovery took place and the BVAD was discontinued. In five recipients intra-aortic balloon pump support was required from 24–48 hours with excellent recovery.

As a result of T_3 therapy to both donor and recipient we were able to use 43 donors (28%) who were considered unacceptable for cardiac transplantation purposes. We therefore strongly recommend T_3 therapy to both donor and recipient with the objective of enlarging the donor pool and decreasing the number of recipients awaiting transplantation.

Since T_3 is a potent vasodilator, optimal intravascular volume is essential prior to T_3 administration [42]. To prevent hypotension, administration of small doses of vasopressin to the donor is recommended, preferably as an infusion at the beginning of T_3 therapy. This combination has produced no adverse effects on other donor organs. There was no detrimental effect on the functional status of other organs procured from T_3 treated donors. The donor pool was significantly enlarged by the ability to harvest these organs from initially unstable donors [25].

Table 1. The impact of T_3 on the dopamine requirements pre- and post-T_3 therapy. The inotropic difference for each group is indicated. The total T_3 dose of each group is compared with Group 1. There is no significant difference in the cardiac ischaemic times.

Group	Range	n	Dopamine requirement (μg/kg/min)					Cardiac ischaemia time (min)
			Pre T_3	Post T_3	p	Total T_3 dose (μg)	p	
1	0–5	46	1.52 (0.31)	1.24 (0.29)	ns	9.55 (0.78)	–	163.76 (8.32)
2	6–10	53	8.92 (0.19)	5.71 (0.40)	< 0.001	12.07 (0.73)	< 0.02	157.34 (10.29)
3	11–15	12	13.5 (0.48)	6.75 (1.52)	< 0.0003	17.16 (1.49)	< 0.0001	194.63 (7.63)
4	16–20	28	18.69 (0.34)	7.5 (0.69)	< 0.0001	19.76 (1.32)	< 0.0001	99.5 (8.07)
5	≥ 21	15	34.00 (1.48)	7.81 (0.95)	< 0.0001	22.14	< 0.0001	184.85 (18.32)

Values are mean (s.e.m.).

Hypokalaemia frequently follows T_3 administration, and it is not unusual to observe serum potassium levels dropping to 2–2.5 meq/l within a few minutes. Periodic potassium measurements are required as well as aggressive replacement, occasionally up to 150–200 meq/h. This effect is directly related to activation of Na^+,K^+-ATPase. Contrary to conventional thought, arrhythmias have not been observed provided potassium has been replaced adequately.

8. T_3 therapy in the low fT_3 states

The T_3 doses required vary considerably between animal species and underlying conditions. For example, pigs are extremely sensitive to T_3, doses as low as 0.1 μg/kg being sufficient to induce desired haemodynamic responses. By comparison, the baboon requires a dose three times higher, and 5–10 times that needed in the dog. The rat requires up to 100-fold more T_3 than the pig.

T_3 doses for brain-dead human organ donors is 2–6 μg as an initial loading dose followed by pulses at various intervals. In our series of high-risk open heart surgery patients, the T_3 loading dose was 2–3 μg/kg. In patients with low cardiac output after open heart surgery a loading dose of 1 μg/kg was sufficient. In these patients, a continuous infusion was given from several hours up to 5 days [43].

9. Summary

The multifactorial damaging events which result in poor organ function after transplantation begin in the organ donor prior to brain death. The intracranial hypertension which induces brain death precipitates an adrenergic storm. This, coupled with endocrine collapse and decreased thyroid hormone plasma levels, results in the inhibition of cellular metabolic aerobic metabolism. Reperfusion injury occurs following organ procurement and cold preservation [22,24]. Immunological responses can further complicate understanding of the aetiology and subsequent treatment of graft dysfunction.

Hormonal therapy has been beneficial in reversing organ failure in experimental and clinical studies [45,46]. Triiodothyronine seems to be the pivotal element in improving organ function in the donor and recipient, and in other acute haemodynamic events. T_3 replacement is safe and beneficial in acute and chronic conditions exhibiting a low free T_3 state.

The cellular effects of T_3 initially are extranuclear, affecting calcium dependent pathways, and delayed events are related to DNA, RNA and protein synthesis [47]. T_3 has inotropic properties [48] as well as acting as a vasodilator [42]. A primary target for T_3 are mitochondria in which aerobic metabolism and production of high energy phosphates is stimulated [49]. This facilitates pyruvate transfer to the TCA cycle, upregulates the adeninucleotide transferase [50], upregulates β-receptors [51,52], participates in the calcium uptake–calcium release from the sarcoplasmic reticulum [53,54] and activates various ATPases such as Na^+K^+ [55,56] myosin [57] and others. These multiple functions at various cellular levels gives T_3 the key role as a metabolic modulator essential for cellular viability.

Acknowledgements

The author wishes to express his gratitude to SmithKline Beecham for the donation of triiodothyronine used in this clinical application, and for the secretarial support given by Bonnie Heath and Pat Conant, MS ARNP.

References

1. Fragomeni LS and Kaye MP. The Registry of the International Society for Heart Transplantation: Fifth official report. J Heart Transplant 1988; 7: 249–53.
2. Toussaint R-M, Mezghebe HH, Millis RM. Hepatic transplantation in the United States. Transplant Proc 1993; 25: 2481–3.
3. Sharples L, Belcher C, Dennis C, Higenbottam T, Wallwork J. Who waits longest for heart and lung transplantation? J Heart Lung Transplant 1994; 13: 282–91.
4. McClelland J, Steidler K, Cecka JM, et al. Kidney allocation under the UNOS point system: an update. In: Terasaki PI and Cecka JM (eds). Clinical Transplants 1992. UCLA Tissue Typing Laboratory, Los Angeles 1992; pp. 405–511.
5. Bourge RC, Naftel DC, Costanzo-Nordin MR, Kirklin JK, Young JB, Kubo SH, Olivari M-T, Kasper EK, et al. Pretransplantation risk factors for death after heart transplantation: a multiinstitutional study. J Heart Lung Transplant 1993; 12: 549–62.
6. Reemtsma K, Berland G, Merrill J, Arons R, Evans D, Drusin R, Smith CR, Rose EA. Evaluation of surgical procedures, changing patterns of patient selection and costs in heart transplantation. J. Thorac Cardiovasc Surg 1992; 104: 1306–11.
7. Novitzky D, Wicomb WN, Cooper DKC, Frazer R, Barnard CN. Electrocardiographic hemodynamic and endocrine changes occurring during experimental brain death in the Chacma baboon. Heart Transplant 1984; 4: 63–9.
8. Eichbaum FW, and Bissetti PC. Cardiovascular disturbances following increases in intracranial pressure. Cardiovasc Res 1971; 5: 1016–20.
9. Cushing H. Some experimental and clinical observations concerning states of increased intracranial tension. Am J Med Sci 1902; 124: 375–400.
10. Novitzky D, Horak A, Cooper DKC, Rose AG. Electrocardiographic and histolopathological changes developing during experimental brain death in the baboon. Transplant Proc 1989; 21: 2567–9.
11. Novitzky D, Wicomb WN, Cooper DKC, Rose AG, Reichart B. Prevention of myocardial injury during brain death by total cardiac sympathectomy in the Chacma baboon. Ann Thorac Surg 1986; 41: 520–4.
12. Novitzky D, Cooper DKC, Rose AG, Reichart B. Prevention of myocardial injury by pre-treatment with verapamil hydrochloride prior to experimental brain death: efficacy in a baboon model. Am J Emerg Med 1987; 15: 11–18.
13. Novitzky D, Cooper DKC, Wicomb W. Electron microscopy of heart, liver, and kidneys following induction of brain death in rabbits. (submitted)
14. Novitzky D, Wicomb WN, Rose AG, Cooper DKC, Reichart B. Pathophysiology of pulmonary edema following experimental brain death in the Chacma baboon. Ann Thorac Surg 1987; 43: 288–94.
15. Leonard JL, Viseer TJ. Biochemistry of deiodination. In: Henneman G (ed). Thyroid Hormone Metabolism. 1st edn. New York, Marcel Dekker 1986; pp. 189–210.
16. Joergensen EO. Spinalman after brain death. Acta Neurochir (Wien) 1973; 28: 259.
17. Madsen M. The low T_3 state, an experimental study. Medical Dissertations No. 229. 1986. Sweden: Linkoping University.
18. Wartofsky L, Burman KD. Alterations in thyroid function in patients with systemic illness: the 'euthyroid sick syndrome'. Endoc Rev 1982; 3: 164–217.
19. Novitzky D, Wicomb WN, Cooper DKC, Tjaalgard MA. Improved cardiac function following hormonal therapy in brain-dead pigs: relevance to organ donation. Cryobiology 1987; 24: 1–10.
20. Wicomb WN, Cooper DKC, Lanza RP, Novitzky D, Isaacs S. The effects of brain death and hour storage by hypothermic perfusion in donor heart function in the pig. J Thorac Cardiovasc Surg 1986; 91: 896–909.
21. Novitzky D, Cooper DKC, Morrell D, Isaacs S. Change from aerobic metabolism after brain death, and reversal following triiodothyronine (T_3) therapy. Transplantation 1988; 45: 32–6.
22. Hearse DJ. Stunning: a radical review. Cardiovasc Drugs Ther 1991; 5: 853–76.
23. Kinzendorf U, Notter M, Hock H, Distler J, Diamantstein T, Walz G. T cells bind to the endothelial adhesion molecule GMP-140 (P-selectin). Transplantation 1993; 56: 1213–17.
24. Gross GJ, Farber NE, Hardman HF, Warltier DC. Beneficial actions of superoxide dismutase and catalase in stunned myocardium of dogs. Am J Physiol 1986; 58: 148–56.
25. Novitzky D, Cooper DKC, Chaffin JS, Greer AE, Debault LE, Zuhdi N. Improved cardiac allograft function following triiodothyronine (T_3) therapy to both donor and recipient. Transplantation 1990; 49: 311–16.
26. Montero JA, Mallol J, Alvarez F, Benito P, Concha M, Blanco A. Biochemical hypothyroidism and myocardial damage in organ donors: are they related? Transplant Proc 1988; 20: 746–8.
27. Wicomb WN, Cooper DKC, Novitzky D. Impairment of renal slice function following brain death, with reversibility of injury by hormonal therapy. Transplantation 1986; 41: 29–33.
28. Pienaar H, Schwartz I, Roncone A, Lotz A, Hickman R. Function of kidney grafts from brain-dead donor pigs. The influence of dopamine and triiodothyronine. Transplantation 1990; 50: 580–2.
29. Novitzky D, Cooper DKC, Reichart B. Haemodynamic and metabolic responses to hormonal therapy in brain-dead potential organ donors. Transplantation 1987; 43: 852–4.
30. Taniguchi S, Kitamura S, Kawachi K, Doi Y, Aoyama N. Effects of hormonal supplements on the maintenance of cardiac function in potential donor patients after cerebral death. Eur J Cardiothorac Surg 1992; 6: 96–101.
31. Darracott-Cankovic S, Cbiol DW, Cankovic M, English TAH, Well F, Wallwork J. Does hormonal pre-treatment improve myocardial function in the donor? A clinical study of the effect of T_3, cortisol and insulin. J Thorac Cardiovasc Surg.
32. Slag MF, Morley JE, Elson MK. Hypothyroxinemia in critically ill patients as a predictor of high mortality. JAMA 1981; 245: 43–5.
33. Hesch RD, Hesch M, Kodding R, Hoffken B, Mayer T. Treatment of dopamine-dependent show with T_3. Endocr Res Commun 1981; 8: 229–37.
34. Dulchavsky SA, Lucas CE, Ledgewood AM, Grabow D. Triiodothyronine (T_3) improves CV function during hemorrhagic shock. Circ Shock 1993; 39: 67–73.

35. Pederson F, Perrilk H, Rasmussen SL, Skovsted L. 'Low T₃-syndrome' in acute myocardial infarction – relationship to beta adrenergic blockade and clinical cause. Eur J Clin Pharmacol 1984; 26: 69–73.

36. Ceremuzynski L. Hormonal and metabolic reactions evoked by acute myocardial infarction. Circ Res 1981; 48: 767–76.

37. Robuschi G, Medici D, Fesani F, et al. Cardiopulmonary bypass: a low T₄ and T₃ syndrome with blunted thyrotropin (TSH) response to thyrotropin-releasing hormone (TRH). Hormone Res 1986; 23: 151–8.

38. Hamilton MA. Prevalence and clinical implications of abnormal thyroid hormone metabolism in advanced heart failure. Ann Thorac Surg 1993; 56: 548–53.

39. Novitzky D. Triiodothyronine replacement, the euthyroid sick syndrome and organ transplantation. Transplant Proc 1991; 23: 2460–2.

40. Novitzky D, Cooper DKC, Rose AG, Wicomb WN, Becerra E, Reichart B. Early donor heart failure following transplantation from myocardial injury sustained during brain death. Clin Transplant 1987; 1: 108–13.

41. Novitzky D, Rose AG, Cooper DKC, Reichart B. Interpretation of endomyocardial biopsy after heart transplantation. Potentially confusing factors. S Afr Med 1986; 70: 789–92.

42. Klein I. Thyroid hormone and the cardiovascular system. Am J Med 1990; 88: 631–7.

43. Novitzky D, Fontanet H, Snyder M, Coblio N, Smith D, Parsonnet V. Impact of triiodothyronine on the survival of high-risk patients undergoing open heart surgery. Cardiology 1996; 87: 509–15.

44. Kukielka GL, Hawkins KH, Michael L, Manning AM, Youker K, Lane C, Entman ML, Smith CW, Anderson DC. Regulation of intercellular adhesion molecule-1 (ICAMO1) in ischemic and reperfused canine myocardium. J Clin Invest 1993; 92: 1504–16.

45. Novitzky D, Cooper DKC, Swanepoel A. Inotropic effect of triiodothyronine in low cardiac output following cardioplegic arrest and cardiopulmonary bypass: initial experience in patients undergoing open heart surgery. Eur J Cardiothorac Surg 1989; 3: 140–5.

46. Novitzky D, Human P, Cooper DKC. Inotropic effect of triiodothyronine following myocardial ischemia and cardiopulmonary bypass. An experimental study in pigs. Ann Thorac Surg 1988; 45: 50–5.

47. Segal J. In vivo effect of 3,5,3′-triiodothyronine on calcium uptake in several tissues in the rat: evidence for a physiologic role for calcium as the first messenger for the prompt action of thyroid hormone at the level of the plasma membrane. Endocrinology 1990; 127: 17–24.

48. Snow TR, Deal MT, Connelly TS, Yokoyama Y, Novitzky D, et al. Acute inotropic response to rabbit papillary muscle to triiodothyronine. Cardiology 1992; 80: 112–17.

49. Sterling K, Brenner MA, Sakurada T. Rapid effect of triiodothyronine on the mitochondrial pathway in rat liver in vivo. Science 1980; 210: 340–2.

50. Sterling K. Direct thyroid hormone activation of mitochondria: the role of adenine nucleotide translocase. Endocrinology 1986; 119: 292–5.

51. Ginsbert AM, Clutter WE, Shah SD, Cryer PE. Triiodothyronine-induced thyrotoxicosis increases mononuclear leukocyte β-adrenergic receptor density in man. J Clin Invest 1981; 67: 1785–91.

52. Revelli J-P, Pescini R, Muzzin P, Seydoux J, Fitzgerald MG, Fraser CM, Giacobino J-P. Changes in beta₁ and beta₂-adrenergic reception nRNA levels in brown adipose tissue and heart of hypothyroid rats. Biochem J 1991; 277: 625–9.

53. Kim D, Smith T. Effects of thyroid hormone on calcium handling in cultured chick ventricular cells. J Physiol 1985; 364: 131–49.

54. Rudinger A, Mylotte KM, Davis PJ, et al. Rabbit myocardial membrane Ca⁺⁺ ATPase activity: stimulation in vitro by thyroid hormone. Arch Biochem Biophys 1984; 229: 379–85.

55. Segal J. Action of the thyroid hormone at the level of the plasma membrane. Endocrine Res 1989; 15: 619–49.

56. Orlowski A, Lingrel J. Thyroid and glucocorticoid hormones regulate the expression of multiple Na, K-ATPase genes in cultured neonatal rat cardiac myocytes. J Biol Chem 1990; 265: 3462–70.

57. Dill WH. Biochemical basis of thyroid hormones. Am J Med 1990; 88: 626–30.

9 | Perioperative management of the cadaveric donor

DIDIER DOREZ, JEAN JACQUES COLPART AND ALAIN MERCATELLO

1. Introduction

Multi-organ retrieval is a complex, difficult surgical procedure entailing particular care from the anaesthetist. The duration of the procedure (4 h) requires scrupulous perioperative care so as not to compromise the grafts. In some cases the therapeutic objectives for maintaining the quality of the organs to be procured are contradictory (e.g. lungs and kidneys). Perfect coordination between the retrieval teams, the surgical stages and the anaesthetist is indispensable if organs are not to be lost during this period. Rapid organization of the multiple retrieval process and scrupulous implementation are the keys to success.

2. General condition of the multi-organ donor

The multi-organ donor is frequently a young subject, the victim of a traumatic or medical, isolated or clearly predominant cerebral injury, leading rapidly to brain death. The necessity for large blood transfusions in cases of severe trauma and rapid fluid management to correct polyuria or cellular dehydration bring risks of fluid, electrolyte and haemodynamic imbalances and hypothermia. The therapeutic objectives to be achieved for different organs before retrieval are summarized in Table I [1–3].

Table 1. General criteria and major therapeutic goals for multiple organs donors.

General criteria
Age compatible with organ
No history of previous disease in that organ
No history of cancer or i.v. drug abuse
No prolonged episodes of hypotension and asystole
Absence of AIDS, sepsis, hepatitis
ABO and donor size compatible with recipient

Major therapeutic goals
Systolic blood pressure ≥ 100 mmHg
Central venous pressure 10–12 mmHg
  (≤ 10 mmHg if lung or heart–lung retrieval)
Dopamine and dobutamine ≤ 15 μg/kg/min
Urinary output > 1 ml/kg/h
Donor's core temperature > 35°C
BUN and creatinine within normal range
Urine analysis normal for circumstances of the donor
Coagulation studies within normal range
Platelets count $\geq 50 \times 10^9$/l
Haematocrit level above 30%
Electrolyte levels and acid–base balance within normal range
$PaO_2 \geq 100$ mmHg on $FiO_2 \leq 0.4$ (PEEP below 5 cm H_2O)
Liver enzymes and bilirubin within normal range

G.M. Collins, J.M. Dubernard, W. Land and G.G. Persijn (eds). Procurement, Preservation and Allocation of Vascularized Organs 69–72
© 1997 Kluwer Academic Publishers.

2.1. Fluid and electrolyte balance

Metabolic disorders characteristic of brain death, such as hypernatraemia, hypokalaemia, hypophosphoraemia and hyperglycaemia, must be corrected before beginning the retrieval [2,4]. Normalization of these parameters must be ascertained by laboratory data just before transfer of the donor to the operating theatre in order to optimize peroperative electrolyte levels. Hypokalaemia brings the risk of ventricular fibrillation. Hypernatraemia is a sign of cellular dehydration resulting from the treatment of cerebral oedema before the brain death stage. It is corrected by administration of 2.5% dextrose in order not to increase hyperglycaemia or cause uncontrolled osmotic diuresis. If urinary output is insufficient, a low-dose Furosemide injection is given to increase natriuresis. Hypophosphoraemia, incriminated in instances of acute heart failure, must be vigorously corrected. Hypocalcaemia, assessed by measurement of ionized calcium, is also frequent, due to the large transfusions administered during initial takeover. The therapeutic objective in this preoperative stage is to obtain an hourly urine flow of 150–300 ml whilst normalizing the ionogram. Urine flow must be monitored at least hourly. If urine flow exceeds 300 ml/h, one must refrain from reducing it by desmopressin injection just before installation for retrieval. There is, in fact, a distinct peroperative reduction of flow as result of increased fluid loss through evaporation (approx. 15 ml/kg/h) and by renal vasoconstriction induced by operative traction on the peritoneum [5].

2.2. Temperature

Loss of thermoregulation, fluid and blood supplies leads to hypothermia. This reduces the action of inotropic agents and increases the risk of ventricular arrythmia. Continuous temperature monitoring (oesophageal, rectal probe or Swan-Ganz catheter thermistance) is essential. A thermal mattress and a humidifier in the respirator circuit are indispensable for preventing this hypothermia. Where appreciable parenteral fluids are administered (≥ 500 ml/h) an efficient perfusions heating system is necessary. The objective is to maintain a central temperature of between 35 and 37°C up to the time of cannulation.

2.3. Haemodynamics

Haemodynamic instability must be corrected before the donor is installed on the operating table. Haemodynamic monitoring requires a central venous catheter with hourly central venous pressure (CVP)

measurement and continuous blood pressure measurement, either non-invasively or (better) by arterial cannulation, preferably of the radial artery since the femoral site hinders surgical asepsis, retrieval of the aortic graft and interpretation of measurements during cannulation of the abdominal aorta. If a Swan-Ganz catheter has been inserted to guide preoperative care or to assess cardiac function it must be maintained until the arrival of the cardiac retrieval team. More recently, transoesophageal echocardiography has been used to assess the function of the future cardiac graft and, if need be, to guide fluid management. The objective is to maintain a systolic arterial pressure (SAP) > 100 mmHg [6]. First-line treatment consists of blood products, albumin solution, crystalloids, hydroxyethyl starch, as required by CVP parameters, ionogram results and the blood count [7]. If, despite the infusion and with a central venous pressure of 10–12 mmHg, the SAP remains lower than 100 mmHg, dopamine is given (5 μg/kg/min). The doses should be progressively increased by 2 μg/kg/min without exceeding 10–12 μg/kg/min. If this fails, giving dobutamine (same therapeutic schema) is preferable to giving epinephrine or norepinephrine, especially for intraabdominal organs, since the latter is too vasoconstrictive for splanchnic vessels. If associated pulmonary retrieval is planned, it is necessary to minimize infusion pressures and rigorously monitor the balance of products injected whilst trying, during retrieval, to obtain a slightly negative balance [8]. Recourse to vasopressor agents is then more frequent.

2.4. Assisted ventilation

Mechanical ventilation is indispensable and must enable normocapnoea to be obtained in order to avoid respiratory alkalaemia, which reduces cardiac inotropism and increases hypokalaemia and polyuria [2] The objective of oxygenation is $PaO_2 \geq 100$ mmHg and $FiO_2 \leq 0.4$ ($PaO_2/FiO_2 \geq 250$). $FiO_2 > 0.6$ contraindicates pulmonary retrieval. Blood gas measurement, facilitated by arterial cannulation, must be performed frequently. Continuous monitoring by pulse oximetry is currently the rule. If pulmonary retrieval is intended, positive end-expiratory pressure (PEEP) of 3–5 cm H_2O must be introduced and maintained peroperatively to prevent the microatelectasia encountered with mechanical ventilation. Tracheal suctioning must be frequent, atraumatic and sterile. The endotracheal probe cuff must be positioned immediately below the vocal chords to avoid lesions to the tracheal mucosa and the cuff pressure must be regularly monitored, and not exceed 25 mmHg. A gastric tube is indispensable to minimize the risk of aspiration. It can be maintained in gentle suction at the time of retrieval to facilitate intra-abdominal dissection, and the volume drained must be included in the input/output balance.

2.5. Coagulation

Haemodilution associated with the perfusion of crystalloids, hydroxyethyl starch or albumin solution must not reduce the haematocrit to below 30%. Similarly, the platelet count must be higher than $50 \times 10^9/l$ and compensated, if necessary [6]. The prothrombin time is maintained above 50%, if necessary by transfusion of *viro-inactivated* fresh frozen plasma. Disseminated intravascular coagulation is diagnosed by levels of fibrin degradation products which, if significantly high, may contraindicate pulmonary retrieval.

2.6. Antisepsis

Strict aseptic precautions apply to all the procedures carried out on the donor [3]. Where this is documented prior to brain death, it is the rule to continue relevant antibiotic therapy. Prophylaxis is begun when brain death is diagnosed followed by repeated injections at the time of installation in the operating theatre. Although there is no research to show the effectiveness of any particular class of antibiotic, it seems logical to use the prophylaxis scheme used in abdominal surgery. Many retrieval centres apply β-lactamin and metromidazol in combination. Digestive tract decontamination is practised by at least one team. Nothing has been published to justify this precaution in brain-dead patients.

3. In the operating theatre

3.1. Verifications

The equipment needed by the anaesthetist responsible for peroperative care is given in Tables 2 and 3 [1,2,9,10]. Before retrieval begins, he must ascertain the full availability of the surgical teams, so that the donor, monitoring and theatre can be organized under optimum conditions, and no time is wasted between setting up and surgical intervention. The anaesthetist ensures observation of aseptic conditions often neglected through urgency and as a result of the large number of participants in a multiorgan retrieval procedure. The availability of preserving fluids for the organs and sterile ice used for *in situ* and *ex vivo* chilling must also be verified. The medical records and

Table 2. Operating room equipment.

Heating blanket on table
Ventilator (with PEEP-valve and heated humidifier) in order
Electrocardioscope with alarms (arrythmias)
Invasive arterial blood pressure monitor (in upper extremity) or automatic non-invasive blood pressure monitored every 3 minutes
CVP line or *PA catheter* in place and monitored
Oesophageal probe temperature monitored
Pulse oximeter
Foley catheter and urimeter in place
Nasogastric tube (suction line)
End-tidal CO₂ monitor
Transoesophageal echocardiograph
Central venous catheter and 2 large-bore i.v. lines (in upper extremity), in place
Defibrillator with external and internal electrodes
Pressure bags for rapid infusion

Optional equipment in italic.

Table 3. Checklist for drug availability.

Blood ABO-checked and ready for transfusion
Crystalloids, hydroxyethyl starch, serum albumin
Dopamine, dobutamine, epinephrine and norepiniphrine
Electrolytes
Organ preservation solutions
Pancuronium bromure or vecuronium bromure or atracurium
Furosemide, mannitol 20%
Sodium nitroprusside
Heparin, PGE₁ (Prostin®)

results of all paraclinical examinations enabling the quality of the different grafts to be assessed are assembled by the anaesthetist close to the operating theatre.

3.2. Position of the donor

The donor is installed on the operating table equipped with a thermal mattress. The right arm is usually kept straight along the body so as not to hinder the thoracic retrieval team. The left arm is held in hyperabduction on a support and supports equipment for non-invasive arterial pressure measurement or radial arterial cannula. A pulse oximeter is installed on the same arm or attached via an ear sensor. One or two large-diameter peripheral venous routes are kept operational in case of high flow perfusion, and the central venous route (the best is the inner right jugular) is fixed for rapid withdrawal the moment the upper vena cava is cut. Central venous pressure is measured regularly. Cardioscopic monitoring electrodes are installed on the medio-axillary line and covered with a waterproof adhesive plaster. The urinary collector is installed to allow twice-hourly monitoring of urinary flow. Corneal irrigation by regularly administered artificial tears is set up, along with complete palpebral occlusion, so as not to compromise corneal retrieval, usually carried out later.

3.3. Peroperative care

Suppression of all reflex muscular activity is ensured by injecting long-acting, non-depolarizing curare before the surgical teams are in position. After performing disinfection from the subclavicular hollows to the top of the thighs and as far as the posterior axillary line, the operating fields must be established to allow the anaesthetist to monitor the operating field. He must monitor especially blood loss (abdominal and chest walls and particularly sternotomy) and the presence of pathological fluids (pleura, pericardium, peritoneum), which are sampled for direct examination, bacteriological culture and cytochemical analysis. The rules for care are the same as for the preoperative period, in particular, the haematocrit must be maintained between 30 and 35% to ensure a sufficient supply of oxygen right to the end of the procedure. Finally, the anaesthetist must regularly inform the surgical teams of the donor's haemodynamic situation.

Systemic heparin (3 mg/kg) is administered 15–20 minutes before cardioplegia. In the case of pulmonary retrieval, furosemide is given about 30 minutes before, sometimes combined with prostacyclin, which may cause an appreciable fall in blood pressure as a result of systemic vasodilation. The ventilator is stopped at the moment of cardioplegia to reduce venous return and facilitate chilling. Some teams recommend high volume insufflation flowing at the moment of tracheal clamping [11]. Finally, the anaesthetist checks that the perfusion flow rate of the preserving fluids is correct.

Peroperative perfusion of substances such as manritol or thyroid hormones and administration of calcium blocker or natriuretic atrial factor have been described, but there is no consensus on their use.

3.4 Complications

Blood losses during multi-organ retrieval may be considerable, because of the sterno-pubic incision, insufficient wall clamping, haemorrhagic suffusion and retroperitoneal haematoma. In these cases, red cells perfusion must be carried out. Aortic cannulation can cause a sudden rise in the post charge of the left ventricle and precipitate heart failure which is difficult to reverse. Its installation must be carefully monitored by the anaesthetist, as are manipulations of the liver, which may cause de-priming of the right ventricle. A congested appearance to the hepatic parenchyma prompts verification of central venous pressure and a reduction in the flow of perfusions. If, despite correct surgical procedures, haemodynamic instability or cardiac rhythm problems appear, the cannulation procedures of the various surgical teams must be speeded up. Fine dissection of the organs must be performed after perfusion of the preserving fluids.

Operating theatre equipment is regularly checked and replenished after each retrieval.

Multi-organ retrieval is a complex surgical procedure requiring extensive perfectly adapted anaesthetist support if one wishes to preserve organs of quality and increase the number of available grafts. The anaesthetist is the co-ordinator for the surgical teams carrying out the retrieval and he must have considerable experience in order to know how to speed up procedures if haemodynamic instability develops, to avoid losing all the organs.

References

1. Bodenham A, Park GR. Care of the multiple organ donor. Intensive Care Med 1989; 15: 340–8.
2. Lang P, Houssin D. Le Prélèvement d'Organes. Paris, Masson 1992.
3. Soifer BE, Gelb AW. The multiple organ donor: identification and management. Ann Intern Med 1989; 110: 814–23.
4. Masson F, Thicoïpe M, Maurette M, Pinaquy C, Léger A, Erny P. Haemodynamic, haemostatic and glycoregulatory changes related to brain death. Ann Fr Anesth Reanim 1990 9: 115–22.
5. Gramm HJ, Zimmermann J, Meinhold H, Dennhardt R, Voigt K. Hemodynamic responses to noxious stimuli in brain-dead organ donors. Intensive Care Med 1992; 18: 493–5.
6. Baldwin JC, Anderson JL, Boucek MM, et al. Task force 2: donor guidelines. JACC 1993; 22: 15–20.
7. Dawidson IJ, Sandor ZF, Coorpender L et al. Intraoperative albumin administration affects the outcome of cadaver renal transplantation. Transplantation 1992; 53: 774–82.
8. Wood RP, Shaw BW. Multiple organ procurement. In: Cerilli GJ (ed.), Organ Transplantation and Replacement. Lippincott, Philadelphia 1988: pp. 322–5.
9. Collins GM, Wicomb WN. New organ preservation solutions. Kidney Int 1992; 42: S197–202.
10. Wiberg CA, Prusak BF, Pollack R, Mozes MF. Multi-organ donor procurement. AOR J 1986; 44: 936–43.
11. Puskas JD, Hirai T, Christie N, Mayer E, Slutsky AS, Patterson GA. Reliable thirty-hour lung preservation by donor lung hyperinflation. J Thorac Cardiovasc Surg 1992; 104: 1075–83.

10 | Multiple organ procurement

X. Martin, P. Cloix, M. Dawahra, J. Ninet and J.M. Dubernard

1. Introduction

The sometimes strange behaviour of individual surgeons and the uncoordinated and delayed arrival of procurement teams have created a need for a rapid, effective technique that reduces potential errors during organ procurement and which might allow the removal of organs from unstable donors. The aim is for a single surgeon to take charge of the donation and coordinate the efforts of the respective teams [1].

A technique of multiple organ procurement was first described by Starzl *et al.* in 1984 [2]. Since that time, many modifications have been reported, the most recent being the total abdominal evisceration of Nakazato *et al.* [3]. Controversies still remain concerning the surgical strategies between initial organ perfusion and initial dissection. Some authors prefer minimal dissection, cooling and *en bloc* removal of all organs which are later separated on the back-table; others have advocated thorough mobilization of all organs with their vascular connections prior to their individual removal. It has been suggested that excessive *in situ* dissection of the liver and pancreas is associated with poor graft function [4]. The excellent preservation properties of the University of Wisconsin (UW) solution permits more of the dissection to be performed *ex vivo*. In our institution, we use the technique of organ perfusion before dissection of organs as it seems to be less time consuming, more efficient and it is more easily performed by less experienced surgeons.

G.M. Collins, J.M. Dubernard, W. Land and G.G. Persijn (eds). Procurement, Preservation and Allocation of Vascularized Organs 73–94
© 1997 Kluwer Academic Publishers.

2. Incision (Fig. 1)

The incision can be modified depending on which
organs are to be retrieved. For example, the transverse
subcostal abdominal incision is applicable when only
the pancreas and kidneys are to be procured. The complete midline incision from the suprasternal notch to
the symphisis pubis is the most commonly used, even
when only abdominal organs are to be procured. This
incision allows excellent exposure and convenient
proximal control of the great vessels. In order to avoid
haemodynamic alterations, the sternum is not fully
spread, as it is later for dissection and perfusion of
thoracic organs.

3. Preparation for *in situ* cooling of abdominal organs

Immediately after incision, one must be ready to
procure the maximal number of organs in case cardiac
arrest occurs. It is therefore necessary to be ready for
immediate perfusion and cooling of the abdominal and
thoracic organs.

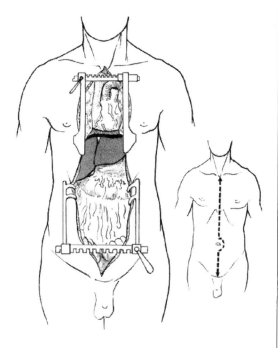

Figure 1. Xyphopubic and sternotomy incisions for
multiorgan donation.

3.1. Isolation of the distal aorta and inferior vena cava (IVC)

Access to the distal aorta, vena cava and ureters is
obtained by medial mobilization of the right and left
colon and the distal part of the small bowel after incision of the white line of Toldt (Fig 2A). A Kocher
manoeuvre is outlined to free the duodenum and the
head of the pancreas is mobilized by blunt dissection
(Fig. 2B, C). On the left side, a defect is created in the
sigmoid mesocolon by ligation and division of the
inferior mesenteric vessels. The left and right ureters
can then be identified; both are dissected distally and
looped. The distal part of the aorta and IVC are dissected free and encircled (Fig. 3A, B). Two or three
sets of lumbar branches have to be ligated and divided
to minimize loss of the preservation solution. Upward
dissection of the anterior surface of the aorta is continued until the left renal vein is encountered crossing
the aorta from left to right. Above the trunk of the left
renal vein, the superior mesenteric artery can be felt as
a taut strand passing almost directly anteriorly, provided the intestines are retracted anteriorly and
superiorly. The aorta is looped at the level of the
inferior mesenteric artery, as is the vena cava below
the entry of the renal veins. At this time, aortic cannulation is performed to allow emergency cooling if
cardiovascular instability develops. Sometimes,
accessory arteries to the lower renal pole originate
from the iliac artery and some authors dissect and loop
common iliac arteries and perform the aortic cannulation through the right iliac artery in order to
provide perfusion of such anomalous arteries.

In an older donor with severe atherosclerotic occlu-
sive disease of the distal aorta, conventional aortic cannulation may be impossible. An alternative aortic flush
method is to cannulate the descending thoracic aorta
after the left pleura and left lung have been discarded.
Flushing is initiated via the proximal aorta and the
distal aorta is clamped below the renal arteries [5].

3.2. Isolation of the coeliac axis and proximal aorta (Fig. 4)

After the lateral portion of the left triangular ligament
of the liver has been taken down, the aorta is mobilized
as it passes through the crura of the diaphragm and
coeliac lymphatic structures, which are divided usually
with electrocautery. The aorta superior to the coeliac
axis must be individualized in order to be clamped. Its
dissection begins on its right side in the avascular
space. In approximately 20% of donors, an aberrant
branch from the left gastric artery supplies the left lobe

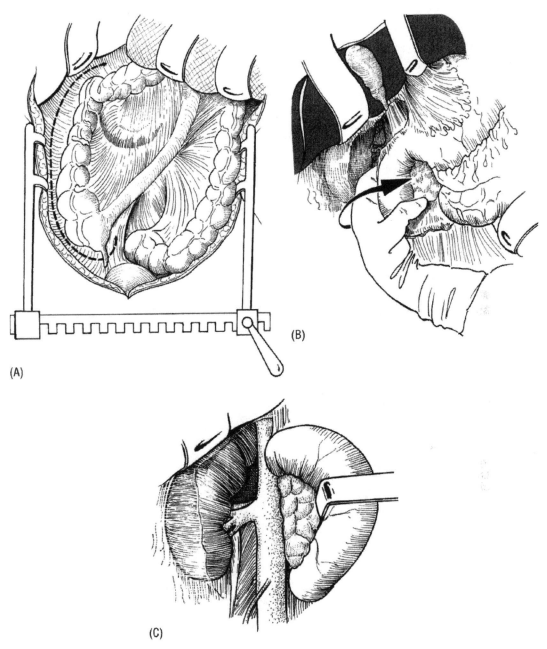

Figure 2. (A) Access to the retroperitoneal space and manoeuvre by incision of right told fascia. (B) Outlining of a Kocher's cartouches. (C) Dissection of aorta and vena cava.

of the liver [6]. If a left replaced hepatic artery is present, the dissection is performed on the left side of the oesophagus and aorta to prevent damage to liver vascularization. (Fig. 4).

A more rapid method is to perform a trans-diaphragmatic dissection of the distal descending supradiaphragmatic aorta. This avoids injury to an anomalous left hepatic artery if the subdiaphragmatic

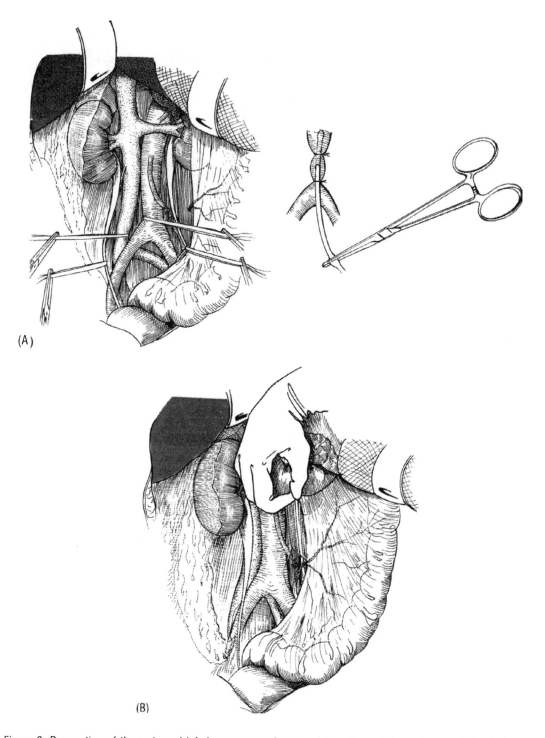

(A)

(B)

Figure 3. Preparation of the aorta and inferior vena cava for cannulation (immediate aortic cannulation in case of conor cardiovascular instability).

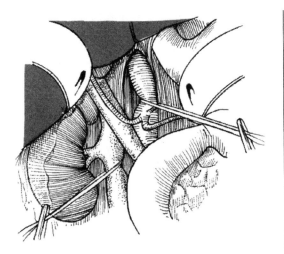

Figure 4. Isolation of the proximal aorta and coeliac axis.

area is surgically difficult, for example in an obese donor.

3.3. Preparation of the liver

The first step is to delineate any aberrant right hepatic artery. Aberrant branches to the right lobe frequently arise from the superior mesenteric artery and pass behind the common duct and portal vein to the right lobe. A right hepatic artery is observed in up to 13% of cadaver organ donors [7] and has long been a contraindication for simultaneous whole pancreas procurement. The right hepatic artery can be found by dissecting the tissue posterior to the surface of the superior mesenteric artery or exploring the right lateral aspect of hepatic pedicle (Fig. 5A). For this the liver is retracted upward and the stomach downward to the donor's left. It is important to avoid extensive retraction of the liver at this point as this may cause cardiovascular instability.

3.3.1. *Division of the common duct and lavage of the gallbladder (Fig. 5B)*

The common duct is identified and divided close to the pancreas. This provides an optimal length of donor common duct for subsequent anastomosis. A longitudinal incision is made in the inferior surface of the fundus of the gallbladder. The biliary tree is flushed with saline through the gallbladder or through the common bile duct after ligation of the cystic duct. This manoeuvre prevents necrosis of the biliary mucosa associated with bile stasis and also demonstrates the patency of the cystic duct–common duct axis [8].

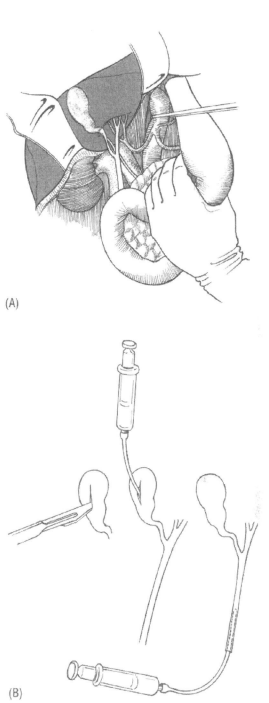

(A)

(B)

Figure 5. (A) Preparation of the liver dissection of the hepatic pedicle. (B) Division of the common duct with lavage of the gallbladder and of the bile duct.

Some authors suggest that the liver should be simultaneously core-cooled with portal infusion and aortic perfusion. For this, a cannula is inserted in the portal vein through a transverse venotomy made in either the splenic or the superior mesenteric vein (SMV) (Fig. 6). The superior mesenteric vein is preferred to the inferior mesenteric vein because of its larger size [9]. If the pancreas is to be harvested special care should be paid to preventing excessive pressure in the pancreatic veins. Therefore the superior mesenteric vein cannula must be placed above the pancreas to avoid back-flow in the splenic vein and oedema to the pancreas. Decompression of the pancreas can also be performed by transection of the inferior mesenteric vein or the portal vein itself; in this case the cannula is fastened to the upper part of the portal vein with a suture.

Cooling of the liver can also be achieved by exclusive aortic cannulation. The latter method has several advantages, including decreased risks of graft loss in

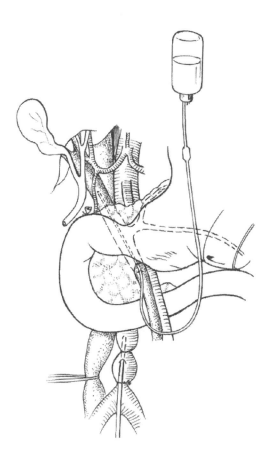

Figure 6. Cannulation of the portal vein.

unstable donor and limited warm ischaemia and intraoperative haemorrhage or hepatic artery injury; moreover, with this latter technique, excessive pressure in the portal system does not occur, thus allowing the pancreas to be harvested in good conditions. Immediate functioning of grafts harvested using this technique have been excellent in animal and clinical studies [10,11].

3.4. Preparation of the pancreas

Adequacy of the vascularization of the head of the pancreas and duodenum is tested by the absence of discoloration of the duodenum and the head of the pancreas after temporary closure of the gastroduodenal artery by a vascular clamp.

3.4.1. *Dissection of the spleen and distal pancreas*
The gastrocolic ligament is separated from the pylorus to the splenic flexure of the colon. The branches of the gastroepiploic vessels are ligated or clipped before division. The dissection is facilitated by upward retraction of the stomach and inferior retraction of the transverse colon. This manoeuvre allows the lesser sac to be entered and provides access to the anterior portion of the spleen (Fig. 7A). The short gastric vessels are ligated and divided, as is the lienocolic ligament. The posterior aspect of the spleen is dissected (Fig. 7B). The spleen is used as a handle to expose the lienophrenic ligament, which is divided (Fig. 7C). After the spleen is freed, the small vessels between the mesocolon and the retroperitoneum are divided. Dissection can then be conducted from the left to the right and separation of the tail of the pancreas from the retroperitoneum is performed. At this point identification of the splenic vein that runs along the posterior aspect of the tail of the pancreas will help to guide the dissection on the right. Dissection is then conducted to the neck of the pancreas. The splenic artery can be localized at the superior aspect of the neck of the pancreas while retracting the pancreas inferiorly (Fig. 8).

3.4.2. *Dissection of a whole pancreas*
When a whole pancreas is harvested the surgical procedure is the same with respect to dissection of the spleen and distal pancreas. The superior mesenteric vessels are identified at the inferior margin of the pancreas and a loop is passed around the vein proximal to the mesocolic branches and around the artery distal to the inferior pancreatico-duodenal artery. A loop is placed on the duodenum at the pyloro duodenal junction and at the duodenojejunal angle (Fig. 9).

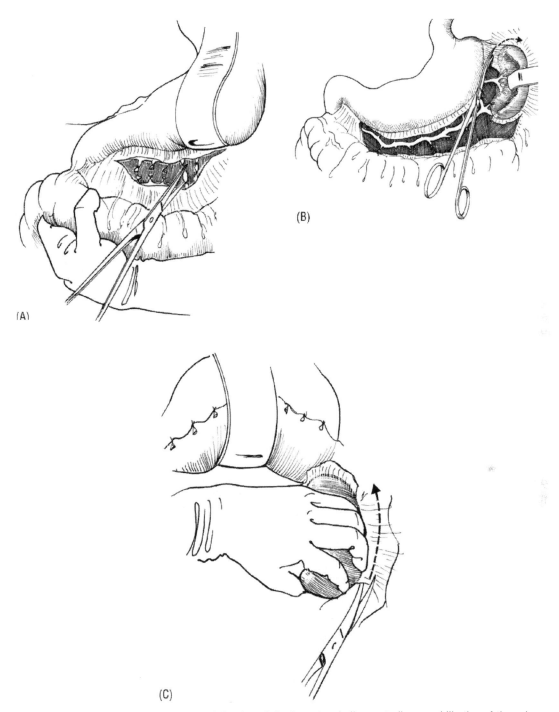

Figure 7. (A) Opening of the lesser sac. (B) Section of the lienophrenic ligament allows mobilization of the spleen. (C) Dissection of the spleen freed from its posterior attachments.

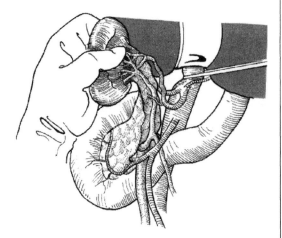

Figure 8. Dissection of the tail of the pancreas using the spleen as a handle.

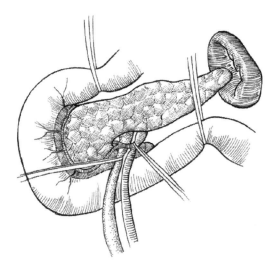

Figure 9. Individualization of mesenteric vessels and the duodeno-jejunal angle.

4. Preparation of thoracic organs

4.1. Mobilization of the heart

Following dissection through the mediastinal fascia and thymus, the pericardial sac is opened vertically from the diaphragm to the innominate vein and fixed to the wound edges with sutures (Fig. 10). At this time, the heart is inspected to provide a final assessment of its suitability as an allograft; in particular its contractility is evaluated and the coronary arteries are assessed.

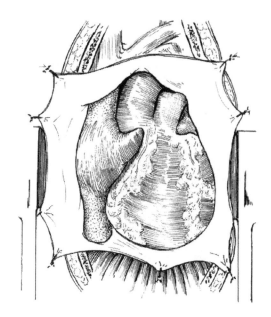

Figure 10. Opening of pericardium.

It is advisable to place the monitoring catheter of arterial blood pressure on the left side in the radial or humeral artery.

The great vessels are mobilized widely to allow for expeditious removal of the organ. The superior and the inferior vena cava are dissected free and encircled just proximal to their junction with the right atrium. A purse-string suture is placed on the anterior portion of the ascending aorta, allowing a catheter to be inserted for subsequent administration of cardioplegic solution. (Fig. 11).

4.2. *En bloc* heart–lung preparation

Dissection begins as for isolated heart excision with mobilization of the vena cava. The superior vena cava is dissected free as far as the azygous vein, which is divided near the right hilum (Fig. 12). The innominate vein is divided between ligatures for better exposure of the innominate artery. The innominate artery is completely mobilized as far as the origin of the right carotid artery. It is divided between two ligatures for exposure of the trachea. The aortic arch is encircled between the innominate and left carotid trunk and the dissection is pursued along the aorta forward to its root. Finally, the pulmonary artery is mobilized as far as the origin of the right and left main pulmonary arteries and separated from the aortic root (Fig. 13). Tracheal mobilization is restricted to the upper medi-

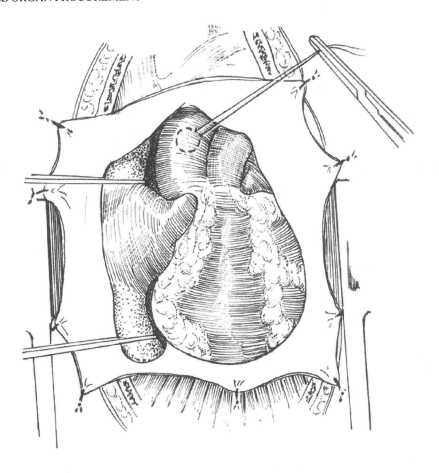

Figure 11. Mobilization of great vessels.

astinal trachea at a level which lies five or six rings above the carina and usually at the level of the innominate artery. Between this latter point and the carina no dissection is performed laterally as it is desirable to leave as intact as possible the paratracheal areolar tissue around that segment of the airway which will be used later. Purse-string sutures are placed in the ascending aorta and the main pulmonary artery and catheters are inserted through the purse-strings.

5. Cooling procedure

When preparation of the organs is completed, cooling and perfusion with preservation solution can be done, and organ procurement can be performed. The preferred sequence of removal is heart or heart/lung first, liver and/or pancreas second and kidneys last. The abdominal organs are often separate in *in vivo* conditions. However an *en bloc* specimen of abdominal organs can be harvested after preservation fluid flush, with separation of the organs on the back-table.

The thoracic and abdominal teams then coordinate cardiopulmonary arrest. The cardioplegic cannula is placed between the aortic root and the aortic clamp and connected to a high-pressure flush system; a total amount of 0.5–1 l is required depending on heart weight. At the same time the pneumoplegia solution is infused via the cannula placed in the main pulmonary artery. The previously cannulated distal abdominal aorta is connected to a gravity flush system containing preservation solution. The abdominal team ligates the isolated distal abdominal inferior vena cava and perfusion of the abdominal organs via the aortic cannula is performed. Slushed iced saline is also poured into the peritoneal cavity and the pericardial sac to complete the cooling process. For adult patients, a total of 3.0 l of preservation fluid is flushed through the aortic and superior mesenteric vein cannula (respectively 2 l and 0.5–1 l) before even attempting to begin extraction of

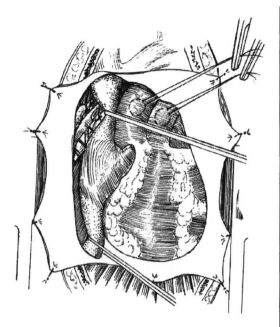

Figure 12. En bloc heart–lung preparation. Division of azygos vein.

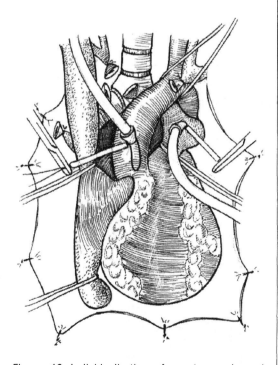

Figure 13. Individualization of great vessels and cannulation of aorta and pulmonary artery.

the organs. This allows the abdominal organs to be generously cooled and flushed while also assisting the thoracic team in removing the heart and lungs. The amount of preservation solution required is variable and guided by decolouration of the organs and cooling, which is judged by touch and sight. The intestines and pancreas often still become chilled and bloodless while the liver remains discoloured and still feels warm. Many institutions have reported graft pancreatitis caused by excessive *in situ* flushing of the donor pancreas and have suggested restricting the flushing volume to 2–3 l [12]. Depending on the speed of the thoracic team's cardioplegia and removal of the heart and lungs, this cooling process is prolonged to about 5–15 minutes. The suprahepatic inferior vena cava is also opened as soon as possible as an extra precaution against overdistension of the liver.

6. Removal of organs

6.1. Thoracic organs

6.1.1. *Isolated excision of the donor heart*
Division of venous inflow: Immediately after aortic cross-clamping the superior vena cava is ligated and divided and the intrapericardial inferior vena cava is clamped (Fig. 14). Excision begins with division of the venous inflow. To avoid the area of the sinus nodes, the superior vena cava is divided 2 cm proximal to its

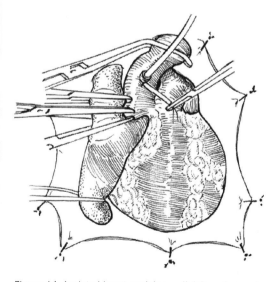

Figure 14. Isolated heart excision – division of superior vena cava.

junction with the right atrium at a level beginning just inferior to the azygos vein. The IVC should be divided with the atrium so that its longest possible length is left attached to the liver. Once the venous inflow is eliminated the heart is rapidly emptied of blood. Incision of the right pulmonary vein provides relief for the left heart while continuing artificial respiration.

Division of outflow (Fig. 15): The aorta is divided just proximal to the aortic cross-clamp. The proximal aorta may be left opened or even stapled with the TA-30 stapling device if an iterative cardioplegia perfusion is required. The main pulmonary artery and its right and left divisions are identified and the pulmonary artery is mobilized as it passes under the aortic arch. This requires division of the ductus. The pulmonary artery main branches are divided as far as possible, leaving the heart attached only by the pulmonary veins.

Division of pulmonary veins (Fig. 16): As a last step in the excision, the heart is elevated from the pericardial sac and the individual pulmonary veins are divided at the level of their respective pericardial reflections. The adventitial tissue at the roof of the left atrium and on the posterior aspect of the pulmonary artery is carefully divided, completing removal of the heart.

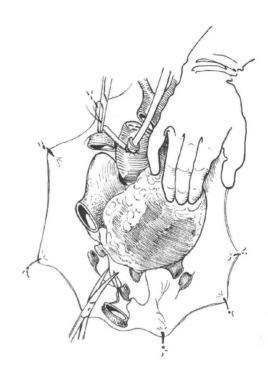

Figure 16. Isolated heart excision – division of pulmonary veins.

6.1.2. En bloc *heart–lung and double lung removal* [13]

The lungs can be procured *en bloc* with the heart for heart–lung transplantation or separated on the backtable. Venting of the left heart is different to that in the isolated heart removal: it is accomplished by amputation of the left atrial appendage (Fig. 17).

Heart–lung extraction: After cardioplegia and pneumoplegia have been performed, the aorta, superior vena cava and the inferior vena cava are divided as for simple heart excision. The ascending aorta is retracted. After the orotracheal tube has been withdrawn the trachea is transected with an automatic stapling device (Fig. 18). This allows collapse of the lung and subsequently facilitates surface cooling of the organs as well as surgery in the recipient. The tracheal mobilization is restricted to the upper mediastinal trachea at a level which lies five or six rings above the carina and usually at the level of the inominate artery [14]. The pericardium is divided transversely above and below. The upper transverse line of division is on a line parallel with the superior vena cava at the level of the azygos vein. The inferior line of adivision lies just at its point of attachment to the diaphragm on each side.

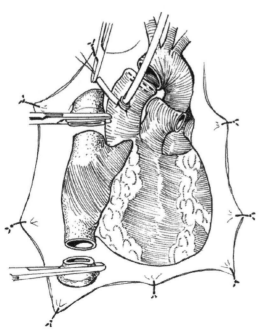

Figure 15. Isolated heart excision – division of outflow.

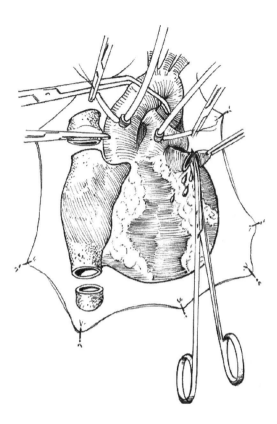

Figure 17. *En bloc* heart–lung excision – venting of left heart is accomplished by amputation of the left arterial appendage.

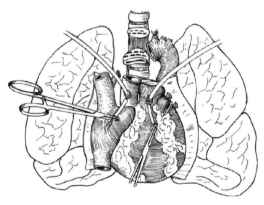

Figure 18. *En bloc* heart–lung excision – division of trachea.

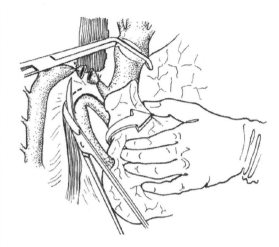

Figure 19. *En bloc* heart–lung excision (right side) retropericardial dissection.

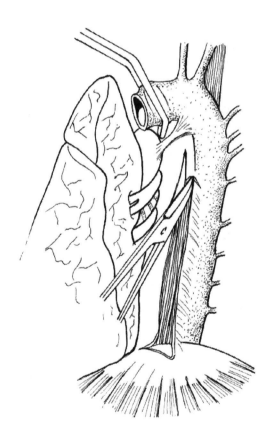

Figure 20. *En bloc* heart–lung excision (left side) division of left triangular ligament.

Mobilization of the heart–lung block consists of retropericardial dissection from the carina to the diaphragm (Fig. 19). With division of the inferior pulmonary ligament (Fig. 20) the entire heart–lung block can be excised away from the descending aorta and the oesophagus by applying gentle traction on the divided trachea from above and the diaphragmatic pericardium from below. This dissection has to be performed with electrical cauterization to avoid haemorrhagic problems in the recipient.

After procurement of the heart–lung block each organ can be separated on the back-table.

6.2. Abdominal organs

6.2.1. *Liver retrieval*

The hepatic artery is identified within the gastrohepatic ligament down to the lymph node at the superior margin of the pancreatic head. The main trunk is followed to the left to the origin of the coeliac axis. For isolated liver retrieval the coeliac axis is kept with an aortic patch (Fig. 21). In donors weighing more than 30 kg, procurement of the aortic patch is not always necessary; however, this technique can be used in small children or in retransplants where the aortic patch is used as an arterial conduit [12]. The gastro-

duodenal artery and the right gastric branch of the hepatic artery are divided close to their origin to maintain the vascularization of the head of the pancreas through the superior pancreaticoduodenal arcade if the whole pancreas is simultaneously harvested. The splenic artery is identified at the origin during the dissection of the hepatic artery and divided.

The liver is mobilized by incision of its ligamentous attachments to the diaphragm (Fig. 22). Initially, the liver is retracted to the patient's left and the right triangular ligament is divided. The liver is then retracted to the right and the left ligament is totally divided. Finally the ligamentum teres is divided. If reduced-sized liver transplantation is planned the entire ligamentum teres is preserved because it can be used to partially cover the cut surface of the liver. These ligaments can be left long for subsequent attachment to the diaphgram of the recipient. The superior aspect of the liver is dissected free by incising the anterior diaphragm back to the suprahepatic inferior vena cava. A rim of diaphragm is left attached to the suprahepatic vena cava. While dissecting the inferior vena cava, it is convenient to insert a finger in the suprahepatic vena cava lumen (Fig. 23). There are usually three phrenic veins and each is individually identified. ligated and divided. Particular care is needed to ensure ligation of the posterior phrenic vein; inattention to this point could result in bleeding in an inaccessible location after the transplantation is completed.

The inferior vena cava is divided proximal to the entrance of the renal veins. The liver is retracted upward and the right adrenal vein is identified, ligated and

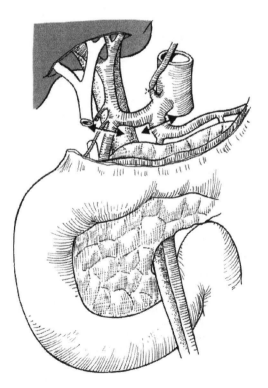

Figure 21. Isolated hepatic procurement: coeliac axis is kept with an aortic patch.

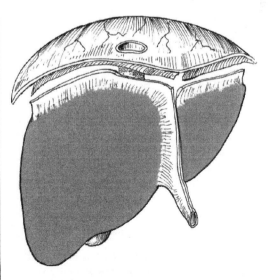

Figure 22. Division of triangular ligaments.

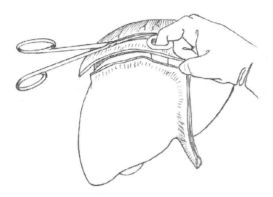

Figure 23. Section of the suprahepatic inferior vena cava. A rim of diaphragm is left attached with the suprahepatic vena cava.

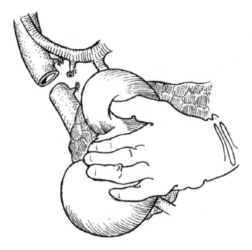

Figure 25. Pancreas procurement–division of portal vein.

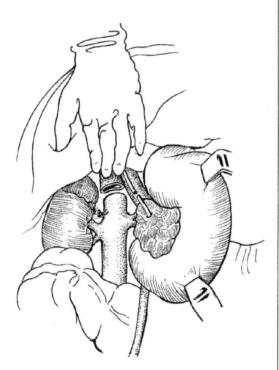

Figure 24. Section of the sub-hepatic inferior vena cava.

divided. If the right adrenal vein cannot be easily isolated at this time, it can be divided later as the liver is removed (Fig. 24).

6.2.2. *Pancreas retrieval*
A Kocher manoeuvre is performed to mobilize the duodenum and the head of the pancreas. The supraduodenal portal vein is divided just below to the

coronary vein (Fig. 25). If the portal vein is too short, subsequent lengthening using a tubular venous graft is possible. The remnant of tissue is trimmed along the superior border of the pancreas and common hepatic artery and near the stumps of the superior mesenteric artery and splenic artery. The segment of duodenum corresponding to the head of the pancreas is transected using a GIA automatic stapling device (Fig. 26). In order to reduce the risks of fungal contamination, antifungic solutions can be injected in the duodenal segments via the gastric catheter. If simultaneous procurement of liver and total pancreas is being performed three situations may occur (Fig. 27A,B,C).

If vascularization of the liver is normal, the arterial supply of the pancreatic graft is represented by the coeliac axis via the splenic artery and superior mesenteric artery on the same aortic patch. The liver is taken with the common hepatic artery (Fig. 27A).

If a left hepatic artery is present, the coeliac axis is left in continuity with the common hepatic artery and the left gastric artery. The pancreatic graft will be vascularized by the superior mesenteric artery and splenic artery. Both vessels can be elongated using the iliac bifurcation as a Y plasty (Fig. 27B).

When an aberrant right hepatic artery originating from the origin of the superior mesenteric artery is present, the initial portion of the superior mesenteric artery is reserved for the hepatic team. The distal portion of the superior mesenteric artery can be revascularized retrogradely by an arterial graft. If vascularization of the total graft is compromised it may be preferable to harvest a segmental graft (Fig. 27C).

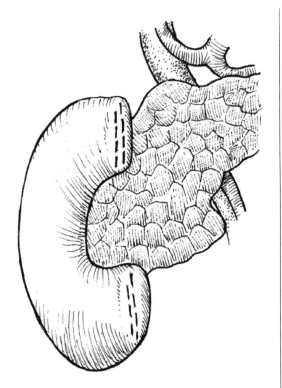

Figure 26. Stapling of the duodenal segment.

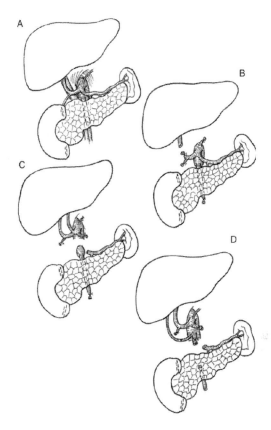

Figure 27. Combined liver and pancreatic procurement. (A) Normal distribution. Pancreas is procured with a patch containing coeliac axis and superior mesenteric artery. (B) Left hepatic artery. (C) Aberrant right hepatic artery.

Segmental pancreas with liver procurement: The pancreatic neck is freed from the portal vein by blunt dissection. A clamp is placed on the head of the gland as close as possible to the duodenum. The pancreas is divided distal to the clamp with a knife. The coeliac axis is abandoned to the liver team (Fig. 28). The portal vein is divided as high as possible and the graft is removed. The splenic artery is prolonged by an external iliac graft; if the portal vein is too short, it also can be lengthened with a patch of iliac vein. [6].

6.2.3. *Isolation of the intestinal component for combined hepatic–intestinal transplantation [15]*

The vessels within the mesentery of the terminal ileum and right colon are divided, sparing the ileal branches of the ileocolic artery. Division of the ileum at the ileocecal valve is deferred as long as possible to allow spontaneous passage of intestinal contents into the colon throughout the dissection. The proximal jejunum is transected close to the ligament of Treitz and the highest jejunal arcades are dissected, taking care not to damage the blood supply to the proximal end of the intestinal graft. Marking this end with a long suture facilitates bowel orientation at the time of exposure. The colon is eliminated by dividing the transverse meso-

colon near its root and rotating the right and transverse colons to the left and out of the field. The portal and superior mesenteric veins are exposed by transecting the pylorus and neck of the pancreas (Fig. 29). Stripping the pancreas and duodenum from the specimen requires ligation of numerous small venous tributaries entering the lateral and posterior walls of the superior mesenteric vein and arteries emanating from the superior mesenteric artery. Further liberation of the skeletonized superior mesenteric vein from the uncinate process and duodenum is best done on the back-table. By using a substantial (> 1.5 cm) splenic vein stump, a branch point is left that can later be clamped separately and anastomosed to the recipient portal vein without interruption of the venous outflow from the intestinal allograft. Severance of the donor aorta from the double arterial stem of the graft is the crucial final step and can ruin the graft if improperly performed.

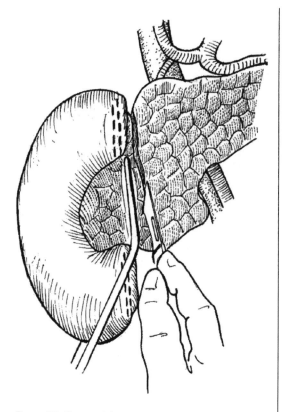

Figure 28. Segmental pancreas procurement.

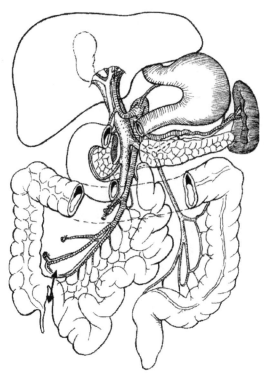

Figure 29. Hepatic-intestinal removal. General disposition.

When taking the arterial pedicle for the liver–intestinal graft, the blood supply to the kidneys that are left behind can be impaired. It is important to check the origin of the renal arteries, looking for them from inside the aorta as it is open to cut the Carrel patch containing the origins of the coeliac axis and superior mesenteric artery. The right renal artery is usually only 1 or 2 mm from the right margin of the Carrel patch. The remainder of the procurement is identical to the standard multiple organ procedures. The excised liver–small bowel graft is placed first in an ice basin and then in a plastic bag containing cold UW solution. No effort is made to wash out the intestine, which was stapled shut at its upper and lower ends at the appropriate stages of the dissection. On the back-table, the Carrel patch of the graft can be given length by anastomosing it to a donor aortic conduit. This technique of liver–small intestine procurement precludes whole-organ pancreas retrieval.

6.2.4. *Removal of the kidneys*

The cannulae in the inferior vena cava and aorta as well as the ureters marked with loops are gently re-

tracted anteriorly, keeping track of these four structures while dissecting the kidneys. Posterior attachments of the kidneys are cut, staying close to the posterior ligaments and muscles covering the vertebral bodies and continuing until the proximal aorta and inferior vena cava are reached (Fig. 30).

Once the posterior dissection is completed, the residual attachments between the gastrointestinal tract and the anterior surface of the specimen are divided. The kidneys are taken out *en bloc* and placed in an ice basin on a back-table. When separating the kidneys, it is most convenient to turn the specimen over. The posterior wall of the aorta is incised allowing a perfect view of renal arterial branches from inside the lumen. The left renal vein is transected close to the inferior vena cava (Fig. 31).

If desired, while still *in situ* and after the left renal vein has been transected and retracted laterally, the anterior aorta may be incised longitudinally and anteriorly, the vessel orifices inspected from within and the kidneys are removed separately rather than *en bloc*. All tissue between the vena cava and the hilum of the right kidney remains and all tissue between the adrenal and

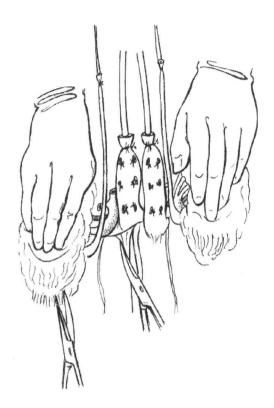

Figure 30. Kidney removal – section of posterior attachments.

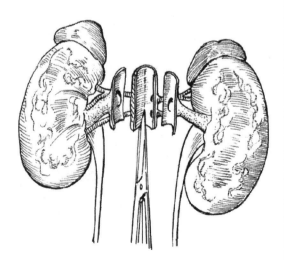

Figure 31. Kidney separation on the back-table. Longitudinal incision of aorta and vena cava.

spermatic/ovarian vein and the left hilum remains with the graft.

When kidneys are retrieved from cadaver donors without the procurement of other visceral organs, only 1 l of perfusate is needed in adults. Maley *et al.* [16] have described a useful procedure with simple instrument occlusion of the anterior visceral branches of the aorta. Two tunnels along both sides of the pedicle containing the coeliac axis and the SMA are created, the jaws of a large Debakey or Satinsky clamp are placed through the tunnels over the renal veins and under the duodenum and pancreas to occlude the two pedicles after perfusion has been started. This modification decreases the procurement time and improves *in situ* cooling of the kidneys by maximizing the amount of cold perfusate in the kidneys.

An important point is to vent the venous outflow as the flush begins. If the heart has been removed, the vena cava can be divided at the entrance to the heart, then the blood can also be shunted to the right chest and out of the way. In the other cases a cannula inserted in the inferior vena cava is used to eliminate the outflow of perfusate.

Excessive perirenal fat should be removed from the kidneys allowing them to be inspected to rule out areas of ischaemia or superficial tumours.

6.2.5. *Total abdominal evisceration procedure*

The total abdominal evisceration procedure was described by Nakazato *et al* [3]. All the abdominal organs are removed *en bloc* after flushing and placed in a chilled saline bath for *ex vivo* dissection. The differences with the standard technique of multi-organ procurement are the boundaries of the *en bloc* specimen: the peripheral diaphragm is cut laterally and posteriorly, to release it from the chest wall and from the midline, the thoracic oesophagus is transected just proximal to the gastro-oesophageal junction (the stomach will be removed on the back-table). Then in a clockwise manner, the surgeon cuts the small bowel to the desired transplant organ system (usually just distal to ligament of Treitz). Next, the jejunal–ileal mesentery is cut towards the ileal–cecal junction as close to the root of the mesentery as possible so that the surgeon can reach the ileal–cecal area in two to three cuts. This *in vivo* dissection is completed when the abdominal aorta and the abdominal IVC are transected just below the cannulae and when the cannulae are disconnected from the perfusion systems and Foley bag.

6.2.6. *Vascular allograft removal*

The segments of the iliac arteries and veins and, sometimes the thoracic arteries, are routinely removed and placed in a cold tissue culture solution for refrigeration. Such grafts can be life-saving in the event of unexpected technical problems in the recipient and for any given graft. Spleen and mesenteric lymph nodes are also removed for tissue typing and other immunological studies.

6.2.7. *Procurement of other tissues*
Other human tissues can be procured including bone, cornea and skin. These tissues are procured after the vascularized organs.

7. Back-table preparation of organs

7.1. Preparation of heart for transplantation (Fig. 32A, B)

The excised heart is immersed in cardioplegia solution at 4°C and immediately prepared for implantation in the recipient so that only final adjustment of the heart to the exact dimensions of the recipient vessels remains to be made. The cannula in the ascending aorta used for cardioplegia can be left in place within the lumen of the stapled aorta. The divided pulmonary trunks are prepared. The staple-ligated superior vena cava can be opened at a safe distance from the sinus node of the donor heart; the inferior vena cava orifice is left open.

The orifices of the individually divided pulmonary veins are connected with dissecting scissors to create a cuff of left atrial tissue for anastomosis to the recipient atria. The donor heart is ready for implantation.

7.2. Preparation of the lungs

7.2.1. *Double lung block*
After removal of the heart–lung block, the main pulmonary artery is divided midway between the pulmonary valve ring and the bifurcation in its intrapericardial segment to ensure an adequate cuff for both subsequent cardiac and pulmonary transplantation. The ascending aorta is then separated from its posterior attachment with the right pulmonary artery. At this time the heart is only attached by the left atrium. The left atrium is divided midway between the atrioventricular groove and the confluence of pulmonary veins, care must be taken to leave a cuff of left atrium away from the circumflex artery. The heart and the double lung block can then be conditioned.

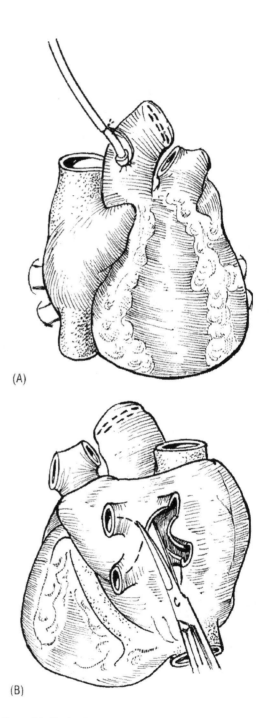

(A)

(B)

Figure 32. Back-table preparation of the heart. (A) Preparation of the pulmonary artery. (B) Preparat on of the left atrium.

7.2.2. *Single lung preparation (Fig. 33)*

When a double lung block has been harvested the two lungs can be simply separated on the back-table by dividing the posterior wall of the left atrium into right and left atrial cuffs. The main distal pulmonary artery is divided vertically and the left main bronchus is stapled and cut near the carina. Each lung can be used for a single lung transplantation.

7.3. Preparation of liver and pancreas allografts for transplantation

Arterial reconstructions of pancreatic (and liver) allografts have been described for combined whole pancreas and liver retrieval in case of replaced hepatic artery and/or if the donor has atherosclerosis or damage occurs to the vessel at the time of procurement.

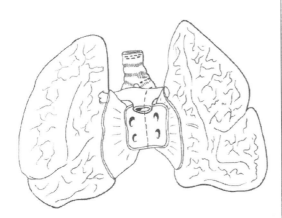

Figure 33. Single long preparation.

7.3.1. *Pancreas*

For the whole pancreas allograft, when no Carrel patch is left with each artery, the method used is a Y graft consisting of common iliac artery, internal iliac artery and external iliac artery anastomosed to the superior mesenteric artery and the splenic artery [17]. In general, because of better size match, the internal iliac artery is anastomosed end-to-end to the splenic artery and the external iliac artery is anastomosed end-to-end to the superior mesenteric artery (Fig. 34).

When a Carrel patch is attached to the superior mesenteric artery, Fernandez-Cruz *et al.* have reported the reconstruction of the arterial supply to the pancreas by end-to-end anastomosis between the proximal splenic artery and the distal end of the superior mesenteric artery [18]. The splenic artery can also be anastomosed to the superior mesenteric artery in an end-to-side fashion [19].

When the duct obstruction technique is chosen (segmental graft), a small blunt-tip catheter is inserted into the main pancreatic duct. Two forceps are placed at the extremities of the cut edge of the gland and a n° 2 silk suture is placed around them to prevent back-flow of the neoprene. Between 3 and 6 ml of neoprene are usually enough to fill the collecting system of the segmental pancreas. This synthetic material progressively solidifies when in contact with the pancreatic juice. When the catheter is removed the duct is ligated with a 4-0 prolene suture (Fig. 35).

After preparation of the gland, reperfusion is performed to check for leakage of vessels that could cause subsequent haemorrhage after revascularization.

Venous reconstructions of the pancreas allograft is sometimes required when the portal vein is too short (Fig. 36).

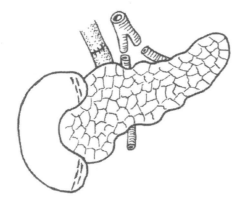 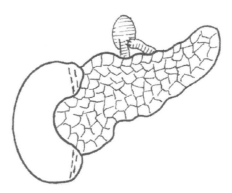

Figure 34. Reconstruction of pancreas vessels in case of combined pancreas removal. Use of iliac vessels – lengthening of portal vein.

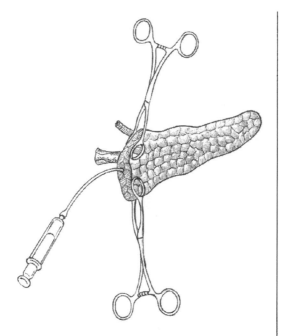

Figure 35. Introductal injection of neoprene.

7.3.2. *Liver*

Arterial reconstructions are rather similar: when both a right and left hepatic artery are present, arterial reconstruction of the liver allograft consists of direct end-to-end anastomosis between the replaced left hepatic artery and the donor gastroduodenal artery. A donor iliac artery bifurcation is then anastomosed to the donor common hepatic artery and replaced right hepatic artery [7] (Fig. 37).

When a right hepatic artery is present, three reconstruction models have been described. (1) After dissec-

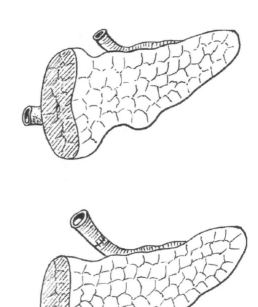

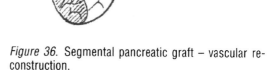

Figure 36. Segmental pancreatic graft – vascular reconstruction.

tion of the coeliac arterial trunk to the branches of the left gastric, splenic, and proximal common hepatic arteries, the proximal splenic artery is transected close to its origin, leaving a rim of proximal splenic artery which can be oversewn and closed or used to anastomose an anomalous right hepatic artery in an end-to-end fashion. (2) Arterial reconstruction of the hepatic allograft can be performed by direct end-to-end anasto-

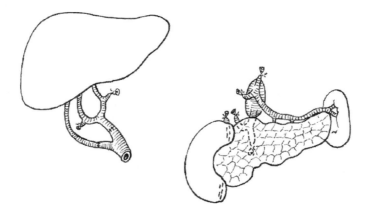

Figure 37. Liver. Arterial reconstruction in cases with both left and right aberrant arteries.

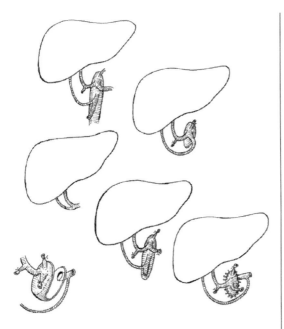

Figure 38. Liver arterial reconstruction in patients with right aberrant artery.

mosis between the right hepatic artery and the gastro-duodenal artery stump (Fig. 38). (3) Gordon *et al.* have accomplished the 'foldover technique': a patch of anterior aorta including the origins of the coeliac axis and superior mesenteric artery is removed. Folding of the aortic patch permits safe anastomosis of the coeliac axis to the mesenteric artery. The superior mesenteric artery distal to the right hepatic artery is used for anastomosis to the recipient artery [20].

7.4. Preparation of the kidneys

Preparation of the kidneys simply consists of removing most of the fat around the peripheral part of the kidney and in the hilum. Care must be taken to avoid extensive dissection of the vessels in the hilum as small arterial branches supplying the ureter may be damaged. This is especially true if an inferior polar artery is present. In case of polar arteries, the best situation is completed if an aortic patch is present. In the absence of an aortic patch, polar arteries have to be replanted in the main renal artery. Kidneys from very young donors can be prepared and grafted *en bloc* [21]. The lumbar vessels of the aorta and IVC are controlled with vascular sutures. The cephalad vena cava is closed at the level of the renal veins taking care to avoid cul-de-sac as well as narrowing of the renal veins. The distal VC

and aorta are kept as long as possible for suture to recipient vessels.

References

1. Margreiter R, Königsrainer A, Schmid Th, Takahashi N, Pernthaler H, Ofner D. Multiple organ procurement – a simple and safe procedure. Transplant Proc 1991; 23: 2307–8.
2. Starzl TE, Hakala TR, Shaw BW Jr, Hardesty RL, Rosenthal TJ, Griffith BP, Iwatsuki S, Bahnson HT. A flexible procedure for multiple cadaveric organ procurement. Surg Gynecol Obstet 1984; 158: 223–31.
3. Nakazato PZ, Concepcion W, Bry W, Limm W, Tokunaga Y, Itasaka H, Feduska N, Esquivel CO, Collins GM. Total abdominal evisceration: an *en bloc* technique for abdominal organ harvesting. Surgery 1992; 111: 37–47.
4. D'Alessandro AM, Stratta RJ, Southard JH, Kalayoglu M, Belzer FO. Agonal hepatic arterial vasospasm: demonstration, prevention, and possible clinical implications. Surg Gynecol Obstet 1989; 169: 324–8.
5. Fukuzawa K, Schwartz ME, Katz E, Mor E, Emre S, Acarli K, Miller CM. An alternative technique for *in situ* arterial flushing in elderly liver donors with atherosclerotic disease. Transplantation 1993; 55: 445.
6. Dubernard JM, Sutherland DER. International Handbook of Pancreas Transplantation. Kluwer Academic Publishers, Dordrecht 1989; pp. 71–130.
7. Shaffer D, Lewis WD, Jenkins RL, Monaco AP. Combined liver and whole pancreas procurement in donors with a replaced right hepatic artery. Surg Gyn Obstet 1992; 175: 204–7.
8. Ascher NL, Bolman RM, Sutherland DER. Multiple organ donation from a cadaver. In: Simmons RL, Linch ME, Ascher NL, Najarian JS (eds). Manual of Vascular Access, Organ Donation and Transplantation. Springer-Verlag, New York, 1984; p. 119.
9. Nghiem DD, Cottington EM. Pancreatic flush injury in combined pancreas–liver recovery. Transplant Int 1992; 5: 19–22.
10. Bittard H, Chiche L, Mouzarkel M, Douguet D, Benoit G. Study of kidney and liver viability in the rat after exclusive aortic perfusion using intracellular ATP measurement. Urol Res 1992; 20: 415.
11. Boillot O, Benchetrit S, Dawahra M, Porcheron J, Martin X. Early graft function in liver transplantation: comparison of two techniques of graft procurement. Transplant Proc 1993; 25: 2642.
12. Nghiem DD. Simultaneous recovery of whole pancreas without arterial reconstruction in the multiple organ liver donor. Transplant Proc 1990; 22: 614–15.
13. Raju S, Heath BJ, Warren ET, Hardy JD. Single- and double-lung transplantation: problems and possible solutions. Ann Surg 1990; 211: 681.
14. Cooper JD. The evolution of techniques and indications for lung transplantation. Ann Surg 1990; 212: 249.
15. Casavilla A, Selby R, Abu-Elmagd K, Tzakis A, Todo S, Reyes J, Fung J, Starzl TE. Logistics and technique for combined hepatic-intestinal retrieval. Ann Surg 1992; 216: 605–9.
16. Maley WR, Melville Williams GM, Colombani P, Perler BA, Burdick JF. Simple instrument occlusion of the anterior visceral branches of the aorta during *en bloc* renal allograft procurement. Surg Gynecol Obstet 1988; 167: 442–4.
17. Faure JL, Takvorian Ph, Champetier P, Neidecker J, Recio H, Villalonga J, Sanseverino R, Camozzi L. Combined liver and pancreas harvesting from cadaveric donors: techniques according to blood supply. Diabetes 1988; 38 (suppl. 1): 232–3.
18. Fernandez-Cruz L, Astudillo E, Sanfey H, Llovera JM, Saenz A, Lopez-Boado MA, Bagur C. Combined whole pancreas and liver retrieval: a new technique for arterial reconstruction of the pancreas graft. Br J Surg 1992; 79: 239–40.

19. Marsh CL, Perkins JD, Hayes DH, Munn SR, Sterioff S. Combined hepatic and pancreaticoduodenal procurement for transplantation. Diabetes 1988; 38 (Suppl. 1): 231.

20. Gordon RD, Shaw BW, Iwatzuki S, Todo S, Starzl TE. A simplified technique for revascularization of homograft of the liver. Surg, Gynecol Obstet 1985; 160: 475–6.

21. Ngheim DD. *En bloc* transplantation of kidneys from donors weighing less than 15 kg into adult recipients. J Urol 1991; 145: 14.

11 | The contribution of the non-heart-beating donor to the solution of the shortage of kidneys

G. Kootstra, M.H. Booster, R.M.H. Wijnen, H. Bonke and E. Heineman

1. Introduction

With the improvements in quality of life and patient survival following kidney transplantation, the discrepancy between demand and supply of organs is increasing. The Eurotransplant figures from the annual report 1992 indicate four times as many patients on the waiting list as there are kidneys transplanted [1]. It is therefore necessary to look for sources of kidneys other than living related and heart-beating (HB) cadaver donors. Kidneys from living related donors offer a major contribution to successful transplantation, with excellent graft survival, but their number is restricted. Procurement of kidneys from heart-beating cadavers is inhibited by a high incidence of refusal by relatives [2]. The criteria for post mortem organ donation are gradually being liberalized, an example of which is the introduction of the notion 'borderline or marginal donor' [3].

The non-heart-beating (NHB) patient represents a category of kidney donor that has only occasionally been used. Such donors have sustained cardiac arrest inside or outside the hospital, and resuscitation has been unsuccessful. These donors are not used for multi-organ procurement, although there are encouraging prospects for liver donation. It is possible that with some more study and experience this donor source will prove useful since both the liver and the kidney have excellent tolerance for warm ischaemia.

This chapter discusses the role of the non-heart-beating donor as a source of transplantable cadaver kidneys.

2. Definition

A NHB donor (also called asystolic donor) is one who has sustained cardiac arrest and in whom resuscitation has been unsuccessful. A distinction can be made between controlled and uncontrolled NHB donors: the former have sufferd cardiac arrest, while monitored and are awaiting nephrectomy in the Intensive Care Unit. Resuscitation is immediately started under ideal circumstances. The uncontrolled NHB donor usually sustains cardiac arrest outside the hospital. Resuscitation has to take place under less ideal circumstances and there may well be an interval between the time of cardiac arrest and start of resuscitation. Donor criteria are listed in Table 1.

Table 1. Donor criteria.

Total duration of circulatory arrest < 30 min, excluding time of effective resuscitation
Effective resuscitation for ≤ 2 h
Age ≤ 60 years
No history of kidney disease, severe hypertension, diabetes mellitus type 1 or malignancies other than primary (non-metastasizing) CNS tumours
No systemic signs of infection or evidence of sepsis
No signs of i.v. drug abuse

G.M. Collins, J.M. Dubernard, W. Land and G.G. Persijn (eds), Procurement, Preservation and Allocation of Vascularized Organs 95–99
© 1997 Kluwer Academic Publishers.

3. Procurement procedure

The successful procurement of kidneys from NHB donors is based on two principles. First, cardiac massage and ventilation of the lungs with oxygen are continued after the pronouncement of cardiac death, in order to provide the organs with oxygenated blood as much as possible. Second, a double balloon triple lumen (DBTL) catheter is placed for *in situ* preservation of the kidneys to limit the warm ischaemic interval.

In The Netherlands, consent from relatives is required before any procedure related to donor nephrectomy, including introduction of a cooling catheter, can be started. We therefore continue to perform external cardiac massage and ventilation until this permission has been received. The catheter is then introduced which, when in proper position, provides *in situ* cooling for the kidneys up to 12–15°C. The 'Maastricht DBTL catheter' is produced by the Porges company (Palaiseau, France) and is designed to block the aorta at its bifurcation and at the level of the diaphragm by means of two balloons. Selective perfusion of the part of the aorta where the renal arteries take their origin is hereby obtained (Fig. 1). The size of the catheter is 16 French, its total length is 90 cm and the distance between the two balloons is 22 cm. Each balloon can contain 30 ml of fluid. The diameter of a fully inflated balloon is 40 mm. The catheter is made out of polyurethane which is radio-opaque, and allows

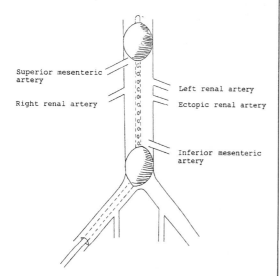

Superior mesenteric artery

Right renal artery

Left renal artery

Ectopic renal artery

Inferior mesenteric artery

Figure 1. Schematic representation of the double balloon triple lumen catheter when inserted into the abdominal aorta.

the position of the two balloons to be checked with a simple X-ray. We prefer to fill the balloons with radio-opaque contrast fluid.

3.1. Insertion of the catheter

For a right-handed surgeon it is preferable to insert the DBTL catheter in the right groin. The insertion area is shaved and disinfected and sterile drapes are applied. A longitudinal incision over the femoral vessels is made between approximately 5 cm above to 10 cm below the inguinal ligament. This incision provides rapid access to and good exposure of the femoral vessels. The femoral artery is identified and blood samples for blood group typing, blood oxygen supply evaluation and biochemical (urea, creatinine, cholesterol) and virological (HbSAg, HIV, CMV) diagnostic tests are obtained. After arteriotomy, the DBTL catheter is introduced as far as possible into the common iliac artery and aorta. The caudal balloon is inflated with 10 ml sterile radio-opaque contrast fluid. To hook the balloon onto the bifurcation of the aorta, the catheter is retracted as far as possible, and an additional 5 ml of radio-opaque contrast fluid is administered to obtain maximal expansion of the balloon. The cranial balloon is then inflated with 15 ml radio-opaque contrast fluid. The catheter is connected to the cold (4°C) preservation solution and *in situ* perfusion of the kidney is started. Care should be taken to ensure that all air is removed from the perfusion system. Immediately after the start of perfusion venotomy of the femoral vein is performed to facilitate venous outflow. A 18 French urinary catheter connected to a sterile urine bag is used to collect the outflowing blood and preservation fluid. Abdominal X-ray is performed to check the position of the balloons. The upper balloon is situated in the thoracic aorta.

Meanwhile the operating staff are notified and an operating room is prepared. In our protocol [4] *in situ* preservation times (the time interval between commencement of *in situ* perfusion and subsequent nephrectomy) of up to 2 h are tolerated.

4. Retrospective analysis

Over a period of 10 years (1982–1991), in our procurement area (with a population of 0.74 million inhabitants) nephrectomy was performed in 53 NHB donors, resulting in 74 transplanted kidneys, of which 33 were transplanted within The Netherlands. In a retrospective analysis we studied the short and long term results of the recipients of these 33 kidneys, compared with a matched control group of HB donor kidney recipients. For each NHB donor kidney recipient, two HB donor kidney recipients were selected. Both groups were matched for the time period in which the transplantation took place; first, second, or third transplantation; the highest and latest level of panel reactive antibodies (PRA); immunosuppressive therapy; donor and recipient age; and the preservation solution used. All kidneys were preserved by simple cold storage. In order to ascertain the adequacy of randomization for the donor population and to check for any relevant differences in patient characteristics between the two recipient populations, statistical analysis of donor and recipient demographics was conducted. Differences were evaluated by using the Mann–Whitney U-test for continuous variables and the χ^2 test with Yeats's correction for discrete variables. A p value < 0.05 was considered significant. Graft and patient survival in both groups were analysed using the Kaplan–Meier method. Significance of differences in survival rate were determined with the log-rank method.

4.1. Results

Table 2 shows the donor and recipient demographic characteristics. There was a statistically significant difference between the two groups of donors with respect

Table 2. Donor and recipient demographic characteristics.

	NHB (*n* = 33)	HB (*n* = 66)	*p*
Donor characteristics			
Median age (years)	45	45	NS
Sex			
Male	25 (76%)	39 (60%)	NS
Female	8 (24%)	27 (40%)	NS
Diagnosis			
Trauma capitis	15 (46%)	27 (41%)	NS
CVA	6 (18%)	35 (53%)	< 0.01
Anoxia	11 (33%)	1 (1%)	< 0.01
Other	1 (3%)	3 (5%)	NS
Median first warm ischaemia time (min)	34	0	< 0.01
Preservation solution			
EC	25 (76%)	54 (82%)	NS
HTK	8 (24%)	6 (9%)	NS
UW	0 (0%)	6 (9%)	NS
Recipient characteristics			
Median age (years)	48	50	NS
Sex			
Male	23 (70%)	45 (68%)	NS
Female	10 (30%)	21 (32%)	NS
PRA (highest, %)			
0–5	22 (67%)	41 (62%)	NS
5–85	7 (21%)	18 (27%)	NS
85–100	4 (12%)	7 (11%)	NS
PRA latest (%)			
0–5	26 (79%)	52 (79%)	NS
5–85	6 (18%)	9 (14%)	NS
85–100	1 (3%)	5 (7%)	NS
Prior transplants			
0	29 (88%)	53 (80%)	NS
> 1	4 (12%)	13 (20%)	NS
Median cold ischaemia time (h)	30	27	NS
Median second warm ischaemia time (min)	34	35	NS
Immunosuppression			
CyA/steroids	21 (64%)	47 (71%)	NS
AZA/steroids	10 (30%)	15 (23%)	NS
CyA/AZA/steroids	2 (6%)	4 (6%)	NS

to cause of death and median length of the first warm ischaemia time. The high incidence of anoxia in the NHB donor group is due to the large uncontrolled NHB donor population which usually consists of patients admitted to the emergency room suffering from electromechanical dissociation and eventual cardiac arrest due to myocardial infarction. No differences in demographic variables among recipients were seen.

Table 3 shows the post-transplant outcome of the 33 kidneys obtained from NHB donors and the matched group of 66 HB donor kidneys. In the NHB donor kidney group immediate life-sustaining function was relatively rare, and a higher proportion of kidneys showed delayed function or never functioned.

There were, however, no statistically significant differences between the two groups with respect to overall graft and patient survival (Figs 2, 3).

4.2. Discussion

Our study revealed no statistical difference in long term function of kidneys obtained from NHB donors and a matched group of HB donors. However, the higher proportion of delayed function in the period

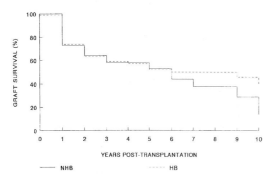

Figure 2. Overall graft survival (%) in the NHB and HB donor kidney groups. Numbers at risk at the time of transplantation; NHB, *n* = 33; HB, *n* = 66.

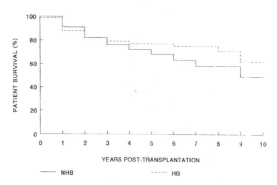

Figure 3. Overall patient survival (%) in the NHB and HB donor kidney groups. Numbers at risk at the time of transplantation; NHB, *n* = 33; HB, *n* = 66.

immediately following the transplantation of kidneys from NHB donors, and the unacceptably high level of never functioning kidneys in the NHB donor group represent major drawbacks to the use of such kidneys. Improved preservation using continuous perfusion preservation (machine preservation) might be a solution. Continuous perfusion has the advantage of allowing delivery of oxygen and nutrients and the removing of waste products [5]. Furthermore, machine preservation might enable tests to be performed which facilitate identification of non-viable kidneys before they are transplanted. Initial results are promising. Kozaki *et al.* [6] compared cold storage with machine perfusion by preserving each of the two kidneys from five NHB donors by a different method. In all cases kidneys preserved on the machine had better post-transplant function.

Implementation of a NHB donor programme has increased our procurement effectiveness by 20% [7]. The major restriction so far has been the fact that it is illegal to perform any medical procedure on a cadaver without consent of the relatives. Therefore, if relatives cannot be located in time the procedure has to be cancelled. In the near future the Dutch law will be altered

Table 3. Post-transplant function of 33 kidneys from non-heart-beating donors versus a matched population of 66 kidneys from heart-beating donors.

	Non-heart-beating donor kidneys (*n* = 33)	Heart-beating donor kidneys (*n* = 66)
Immediate function (%)	21 (*n* = 7)	55 (*n* = 37)*
Delayed function (%)	61 (*n* = 20)	40 (*n* = 26)**
Never function (%)	18 (*n* = 6)	5 (*n* = 3)**

Two-sample χ^2 test with Yeats's correction.)
* $p < 0.01$; ** $p < 0.05$

so that it will be permissible to introduce a DBTL catheter into the femoral artery of any NHB donor to start cooling of the organs as soon as possible. Actual procurement of the organs will only take place if permission of the relatives is obtained. In case of an unnatural death, such as a traffic accident, additional permission of the legal authorities is necessary.

The combination of this juridical breakthrough and developments in organ preservation will make the NHB donor an important source of organs in the next decade, when the need for transplant organs will become more urgent than ever before.

References

1. Eurotransplant Annual Report 1992. Cohen B and Persijn G, ed. Eurotransplant foundation Leiden 1992; p. 31.
2. Buckley PE. The delicate question of the donor family. Transplant Proc 1989; 21: 1411.
3. Alexander JW, Vaughn WK, Carey MA. The use of marginal donors for organ transplantation: the older and younger donors. Transplant Proc 1991; 23: 905–9.
4. Booster MH, Wijnen RMH, Vroemen JPAM, van Hooff JP, Kootstra G. *In situ* preservation of kidneys from non-heart-beating donors: proposal for a standardized protocol. Transplantation 1993; 56: 513–17.
5. Belzer FO, Ashby BS, Dumphy JE. 24- and 72-hour preservation of canine kidneys. Lancet 1967; 2: 536.
6. Kozaki M, Matsuno N, Tamaki T, *et al.* Procurement of kidney grafts from non-heart-beating donors. Transplant Proc 1991; 23: 2575–8.
7. Kootstra G, Wijnen RMH, van Hooff JP, van der Linden CJ. Twenty percent more kidneys through a non-heart-beating donor program. Transplant Proc 1991; 23: 910–11.

Section II
Organ Preservation

12 | Biochemistry and cell physiology of organ preservation

JAMES H. SOUTHARD

1. Introduction

The enormous success of organ transplantation is due in part to the development of methods to preserve organs from the time they are donated until they are transplanted. Preservation has the goal of maintaining the viability of organs *ex vivo* for a period of time that will allow maximal utilization of all cadaveric organs. Over the past 25 years of organ transplantation it has become clear that most organs can be transported to an appropriate recipient within about 24 h after procurement. To give a margin of safety and to maximize utilization of all organs, ideal preservation times would be at least two to three times this clinical minimum (48–72 h).

In the past, methods of organ preservation were studied mostly on the basis of trial and error experimentation. The experiments were designed on the basis of what was then known about how ischaemia and hypothermia affected metabolism and what agents might theoretically improve preservation. These methods did result in the development of successful preservation solutions and methods, but improved preservation requires a more detailed understanding of the biochemical mechanisms of injury to the organs. With this knowledge, appropriate therapeutic approaches can be systematically applied to improve preservation quality and duration.

2. Factors that affect organ preservation

Once removed from the body, an organ begins to die; slowing down the biochemical processes that lead to cell death is the goal of organ preservation. However, the rate of cell death and the optimization of preservation of organs is complicated by the myriad factors – donor, preservation and recipient – that can affect successful organ preservation (Table 1).

The ideal is to obtain an organ in perfect condition from the donor; this can be done in laboratory studies, but is less likely in the clinical situation. Most donors are brain dead, often have reduced heart functions, and have been maintained haemodynamically with ionotropes and fluid administration. Despite continuous perfusion of the donor organs, the trauma of

Table 1. Factors that affect successful organ preservation.

Donor factors	Cause of death
	Length of time in hospital
	Adequacy of nutritional support
	Haemodynamic stability
	Drugs used to sustain donor
Preservation factors	Method of preservation
	Cold storage
	Continuous perfusion
	Composition of preservation solution
	Time of preservation
Recipient factors	Age
	Health at time of transplant
	Reperfusion injury
	Pharmacological agents used post-transplant

G.M. Collins, J.M. Dubernard, W. Land and G.G. Persijn (eds). Procurement, Preservation and Allocation of Vascularized Organs 103–113
© 1997 Kluwer Academic Publishers.

brain death causes metabolic imbalances as a result of hypotension and altered hormonal control of metabolism; these could affect the tolerance of the organ to cold preservation. Furthermore, if the donor is haemodynamically unstable the organs may be exposed to various periods of hypoxia resulting from inadequate perfusion. Drugs used to stabilize these patients can affect the tolerance of the organ to preservation.

Some studies have suggested a correlation between length of time the potential donor is in the terminal phase and the success of subsequent liver transplantation

Table 2. Composition of commonly used cold storage solutions.

Solution		Components	Concentration
UW[1]	Na 25 mM; K 125 mM pH 7.4 320 mOsm/l	Lactobionate KH_2PO_4 $MgSO_4$ Raffinose Glutathione Adenosine Allopurinol Starch (HES)	100 mM 25 mM 5 mM 30 mM 3 mM 5 mM 1 mM 50 g/l
Collins'[2]	Na 10 mM; K 115 mM pH 7.0 320 mOsm/l	KH_2PO_4 K_2HPO_4 KCl $NaHCO_3$ Glucose $MgSO_4$	15 mM 42.5 mM 15 mM 10 mM 139 mM 30 mM
Hypertonic citrate (HOC)[3]	Na 80 mM; K 80 mM pH 7.1 400 mOsm/l	NaCitrate KCitrate $MgSO_4$ Mannitol	80 mM 80 mM 70 mM 150 mM
Phosphate buffered sucrose (PBS)[4]	Na 60 mM; K 0 mM pH 7.4 300 mOsm/l	$NaHPO_4$ Na_2HPO_4 Sucrose	10 mM 25 mM 140 mM
Histidine-tryptophan-ketoglutarate (HTK)[5]	Na 15 mM; K 9 mM pH 7.0 300 mOsm/l	Ketoglutarate Tryptophan $MgCl_2$ KCl NaCl Histidine Mannitol	1 mM 2 mM 4 mM 9 mM 15 mM 198 mM 38 mM

[1] UW solution was developed for preservation of the pancreas, kidney, and liver in 1987 [10, 11, 13]. HES is hydroxyethyl starch (pentafraction) with an average mol. wt of 250 kDa.

[2] Collins' solution was developed for cold storage of the kidney in 1969 [5] and was later modified (EuroCollins' solutions) by removal of magnesium, which precipitated as a phosphate salt in the original Collins' solution. This solution was effective for 30 h storage of the kidney, but only about 4–9 h storage of other organs. This solution is used by some centres for the kidney.

[3] Hypertonic citrate developed by Ross *et al.* in 1973 [40] was found to equal Collins' solutions for kidney preservation, but was not particularly good for other organs. Other versions of this solution have been developed (isoosmotic versions) that work as well as the hypertonic versions. This solution is used for kidney preservation in the UK and Australia.

[4] PBS was originally described and studied by Andrews and Coffey [41] and shown to effectively preserve the morphology of ischaemically stored kidneys. Lam *et al.* [42] used this solution for effective experimental and clinical Kidney preservation. It has not been particularly effective for preservation of other organs.

[5] HTK was originally designed as a cardioplegic solution and used clinically. Its use in liver and kidney preservation has resulted in some degree of success, but direct comparisons with UW solution suggest that HTK is not as good [43].

[1,2]. This has led to the concept that nutritional (glycogen) depletion sensitizes the liver to preservation injury [3,4]. In general, donor factors that may affect outcome of transplantation become more important if the organs are exposed to long periods of preservation. Thus, the combination of preservation time and donor factors must be considered in evaluating clinical outcome.

Preservation factors include methods of preservation, the most common of which is simple cold storage (cold static storage, cold ischaemic storage). The organ is flushed out with a cold storage solution, placed in a sterile container containing additional cold storage fluid, and refrigerated at 0–4°C [5]. This method is used for all organs. Another method, used successfully for clinical kidney preservation, is continuous machine perfusion [6,7], which has also been used for successful liver [8] and heart [9] preservation in the laboratory. Continuous perfusion might ultimately be a superior method to preserve organs. Because some consider this method more cumbersome than cold static storage, however, only a few transplant centres use this method for the kidney.

The composition of the preservation solution appears critically important to obtain successful preservation for times necessary for optimal use of most organs. Simple solutions such as Ringer's lactate, saline or whole blood are suitable for short periods (generally 4 h or less). Longer periods of preservation, however, require specifically designed preservatives. For the kidney, successful cold storage has been obtained with several types of solutions (Table 2). Only the University of Wisconsin (UW) solution has been shown to be effective for long-term liver [10], kidney [11], heart [12] and pancreas [13] preservation, and it is used world-wide for clinical preservation of these organs. For continuous perfusion of kidneys a gluconate-based solution [14], also developed at the University of Wisconsin, has been shown to be successful in the laboratory for up to 7 days. It is used clinically [15].

Recipient factors also affect the success of organ transplantation, although these have not been well studied. Liver and heart transplant recipients can be very ill immediately prior to transplantation because of failure of their own organs. Outcome can be influenced by a combination of quality of the organ and general health of the recipient. Kidney and pancreas recipients' health can be relatively well maintained by dialysis or insulin. One-year graft survival for most organs is currently around 90%. The other 10% are usually lost due to immunological rejection, although there is some poor organ function resulting from factors such as inadequate preservation and ischaemic/reperfusion injury (Table 3). (In clinical consideration of the adequacy of preservation, it is preferable to consider 1-month graft survival, for preservation injury that leads to graft failure should be discernible within this period of time.) For the liver and kidney, a longer duration of preservation carries a greater chance of delayed graft function (kidney and liver) or primary non-function (liver). The exact relationship between these occurrences and preservation quality is not fully known since outcomes in kidney and liver transplantation vary considerably between centres. For the heart, lung and intestine, preservation times are kept short; maximal successful time is thought to be about

Table 3. Current problems in organ preservation.	
Organ	Problems
Kidney (Cold storage max 72 h)	Delayed graft function (10–50%)
	Delayed graft function more likely with longer preservation times (optimal ~ 24–30 h)
	Poor preservation of kidneys from non-heart beating donors (warm ischaemia > 30 min)
	Preservation injury may lead to greater long term graft loss (5–10 years)
Liver (Cold storage max 24–30 h)	Primary and initial poor function (5–15%)
	Greater injury with longer storage
	Bile duct strictures
	Preservation injury may lead to more rejection episodes and greater long-term graft loss (5–10 years)
Heart, lung, intestine (Cold storage ~ 8 h)	Inadequate preservation time for optimal utilization
Pancreas (Cold storage ~ 24–30 h)	Preservation basically adequate

8 h for these organs preserved in UW solution. It would seem then that some problems in organ transplantation can be mitigated by improved organ preservation.

3. Current understanding of preservation

Understanding why the current methods of preservation are successful may help us to understand some of the mechanisms underlying preservation injury and, therefore, their avoidance. Three factors important in organ preservation are hypothermia, the physical environment, and the biochemical environment (Table 4).

Hypothermia is a critical factor in preserving organs. Lowering the temperature suppresses injury caused by ischaemia in most organs. Collins *et al.* [5] used this knowledge successfully to preserve dog kidneys for 30 h. Under conditions of warm ischaemia most organs lose viability within about 1–2 h (except the brain and heart, which lose viability in 10–30 min). Lowering the temperature of the organ to 0–4°C extends tolerance to ischaemia. The kidney can be preserved for about 12 h when flushed out with cold blood [16]. Cooling the organ itself slows metabolism and suppresses the rate of degradation of cellular components necessary for viability. Exactly which cellular reactions are slowed down and allow extended viability of the organ is not known.

The physical environment important in organ cold storage is that created by the components of the flushing and storage solutions. In particular, these solutions are designed to suppress cell swelling, often have high concentrations of K, sometimes a colloid, and always a hydrogen ion buffer.

Suppression of cell swelling appears to be one of the most important roles of cold-storage solutions. Under conditions of cold ischaemia metabolic (energy-requiring) reactions, including the energy-driven

Table 4. Factors important in organ preservation by cold storage.

Hypothermia (0–4°C)	Cooling by vascular flushout with cold solution
	Organ stored at 0–4°C suspended in cold solution
	Metabolism is slowed by about half for each 10°C decrease in temperature (at 0°C, metabolism slowed to one-eighth that at 37°C)
Physical environment	Created by agents in the flushing solution
	Exchange with the normal vascular and interstitial fluids
	Agents used to affect:
	Osmotic pressure (suppress cell swelling)
	Saccharides (mannitol, glucose, sucrose, raffinose)
	Anions (lactobionate, gluconate, phosphate, citrate, sulphate)
	Electrolytes (sodium, potassium, histidine)
	Oncotic pressure (suppress cell swelling)
	Hydroxyethyl starch
	Dextrans
	Polyethylene glycols
	Hydrogen ion buffers
	Phosphate
	Histidine
	Electrolytes (maintain structural integrity)
	Sodium and potassium
	Calcium and magnesium
Biochemical environment	Created by agents in the flushing solutions
	Ideally enter the cell and affect rates of metabolism
	Agents include:
	Purine nucleotides precursors (adenine, ribose, phosphate)
	Antioxidants (glutathione, vitamin E, desferioxime)
	Enzyme inhibitors (allopurinol, chlorpromazine)
	Metabolizable substrates (fructose, Krebs cycle intermediates, etc.)

membrane-bound ion pumps, are slowed down. There is, therefore, a tendency for equilibration of permeable electrolytes (and other permeable substances) across the plasma membrane. This results in the loss of K^+ from the cell unless the cold storage solution contains a high content of K^+. The need for a high K^+ content in cold storage solutions is debated; excellent preservation of most organs has been achieved with preservatives containing high levels of Na^+ [17].

Cells also have a tendency to gain water. This is the result of higher levels of impermeants inside the cell (intracellular proteins, phosphorylated compounds, etc.) that create an osmotic (oncotic) force that pulls water inside to equilibrate the osmolality across the cell membrane. Suppression of cell swelling under conditions of cold storage is achieved by adding impermeants to the preservative: these include saccharides (glucose, mannitol, sucrose, raffinose), colloids (hydroxyethyl starch, polyethylene glycols, dextrans), and anions (gluconate, phosphate, citrate, sulphate, lactobionate). Some impermeants appear more suitable than others for preservation of the different organs. Lactobionate (mol. wt 358 kDa) is derived from lactose and is relatively impermeable to cells of most hypothermically stored organs studied to date. This is a primary component of the successful UW organ preservation solution. Lactobionate appears to have characteristics other than the suppression of hypothermically induced cell swelling that render it ideal for preservation of most organs. The nature of these other attributes is not clear, but they may be related to calcium and iron chelation. Replacement of lactobionate with other impermeant anions (gluconate, phosphate, etc.) has not yielded preservatives as efficacious as those containing lactobionate.

Another aspect of the physical environment affected by the preservation solution is the pH, which is regulated by the type of hydrogen ion buffer. Most preservatives utilize phosphate, although there is some evidence that high concentrations of histidine may be helpful for preservation of some organs [18].

The biochemical environment is created by additives that directly affect metabolism at hypothermia or upon reperfusion. These are agents that can be metabolized by the tissue or that act as specific inhibitors, and include: allopurinol (inhibitor of xanthine oxidase), glutathione, adenosine, dexamethasone, co-enzyme Q10, vitamin E, calcium channel blockers, phospholipase inhibitors, vasoactive agents and prostanoids. The beneficial effects or lack thereof of some of these agents has allowed speculation concerning the biochemical events involved in organ preservation.

Organ preservation by simple cold storage appears to be successful, therefore, because the organs are stored cold, in solutions that suppress cell swelling and contain agents that may facilitate restoration of biochemical integrity upon reperfusion. The UW solution, and others, are used quite commonly for preservation of most organs and appear to satisfy most clinical needs at this time. However, improvements in length and safety of preservation time, decreased preservation injury to the tissue and utility for all organs (including heart and lung) are goals not yet completely satisfied. These require a more comprehensive understanding of the biochemical and physiological events that occur during preservation of organs.

4. Biochemistry of organ deterioration

The biochemistry of preservation and reperfusion damage has been well described in several excellent comprehensive reviews on kidney [19] and liver [20] preservation. Other reviews of more specific topics related to organ preservation/reperfusion are also available [21–24].

The biochemical injuries that cause loss of organ viability take time (hours to days) to develop. Most organs stored at $4°C$ for 4–8 h regain function relatively rapidly after transplantation. Little biochemical damage occurs until after longer periods of storage. This suggests that biochemical (or physical) degradative processes go on within the organ and, at some point in time, cause irreversible injury to the organ. The causes of injury are not known, but there is probably not a single cause of damage. Instead, multiple alterations probably take place in the organ, contributing to loss of viability. Understanding the mechanisms of organ preservation injury is, therefore, difficult and involves determining the number of different pathways and events contributing to irreversible injury. Furthermore, suppressing damage during preservation may require a multifaceted approach.

The biochemical changes that lead to injury to cold-stored organs generally take place during the period of storage. The manifestations of the injury are observed upon transplantation and reperfusion of the organ. Reperfusion can exacerbate injury by stimulating metabolic events that cause direct injury to the organ as a result of the increase in temperature and exposure to oxygen (and calcium), leading to activation of enzymes and generation of oxygen free radicals. Thus, there are two places in organ transplantation where improvements in preservation/reperfusion understanding must be made. One is suppression of the changes that take place during the period of cold storage; the other is suppression of the injurious events that are the result of reperfusion (reperfusion injury).

4.1. Biochemical phenomena during storage and reperfusion

Among the events that occur in the donated organ *ex vivo* and during reperfusion are four that must be better understood: energy metabolism, production of oxygen free radicals, activation of certain enzymes and disturbances of the microcirculatory system. Understanding the biochemical and physiological impacts and interactions of these phenomena is essential to an objective approach to improved organ preservation.

4.1.1. *Energy metabolism*
Hypothermic storage delays the breakdown of high-energy compounds (adenine nucleotides). However, without oxygen there is a relatively rapid loss of ATP from the liver and kidney: within about 4 h nearly 95% of ATP has disappeared. The heart, by contrast, retains nearly 80% of its ATP during 12–15 hours of cold storage as a result of effective utilization of glycogen by anaerobic glycolysis in the heart and the production of ATP. Glycolysis occurs in the liver during cold storage, but not fast enough to maintain a high ATP content. The ATP is consumed by energy-requiring reactions (mostly by various ATPases) that produce ADP and phosphate. ADP is rephosphorylated by either glycolytic reactions or adenylate kinase, which couples two ADPs to yield one ATP and one AMP. Accumulation of AMP initiates purine nucleotide catabolism (Fig. 1), leading to the formation of inosine monophosphate, inosine, adenosine, hypoxanthine, xanthine and uric acid. The oxypurines are readily permeable across the plasma membrane and diffuse out of the cells when the organ is reperfused. This leads to a reduction in the total pool of ATP precursors available for regeneration of ATP when reperfusion is initiated and a concomitant energy crisis for the transplanted organ.

The loss of ATP (and other adenine nucleotides), methods by which this can be suppressed and the relationship between ATP and organ viability have been the focus of much research in organ preservation. Various methods have been used to suppress adenine nucleotide catabolism during organ storage, but without much success. Precursors of ATP regeneration have been used in organ storage solutions and in the organ prior to transplantation. Although these methods stimulate ATP production upon rewarming and re-

oxygenating (transplantation) of the stored tissue, no direct correlation has been established between ATP content and transplant viability.

The loss of ATP, however, may be the critical event in initiating the cascade of events that eventually lead to cell death. Certainly, cells and tissues can tolerate very low concentrations of ATP for many hours without dying. Cold-stored livers and kidneys contain less than 5% of the normal ATP levels, yet remain viable when stored for up to 3 days. Loss of ATP, however, causes the cell to lose control over its metabolism; ATP-requiring synthetic reactions stop while catabolic reactions (catalysed by phospholipases, lipases, proteases, endonucleases and other enzymes) continue. ATP may also be necessary for maintenance of the integrity of cellular and subcellular (mitochondrial, lysosomal) membrane systems. These catabolic reactions are quite slow at low temperatures; cell death resulting from these reactions, therefore, takes a relatively long time. However, during the period of cold storage there may be a slow but continual synthesis and breakdown of ATP, derived from anaerobic pathways such as glycolysis in the liver and kidney medulla. This limited production of ATP in some cold-stored tissues may be critical for maintenance of tissue viability. The role of this anaerobically generated ATP in sustaining cell viability is not known, but it may be related to the maintenance of the structural integrity of the tissue.

4.1.2. *Production of oxygen free radicals*
Production of oxygen free radicals jeopardizes the viability of the transplanted reperfused organ Metabolites produced by the reduction of oxygen include the superoxide anion, which can dismutate to hydrogen peroxide and be converted to highly cytotoxic hydroxyl radicals. These metabolites of oxygen are highly reactive (enhancing the difficulties encountered in measuring them in tissues) and cause changes in proteins, nucleotides, lipids and cell membranes which can lead to cell injury and cell death (Fig. 2).

The cytotoxic products of oxygen reduction are continually produced in oxygen-consuming cells, but are not normally injurious because the cell controls their rate of formation and contains a series of enzymatic pathways for degrading these potential cytotoxins to innocuous substances. Phenomena that injure organs and cells (such as warm or cold ischaemia) can stimulate the rate of production of oxygen free radicals, reduce their rate of metabolism, or initiate anti-inflammatory response in the tissue and attract cells (macrophages, etc.) that generate oxygen free radicals as part of their response to injury. Each of

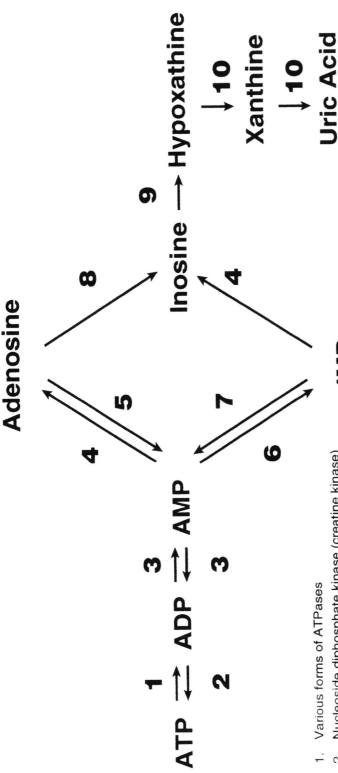

1. Various forms of ATPases
2. Nucleoside diphosphate kinase (creatine kinase)
3. Adenylate Kinase
4. 5' – Nucleotidase
5. Adenosine Kinase
6. AMP Deaminase
7. Adenylosuccinate synthase and lyase
8. Adenosine deaminase
9. Purine nucleoside phosphorylase
10. Xanthine oxidase

Figure 1. Pathway of adenine nucleotide catabolism in ischaemia. The pathway for the breakdown of adenine nucleotides follows the scheme shown in the figure. There are some differences, however, in different tissues. For instance, in the liver it appears that the breakdown of AMP to inosine occurs primarily through IMP. In the kidney the breakdown of AMP appears to go through adenosine to inosine.

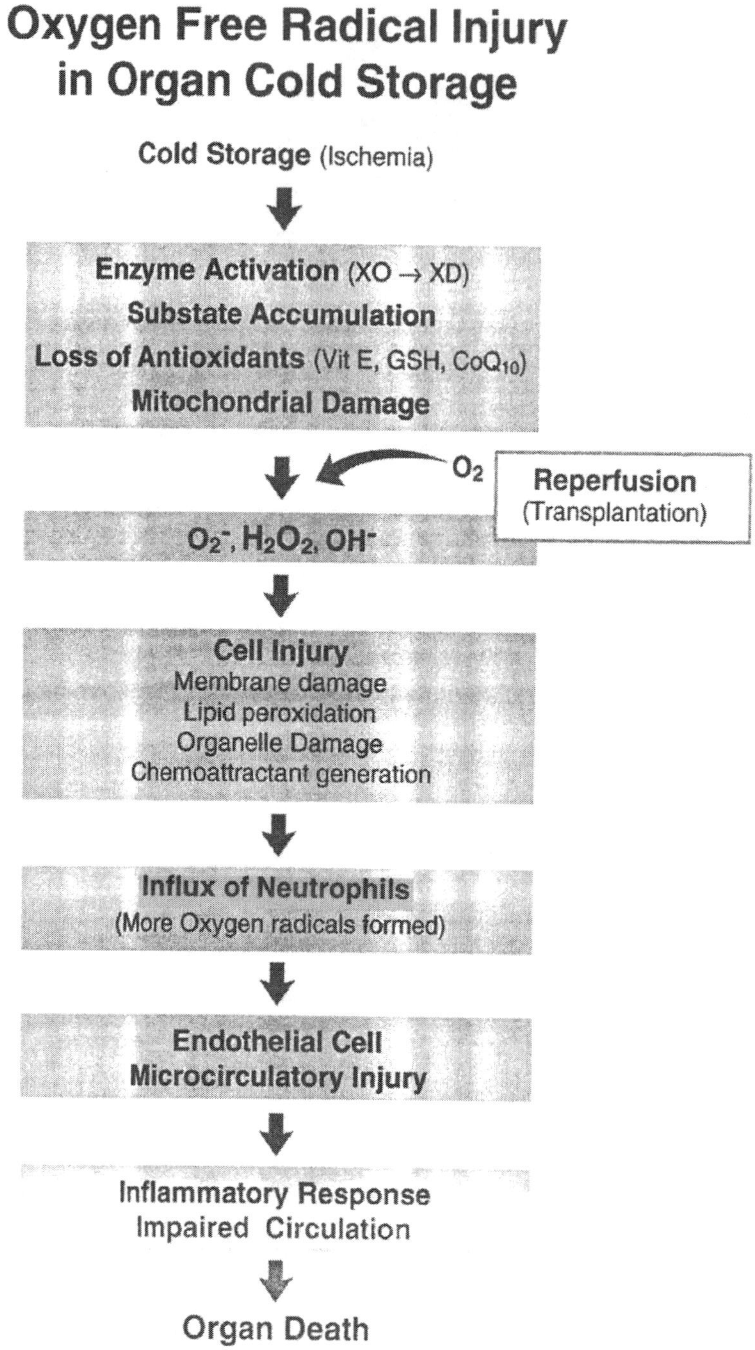

Oxygen Free Radical Injury in Organ Cold Storage

Cold Storage (Ischemia)

⬇

Enzyme Activation (XO → XD)

Substate Accumulation

Loss of Antioxidants (Vit E, GSH, CoQ_{10})

Mitochondrial Damage

⬇ ⬅ O_2 **Reperfusion** (Transplantation)

O_2^-, H_2O_2, OH^-

⬇

Cell Injury
Membrane damage
Lipid peroxidation
Organelle Damage
Chemoattractant generation

⬇

Influx of Neutrophils
(More Oxygen radicals formed)

⬇

Endothelial Cell Microcirculatory Injury

⬇

Inflammatory Response Impaired Circulation

⬇

Organ Death

Figure 2. Oxygen free radical injury in cold storage. This is a generalized pathway for oxygen derived free radical injury. Reperfusion exposes the damaged tissue to oxygen and normothermia. Superoxide anion hydrogen peroxide and hydroxyl radicals are produced through many cellular reactions and if not scavenged will lead to cell injury through various potential mechanisms.

these possibilities has been suggested as a cause of reperfusion injury in preserved organs [25,26].

A role of oxygen free radicals in reperfusion injury is best seen under conditions of warm ischaemia and reperfusion and appears to be a greater problem in some organs (intestine, heart, lung, liver) than in others. Furthermore, the extent of oxygen free radical injury caused by hypoxia or ischaemia may be species-dependent; rats and mice appear to be more susceptible to this form of injury than do higher species. The evidence for free radical injury as a major cause of organ failure after preservation and transplantation is controversial. Oxygen free radicals do appear to be produced following reperfusion of cold-stored organs. This has been shown by trapping free radical species in the liver [27], measuring the end-products of free radical metabolism (malondialdehyde, conjugated dienes, etc.) [28] in reperfused organs and by showing that the presence of oxygen free radical scavengers improves the rate of recovery of at least some measures of biochemical or physiological integrity following reperfusion [29]. Although it is clear that oxygen free radicals are produced, how they cause injury, and whether scavengers are a panacea for organ transplantation are not known.

There are many types of oxygen free radical scavengers: scavengers of superoxide anions (superoxide dismutase), hydroxyl radicals (mannitol, dimethyl-thiourea), inhibitors of enzymes that generate oxygen free radicals (allopurinol), chelators of iron (des-ferrioxamine) and naturally occurring scavengers (glutathione, vitamin E, co-enzyme Q). Many of these have been used for pretreatment of the donor, incorporated into the cold storage solution, given to the recipient, or used in a combination of these three methods, as well as being included in a final rinse of the organ prior to transplantation [30]. Despite evidence that some of these scavengers are beneficial, none has been universally accepted for clinical use.

4.1.3. Activation of degradative enzymes

During ischaemia, the lack of ATP and delivery and removal of substrates could lead to activation of enzymes that cause degradation of structural or functional components of the cell. Lysosomal hydrolyses, phospholipases [31,32], proteases [33] and endonucleases can cause disruption of structural components of the cell and cause irreversible damage. Evidence in support of this hypothesis is in general derived from the improvement in preservation of organs achieved by the addition of inhibitors of phospholipases or proteases. The difficulty in interpreting this data, however, is related to the multiplicity of actions of many of these inhibitors. Although beneficial to the transplanted or reperfused organ, their action may be more related to improved flow and delivery of oxygen than to inhibition of a specific enzyme.

Phospholipase inhibitors have been shown to improve preservation of the liver [34] and kidney [31,32]. A mechanism has been developed that involves the activation of phospholipases that hydrolyse membrane-bound phospholipids, causing alterations in the permeability characteristics of the membrane and the generations of potentially cytotoxic end-products (lysophosphatides and free fatty acids). However, it is clear that phospholipase inhibitors are not needed for relatively long term preservation of the liver and kidney, suggesting that the activation of these enzymes may be dependent upon the storage conditions used. Furthermore, no decrease in phospholipids is detected during long term storage of the liver [35], although there is an accumulation of free fatty acids. The origin of these free fatty acids is not known, but they could lead to injury to the preserved/reperfused organ. Removal of free fatty acids by flushing the liver with a solution containing serum albumin has been shown to improve liver function [36].

Evidence for protease activation and the degradation of proteins in cold-stored organs is not well developed. Some have shown improved preservation of the liver with protease inhibitors. Recently, Gores [37] has shown increased proteolysis in cold-stored livers.

The role of phospholipases and proteases in ischaemic injury to organs derives from studies related to warm ischaemia. It appears that under conditions of warm (37°C) ischaemia, proteases and phospholipases are active and can lead to cellular injury. However, hypothermia is an effective inhibitor of enzyme activity and phospholipase and protease degradation of the tissue may be a minor component of the injury during the period of cold storage. It is possible, however, that these enzymes become active upon reperfusion and rewarming of the organ, causing tissue degradation and irreversible injury.

5. Disturbances of the microcirculatory system

From the beginning of studies on organ preservation it was recognized that successful preservation would require maintenance of the integrity of the microcirculatory system. If tissue injury caused by hypothermic storage is to be repaired after transplantation it is essential that blood flow to the organ is nearly optimal and that areas of hypoxia or ischaemia do not develop. However, injury to the vascular system caused by long term storage of organs could lead to reperfusion injury. Damaged cells can release substances that elicit an inflammatory response, which recruits cells such as macrophages which in turn induce further injury to the microcirculatory system or parenchymal cells of the organ. Endothelial cells can slough off or round up and expose collagen of the basement membrane to circulating cells, causing adherence of platelets. These clog the microcirulatory system and restrict flow to various parts of the organ. In the liver, Kupffer cells can be activated by hypothermic storage, and can generate cytotoxic products that lead to cellular injury or injury to the microcirculatory system.

Evidence for microcirculatory disturbances has been obtained by microscopic studies of the effects of preservation on the liver and kidney. These studies show intact parenchymal cells but disrupted vascular endothelial cells after injurious preservation periods. Strasberg's group [38] has demonstrated injury to the sinusoidal lining cells of the rat liver after cold-preservation. They consider this injury to be the limiting factor in successful organ preservation. Thurman and Lemasters [39] have also implicated sinusoidal lining cells, in particular, Kupffer cells, as a limiting feature to successful liver preservation. Their studies suggest that Kupffer cells are activated after reperfusion of cold-stored livers, resulting in the generation of cytotoxic metabolites that cause injury to the microvasculature or hepatocellular functions.

6. Observations

Numerous biochemical changes occur in organs exposed to cold ischaemia. Which are responsible for the loss of viability is not clear. It is likely that when cold storage is the method of preservation, little can be done to alter the rate of cell death. Suppressing cell swelling certainly increases the duration of tolerance to preservation injury. Other preservation techniques used in the laboratory, such as the use of various pharmacological agents, can increase preservation tolerance by a small amount (12–24 h).

The limits of cold storage of organs remain at about 48–72 h. Organs stored for this length of time are, no doubt, damaged, but the damage can be reversed after reperfusion (transplantation). This period of time (24–72 hours) is sufficient to allow utilization of almost all cadaveric organs not injured prior to procurement. Longer periods of preservation are not necessary, but are desired.

Static cold storage, then, is a method of limited utility for high quality and long term organ preservation because catabolic metabolism continues even in the cold. Improved preservation could be obtained if catabolism were suppressed and anabolic metabolism stimulated. This can be accomplished by continuous hypothermic perfusion of organ. This method appears to give the best quality and longest preservation of the liver [4], kidney [15] and heart [9]. Our current ability to understand and control the biochemistry and cell physiology of organ preservation may, therefore, suggest further development and utilization of continuous perfusion as the method of choice.

References

1. Greig PD, Forster J, Supezina RA, Strasberg SM, Mohamed M, Blendis LM, Taylor BR, Levy GA, Langer B. Donor-specific factors predict graft function following liver transplantation. Transplant Proc 1990; 22: 2072–3.
2. Cywes R, Mullen JBM, Stratis MA, Greig PD, Levy GA, Harvey PRC, Strasberg SM. Prediction of the outcome of transplantation in man by platelet adherence in donor liver allografts. Evidence of the importance of prepreservation injury. Transplantation 1993; 56: 316–23.
3. Adam R, Reynes M, Bao YM, Astrazcioglu I, Azoulay D, Chiche L, Bismuth H. Impact of glycogen content of the donor liver in clinical liver transplantation. Transplant Proc 1993; 25: 1536–7.
4. Boudjema K, Lindell SL, Southard JH, Belzer FO. The effects of fasting on the quality of liver preservation by simple cold storage. Transplantation 1990; 50: 943–8.
5. Collins GM, Bravo-Shugarman MB, Terasaki PI. Kidney preservation for transplantation: initial perfusion and 30 hour ice storage. Lancet 1969; 2: 1219–25.
6. Belzer FO, Ashby BS, Dumphy JE. 24- and 72-hour preservation of canine kidneys. Lancet 1967; 2: 536–9.
7. Belzer FO, Ashby BS, Gulyassy PF, Powell M. Successful seventeen-hour preservation and transplantation of human-cadaver kidney. N Engl J Med 1968; 278: 608–10.
8. Pienaar BH, Lindell SL, van Gulik TM, Southard JH, Belzer FO. Seventy-two-hour preservation of the canine liver by machine perfusion. Transplantation 1990; 49: 258–60.
9. Wicomb WN, Cooper DKC, Barnard CN. Twenty-four-hour preservation of the pig heart by a portable hypothermic perfusion system. Transplantation 1982; 34: 246–50.
10. Jamieson NV, Sundberg R, Lindell S, Southard JH, Belzer FO. Preservation of the canine liver for 24–48 hours using simple cold storage with UW solution. Transplantation 1988; 46: 517–25.
11. Ploeg RJ, Goossens D, NcAnulty JF, Southard JH, Belzer FO. Successful 72-hour cold storage of dog kidneys with UW solution. Transplantation 1988; 46: 191–6.
12. Jeevanandam V, Auteri JS, Sanchez JA, Hsu D, Marboe C, Smith CR, Rose EA. Cardiac transplantation after prolonged graft preservation with the University of Wisconsin solution. J Thorac Cardiovasc Surg 1992; 104: 224–8.
13. Wahlberg JA, Love R, Landegaard L, Southard JH, Belzer FO. 72-hour preservation of the canine pancreas. Transplantation 1987; 43: 5–10.
14. McAnulty JF, Vreugdenhil PK, Lindell S, Southard JH, Belzer FO. Successful seven-day perfusion preservation of the canine kidney. Transplant Proc 1993; 25: 1642–44.
15. Henry ML, Sommer BG, Ferguson RM. Improved immediate function of renal allografts with Belzer perfusate. Transplantation 1988; 45: 73–5.

16. Calne, RY, Pegg DE, Pryse-Davis J, Leigh-Brown F. Renal preservation by ice cooling. An experimental study relating to kidney transplantation from cadavers. Br Med J 1963; 2: 651–4.

17. Moen J, Claesson K, Pienaar BH, Ploeg RJ, McAnulty JF, Vreugdenhil P, Lindell S, Southard JH, Belzer FO. Preservation of dog liver, kidney, and pancreas using the Belzer–UW solution with a high-sodium and low-potassium content. Transplantation 1989; 47: 940–5.

18. Sumimoto R, Lindell SL, Southard JH, Belzer FO. A comparison of histidine-lactobionate and UW solution in 48 hour dog liver preservation. Transplantation 1992; 54: 610–14.

19. Bonventre JV, Weinberg JM. Kidney preservation *ex vivo* for transplantation. Annu Rev Med 1992; 43: 523–53.

20. Clavien P, Harvey PRC, Strasberg SM. Preservation and reperfusion injuries in liver allografts. An overview and synthesis of current studies. Transplantation 1992; 53: 957–8.

21. Blankensteijn JD, Terpstra OT. Liver preservation: past and the future. Hepatology 1991; 13: 1235–50.

22. Chueng JY, Bonventre JV, Malis CD, Leaf A. Calcium and ischemic injury. N Engl J Med 1986; 314: 670–6.

23. Bienvenu K, Granger DN. Leukocyte adhesion in ischemia reperfusion. Blood Cells 1993; 19: 279–89.

24. Weinberg JM. The cell biology of ischemic renal injury. Kidney Int 1991; 39: 476–500.

25. Bulkley GB. Free radicals and other reactive oxygen metabolites: clinical relevance and the therapeutic efficacy of antioxidant therapy. Surgery 1993; 113: 479–83.

26. Parks DA, Bulkley GB, Granger DN. Role of oxygen free radicals in shock, ischemia, and organ preservation. Surgery 1983; 94: 428–32.

27. Connor HD, Gao W, Nukina S, Lemasters JJ, Mason RP, Thurman RG. Evidence that free radicals are involved in graft failure following orthotopic liver transplantation in the rat – an electron spin paramagnetic resonance spin trapping study. Transplantation 1992; 54: 199–204.

28. Fuller BJ, Gower JD, Green CJ. Free radical damage and organ preservation: fact or fiction? A review of the interrelationship between oxidative stress and physiological ion disbalance. Cryobiology 1988; 25: 377–93.

29. Hoshino T, Maley WR, Bulkley GB, Williams GM. Ablation of free radical-mediated reperfusion injury for the salvage of kidneys taken from non-heartbeating donors. Transplantation 1988; 45: 284–9.

30. Gao W, Takei Y, Marzi I, Lindert KA, Caldwell-Kenkel JC, Currin RT, Tanaka Y, Lemasters JJ, Thurman RG. Carolina rinse solution – a new strategy to increase survival time after orthotopic liver transplantation in the rat. Transplantation 1991; 52: 417–24.

31. Tokunaga Y, Wicomb WN, Concepcion W, Nakazato P, Cox KL, Esquivel CO, Collins GM. Improved rat liver preservation using chlorpromazine in a new sodium lactobionate sucrose solution. Transplant Proc 1991; 23: 660–1.

32. McAnulty JF, Vreugdenhil PK, Southard JH, Belzer FO. Improved survival of kidneys for seven with a phospholipase inhibitor. Transplant Proc 1991; 23: 691–2.

33. Takei Y, Marzi I, Kauffman FC, Currin RT, Lemasters JJ, Thurman RG. Increase in survival time of liver transplants by protease inhibitors and a calcium channel blocker, nisoldipine. Transplantation 1990; 50: 14–20.

34. Anaise D, Ishimaru M, Madariaga J, Irisawa A, Lane B, Zeidan B, Sonoda K, Shabtai M, Waltzer WC, Rapaport FT. Protective effects of trifluoperazine on the microcirculation of cold-stored livers. Transplantation 1990; 50: 933–9.

35. Hamamoto I, Nemoto EM, Evans RW, Mischinger H, Fujita S, Murase N, Todo S. Rat liver lipids during *ex vivo* warm and cold ischemia and reperfusion. J Surg Res 1993; 55: 382–9.

36. Kim S, Belzer FO, Southard JH. The loss of mitochondrial respiratory function and its suppression during cold ischemic preservation of rat livers with UW solution. Hepatology 1992; 16: 742–8.

37. Ferguson D, Gores GJ, Krom R. Cytosolic protease activity is increased during liver storage and is inhibited by glutathione. Transplant Proc 1991; 23: 1552–3.

38. McKeown CMB, Edwards V, Phillips MJ, Harvey PRC, Petrunka CN, Strasberg SM. Sinusoidal lining cell damage: the critical injury in cold preservation of liver allografts in the rat. Transplantation 1988; 46: 178–91.

39. Caldwell-Kenkel JC, Thurman RG, Lemasters JJ. Selective loss of nonparenchymal cell viability after cold ischemic storage of rat livers. Transplantation 1988; 45: 834–7.

40. Ross H, Marshall VC, Escott ML. 72-hr canine kidney preservation without continuous perfusion. Transplantation 1976; 21: 498–501.

41. Andrews PM, Coffey AK. Factors that improve the preservation of nephron morphology during cold storage. Lab Invest 1982; 46: 100–20.

42. Lam FT, Ubhi CS, Mavor AID, Lodge JPA, Giles GR. Clinical evaluation of PBS140 solution for cadaveric renal preservation. Transplantation 1989; 48: 1067–8.

43. Van Gulik TM, Nio CR, Cortissos E, Klopper PJ, van der Heyde MN. Comparison of HTK solution and UW solution in 24- and 48-hour preservation of canine hepatic allografts. Transplant Proc 1993; 25: 554.

13 | Preservation by simple hypothermia

Vernon Marshall

1. Introduction

The major importance of cold in extracorporeal storage of transplantable vascularized organs was recognized early in the history of transplantation. Hypothermia was first applied by simple surface cooling of the organ. Cooling was enhanced by flushing the blood from the organ by a chilled preserving solution – such solutions initially mimicked extracellular fluid or plasma. A major breakthrough occurred in the late 1960s when Collins demonstrated that a crystalloid preserving solution containing high concentrations of potassium and phosphate (an 'intracellular' solution) improved preservation markedly [1]. Subsequent modifications and alternatives to Collins' solution showed that several flushing solutions, widely varying in their content, could give approximately equivalent results for simple hypothermic storage of kidneys and other vascularized organs [2]. Search for an optimal flushing solution applicable to all organs received a further major stimulus in the late 1980s with the advent of Belzer's University of Wisconsin (UW) solution. This multi-component solution extended storage times even further, particularly of pancreas and liver, and was also applicable to kidney, heart, lung and small bowel grafts [3].

Simple hypothermic storage after a cold intravascular flush is now applied as standard clinical practice for all types of vascularized organ grafts in most centres world-wide. The importance of individual components, variations between solutions required for different organs, optimal conditions of storage and storage temperatures in regard to protection of parenchymal and non-parenchymal cells, the benefits or otherwise of reflushing the organ before revascularization, and the proportional damage induced by cold

G.M. Collins, J.M. Dubernard, W. Land and G.G. Persijn (eds). Procurement, Preservation and Allocation of Vascularized Organs 115–129
© 1997 Kluwer Academic Publishers.

storage and by subsequent vascular reperfusion, continue to be important matters for experimental and clinical investigation. Although much progress has been made, and a reasonable degree of order has been restored to most clinical organ grafts by these means, we need to remember that organ preservation by hypothermic static storage still only slows and ameliorates extracorporeal ischaemic/hypoxic damage rather than reversing such damage. The latter remains a future goal of great importance in view of the continuing shortage of ideal brain-dead cadaver donors, and the concomitant increased utilization of organs from less optimal donors presenting with cardiac arrest (asystolic or non-heart-beating cadavers). For preservation of organs from these latter group of donors continuous hypothermic machine perfusion preservation (the second major technique of organ storage – see Chapter 11), has a continuing major role.

When organs are removed from brain-dead, heart-beating cadavers static storage is simpler, safer, more economical and in most instances equally effective. A carefully performed intravascular cold flush combined with surface cooling is the first step in all cases of organ procurement for transplantation. Only rarely is subsequent machine perfusion obligatory. After organ washout, sterile packaging and appropriate maintenance of hypothermia during storage, no further complications or side-effects exist. If organ function in the donor has been satisfactory and warm ischaemia minimal prior to organ removal, and if implantation is expeditiously performed without technical problems within the limits of safe storage times for individual organs, then good initial function can be confidently expected unless immunological problems prevent this.

2. The ischaemic/anoxic organ

Cells of normally functioning vascularized organs derive their energy via an adequately maintained circulation. Oxidation of substrates obtained from circulating blood (glucose, fatty acids, amino acids, ketones) provides the energy for life-sustaining cellular, tissue and organ function. In the liver energy is additionally obtainable from breakdown of endogenous stores of glycogen. Energy production within cells is created by phosphate bonds of adenosine triphosphate (ATP), creatine phosphate and other nucleotides. Cellular homeostasis is maintained by numerous enzymic reactions proceeding in concert under the direction of hormones or key compounds such as cyclic adenosine monophosphate (cAMP) and cyclic guanosine monophosphate (cGMP). Ischaemia causes

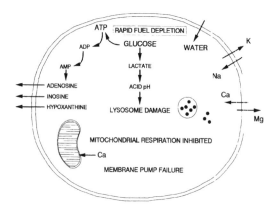

Figure 1. The ischaemic/anoxic cascade of cellular damage following ischaemia at body temperature: rapid fuel depletion, membrane and organelle damage, cell swelling and death.

depletion of oxygen and nutrients. Continuing metabolic activity of the organ's parenchymal and non-parenchymal cells causes an ischaemic/anoxic cascade, leading ultimately to irreversible cell damage and death (Fig. 1). Anaerobic metabolism rapidly depletes high-energy phosphate bonds. Anaerobic glycolysis can generate only two molecules of ATP per glucose molecule metabolized, compared with 38 molecules of ATP generated during aerobic metabolism. Dephosphorylation of nucleotides increases cellular levels of adenosine, inosine and hypoxanthine and depletes the total nucleotide pool available for rephosphorylation once blood flow is restored. Fuel depletion inactivates the enzyme system controlling the sodium pump of the cell membrane (Na^+, K^+-ATPase); thus chloride and sodium (permeable electrolytes which are normally actively extruded from the cell) diffuse into the cell down concentration gradients, and potassium diffuses out. Water also enters the cell and causes harmful cellular swelling and oedema. Ca^{2+}, Mg^--ATPase is also inactivated, inhibiting mitochondrial respiration. Calcium enters the cytosol and mitochondria, activating phospholipase, an enzyme which lyses cellular and intracellular membranes; and cellular magnesium is depleted. Anaerobic metabolism also generates lactic acid leading to progressive intracellular acidosis. Intracellular acidosis, although partly serving as an autoregulatory protective mechanism [4], also activates lysosomal enzymes [5], whose release leads to cellular autolysis. Parenchymal cells of most transplantable organs are generally similar in their tolerance to ischaemic/anoxic damage. Most parenchymal organ cells can tolerate ischaemic hypoxia for 30–60 min without permanent damage. Rapidly metabolizing tissues are less tolerant. Most organs are irreversibly damaged by 120 min of ischaemia at body temperatures. Vascular damage occurs along with the parenchymal effects – the cells of the vascular endothelial lining bear the brunt of this injury, particularly affecting the microvasculature. These harmful effects are slowed, but not reversed, by cooling.

3. Reperfusion injury

Reperfusion injury is an additional hazard contributing to organ damage upon revascularization after prolonged ischaemia. Accumulation of metabolic endproducts such as hypoxanthine under anaerobic conditions can set the stage for reperfusion injury. When blood flow is restored oxygen influx leads to formation of toxic compounds such as hydrogen peroxide, and superoxide and hydroxyl radicals (Fig. 2). These active free radicals of oxygen produce further cellular, membrane and microvascular injury [6]. Under normal circumstances these harmful radicals are short lived and are rapidly cleared by endogenous scavenging mechanisms. Ischaemia and prolonged organ storage deplete endogenous mediators, rendering the organ more prone to reperfusion damage.

4. Effects of hypothermia: principles of static cold storage

Organ preservation techniques begin with cooling: this remains the most important method of diminishing the

detrimental effects of ischaemic anoxia. Cooling diminishes metabolic activity and curtails the oxygen demand of the preserved organ. However metabolism still persists during hypothermia, even in ice at 0°C [7]. Oxygen consumption decreases exponentially, to 10% of normal at 10°C, 5% at 5°C and 3% at 0°C [8]. Cooling from 37°C (body temperature) to around 0–5°C (storage temperatures) extends the tolerance of most organs to ischaemia from 1–2 h to about 12 h. Hypothermia alone is only a partial solution, however. Unfortunately cold does not slow all biological functions uniformly and a variety of metabolic processes become discordant when the organ is cooled. Transmembrane passive diffusion of ions is not appreciably affected by hypothermia, while active transport mechanisms such as those governed by Na^+,K^+-ATPase and $Ca^{2+}Mg^+$-ATPase are inhibited below 10°C [9]. Hypothermia alone does not, therefore, prevent deleterious cell swelling during storage (Fig. 3). The challenge is thus to develop stable cold solutions which will enhance the rapidity and uniformity of cooling by a simple intravascular gravity flush and will also provide solutes which improve preservation of vasculature, parenchyma and interstitium. It was early recognized that blood was not the ideal flushing solution; cold blood adds rheological problems of greater viscosity and sluggish flow. Simple balanced electrolyte solutions mimicking extracellular fluid, such as Ringer's lactate solution or saline, were also shown to be unsatisfactory as organ-preserving solutions, exacerbating interstitial and cellular oedema. Attention was then directed at plasma-like solutions containing albumin, dextrans or other colloids (combined with extracellular electrolyte levels) to provide oncotic support and to prevent

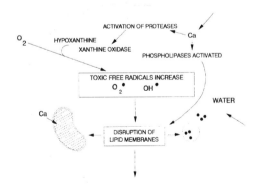

Figure 2. Reperfusion damage when oxygen supply is restored after prolonged ischaemia, due to formation of toxic free radicals.

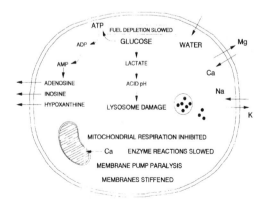

Figure 3. Effects of cooling on the cellular ischaemic/anoxic cascade: fuel depletion slowed, cold-induced membrane pump paralysis, gradual cell swelling.

interstitial oedema. Collins ushered in a new era of cold storage preservation by showing that a solution of crystalloid solutes alone, with a composition more resembling 'intracellular' than 'extracellular' fluids and quite free of colloid, could extend renal preservation reliably for 48 h or more [1]. Collins' solution contained high concentrations of glucose and phosphate (relatively impermeable solutes to cellular membranes). Phosphate (and bicarbonate) could additionally act as buffers to counter intracellular acidosis, and high levels of potassium were included to resist potassium loss from cells.

Subsequent studies confirmed that a major requirement for any cold flushing solution is inclusion of an impermeable molecule to provide an extracellular osmotic force opposing the development of cellular oedema, which is otherwise progressive and inevitable after hypothermic paralysis of the cellular membrane pumps. Large anions in particular, such as lactobionate (mol. wt 358 kDa) or gluconate (mol. wt 195 kDa), or non-electrolytes such as the non-metabolizable saccharides raffinose (505 kDa) or sucrose (342 kDa), or chelates of citrate and magnesium (approximately 1000 Da), or larger molecules such as polyethylene glycol (20 000 Da), or protein (70 000 Da) can achieve this. An effective buffer (phosphate, bicarbonate, citrate, histidine) to counter intracellular acidosis was identified as a second major requirement. The ionic electrolyte composition of flushing solutions is of lesser importance, and can vary widely. Freely diffusible anions such as chloride are preferably replaced by an impermeable ion or solute (lactobionate, gluconate, chelated citrate, sucrose, polyethylene glycol, histidine or other agent). Flushing solutions often have high potassium and low sodium concentrations, with potassium 100–130 mM and sodium 10–30 mM. High potassium concentrations are potentially cardiotoxic and certainly vasoconstrictive; they thus slow flushing rates and rates of organ cooling. Solutions containing high potassium also need to be removed from large organs such as the liver prior to revascularization to prevent delivery of a cardioplegic bolus of potassium on release of clamps. Solutions with the sodium/potassium ratios reversed (Na 130 mM, K 10–30 mM) have been shown to be virtually as effective, provided chloride concentration is kept low and there are suitable impermeants and buffers in the solution [10]. Magnesium is a useful additive in many solutions since it chelates with lactobionate and citrate to form large solutes which cannot pass through membranes. Calcium also chelates with these anions, but calcium in flushing solutions is usually kept at low level or excluded since cell damage is associated with calcium

influx. Calcium (and magnesium) can precipitate in unstable solutions. Colloids can act as alternative impermeable solutes, but colloids are not obligatory or necessary for simple hypothermic storage. The multiple factors influencing the effectiveness of preservation were analysed by Belzer and Southard in producing the University of Wisconsin solution. This contained an impermeable anion (lactobionate), a saccharide (raffinose), a buffer (phosphate), free radical inhibitors and scavengers and metabolic inhibitors (glutathione, allopurinol), energy precursors (adenosine), vasoactive agents and hormones (steroids, insulin) and a colloid (hydroxyethyl starch; HES). This complex solution was markedly more effective than other solutions used for liver and pancreas preservation and was also very effective for kidney and heart.

In addition to the major constituents aimed at diminishing cellular swelling and intracellular acidosis, a host of additional agents with biochemical, pharmacological and vascular effects have been added to flushing solutions. These include other energy sources and precursors, calcium channel blocking agents, metabolic inhibitors, antagonists of cytokines, phenothiazides, protease inhibitors, prostaglandins and other vasoactive agents. These will be further considered in relation to individual solutions and organs.

Preservation by static hypothermic storage is limited ultimately by exhaustion of nutrients and accumulation of waste products. Preservation of kidneys by simple storage could be extended to 3 days using Collins', citrate and sucrose solutions; and subsequently to 5 days by derivatives of UW solution [11]. Preservation of liver and pancreas was not consistently extended to beyond 24 h until the advent of UW solution [12]. Heart, lung and small bowel still have short preservation times compared with other organs.

Static organ storage is most effective when normothermic ischaemic damage prior to cold flushing is kept to a minimum. The world-wide use of brain-dead heart-beating cadaver donors for multiple organ procurement thus facilitated markedly simple hypothermic organ storage. Additional normothermic ischaemic damage before organ removal markedly diminishes the tolerated storage time. Addition of 30 min of normothermic warm ischaemia (WI) is more harmful than an additional 24 h of cold storage to a kidney [13].

5. Flush solutions for simple hypothermic storage

The composition of various flush solutions differs significantly, but each has components aimed at preventing cellular swelling, and each contains a buffer. Adjuvant biochemically active solutes can further enhance preservation.

5.1. Collins' solutions (Table 1)

Prolonged organ preservation became possible after the development of solutions of 'intracellular' electrolyte composition [1,13–16]. However, initial function of kidneys after 72 h cold storage was poor, and any added WI time markedly diminished the efficacy of these solutions [17]. The early Collins' solutions (C2, C3, C4) contained high concentrations of potassium, magnesium, phosphate, sulphate and glucose (120 mM). Precipitation of magnesium phosphate was a problem. Additions of procaine (C3, C4) and of phenoxybenzamine (C4) were found unnecessary and, in the case of procaine, harmful. Subsequently, magnesium, procaine and phenoxybenzamine were omitted from the widely used Euro-Collins' solution, which contains high concentrations of potassium (110 mM), phosphate (60 mM) and increased glucose (180 mM). The higher concentrations of glucose may to some degree reduce the potential efficacy of EuroCollins' solution, or may make it less effective in preservation of organs other than kidney. Glucose is slowly permeable across cell membranes, stimulates cellular anaerobic glycolysis and augments tissue acidosis. These potentially harmful effects become more apparent with prolonged storage times. Replacement of glucose by less permeable and non-metabolizable solutes (sucrose, mannitol) improved the results of renal preservation by Collins' solution in rat [18] and dog kidneys [19]. A significant reduction in post-transplantation renal failure occurred when human kidneys were preserved

in EuroCollins' solution containing mannitol instead of glucose [20]. Replacement of glucose by sucrose may be even more relevant in liver and pancreas grafts, whose cells are more permeable to glucose.

5.2. Citrate solutions (Table 2)

Citrate solution [21,22] was developed as an alternative to Collins' solution. The solution also has high concentrations of potassium and magnesium, but citrate replaces phosphate and mannitol replaces glucose. Citrate provides buffering capacity as well as interacting with magnesium to form impermeable, stable chelates. Isotonic and hypertonic solutions seem to be equally effective; sulphate ion is an unimportant component and can be replaced by other anions. Mannitol can be replaced by sucrose with equivalent results; replacement of mannitol with glucose was detrimental in kidney preservation. An acid pH (6.5)

Table 2. Flushing solutions for hypothermic storage: citrate solutions.

	Hypertonic citrate	Isotonic citrate
Sodium (mmol/l)	78	78
Potassium (mmol/l)	84	84
Magnesium (mmol/l)	40	40
Citrate (mmol/l)	54	54
Sulphate (mmol/l)	40	40
Mannitol (mmol/l)	200	100
Osmolality (mmol/kg)	400	300
pH (at 0°C)	7.1	7.1

Table 1. Flushing solutions for hypothermic storage: Collins' solutions.

	C2	EuroCollins'	EuroCollins' sucrose	EuroCollins' mannitol
Sodium (mmol/l)	10	10	10	10
Potassium (mmol/l)	110	110	110	110
Magnesium (mmol/l)	30	–	–	–
Bicarbonate (mmol/l)	10	10	10	10
Chloride (mmol/l)	14	15	15	15
Phosphate (mmol/l)	47	60	60	60
Sulphate (mmol/l)	30	–	–	–
Glucose (mmol/l)	126	180	–	–
Mannitol (mmol/l)	–	–	–	180
Sucrose (mmol/l)	–	–	180	–
Osmolality (mmol/kg)	320	340	340	340
pH (at 0°C)	7.0	7.3	7.2	7.2

also proved deleterious. Solutions of pH 7.1–7.8 were equally effective [23]. Citrate solutions gave results comparable to those of Collins' solutions for kidney, liver and pancreas grafts.

5.3. Sucrose solutions (Table 3)

The demonstration that sucrose improved efficacy of preserving solutions [18] led to formulation of a simple isosmolar sodium phosphate-buffered sucrose solution. This solution gave excellent preservation of rat, pig, dog and human kidneys [24–27]. Sucrose-based solutions, optimally at a sucrose concentration of around 140 mM, are also effective in the preservation of other organs.

5.4. Bretschneider's HTK solution (Table 4)

This solution was initially developed for cardioplegia in open heart surgery, and was subsequently shown to be effective in experimental and clinical preservation of kidney and liver [28]. It contains large and relatively impermeable solutes: histidine (200 mM), mannitol (30 mM) and additives of tryphophan and α-keto-

glutaric acid, with low concentrations of sodium, potassium and magnesium. Histidine is an excellent buffer and tryptophan, histidine and mannitol can act as free radical scavengers. The solution is associated with a low incidence of delayed function in kidney transplantation clinically, and was shown to be better than EuroCollins' solution in kidney transplantation in a prospective randomized clinical trial [29].

5.5. University of Wisconsin solution (Table 5)

This complex flushing solution was originally developed for use in transplantation of the pancreas [5]. Its components include impermeable solutes and buffering agents, colloid, electrolytes, adenosine, allopurinol, glutathione, insulin and steroids. Subsequently, UW was effectively applied experimentally and clinically to liver, kidney, heart and small bowel preservation. The clinical success of UW solution and its variants in heart and lung, liver, pancreas, kidney, small bowel, and organ cluster grafts has made it the preferred solution and gold standard for multiple organ harvest in the 1990s [2,28,30–32]. A multicentre trial in Europe comparing UW with EuroCollins' showed that the former gave more rapid recovery of renal function and less post-transplant dialysis [33]; other studies showed equivalent function of kidneys preserved by UW and Collins' solution in a randomized prospective clinical trial [34]. The UW solution has been shown to diminish trapping of erythrocytes in the microcirculation [35]. The effects of UW solution on protecting nonparenchymal cells in kidney, liver and pancreas

Table 3. Flushing solutions for hypothermic storage: sucrose-phosphate flushing solutions.

	Phosphate-buffered sucrose-120	Phosphate-buffered sucrose-140
Sodium (mmol/l)	170	120
Phosphate (mmol/l)	100	60
Sucrose (mmol/l)	120	140
Osmolality (mmol/kg)	300	310
pH (at 0°C)	7.1	7.2

Table 4. Flushing solutions for hypothermic storage: Bretschneider's HTK solution.

Sodium (mmol/l)	15
Potassium (mmol/l)	9
Magnesium (mmol/l)	4
Chloride (mmol/l)	50
Histidine (mmol/l)	198
Tryoptophane (mmol/l)	2
α-Ketoglutarate (mmol/l)	1
Mannitol (mmol/l)	30
Osmolality (mmol/kg)	310
pH (at 0°C)	7.3

Table 5. Flushing solutions for hypothermic storage: University of Wisconsin solution (UW).

Potassium (mmol/l)	135
Sodium (mmol/l)	35
Magnesium (mmol/l)	5
Lactobionate (mmol/l)	100
Phosphate (mmol/l)	25
Sulphate (mmol/l)	5
Raffinose (mmol/l)	30
Adenosine (mmol/l)	5
Allopurinol (mmol/l)	1
Glutathione (mmol/l)	3
Insulin (units/l)	100
Dexamethasone (mg/l)	8
Hydroxyethyl Starch (g/l)	50
Bactrim (ml/l)	0.5
Osmolality (mmol/kg)	320
pH (at room temperature)	7.4

may be important aspects of its abilities to provide extended preservation, rather than its effect on the more resistant parenchymal cells.

Analysis of the various components of UW solution has demonstrated, both experimentally and clinically, that equivalent results can be obtained by omission of some of the less important components, as discussed below.

5.5.1. *HES*
The synthetic colloid HES confers no advantage in simple hypothermic storage. The additional colloid, apart from being unnecessary, adds to the expense and increases viscosity, thus slowing rates of flushing. HES-free derivatives of UW solution have given equivalent or better results for simple hypothermic storage than those containing HES. Preservation of canine kidneys by simple hypothermic storage was reliably extended to 5 days after a single flush with Monash UW solution, a modified UW solution without HES [11]. Similarly, randomized clinical trials in kidney transplantation have showed equivalent and satisfactory preservation by HES-free UW solution over standard UW solution. Both UW and its colloid-free modification were significantly better than EuroCollins' solution [36].

5.5.2. *Impermeable components*
The major effective component is the impermeable anion lactobionate. Gluconate, which is also impermeable, can substitute for lactobionate. Raffinose can be replaced by sucrose.

5.5.3. *Electrolytes*
Reduction of potassium concentration with reversal of the Na^+/K^+ ratio considerably improves flushing efficiency by removing the vasoconstrictive effect of a high potassium level. This modification has been as effective in preservation of kidney, liver and pancreas, as has standard UW solution [37].

5.5.4. *Other components*
Adenosine and allopurinol are helpful as adjuvants, as is glutathione [38]. Glutathione is unstable in solution, which diminishes its value unless it is freshly added just before use. Glycine may also be a useful additive [39]. Insulin and steroid confer no additional benefit. Organ-specific differences in sensitivity to ischaemic damage and organ-specific requirements for optimal preservation exist [40], and relative sensitivities of parenchymal and endothelial cells may vary between allografts. These variations are outweighed by the globally protective effects across all organs of the major constituents of UW solution.

5.6. Modifications of UW solution

5.6.1. *Sodium lactobionate–sucrose solutions (SLS) (Table 6)*
This simplified HES-free modification of UW solution developed by Collins has as its main components sodium lactobionate (100 mM) with a phosphate buffer (25 mM) and added sucrose (75 mM), to give a lactobionate-sucrose-phosphate based solution with an extracellular cation composition (Na^+ 155 mM, K^+ 5 mM, Mg^+ 5 mM). This solution has been effective in experimental and clinical organ preservation; its efficacy has been enhanced by adjuvants of nisoldipine and chlorpromazine [41].

5.6.2. *Histidine–lactobionate solution*
A modification of Bretschneider's HTK solution, with added lactobionate instead of mannitol, has also been effective experimentally in liver, pancreas and heart transplantation [42].

6. Other modifications of storage conditions

6.1. Storage temperature

Organs surrounded by preserving solution, and stored and transported in a container of crushed ice, maintain a storage temperature of melting ice (0°C). Temperatures above 0°C aim to diminish cold-induced membrane paralysis while maintaining the protective effects of hypothermia. Temperatures above 15–20°C have usually been considerably less effective than 0°C.

The optimal storage temperature of non-parenchymal cells may differ from that required by parenchymal cells, perhaps over quite a narrow range. Storage of rat livers for 48 h was possible by simple

Table 6. Flushing solutions for hypothermic storage: sodium lactobionate-sucrose (SLS).	
Potassium (mmol/l)	5
Sodium (mmol/l)	155
Magnesium (mmol/l)	5
Lactobionate (mmol/l)	100
Phosphate (mmol/l)	25
Sulphate (mmol/l)	5
Sucrose (mmol/l)	75
Glutathione (mmol/l)	3
Osmolality (mmol/kg)	370
pH (at room temperature)	7.4

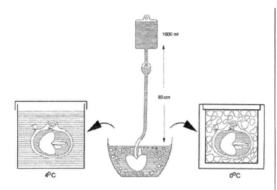

Figure 4. Flush cooling and hypothermic storage at 0°C and 4°C respectively.

hypothermic storage at 4°C but not at 0°C [43]. Differences in effectiveness between various solutions (UW, sucrose, citrate) were less marked during storage at 4°C than at 0°C. If these results, suggesting a greater sensitivity of endothelial cells to cold damage than occurs with parenchymal cells, are confirmed, storage at 4°C may prove the optimal method. Storage at 4°C could be simply obtained by domestic refrigerator storage of organs surrounded by cold liquid rather than ice (Fig. 4).

6.2. Oxygen and substrate supply

Preservation by simple storage normally implies anaerobic conditions. Addition of oxygen during hypothermic storage is possible by continuous bubbling of gas (persufflation), delivered to the stored organ via its artery, vein or drainage system (ureter) [44]. Multiple fine needle punctures on the surface of the organ allow more even diffusion and escape of oxygen during storage. Although persufflation has shown some advantages in kidney storage [45], concerns that damage to the endothelium may be excessive, with a tendency to vascular thrombosis, have meant that the technique has not gained wide acceptance [46]. The role of nutrient substrates added to flushing solutions used for static storage is not clearly established. On the one hand, solutions containing no utilizable metabolizable substrates can give excellent preservation of several organs for 24 h, and in the case of kidneys up to at least 72 hours experimentally with PBS solutions [25]. Precursors of ATP such as adenosine, ATP-magnesium chloride, inosine and other agents added to flushing solutions have been shown to be helpful in some studies, but whether they are acting as fuel sources or as rheological agents is uncertain. Paradoxically, glycogen-depleted livers from fasted rats appear to acquire

resistance to ischaemic injury and show better survival after transplantation [47].

Even with machine perfusion, metabolism of the continuously perfused organ during hypothermia is not fully aerobic [48]. All machine perfusion preservation techniques, however, utilize some form of oxygenation and addition of substrate to maintain hypothermic metabolism. The substrate is usually glucose, sometimes enriched with fructose, pyruvate, amino acids, fatty acids and other metabolites. The advantages of machine perfusion over static storage are seen only with extended preservation times (2–3 days and longer), or when resuscitation of ischaemically damaged organs during preservation requires replenishment of the depleted substrate pool.

6.3. Two-layer interface storage

Storing organs balanced at the interface between two solutions of different physical characteristics can help facilitate oxygen delivery by surface oxygenation, when one of the solutions contains a synthetic perfluorochemical facilitating oxygen transport. The method has been shown to enhance pancreatic storage [49].

6.4. Intermittent normothermic perfusion

This technique has extended preservation times when applied to both hypothermic machine perfusion and static storage [50,51]. The principle in each case has been to interrupt the process of cold storage by a period of rewarming (utilizing normothermic blood perfusion by machine, or by connecting the organ temporarily to the recipient via an arteriovenous shunt). The method serendipitously gives an opportunity during the rewarming process to test organ function (which is difficult to do during cold perfusion and impossible with static storage). It is also possible to deliver immunosuppressive agents during the period of resumed normal metabolic activity.

6.5. Protection of the vasculature: vasoactive agents

The vascular endothelial cells are the first to face reperfusion damage. Inadequacies of machine preservation, in particular, can cause endothelial damage at macrocirculatory and microcirculatory levels during cold perfusion. The liver vasculature, with its complex sinusoidal fenestrated membrane guarded by endothelial cells and by macrophages (Kupffer cells) and its double blood supply, is particularly liable to preservation injury. Vascular complications have also plagued pancreatic transplants. It is therefore not surprising that many additives found to be of value in organ preservation (calcium channel blockers, prostaglandins, cytokine antagonists) have rheological effects which may partially explain their benefit.

6.6. Effects of reflushing during storage

The effects of reflushing during storage are important and complex. Retrieval techniques of abdominal organs utilizing *in situ* vascular cooling with large volumes of balanced electrolyte solution often precede organ removal. This facilitates early core cooling; and is followed by rapid *en-bloc* removal of organs or organ clusters. Bench surgery is performed on the removed and externally cooled organs while the organs are given a definitive cold flush. It is important to realize that Ringer's lactate solution, although a convenient vehicle to institute initial cooling, is quite unsatisfactory as a preserving solution. Definitive cold flushing with an optimal organ preservation solution (UW or one of its precursors or derivatives) is essential before cold storage. Cold reflushing during storage does not improve preservation if the first flush is optimal.

6.7. Effects of prevascularization rinse: Carolina rinse solution

A prevascularization flush or rinse at the conclusion of the storage period, just prior to reimplantation, has two main aims: to remove potentially toxic components of the preservation solution and accumulated waste products (for example, high potassium levels, hydrogen ions, or a large intracardiac bolus of cold fluid), and to smooth the transition between hypothermic storage and isothermic revascularization. Anastomoses can also be tested advantageously prior to revascularization by intravascular wash-out before final clamp release. This

has been most studied in relation to the liver. One method allows blood flow to the liver via portal vein, venting the initial effluent from the infrahepatic vena cava prior to completing this anastomosis, and finally releasing the clamp on the suprahepatic vena cava. Alternatively the organ can be reflushed via the portal vein with cold or warm balanced electrolyte solution (Ringer's lactate) prior to clamp release [52].

Carolina rinse (CR) solution, developed by Lemasters and colleagues at the University of North Carolina, maintains the basic electrolyte composition of Ringer's lactate, but has added components and gave better results than a simple electrolyte rinse in animals and man [53,54]. CR solution combines ECF electrolyte composition with a mildly acidic pH, oncotic support (albumin or HES), antioxidants (allopurinol, glutathione, desferrioxamine), energy substrates (adenosine, glucose and insulin, fructose), vasodilators (calcium channel blockers) and glycine. As with UW solution, it was not clear which of the several components were effective and whether the effects were due to the beneficial effects of the CR solution or the potentially harmful effects of a Ringer's lactate rinse [55].

Analysis of the various components and techniques indicates that the temperature of the rinse solution should be above the cold storage temperature of 0–4°C. Rinses at ambient temperatures (20°C) and at body temperatures (37°C) have given better results. The preferred reaction may be sightly acidic (pH 6.8). Components which seem unnecessary are colloid (HES or albumin), nicardipine and magnesium; glucose, fructose and insulin also do not seem essential. Beneficial agents include adenosine, allopurinol, desferrioxamine, glutathione and glycine, possibly due to their free radical scavenging and quenching effects [54,56–58]. Similarities between these findings and those with UW solution are apparent. Whether a CR rinse has advantages over a prevascularization rinse with a UW-derived low potassium solution is not yet established, nor is the effect of CR on other vascularized allografts.

Table 7. Current status of organ preservation by simple cold storage after a preliminary flush.

	Experimental	Clinical (h)	Optimal flushing solution
Kidney	5 days (120 h)	24 (to 60)	HES-free UW
Pancreas	4 days (96 h)	12 (to 36)	UW and others
Liver	2 days (48 h)	12 (to 36)	UW and others
Small Intestine	2 days (48 h)	8 (to 12)	UW and others
Heart	1 day (24 h)	6 (to 12)	CU
Lung	1 day (24 h)	8 (to 12)	UW and others

7. Hypothermic storage for individual organs

The current status of organ preservation by simple hypothermic storage is shown in Table 7, giving the limits of storage which have been achieved experimentally and clinically using optimal flushing solutions and static cold storage.

7.1. Kidney

Prospective, randomized clinical trials using preservation times averaging 24 h have shown no significant differences in early function or in long term survival between machine preservation and simple cold storage [22,59]. Extended cold storage for up to 2 and 3 days, although still capable of giving satisfactory results, is accompanied by an increased frequency of acute tubular necrosis (ATN) as storage times lengthen beyond 24–48 h. Although in experienced units delayed initial function is compatible with good long term results, the advantages of immediate good renal function with a maintained urine output and rapid correction of azotemia after transplantation are striking. Clinical management is markedly facilitated, with earlier hospital discharge and earlier recognition and treatment of rejection episodes. Kidneys with early ATN, even when this is followed by adequate function, do less well in terms of long term survival than those kidneys which function immediately, raising the likelihood that ischaemically damaged kidneys may be more prone to immunological rejection.

Thus even in kidney transplantation, where dialysis can maintain patient survival in the face of poor early function, good early function remains the paradigm of clinical organ preservation. Simple hypothermic storage can give early function in the majority of grafts. Storage times over 48 h are rarely obligatory except when organs are transplanted over very long distances, for example between continents.

UW-derived solutions (HES-free UW) have proved successful for the static storage of dog kidneys for 5 days (Fig. 5). The gold standard for cadaver kidney preservation thus remains UW solution. Comparable results are achievable by a variety of other solutions when preservation times do not exceed 24 h, so for shorter anticipated preservation periods and for living donor transplantation, UW, sucrose, Collins', citrate and Bretschneider's solutions can give equivalent results.

7.2. Liver

There is general agreement that the introduction of UW solution revolutionized liver transplantation.

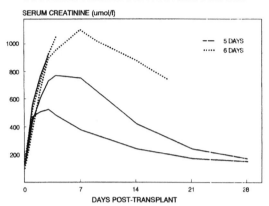

DOG KIDNEY PRESERVATION WITH UMW SOLUTION

SERUM CREATININE (umol/l)

Figure 5. Renal function in beagles after simple hypothermic storage for 5 and 6 days using HES-free UW solution (UMW), reimplantation and immediate contralateral nephrectomy. Survival and recovery to normal function after 5 days' storage; extension to 6 days was unsuccessful.

Previous solutions had given successful preservation for only 8–16 h in canine, porcine or rodent models. UW solution allowed reliable and near 100% successful preservation in dog and in rat livers for 24 h. Extended preservation for 30–48 h was also possible experimentally.

Clinical practice requires immediate function for liver grafts. Currently 80% or more grafts function adequately; about 10% show initially poor graft function (IPF) and about 5% of grafts show permanent non-function (PNF), necessitating life-saving retransplantation. Factors influencing and responsible for poor initial function include fatty change in the donor liver, older donor age, preliminary liver reduction surgery and longer cold storage [2]. Although clinical preservation times of 24–30 h are possible, it is thus preferable to keep storage times to under 12 h for optimal results [60]. Clinical best practice remains hypothermic storage using UW solution. When using high-K UW solution for preservation, a prevascularization rinse with a further washout solution is desirable: Carolina Rinse solutions are preferable to the widely used Ringer's lactate rinse [61]. Important considerations, whatever the composition of the solution, are that a brief rinse should be performed at room or body temperature; and that a basic ECF-like crystalloid composition can be enhanced by addition of adenosine, allopurinol, desferrioxamine and glycine. Glucose, fructose or other nutrients are probably unnecessary in either the cold preserving solutions or the pretransplant rinse. Other additions to UW solution have been pentoxyfilline, chlorpromazine and calcium channel blockers, prostaglandins, eicanosoids and lazaroids. Future modifications may incorporate these together with glycine and reversed Na^+/K^+ content.

7.3. Pancreas

UW solution was originally introduced to improve pancreas preservation, which requires preservation of the essential insulin-producing beta cells. Exocrine cell function can provide a marker of viability in the form of amylase excretion. Another important aim of preservation is to minimize the occurrence of ischaemia-induced acute pancreatitis, which adds morbidity after transplantation. Preservation of the pancreas using Collins' and other solutions proved difficult, and it was not until the advent of UW solution that reliable preservation for 24 h was achieved experimentally and clinically. Experimental preservation has since been extended to 96 h using UW with an added prostanoid inhibitor [62]. Other variations of UW can give satisfactory cold storage, including removal of HES or its replacement with dextran, and combinations of sodium lactobionate with histidine [42,63,64].

The pancreas has also been studied in relation to the benefit of additional oxygen using a two layer storage technique with a perfluorochemical adjacent to UW solution. In small animals, the technique of cold storage, whether surrounded by the preserving liquid or wrapped in moistened gauze, has influenced efficacy of preservation. This may be related to the filamentous and non-encapsulated nature of the pancreas, resulting in a greater tendency for harmful oedema and weight gain to occur during storage [65,66].

Preservation needs to include the associated duodenal segment containing the duodenal papilla and pancreatic ducts. Fortunately the duodenum has not proved to be more sensitive to preservation injury than the pancreas itself.

7.4. Small bowel

Small bowel grafts can be transplanted alone or combined with liver or pancreas. The main site of injury during small bowel preservation has been thought to be the endothelium and basement membrane of the highly vascularized mucosa. The small intestine contains a high concentration of the enzyme xanthine oxidase, rendering it liable to reperfusion injury. Free radical damage has been implicated particularly after prolonged preservation and after warm ischaemic injury. Experimental preservation is possible for up to 48 h in the rat and dog, and the advantages of any one

preservation solution are less obvious than with other organs. Sucrose, Collins', UW and Bretschneider's solutions, and solutions with added dextran and containing free radical scavengers have given more or less equivalent results [67]. Pretransplant rinsing has not been helpful in preventing reperfusion injury. Polyethylene glycol has been suggested as an additive both to enhance preservation and to modify rejection in experimental small bowel, heart and pancreas transplantation [68].

7.5. Heart

Preservation of the vasculature together with myocytes and conductive tissue is vital for optimal cardiac preservation. Simple hypothermic storage has been used for clinical heart transplantation since the earliest days. As most of the energy consumed by the heart fuels contraction of the myofibrils, and as the ischaemic heart continues beating until all its fuel has been depleted, cardioplegic arrest has been an essential feature of heart preservation. The development of heart transplantation from open heart surgery influenced significantly early strategies of heart preservation. The heart was excised after induction of hypothermic cardioplegic arrest by an *in situ* flush with one of several standard cardioplegic solutions. Cardioplegic solutions previously developed for cardiac surgery were applied to cardiac transplantation (Table 8). Stanford, St Thomas's and Bretschneider's solutions provided effective preservation of myocardial function for up to 6–8 h. Flushing solutions used to preserve other organs are also cardioplegic, but generally contain much higher concentrations of potassium (> 100 mM rather than 20 mM); and no calcium. Initial reluctance to use these solutions in heart preservation stemmed from studies which indicated that such levels of potassium were deleterious [69]. A 'calcium paradox' effect in cardiac preservation was also important: cardiac

Table 8. Cardioplegic solutions.

	St Thomas's	Stanford
Sodium (mmol/l)	120	125
Potassium (mmol/l)	16	18
Magnesium (mmol/l)	16	–
Calcium (mmol/l)	1.2	–
Chloride (mmol/l)	160	98
Bicarbonate (mmol/l)	10	25
Osmolality (mmol/kg)	320	400
pH (at 0°C)	7.3	8.2

muscle when incubated in calcium-free medium undergoes severe and irreversible damage when reperfused
with calcium-containing medium due to a massive
influx of calcium. This influx is enhanced by warm
ischaemic damage. Calcium paradox has been seen in
experimental cardiopulmonary bypass, but is possibly
less influential during hypothermia [70].

Following the development of UW solution and its
introduction as a solution appropriate for multi-organ
transplantation, studies of UW and UW-derived solutions were applied to open heart surgery and to heart
transplantation. Experimental models have ranged
from heterotopic transplantation into the abdomen or
neck in small animals, isolated perfused working heart
models, metabolic tissue analysis and histology,
nuclear magnetic resonance spectroscopy and allograft
function in large animals [71–73]. UW solution has
given superior donor heart preservation over that obtained by Stanford or St Thomas's solution in randomized clinical trials [74–76]. Repeated cold flushing
with UW or other solutions was detrimental to hypothermic storage. Generation of oxygen free radicals has
been implicated in ischaemic heart disease and in
reperfusion injury after transplantation. Several agents
have been used to pretreat the donor and as additions
to the preserving solutions. Addition of ATP or its precursors to preserving solutions sometimes improves
cardiac function, but this is not necessarily due to
improved high-energy phosphate levels. Many institutions pre-oxygenate the solution. Other additives
thought to be of importance include adenosine, pyruvate and aspartate, prostaglandins to improve perfusion, pentoxifylline to diminish neutrophil-induced
vascular injury and neutrophil adhesion, and lazaroids
(21-aminosteroids) to prevent lipid peroxidation. Nitric
oxide (NO) is a biological messenger with diverse
effects. Failure of the NO pathway during preservation
and transplantation results in formation of oxygen free
radicals during reperfusion, which quench available
NO. Augmentation of NO by cGMP-dependent
mechanisms can enhance vascular function after
ischaemia and reperfusion [77].

7.5.1. *Columbia University solution* (CU, Table 9)

A novel preservation solution, developed primarily for
cardiac preservation, incorporates many of the salient
features of UW solution (potassium 120 mM, magnesium 5 mM, adenosine 5 mM) and a colloid (dextran
50 g/l). Added components include glucose, verapamil,
cysteine and heparin, together with agents enhancing
vascular homeostatic mechanisms by repleting extra-
cellular/intracellular messengers, and nitroglycerin to
enhance nitric oxide-related mechanisms. This solution

Table 9. Flushing solutions for cardiac preservation Columbia University solution (CU).

Potassium (mmol/l)	120
Magnesium (mmol/l)	5
Gluconate (mmol/l)	95
Phosphate (mmol/l)	25
Glucose (mmol/l)	67
Adenose (mmol/l)	5
N-acetyl cysteine (mmol/l)	0.5
Butylated hydroxyanisole (μmol/l)	50
Butylated hydroxytoluene (μmol/l)	50
Verapamil (μmol/l)	10
Nitroglycerin (mg/ml)	0.1
Dibutyryl cAMP (mmol/l)	2
Heparin (μ/l)	10
Dextran (g/l)	50
Osmolality (mmol/kg)	325
pH	7.6

contains a cAMP analogue and has extended cardiac
preservation beyond that observed with UW alone in
both rat and baboon cardiac transplant models. Primate
hearts have been stored for 24 h in CU solution and
have functioned normally after orthotopic cardiac
transplantation [78].

7.6. Lung and heart–lung

Simple cooling has been used for short term preservation of heart–lung transplants. Lungs were originally flushed with cold EuroCollins' solution via the
pulmonary artery immediately after induction of cardioplegia. Flushing should maintain pressure below
that normally found in the pulmonary artery.
Hyperinflation of the lung prior to storage was shown
to be beneficial [79]. Treatment of the donor with
prostaglandin E_1 followed by a hypothermic flush gave
adequate 6 h preservation [80].

Single lung transplantation is now increasingly
common and lung preservation using a EuroCollins'
flush is successful for only 5–6 h. Progressive deterioration with increased pulmonary vascular resistance and
decreased compliance occurs by 12 h, with interstitial
haemorrhage and oedema by 24 h. The disaccharide
trehalose has been substituted for glucose in
EuroCollins' solution, with advantage [81]. Increasing
experience with lung and heart–lung transplantation
has demonstrated that the lung may be more robust
than previously thought in relation to its tolerance of
extended storage. UW and other solutions have given
successful preservation for 24 h [82]. Additions to the

preserving solution which have been found useful have included prostaglandin E₁, pentoxifylline, verapamil and glutathione. Equivalent results to UW solution have been found with a dextran-based low potassium solution [83].

7.7. Composite tissues, limbs

Reconstructive plastic surgery uses vascularized autografts of composite tissues to fill large defects. Such composite grafts involve skin, subcutaneous fat, muscle, bone, nerves and blood vessels. Severed limbs and digits are also replaced as autografts. These complex operative procedures can take many hours. Storage of the grafts relies predominantly on simple external cooling by refrigerated saline and wrapping the grafts in cold saline-soaked packs during implantation. Supplementary vascular flushing has not been widely used to augment hypothermic storage, for fear of damage to the small vessels requiring microvascular suture. Flushing does not give any significant improvement over simple hypothermic storage in cold preserving liquid. Simple hypothermic storage usually adequately covers the periods (usually less than 12 h) required in clinical practice. Tolerance of the various tissues to ischaemia varies: muscle and nerve are more sensitive than skin and bone. It is prudent to remember that restoration of the circulation to reimplanted limbs or other composite grafts of large bulk may release a bolus of high potassium into the circulation and can induce fatal hyperkalaemic cardiac arrest. After extended storage the contained blood or preservation solution should be flushed out with warm plasma or balanced electrolyte solution prior to release of the clamps.

8. Summary and conclusions

Simple hypothermic storage remains the lynch-pin of preservation for all transplantable organs and composite tissues. Flush solutions of widely different character have given equivalent results across a wide range of transplantable vascularized organs, but a unifying theme relevant to multi-organ preservation by hypothermic storage is apparent. The principles of organ preservation include three major aims. First, rapid cooling of the organ by surface and intravascular flushing to a temperature which protects adequately the vasculature, the cellular parenchyma, interstitium, ducts and lumina. Second, all successful solutions contain agents which minimize cell swelling and oedema during hypothermia. Third, preservation can

be enhanced by a variety of adjuvant metabolically and biochemically effective agents aimed at protecting the organ during storage and upon reperfusion.

Current methods of hypothermic storage now give adequate storage times approaching 24 h for all organs. Antigenic manipulations during storage, with polyethylene glycol and possibly other agents, hold prospects for the future.

References

1. Collins GM, Bravo-Shugarman M, Terasaki PI. Kidney preservation for transportation. Initial perfusion and 30 hours' ice storage. Lancet 1969; 2: 1219–22.
2. Belzer FO. Evaluation of preservation of the intra-abdominal organs. Transplant Proc 1993; 25: 2527–30.
3. Wahlberg JA, Southard JH, Belzer FO. Development of a cold storage solution for pancreas preservation. Cryobiology 1986; 23: 477.
4. Gores GJ, Nieminen AL, Fleishman KE, Dawson TL, Hermann B, Lemasters JJ. Extracellular acidosis delays onset of cell death in ATP-depleted hepatocytes. Am J Physiol 1988; 255: C315.
5. Wattiaux R, Wattiaux-De Conninck S. Trapping of mannitol in rat-liver mitochondria and lysosomes. Int Rev Exp Pathol 1984; 26: 85.
6. Ratych RE, Bulkley GB, Williams GM. Ischemia/reperfusion injury in the kidney. Prog Clin Biol Res 1986; 224: 63–89.
7. Burg MB, Orloff MJ. Active cation transport by kidney tubules at 0°C. Am J Physiol 1964; 207: 983–6.
8. Levy MN. Oxygen consumption and blood flow in the hypothermic, perfused kidney. Am J Physiol 1959; 197: 11.
9. Leaf A. Maintenance of concentration gradients and regulation of cell volume. Ann NY Acad Sci 1959; 72: 396.
10. Collins GM, Wicomb W, Warren R et al. Canine and cadaver kidney preservation with sodium lactobionate sucrose solution (SLS). Transplant Proc 1993; 25: 1588–90.
11. Marshall VC, Howden BO, Thomas AC et al. Extended preservation of dog kidneys with modified UW solution. Transplant Proc 1991; 23: 2366–7.
12. Wahlberg JA, Love R, Landegard L, Southard JH, Belzer FO. 72-hour preservation of the canine pancreas. Transplantation 1987; 3: 5.
13. Sacks SA, Petritsch PH, Kaufman JJ. Canine kidney preservation using a new perfusate. Lancet 1973; 1: 1024–8.
14. Collins GM, Hartley LC, Clunie GJ. Kidney preservation for transportation. Experimental analysis of optimal perfusate composition. Br J Surg 1972; 59: 187–9.
15. Collins GM, Green RD, Halasz NA. Importance of anion content and osmolarity in flush solutions for 48 to 72 hr hypothermic kidney storage. Cryobiology 1979; 16: 217.
16. Hardie I, Balderson G, Hamlyn L, McKay D, Clunie G. Extended ice storage of canine kidneys using hyperosmolar Collins' solution. Transplantation 1977; 23: 282–3.
17. Halasz NA, Collins GM. Forty-eight-hour kidney preservation. A comparison of flushing and ice storage with perfusion. Arch Surg 1976; 111: 175–7.
18. Andrews PM, Bates SB. Improving EuroCollins flushing solution's ability to protect kidneys from normothermic ischemia. Miner Electrolyte Metab 1985; 11: 309–13.
19. Bretan PN, Baldwin N, Martinez A et al. Improved renal transplant preservation using a modified intracellular flush solution (PB-2). Characterization of mechanisms by renal clearance, high performance liquid chromatography, phosphorus-31 magnetic resonance spectroscopy, and electron microscopy studies. Urol Res 1991; 19: 73–80.

20. Grino JM, Castelao AM, Sebate I et al. Low-dose cyclosporine, ALG and steroids in first cadaveric renal transplants. Transplant Proc 1987; 19: 3674–6.

21. Ross H, Marshall VC, Escott ML. 72-hour canine kidney preservation without continuous perfusion. Transplantation 1976; 21: 498–501.

22. Marshall VC, Ross H, Scott DF et al. Preservation of cadaver renal allografts: comparison of ice storage and machine perfusion. Med J Aust 1977; 2: 353–6.

23. Jablonski P, Howden BO, Marshall VC, Scott DF. Evaluation of citrate flushing solution using the isolated perfused kidney. Transplantation 1980; 30: 239–43.

24. Marshall VC, Howden BO, Jablonski P, Tavanlis G, Tange J. Sucrose-containing solutions for kidney preservation. Cryobiology 1985; 22: 622.

25. Lam FT, Mavor AID, Potts DJ, Giles GR. Improved 72-hour renal preservation with phosphate buffered sucrose. Transplantation 1989; 47: 767–71.

26. Lam FT, Ubhi CS, Mavor AID, Lodge JPA, Giles GR. Clinical evaluation of PBS140 solution for cadaveric renal preservation. Transplantation 1989; 48: 1067–8.

27. Lodge JPA, Perry SL, Skinner C, Potts DJ, Giles GR. Improved porcine renal preservation with a simple extracellular solution-PBS140. Comparison with hyperosmolar citrate and University of Wisconsin solution. Transplantation 1991; 51: 574–9.

28. Erhard J, Lange R, Scherer R et al. Comparison of histidine-tryptophane-ketoglutarate (HTK) solution versus University of Wisconsin (UW) solution for organ preservation in human liver transplantation. A prospective, randomized study. Transplant Int 1994; 7: 177–81.

29. Groenewoud AF, Thorogood J. A preliminary report of the HTK randomized multicenter study comparing kidney graft preservation with HTK and EuroCollins solutions. Transplant Proc 1992; 5: 429–32.

30. Belzer FO, D'Alessandro AM, Hoffman RM et al. The use of UW solution in clinical transplantation. A 4-year experience. Ann Surg 1992; 215: 579–83.

31. Stein DG, Drinkwater DC, Laks H. Cardiac preservation in patients undergoing transplantation. A clinical trial comparing UW solution and Stanford solution. J Thorac Cardiovasc Surg 1991; 102: 657–65.

32. D'Alessandro AM, Reed A, Hoffman RM et al. Results of combined hepatic, pancreaticoduodenal, and renal procurements. Transplant Proc 1991; 23: 2309–11.

33. Ploeg RJ, van Bockel JH, Langendijk PT et al. Effect of preservation solution on results of cadaveric kidney transplantation. The European Multicentre Study Group. Lancet 1992; 340: 129–37.

34. Hefty T, Fraser S, Nelson K, Bennett W. Comparison of UW and EuroCollins solutions in paired cadaveric kidneys. Transplantation 1992; 53: 491–2.

35. Jacobsson J, Tufveson G, Odlind B, Wahlberg J. The effect of type of preservation solution and hemodilution of the recipient on postischemic erythrocyte trapping in kidney grafts. Transplantation 1989; 47: 876–9.

36. Baatard R, Pradier F, Dantal J et al. Prospective randomized comparison of University of Wisconsin and UW-modified, lacking hydroxyethyl-starch, cold-storage solutions in kidney transplantation. Transplantation 1993; 55: 31–5.

37. Moen J, Claesson K, Pienaar H et al. Preservation of dog liver, kidney, and pancreas using the Belzer-UW solution with a high-sodium and low potassium content. Transplantation 1989; 47: 940–5.

38. Biguzas M, Jablonski P, Howden BO et al. Evaluation of UW solution in rat kidney preservation. II. The effect of pharmacological additives. Transplantation 1990; 49: 1051–5.

39. den Butter G, Lindell SL, Sumimoto R, Schilling MK, Southard JH, Belzer FO. Effect of glycine in dog and rat liver transplantation. Transplantation 1993; 56: 817–22.

40. Zhu Y, Furukawa H, Nakamura K et al. Sodium lactobionate sucrose solution for canine liver and kidney preservation. Transplant Proc 1993; 25: 1618–19.

41. Tokunaga Y, Collins GM, Esquivel CO, Wicomb WN. Calcium antagonists in sodium lactobionate sucrose solution for rat liver preservation. Transplantation 1992; 53: 726–30.

42. Sumimoto R, Dohi K, Urushihara T et al. An examination of the effects of solutions containing histidine and lactobionate for heart, pancreas and liver preservation in the rat. Transplantation 1992; 53: 1206–10.

43. Marshall VC, Howden BO, Jablonski P. Effect of storage temperature in rat liver transplantation: 4°C is optimal and gives successful 48h preservation. Transplant Proc 1994; 26: 3657–8.

44. Fischer JH, Czerniak A, Hauer U, Isselhard W. A new simple method for optimal storage of ischemically damaged kidneys. Transplantation 1978; 24: 43–9.

45. Rolles K, Foreman J, Pegg DE. Preservation of ischemically injured canine kidneys by retrograde oxygen persufflation. Transplantation 1984; 38: 102–6.

46. Ross H, Escott ML. Renal preservation with gaseous perfusion. Transplant Proc 1982; 13: 693–5.

47. Sumimoto R, Southard JH, Belzer FO. Livers from fasted rats acquire resistance to warm and cold ischemia injury. Transplantation 1993; 55: 728–32.

48. Pegg DE, Wusterman MC, Foreman J. Metabolism of normal and ischemically injured rabbit kidneys during perfusion for 48 hours at 10°C. Transplantation 1981; 32: 437–43.

49. Kuroda Y, Tanioka Y, Morita A et al. Protective effect of preservation of canine pancreas by the two-layer (University of Wisconsin solution/perfluorochemical) method against rewarming ischemic injury during implantation. Transplantation 1994; 57: 658–61.

50. Rijikmans B, Buurman WA, Kootstra G. Six day canine kidney preservation. Hypothermic perfusion combined with isolated blood perfusion. Transplantation 1984; 27: 130–4.

51. Gaber AO, Yang HC, Haag BW et al. Intermediate normothermic hemoperfusion doubles safe cold preservation of rat kidneys. Transplant Proc 1987; 9: 1369–71.

52. Emre S, Schwartz ME, Mor E et al. Obviation of pre-reperfusion rinsing and decrease in preservation/reperfusion injury in liver transplantation by portal blood flushing. Transplantation 1994; 57: 799–803.

53. Gao W, Takei Y, Marzi I et al. Carolina rinse solution: a new strategy to increase survival time after orthotopic liver transplantation in the rat. Transplantation 1991; 52: 417–19.

54. Gao W, Hijioka T, Lindert K, Caldwell-Kenkel J, Lemasters J, Thurman R. Evidence that adenosine is a key component in Carolina rinse responsible for reducing graft failure after orthotopic liver transplantation in the rat. Transplantation 1991; 52: 992–8.

55. Egawa H, Esquivel CO, Wicomb WN, Kennedy RG, Collins GM. Significance of terminal rinse for rat liver preservation. Transplantation 1993; 56: 1344–7.

56. Bachmann S, Caldwell-Kenkel JC, Currin RT et al. Protection by pentoxyifylline against graft failure from storage injury after orthotopic rat liver transplantation with arterialization. Transplant Int 1992; 5: 345–50.

57. Post S, Palma P, Rentsch M, Gonzalez AP, Otto G, Menger MD. Importance of rinse solution vs preservation solution in prevention of microcirculatory damage after liver transplantation in the rat. Transplant Proc 1993; 25: 1607.

58. Gonzalez AP, Post S, Palma P, Rentsch M, Menger MD. Essential components of Carolina rinse for attenuation of reperfusion injury in rat liver transplantation. Transplant Proc 1993; 25: 2538–9.

59. Heil JE, Canafax DM, Sutherland DER, Simmons RL, Dunn M, Najarian J. A controlled comparison of kidney preservation by two methods: matching perfusion and cold storage. Transplant Proc 1987; 19: 2046.

60. Adam R, Bismuth H, Diamond T *et al.* Effect of extended cold ischaemia with UW solution on graft function after liver transplantation. Lancet 1992; 340: 1373–6.

61. Sanchez-Urdazpal L, Gores GJ, Lemasters JJ *et al.* Carolina rinse solution decreases liver injury during clinical liver transplantation. Transplant Proc 1993; 25: 1574–5.

62. Kin S, Stephanian E, Gores P *et al.* Successful 96-hr cold storage preservation of canine pancreas with UW solution containing the thromboxane A2 synthesis inhibitor OKY046. J Surg Res 1992; 52: 577–82.

63. Urushihara T, Sumimoto R, Sumimoto K *et al.* A comparison of some simplified lactobionate preservation solutions with standard UW solution and EuroCollins solution for pancreas preservation. Transplantation 1992; 53: 750–4.

64. Morel P, Moss A, Schlumpf R *et al.* 72-hour preservation of the canine pancreas: successful replacement of hydroxy-ethylstarch by dextran-40 in UW solution. Transplant Proc 1992; 24: 791–4.

65. Urushihara T, Sumimoto K, Ikeda M, Hong HQ, Fukuda Y, Dohi K. A comparative study of two-layer cold storage with perfluorochemical alone and University of Wisconsin solution for rat pancreas preservation. Transplantation 1994; 57: 1684–6.

66. Howden BO, Jablonski P, Marshall VC. A novel approach to pancreas preservation: does the gaseous milieu matter? Transplant Proc 1992; 24: 795–6.

67. Muller AR, Nalesnik M, Platz KP, Langrehr JM, Hoffman RA, Schraut WH. Evaluation of preservation conditions and various solutions for small bowel preservation. Transplantation 1994; 57: 649–55.

68. Itasaka H, Burns W, Wicomb WN, Egawa H. Collins G, Esquivel CO. Modification of rejection by polyethylene glycol in small bowel transplantation. Transplantation 1994; 57: 645–8.

69. Harjula A, Mattila S, Mattila I *et al.* Coronary endothelial damage after crystalloid cardioplegia. J Thorac Cardiovasc Surg 1984; 25: 147–52.

70. Alto LE, Dhalla NS. Hypothermia appears to protect against calcium paradox role of changes in microsomal calcium uptake in the effects of reperfusion of calcium-deprived hearts. Circulation Res 1981; 48: 17–24.

71. Stringham JC, Paulsen KL, Southard JH, Mentzer RM Jr, Belzer FO. Prolonging myocardial preservation with a modified University of Wisconsin solution containing 2, 3-butanedione monoxime and calcium. J Thorac Cardiovasc Surg 1994; 107: 764–75.

72. Lasley RD, Mentzer RM Jr. The role of adenosine in extended myocardial preservation with the University of Wisconsin solution. J Thorac Cardiovasc Surg 1994; 107: 1356–63.

73. Mertes PM, Burtin P, Carteaux JP *et al.* Changes in hemo-dynamic performance and oxygen consumption during brain death in the pig. Transplant Proc 1994; 26: 229–30.

74. Demertzis S, Wippermann J, Schaper J *et al.* University of Wisconsin versus St Thomas's Hospital solution for human donor heart preservation. Ann Thorac Surg 1993; 55: 1131–7.

75. Stein DG, Drinkwater DC Jr, Laks H *et al.* Cardiac pre-servation in patients undergoing transplantation. A clinical trial comparing University of Wisconsin solution and Stanford solution. J Thorac Cardiovasc Surg 1991; 102: 657–65.

76. Jeevandandam V, Barr ML, Auteri JS *et al.* University of Wisconsin solution versus crystalloid cardioplegia for human donor heart preservation. A randomized blinded prospective clinical trial. J Thorac Cardiovasc Surg 1992; 103: 194–8.

77. Pinsky DJ, Oz MC, Koga S *et al.* Cardiac preservation is enhanced in a heterotopic rat transplant model by sup-plementing the nitric oxide pathway. J Clin Invest 1994; 93: 2291–7.

78. Oz MC, Pinski DJ, Koga S *et al.* Novel preservation solution permits 24-hour preservation in rat and baboon cardiac transplant models. Circulation 1993; 88: II291–7.

79. Puskas JD, Hirai T, Christie N, Mayer E, Slutsky AS, Patterson GA. Reliable thirty-hour lung preservation by donor lung hyperinflation. J Thorac Cardiovasc Surg 1992; 104: 1075–83.

80. Kirk AJ, Colquhoun IW, Dark JH. Lung preservation: a review of current practice and future directions. Ann Thorac Surg 1993; 56: 990–1000.

81. Hirata T, Yokomise H, Fukuse T *et al.* Effects of trehalose in preservation of canine lung for transplants. J Thorac Cardiovasc Surg 1993; 41: 59–63.

82. Kawahara K, Itoyanagi N, Takahashi T, Akamine S, Kobayashi M, Tomota M. Transplantation of canine lung allografts preserved in UW solution for 24 hours. Transplantation 1993; 55: 15–18.

83. Steen S, Kimblad PO, Sjoberg T, Lindberg L, Ingemansson R, Massa G. Safe lung preservation for twenty-four hours with Perfadex. Ann Thorac Surg 1994; 57: 450–7.

14 | Pulsatile preservation in renal transplantation

MITCHELL L. HENRY

1. Introduction

A subtle but important part of the success of cadaveric renal transplantation has been effective and prolonged organ preservation. During the early 1970s, pulsatile perfusion for preservation of kidneys was used by the majority of centres in the United States. This gradually changed later in the decade to a predominance of simple cold storage. There were a number of reasons for this change, including reports demonstrating few or no benefits of pulsatile perfusion over cold storage, as well as the perception that cold storage was significantly easier to accomplish from a technical standpoint and was less expensive. Interestingly, there now appears to be a trend towards pulsatile perfusion.

Advantages of pulsatile perfusion include (1) lower incidence of early dysfunction (i.e. ATN), (2) better preservation over longer periods of time (especially > 24 h), (3) the ability to monitor flow rates and pressures, thus intrarenal resistance during perfusion, (4) decreased intrarenal vasospasm, (5) ability to provide metabolic support during perfusion and (6) potential to manipulate flow pharmacologically during perfusion. Potential disadvantages include increased costs, endothelial injury, and equipment failure.

It is becoming clear that one of the most important determinants of early graft outcome (i.e. one year survival) is the quality of the organ at the time of transplantation. Preservation injury, or lack of it, can affect early graft outcome. Several studies have shown that patients requiring dialysis after transplantation (early dysfunction) have significantly poorer graft survival at 1 year than do those with good early graft function [1–5]. This can be as significant as a 20% decline in

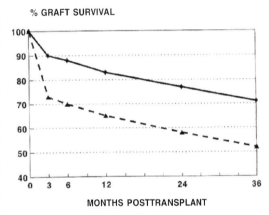

Figure 1. Differential graft survival in patients demonstrating early graft function (no dialysis, ♦) or early dysfunction (dialysis, ▲).

graft survival at 1 year (Fig. 1) [5]. This concept can be reinforced by comparing the outcomes of three categories of recipients (as demonstrated by Terasaki [6]) all with minimal preservation times, but differing graft survival as presented classically. These are (1) living related haploidentical recipients (2) non-related living donor/recipient combinations and (3) recipients of cadaveric kidneys with less than 6 h preservation time (Fig. 2). There is essentially no difference in 1-year graft survival in these patients as the variable of preservation is essentially removed, although survival might classically be thought better in the living related recipient, with the non-related living donor recipient in the middle and the cadaveric recipient with the worst survival of the three categories. If, in fact, organ

G.M. Collins, J.M. Dubernard, W. Land and G.G. Persijn (eds). Procurement, Preservation and Allocation of Vascularized Organs 131–135
© 1997 Kluwer Academic Publishers.

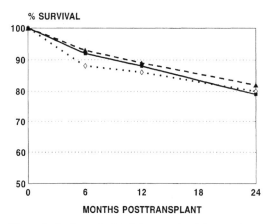

Figure 2. Graft survival in living unrelated (■, *n* = 282), haploidentical living related (▲, *n* = 3039) or mismatched cadaver (preservation < 6 h) (◇, *n* = 245) donor–recipient combination.

quality is an important predictor of outcome, pulsatile preservation might be able to improve graft survival.

2. Costs

One of the previously identified disadvantages associated with pulsatile preservation was the cost, compared with simple cold storage. Initial costs associated with the mechanical equipment, as well as the costs of disposable items (perfusion cassettes) and technician time can make pulsatile preservation appear to consume significantly more resources. However, if pulsatile perfusion can really decrease the rate of early dysfunction of transplanted kidneys, considerable cost saving can be realized both in terms of hospital dollars (initial hospital stay) and fewer graft losses. Graft losses are expensive as the patient is returned to dialysis without the benefit of the costs of the transplant procedure and are less likely to be successfully retransplanted, furthering the reliance on expensive long term maintenance dialysis. As previously noted, kidneys suffering from early dysfunction have significantly poorer 1 year graft survival than those with immediate function. In our programme initial hospital costs for a primary renal transplant are increased by 57% in patients with early dysfunction compared with those with immediate function, and increase even further (by 65%) for a retransplant with early dysfunction (not published). Rosenthal *et al.* [7] also found that average hospital charges for primary adult renal cadaveric recipients were nearly $32 000 more for recipients with delayed graft function compared with those with immediate

function, with an increase in the mean hospital stay of almost 10 days. Johnson [8] showed that initial hospital costs of patients with delayed graft function were significantly higher than those for patients with immediate function treated either with ALG induction therapy or immediate cyclosporine. Decreasing the incidence of delayed graft function with pulsatile preservation (even minimally) can, therefore, produce large cost savings.

3. Mechanics

Several important features of the perfusion device make pulsatile perfusion unique. The pump primarily generates pressure and, secondarily, a pulsatile fluid wave that allows perfusion of the renal vasculature. A pressure transducer placed in line with the tubing monitors pressures continuously. The heat exchanger provides for continuous cooling of the preservation fluid by circulating cold fluid in close proximity to the preservation solution. Closely associated is ongoing temperature monitoring by a temperature probe. Membrane oxygenators allow for passive diffusion of high local oxygen concentration to the passing preservation solution.

The overall setup of the device is shown in Figure 3. In general, most of the perfusate resides in a dependently placed reservoir. Proximal tubing leaves the reservoir and the perfusate is propelled via the pump, past the heat exchanger, to a proximal perfusate chamber (where medications can be injected), to the chambers where the kidneys are housed. The kidneys are attached either separately via the renal artery or *en bloc* via the aorta by special cannulae attached to this proximal tubing. The perfusate effluent then drains through a filter and into graduated reservoirs (one for each of the two perfusion chambers) in order to measure each renal perfusate flow (ml/min). This then drains past the membrane oxygenator back to the main reservoir for recirculation.

The mechanics allow manipulation of either the renal vasculature or the perfusate. We routinely infuse vasodilators directly into the efferent limb of the system when intrarenal resistance has been identified as being elevated. The use of calcium channel blocking agents (e.g. verapamil), papaverine or priscoline have allowed effective dilation of constricted renal vasculature under many circumstances (data not published). Zucker *et al.* [9] have suggested that the quantitative load of hepatitis C virus transplanted in a kidney from a hepatitis C-positive donor can be diminished significantly by simple pulsatile perfusion of that

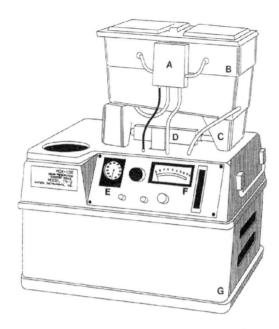

Figure 3. Perfusion chamber. (A) Proximal perfusate chamber; (B) chamber housing kidneys; (C) perfusate reservoir; (D) pulsatile pump; (E) pressure monitor; (F) temperature monitor; (G) base of transport module (Courtesy Waters, Inc., Rochester, MN).

kidney. Strategies for insertion of in-line filters to trap infectious particles may be an important use of pulsatile preservation in the future.

4. Preservation solutions

Preservation solutions have matured in the recent past. Cryoprecipitated plasma was used widely in the early days of pulsatile preservation, but because of inter-batch variability, complex preparation techniques and potential transmission of disease, fell from favour. Other alternative solutions arose such as human serum albumin (HSA), plasma protein fraction (PPF), and silica gel fraction (SGF). The Belzer perfusate was developed at the University of Wisconsin and has gained favour for pulsatile preservation in many American centres. It has been used in two forms, differing primarily only in the colloid fraction. The first was an albumin-based solution, but the more recent form is pentastarch based. Both have provided excellent clinical outcome, with the latter demonstrating superior results in some centres [10,11] (Table 1). Colloid support in the perfusate is mandatory to prevent interstitial oedema during pulsatile preservation. Other important components of

Table 1. Outcome as a function of preservation solution.		
Study	Albumin	HES
Hoffman [10]	14.9%	8.6%
Barber [11]	19%	13%
Ohio State	10%	3%

these solutions include gluconate to prevent cell oedema, glutathione and elevated potassium to prevent losses of these components from inside the cell, and adenosine and phosphate to allow for maintenance of intracellular high-energy phosphate molecules.

5. Outcome

Conclusions from studies directly comparing the outcome of simple cold-stored kidneys versus those preserved using pulsatile perfusion are somewhat difficult to make. Small prospective studies have been performed, and larger retrospective investigations are also available for review. Table 2 lists many of these for comparison. Those that demonstrate differences in early function associated with method of preservation tend to favour pulsatile perfusion. Of the five randomized prospective trials, three demonstrated significantly improved immediate function with pulsatile preservation while two showed statistically insignificant differences favouring simple cold storage. The two studies with the largest patient populations are neither prospective nor randomized, but each demonstrates at least a 10% improvement in early function with pulsatile perfusion [11,17]. Those studies that compared length of perfusion consistently found that immediate function was improved in the pulsatile perfusion group under conditions of prolonged preservation [11,17]. It has also been shown that 'imported' kidneys previously stored on ice and pump perfused secondarily can have excellent immediate function (with prolonged storage times) when compared with those subjected to immediate pulsatile preservation [18].

Some reports suggest that the characteristics of pulsatile perfusion can help identify those kidneys likely to show early dysfunction and help with decision making as to their use. Henry [19] has shown that kidneys with significantly elevated intrarenal resistances during perfusion are at an increased risk to develop delayed graft fraction. Tesi [20] has demonstrated that secondary pulsatile perfusion in imported kidneys from marginal donors (previously cold stored)

Table 2. Summary of studies of simple cold storage versus pulsatile preservation.

Study		n	DGF Iced	DGF Pumped	p
Alijani [12]	a	29	63%		
	b	29		17%	< 0.01
Merion [13]	a	51	31%		
	b	51		41%	NS
Halloran [14]	a	90	44%		
		91		31%	0.003
Mendez [15]	a	26	65%		
	b	26		35%	not reported
Heil [16]	a	27	41%		
	b	27		52%	NS
Barber [11]		346	29%		
		290		19% (alb)	
		188		13% (HES)	0.0001
Koyama [17]		18 637	27%		
		2 944		16%	< 0.01
Johnson [8]		18	17%		
		82		4%	NS

a prospective, randomized trial.
b paired kidney 1 simple cold stored, 1 pulsatile perfused.

may help identify organs which are likely to perform poorly by following perfusion characteristics.

While immediate function is clearly a multifactorial process, we believe that pulsatile machine preservation is very important in providing a low incidence of early graft dysfunction. We have recently reviewed the results of pulsatile perfusion at Ohio State over the last 11 years. Overall, 4.4% of patients receiving a total of 1513 kidneys required post-transplant dialysis. All organs were preserved with pulsatile perfusion either primarily or secondarily (following a period of simple cold storage). All patients received polyclonal or monoclonal induction therapy followed by a delayed cyclosporine-based maintenance immunotherapy. The average length of preservation was 18.6 h for those primarily perfused ($n = 1040$) and > 33 h in the secondarily perfused group ($n = 473$). While there was no control group for simple cold storage, we feel this is strong support for the efficacy of pulsatile perfusion.

6. Summary and conclusions

Short and long term graft survival is significantly improved when a graft functions immediately (as opposed to early dysfunction requiring dialysis), emphasizing the need for efforts directed at this post-transplant variable. Studies of outcomes with kidneys preserved by pulsatile preservation almost all demonstrate very low rates of early dysfunction post-transplant. Many have discounted mechanical perfusion as too expensive; however, reports show that overall costs in dollars, as well as costs reflected by graft loss, when considered globally, are reduced by the use of pulsatile preservation for renal transplantation. Current preservation solutions (primarily the Belzer perfusate) have contributed to the improvement in outcome with machine perfusion, and positive improvements with the heptastarch based solutions have been demonstrated. Several small, prospective studies have compared pulsatile preservation with simple cold storage. While not definitive, the trend favours improved graft quality with machine preservation. This is reinforced strongly by larger retrospective and single centre experiences. The trend back toward the use of pulsatile preservation appears to be justified by the existing data. With the prospect of longer duration of cold ischaemia mandated by various organ sharing proposals, along with the increasing use of the marginal and non-heart beating donor, pulsatile perfusion may actually improve the quality of the organ during preservation and allow for excellent preservation and early post-transplant graft function.

References

1. Sanfilippo F, Vaughn WK, Spees EK, Lucas BA. The detrimental effects of delayed graft function in cadaver donor renal transplantation. Transplantation 1984; 38: 643-8.
2. Halloran PF, Aprile MA, Farewell V et al. Early function as the principal correlate of graft survival. Transplantation 1988; 46: 223.
3. Lim EC, Terasaki PI. Early graft function. In: Terasaki P, Cecka JM, (eds.), Clinical Transplants 1991. UCLA Tissue Typing Laboratory, Los Angeles 1992; pp. 401-7.
4. Ferguson RM and the Transplant Information Share Group (TISG). A multicenter experience with sequential ALG/ cyclosporine therapy in renal transplantation. Clin Transplant 1988; 2: 285.
5. Cecka JM, Terasaki PI. The UNOS Scientific Renal Transplant Registry – 1990. In: Terasaki P (ed.), Clinical Transplants 1990. UCLA Tissue Typing Laboratory, Los Angeles 1991; p. 1.
6. Terasaki PI, Cecka JM, Lim E, Takemoto S, Cho Y Gjertson D, Ogura K, Koyama H, Mitsuishi Y, Yuge J, Cohn M. Overview. In: Terasaki P (ed.), Clinical Transplants 1991. UCLA Tissue Typing Laboratory, Los Angeles 1992; p. 416.
7. Rosenthal JT, Danovitch GM, Wilkinson A, Ettenger RB. The high cost of delayed graft function in cadaveric renal transplantation. Transplantation 1991; 51: 1115-39.
8. Johnson CP, Roza AM, Adams MB. Local procurement with pulsatile perfusion gives excellent results and minimizes initial cost associated with renal transplantation. Transplant Proc 1990; 22: 385-7.

9. Zucker K, Cirocco R, Roth D *et al.* Depletion of hepatitis C virus from procured kidneys using pulsatile perfusion preservation. Transplantation 1994; 57: 832–40.

10. Hoffmann RM, Stratta RJ, D'Alessandro AM *et al.* Combined cold storage-perfusion preservation with a new synthetic perfusate. Transplantation 1989; 47: 32–7.

11. Gruessner RW, Nakhleh R, Tzardis P *et al.* Rejection in single versus combined pancreas and kidney transplantation in pigs. Transplantation 1993; 56: 1053–62.

12. Alijani MR, Cutler JA, DelValle CJ *et al.* Single-donor cold storage versus machine perfusion in cadaver kidney preservation. Transplantation 1985; 40: 659–61.

13. Merion RM, Oh HK, Port FK, Toledo-Pereyra LH, Turcotte JG. A prospective controlled trial of cold-storage versus machine-perfusion preservation in cadaveric renal transplantation. Transplantation 1990; 50: 230–3.

14. Halloran P, Aprile M. A randomized prospective trial of cold storage versus pulsatile perfusion for cadaver kidney preservation. Transplantation 1987; 43: 827–32.

15. Mendez R, Mendez RG, Koussa N, Cats S, Bogaard TP, Khetan U. Preservation effect on oligo-anuria in the cyclo-sporine era: a prospective trial with 26 paired cadaveric renal allografts. Transplant Proc 1987; 19: 2047–50.

16. Heil JE, Canafax DM, Sutherland DER, Simmons RL, Dunning M, Najarian JS. A controlled comparison of kidney preservation by two methods: machine perfusion and cold storage. Transplant Proc 1987; 19: 2046.

17. Koyama H, Cecka JM, Terasaki PI. A comparison of cadaver donor kidney storage methods: pump perfusion and cold storage solutions. Clin Transplantation 1993; 7: 199–205.

18. Henry ML, Sommer BG, Ferguson RM. Improved immediate function of renal allografts with belzer perfusate. Transplantation 1988; 45: 73–5.

19. Henry ML, Sommer BG, Tesi RJ, Ferguson RM. Improved immediate renal allograft function after initial simple cold storage. Transplant Proc 1990; 22: 388–9.

20. Tesi RJ, Elkhammas EA, Davies EA, Henry ML, Ferguson RM. Pulsatile kidney perfusion for evaluation of high-risk kidney donors safely expands the donor pool. Clin Transplant 1994; 8: 134–8.

15 Endothelial cell damage and Kupffer cell activation in reperfusion injury to livers stored for transplantation

John J. Lemasters and Ronald G. Thurman

1. Introduction

Liver transplantation is an accepted therapy that achieves good long-term survival and a return to productive life for children and adults with end-stage liver disease. Scarcity of donor organs and graft dysfunction or failure are major obstacles to more widespread and successful application of liver transplantation surgery. In the USA alone, more than 2000 patients await donor livers, and hundreds die each year because none can be found [1]. In addition, primary non-function of grafts leading to graft failure and retransplantation occurs in 5–15% of patients [2–4]. Initial poor function of transplanted liver grafts occurs in another 20% of patients [5,6]. Since the clinical incidence of primary non-function is strongly dependent on time of cold storage, its aetiology is related to injury associated with graft harvest, storage and reperfusion. Liver damage after cold ischaemic storage is a special instance of the more general phenomenon of ischaemia/reperfusion injury. Recent advances in the understanding of storage/reperfusion injury reveal the many facets of this injury, virtually all of which are applicable to reperfusion injury after warm ischaemia to liver and other organs.

2. Endothelial cell killing and Kupffer cell activation

In rat models, liver reperfusion after prolonged storage produces two prominent effects. The first is the loss of viability of sinusoidal endothelial cells, and the second is the activation of Kupffer cells, the hepatic macrophages (Fig. 1) [7–10]. After storage for 24 h or longer in University of Wisconsin (UW) solution, reperfusion induces loss of endothelial cell viability within minutes (Fig. 2A). Kupffer cell activation also occurs after reperfusion, as evidenced by cell surface ruffling, degranulation, increased phagocytosis, and release of hydrolytic enzymes and oxygen radicals (Fig. 3). Similar non-parenchymal changes are observed in human livers after storage and reperfusion [11,12].

Activated Kupffer cells release several inflammatory mediators in addition to oxygen radicals, including tumour necrosis factor (TNF-α), interleukins (IL) 1 and 6, prostaglandins and nitric oxide (NO). These mediators probably aggravate injury to the transplanted graft and may promote development of the systemic inflammatory response syndrome. Together, endothelial damage and Kupffer cell activation cause marked microcirculatory disturbances within the transplanted liver graft, leading to leucocyte and platelet adhesion, diminished blood flow and a continuation of the ischaemic process [13.14]. In the worst case, these events culminate in inflammation, necrosis and fulminant graft failure requiring emergency retransplantation. However, storage/reperfusion injury occurs to a significant extent in nearly all liver transplantations, as documented by high serum transaminase levels in the first few postoperative days in virtually every liver transplant recipient.

G.M. Collins, J.M. Dubernard, W. Land and G.G. Persijn (eds). Procurement, Preservation and Allocation of Vascularized Organs 137–144
© 1997 Kluwer Academic Publishers.

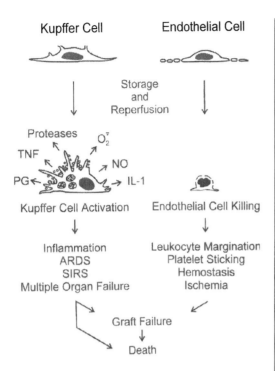

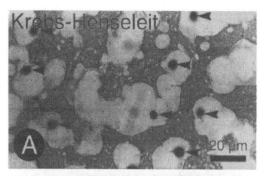

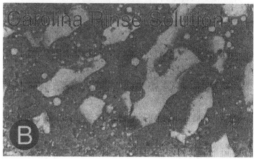

Figure 1. Scheme of storage/reperfusion injury to liver. After storage and reperfusion, endothelial cells lose viability and Kupffer cells swell, ruffle and degranulate, indicating activation. Activated Kupffer cells release several inflammatory mediators, including tumor necrosis factor-alpha (TNF), interleukin-1 (IL-1), proteases, prostaglandins (PG), oxygen radicals (O_2^-), and nitric oxide (NO). Together these changes promote leukocyte margination, platelet sticking, haemostasis and continued ischaemia within the graft, leading to graft failure. In addition, the systemic release of inflammatory mediators promotes the adult respiratory distress syndrome (ARDS), the systemic inflammatory response syndrome (SIRS) and multiple organ failure, all of which culminate in death of the transplant recipient unless retransplantation takes place.

3. The pH paradox of reperfusion injury

The damage caused by storage/reperfusion injury has several causes. One is the stress of restoring normal metabolism after prolonged ischaemia. Tissue pH decreases substantially during both warm and cold ischaemia as a result of ATP hydrolysis and anaerobic glycolysis. Acidotic pH protects against loss of cell viability during ischaemia [15], but the restoration of pH to normal levels during reperfusion accelerates lethal endothelial cell injury in stored livers [16]. Injury may be mediated by activation of latent

Figure 2. Endothelial cell killing after reperfusion of stored rat livers: protection by Carolina Rinse Solution. Rat livers were stored in UW solution for 24 h and reperfused with Krebs–Henseleit bicarbonate buffer (A) or Carolina Rinse Solution (B). Trypan blue was added at the end of reperfusion to identify the nuclei of non-viable cells (arrows).

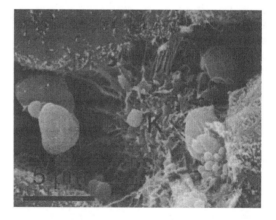

Figure 3. Scanning electron micrograph showing Kupffer cell activation after cold storage and brief reperfusion. Note rounding and ruffling of a Kupffer cell (K).

pH-dependent proteases and phospholipases [17–19]. This worsening of injury when pH returns to normal levels during reperfusion is a 'pH paradox'. The pH paradox has also been observed in hepatocytes and cardiac myocytes and is linked to the recovery of intracellular pH during reperfusion [20–22]. This recovery may promote the onset of a pH-dependent mitochondrial permeability transition caused by opening of high conductance pores in the mitochondrial inner membrane, resulting in mitochondrial depolarization and uncoupling of oxidative phosphorylation [23]. Cyclosporin A blocks conductance through these pores and prevents injury caused by reoxygenation and oxidative stress in several models, including reoxygenated sinusoidal endothelial cells [24–26]. This effect on mitochondria is unrelated to the immunosuppressive action of cyclosporin A.

4. Oxygen-dependent reperfusion injury

In addition to pH-dependent damage, oxygen-dependent reperfusion injury occurs after liver storage. In orthotopic rat liver transplantation, rinsing livers with oxygen-free buffer just prior to implantation decreases liver damage observed 24 h later, suggesting that reactive oxygen species, such as superoxide ($O_2^{\cdot}$), are involved in liver injury [27]. Kupffer cells are probably a major source of such radicals [16,28], but radicals may also be formed by damaged mitochondria and xanthine oxidase [29–31]. $O_2^{\cdot}$ and hydrogen peroxide (H_2O_2) formation initiate a cascade of reactions, including lipid peroxidation and iron-catalysed generation of highly toxic hydroxyl radicals ($OH^{\cdot}$). Consistent with this chemistry, failing liver grafts release a carbon-centred lipid radical detectable by spin-trapping techniques [32]. Stimulated Kupffer cells also synthesize NO [33]. Reaction of NO with $O_2^{\cdot}$ can produce toxic peroxynitrite radicals, which may also contribute to reperfusion injury [34]. Nonetheless, oxygen radicals are not responsible for pH-dependent killing of endothelial cells after storage and reperfusion [16].

5. Kupffer cell function and graft failure

Kupffer cell activation is reduced and graft survival is improved when livers are stored with nisoldipine, a dihydropyridine calcium channel blocker [35]. This finding led to the discovery of voltage-sensitive calcium channels in Kupffer cells [36]. Thus, Kupffer cell activation is the likely consequence of an increase of cytosolic calcium either during storage or after

reperfusion. However, the once widely held notion that increased cytosolic free Ca^{2+} is the major cause of cell death during anoxia is now in doubt and should not be applied universally [37].

Like other macrophages, Kupffer cells synthesize several cytokines. One of these, TNF-α, promotes pulmonary leucocyte infiltration and injury after hepatic ischaemia/reperfusion, and anti-TNF-α antibodies reduce pulmonary injury in models of warm and cold hepatic ischaemia in rats [38,39]. Lipopolysaccharide (LPS) is a potent stimulator of TNF-α formation by Kupffer cells, and agents that suppress LPS-stimulated TNF-α formation by Kupffer cells also reduce graft failure from storage/reperfusion injury [40]. These agents include calcium channel blockers, adenosine, pentoxifylline, prostaglandin E_1 and tirilazad. Suppression of cytokine release by Kupffer cells may be the basis for the beneficial effect of prostaglandin E_1 in clinical liver transplantation [3,41].

Sinusoidal adhesion of leukocytes and platelets increases in failing liver grafts [14,42]. Studies by Jaeschke and co-workers have established the importance of neutrophil infiltration in warm ischaemia/reperfusion injury in liver [43]. Infusion of superoxide dismutase decreases leukocyte margination after both warm and cold ischaemia, indicating that oxygen radicals promote leukocyte sticking to hepatic sinusoids [44,45]. As in endotoxin shock [46], liver storage and reperfusion up-regulates endothelial intercellular adhesion molecules (ICAMs) that mediate sticking of leucocytes [47]. TNF-α produced by activated Kupffer cells may be responsible for increased expression and synthesis of these intercellular adhesion molecules after reperfusion [46].

LPS is one of the most powerful stimulants of cytokine release by Kupffer cells. Small amounts of LPS injected into donors reduce graft survival and increase graft injury after rat liver transplantation, as assessed by serum transaminases [48]. The effect of LPS is to decrease the time that grafts can be successfully preserved. These findings indicate that translocation of bacterial cell wall products across the gut mucosa, which occurs frequently in brain-dead heart beating cadaver donors [49], may be a critical factor contributing to unexplained graft non-function and initial poor function in clinical liver transplantation.

6. Survival of fatty liver grafts

Another factor promoting primary graft non-function in human transplantation is steatosis in livers from obese and alcoholic donors [50]. Failure of experimental fatty liver grafts is associated with increased leucocyte and platelet margination, disturbed microcirculation and formation of a new, antioxidant-insensitive and as yet unidentified carbon-centred free radical [51–54]. Kupffer cells may be the source of this radical. Since many organ donors are ethanol-consuming accident victims, it is important to understand the mechanisms predisposing fatty grafts to primary non-function.

7. Carolina rinse solution

Proof that endothelial cell killing and Kupffer cell activation are indeed trigered by reperfusion comes from the experimental demonstration that modification of the conditions of reperfusion can dramatically reduce these changes. In particular, rinsing livers with warm Carolina rinse solution (Table 1) at the end of storage almost totally abolishes endothelial cell killing (Fig. 2B), suppresses Kupffer cell activation and radical formation, and improves hepatic microcirculation after transplantation [32,55–57]. Moreover, this treatment increases graft survival and reduces graft injury after transplantation (Fig. 4) [56,58,59]. In a

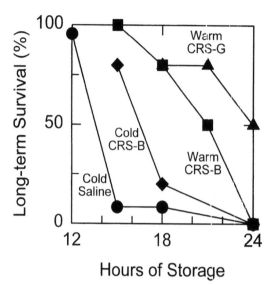

Figure 4. Improvement of long term (30-day) graft survival by rinses at the end of storage. Livers of syngeneic Lewis rats were stored for various times in UW solution and rinsed with cold Ringer's or saline solution, cold or warm Carolina Rinse Solution B or warm Carolina Rinse Solution G containing glycine (see Table 1).

Table 1. Composition of Carolina Rinse Solution G [69].

Component	Concentration
NaCl	115 mM
KCl	5 mM
CaCl$_2$	1.3 mM
KH$_2$PO$_4$	1 mM
MgSO$_4$	1.2 mM
Hydroxyethyl starch	50 g/l
Allopurinol	1 mM
Desferrioxamine	1 mM
Glutathione	3 mM
Fructose	10 mM
Glucose	10 mM
Adenosine	200 μM
Nicardipine	2 μM
Insulin	100 U/l
3-[N] morpholinopropanesulfonic acid (MOPS)	20 mM
Glycine[a]	5 mM
Total Na$^+$	115 mM
Total K$^+$	6 mM
Total Cl$^-$	122 mM
pH	6.5
Osmolarity	290–310 mOsm

[a] Absent in Carolina Rinse Solution B [58].

recent clinical trial, Carolina rinse solution decreased several indicators of graft injury in the early period following liver transplantation, including serum bilirubin, alanine transaminase, alkaline phosphatase and γ-glutamyltranspeptidase (Fig. 5) [60].

Consistent with the multiple mechanisms causing reperfusion injury to stored livers, no single component of Carolina rinse solution accounts entirely for its success. Slightly acidic pH (6.5), adenosine and antioxidants (allopurinol, desferrioxamine and glutathione) are each required for maximal benefit [58,61,62]. Acidotic pH prevents pH-dependent reperfusion injury to endothelial cells, whereas adenosine decreases Kupffer cell free Ca^{2+} and cytokine formation by a cAMP-dependent adenosine A$_2$ receptor mechanism [16,61,63]. Antoxidants probably counter the effects of reactive oxygen species and lipid radicals formed during reperfusion [16,31]. Other potentially important ingredients are substrates to promote glycolytic ATP formation (fructose, glucose and insulin) and a dihydropyridine calcium channel blocker (nicardipine). The calcium channel blocker inhibits an L-type voltage sensitive calcium channel in Kupffer cells and blocks release of TNF by stimulated Kupffer cells [36,40]. Other strategies to down-regulate Kupffer cells also improve graft survival, including storage with nisoldipine mentioned above and recipient

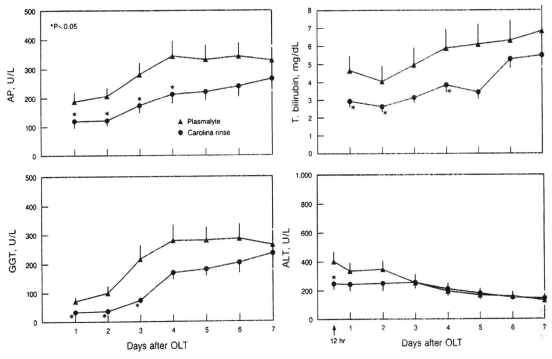

Figure 5. Efficacy of Carolina Rinse Solution B in clinical liver transplantation. During the implantation procedure, the hepatic artery was flushed with 150 ml and the portal vein with 350 ml of either Carolina Rinse Solution B or Plasmalyte at room temperature. Serum chemistries were measured daily for the first 7 days postoperatively. From Ref. 60 with permission.

treatment with pentoxifylline, an agent that suppresses cytokine formation by Kupffer cells [35,50,64].

8. Glycine

Glycine is a cytoprotective amino acid that protects renal tubular cells, hepatocytes and other cells against lethal hypoxic injury [65–67]. Glycine is as effective as Carolina rinse solution in preventing reperfusion-induced endothelial cell death following 24 h of rat liver storage in UW solution [68]. After 48 h of storage, when neither glycine nor Carolina rinse solution protects fully, addition of glycine to Carolina rinse solution restores nearly full protection against endothelial cell killing. Importantly, glycine also improves the efficacy of Carolina rinse solution in orthotopic rat liver transplantation, as documented by increased graft survival and decreased serum transminases postoperatively (Fig. 4) [69]. In these rinse strategies, direct infusion of cytoprotective solutions into liver explants at the end of storage must be performed to achieve significant benefit. Use of glycine as an additive to the storage solution or by systemic

administration to graft recipients provides at best a marginal improvement of graft outcome [70].

9. Conclusions

Clinical and experimental data indicate that both Kupffer cell activation and endothelial damage contribute to storage/reperfusion injury in livers stored for transplantation. Unexpectedly, hepatic parenchymal cells proved quite resistant to storage/reperfusion injury, even after very long periods of storage [7,9,71]. This contrasts with the high vulnerability of hepatocytes to warm ischaemia/reperfusion injury [72], which highlights the temperature dependence of the mechanisms involved [73]. The importance of temperature is underscored by the observation that Carolina rinse solution is more effective when used warm (30°C) than cold (1–4°C) [58] (Fig. 4). Our understanding of the role of sinusoidal cells in storage/reperfusion injury forms the basis for developing new strategies, like Carolina rinse solution, to prolong organ storage, improve initial graft function, reduce failure of normal and fatty grafts, and expand donor availability for life-saving transplantation therapy. The observation that no single component of Carolina rinse solution can account entirely for its success demonstrates that multiple mechanisms contribute to storage/reperfusion injury. Each mechanism must be dealt with if optimal overall success is to be achieved.

Acknowledgements

This work was supported, in part, by NIH Grants DK37034 and AA09156 and NIH Grant P30 DK34987 to the Center for Gastrointestinal Biology & Disease at the University of North Carolina.

References

1. McCartney S. Agonizing choices: people most needing transplantable livers now miss out. Wall St J 1993; 221: 63, A1, A8.
2. Kahn D, Esquivel CO, Makowka L, Machigal-Torres M, Yunis E, Iwatsuki S, Starzl TE. Causes of death after liver transplantation in children treated with cyclosporine and steroids. Clin Transplant 1989; 3: 150–5.
3. Greig PD, Woolf GM, Sinclair SB, Abecassis M, Strasberg SM, Taylor BR, Blendis LM, Superina RA, Glynn MF, Langer B, Levy GA. Treatment of primary liver graft nonfunction with prostaglandin E₁. Transplantation 1989; 48: 447–53.
4. Furukawa H, Todo S, Imventarza O, Casavilla A, Wu YM, Scotti-Foglieni C, Broznick B, Bryant J, Day R, Starzl TE. Effect of cold ischemia time on the early outcome of human hepatic allografts preserved with UW solution. Transplantation 1991; 51: 1000–4.
5. Ploeg RJ, D'Alessandro AM, Knechtle SJ, Stegall MD, Pirsch JD, Hoffman RM, Sasaki T, Sollinger HW, Belzer FO, Kalayoglu M. Risk factors for primary dysfunction after liver transplantation – a multivariate analysis. Transplantation 1993; 55: 807–13.
6. Katz E, Mor E, Patel T, Theise N, Emre S, Schwartz ME, Miller CM. Association between preservation injury and early rejection in clinical liver transplantation: fact or myth? Transplant Proc 1993; 25: 1907–8.
7. Caldwell-Kenkel JC, Thurman RG, Lemasters JJ. Selective loss of non-parenchymal cell viability after cold, ischemic storage of rat livers. Transplantation 1988; 45: 834–7.
8. MeKeown CMB, Edwards V, Phillips MJ, Harvey PR, Petrunka CN, Strasberg SM. Sinusoidal lining cell damage: the critical injury in cold preservation of liver allografts in the rat. Transplantation 1988; 46: 178–91.
9. Caldwell-Kenkel JC, Currin RT, Tanaka Y, Thurman RG, Lemasters JJ. Reperfusion injury to endothelial cells following cold ischemic storage of rat livers. Hepatology 1989; 10: 292–99.
10. Caldwell-Kenkel JC, Currin RT, Tanaka Y, Thurman RG, Lemasters JJ. Kupffer cell activation and endothelial cell damage after storage of rat livers: effects of reperfusion. Hepatology 1991; 13: 83–95.
11. Carles J, Fawaz R, Neaud V, Hamoudi ND, Bernard PH, Balabaud C, Bioulac-Sage P. Ultrastructure of human liver grafts preserved with UW solution. Comparison between patients with low and high postoperative transaminases levels. J Submicrosc Cytol Pathol 1994; 26: 67–73.
12. Carles J, Fawaz R, Hamoudi NE, Neaud V, Balabaud C, Bioulac-Sage P. Preservation of human liver grafts in UW solution. Ultrastructural evidence for endothelial and Kupffer

13. cell activation during cold ischemia and after ischemia–reperfusion. Liver 1994; 124: 50–6.
14. Takei Y, Gao W, Hijioka T, Savier E, Lindert K, Lemasters JJ, Thurman RG. Increase in survival of liver grafts after rinsing with warm Ringer's solution due to improvement of hepatic microcirculation. Transplantation 1991; 52: 225–230.
15. Takei Y, Marzi I, Gao W, Gores GJ, Lemasters JJ, Thurman RG. Leukocyte adhesion and cell death following orthotopic liver transplantation in the rat. Transplantation 1991; 51: 959–65.
16. Gores GJ, Nieminen A-L, Fleishman KE, Dawson TL, Herman B, Lemasters JJ. Extracellular acidosis delays onset of cell death in ATP-depleted hepatocytes. Am J Physiol 1988; 255: C315–22.
17. Caldwell-Kenkel JC, Currin RT, Coote A, Thurman RG, Lemasters JJ. Reperfusion injury to endothelial cells after cold storage of rat livers: protection by mildly acidic pH and lack of protection by antioxidants. Transplant Int 1995; 8: 77–85.
18. Currin RT, Gores GJ, Thurman RG, Lemasters JJ. Protection by acidotic pH against anoxic cell killing in perfused rat liver: evidence for a pH paradox. FASEB J 1991; 5: 207–10.
19. Harrison DC, Lemasters JJ, Herman B. A pH-dependent phospholipase A₂ contributes to loss of plasma membrane integrity during chemical hypoxia in rat hepatocytes. Biochem Biophys Res Commun 1991; 174: 654–9.
20. Bronk SF, Gores GJ. pH-dependent nonlysosomal proteolysis contributes to lethal anoxic injury of rat hepatocytes. Am J Physiol 1993; 264: G744–51.
21. Bond JM, Herman B, Lemasters JJ. Protection by acidotic pH against anoxia/reoxygenation injury to rat neonatal cardiac myocytes. Biochem Biophys Res Commun 1991; 179: 798–803.
22. Kaplan SH, Yang H, Gilliam DE, Shen J, Lemasters JJ, Cascio WE. Hypercapnic acidosis and dimethyl amiloride reduce reperfusion induced cell death in ischemic rabbit ventricular myocardium. Cardiovasc Res 1995; 29: 231–8.
23. Qian T, Nieminen A-L, Herman B, Lemasters JJ. The pH paradox of reperfusion injury to cultured rat hepatocytes is Na⁺-dependent, Cl⁻ and Ca²⁺-independent, and inhibited by glycine. Hepatology, 1994; 20: 176A.
24. Gunter TE, Pfeiffer DR. Mechanisms by which mitochondria transport calcium. Am J Physiol 1990; 258: C755–86.
25. Nazareth W, Nasser Y, Crompton M. Inhibition of anoxia-induced injury in heart myocytes by cyclosporin A. J Mol Cell Cardiol 1991; 23: 1351–4.
26. Imberti R, Nieminen A-L, Herman B, Lemasters JJ. Mitochondrial and glycolytic dysfunction in lethal injury to hepatocytes by t-butyl hydroperoxide: protection by fructose, cyclosporin A and trifluoperazine. J Pharmacol Exp Ther 1993; 265: 392–400.
27. Fujii Y, Johnson ME, Gores GJ. Mitochondrial dysfunction during anoxia/reoxygenation injury of liver sinusoidal endothelial cells. Hepatology 1994; 20: 177–85.
28. Thurman RG, Marzi I, Seitz G, Thies J, Lemasters JJ, Zimmerman F. Hepatic reperfusion injury following orthotopic liver transplantation in the rat. Transplantation 1988; 46: 502–6.
29. Brass CA, Roberts TG. Hepatic free radical production after cold storage: evidence for Kupffer cell dependent and independent mechanisms. Gastroenterology 1995; 108: 1167–75.
30. Chance B, Sies H, Boveris A. Hydroperoxide metabolism in mammalian organs. Physiol Rev 1979; 59: 527–605.
31. Granger DN, Hollwarth ME, Parks DA. Ischemia-reperfusion injury: role of oxygen-derived free radicals. Acta Physiol Scand Suppl 1986; 548: 47–63.
32. Dawson TL, Gores GJ, Nieminen A-L, Herman B, Lemasters JJ. Mitochondria as a source of reactive oxygen species during reductive stress in rat hepatocytes. Am J Physiol 1993; 264: C961–7.
33. Connor HD, Gao W, Nukina S, Lemasters JJ, Mason RP, Thurman RG. Evidence that free radicals are involved in graft

failure following orthotopic liver transplantation in the rat – an electron paramagnetic resonance spin trapping study. Transplantation 1992; 54: 199–204.

33. Gaillard T, Mulsch A, Busse R, Klein H, Decker K. Regulation of nitric oxide production by stimulated rat Kupffer cells. Pathobiology 1991; 59: 280–3.

34. Beckman JS, Beckman TW, Chen J, Marshall PA, Breeman BA. Apparent hydroxyl radical production by peroxynitrite: implications for endothelial injury from nitric oxide and superoxide. Proc Natl Acad Sci USA 1990; 87: 1620–4.

35. Takei Y, Marzi I, Kauffman FC, Currin RT, Lemasters JJ, Thurman RG. Increase in survival time of liver transplants by protease inhibitors and a calcium channel blocker, nisoldipine. Transplantation 1990; 50: 14–20.

36. Hijioka T, Rosenberg RL, Lemasters JJ, Thurman RG. Kupffer cells contain voltage-dependent calcium channels. Mol Pharmacol 1992; 41: 434–40.

37. Kawanishi T, Nieminen A-L, Herman B, Lemasters JJ. Suppression of Ca^{2+} oscillations in cultured rat hepatocytes by chemical hypoxia. J Biol Chem 1991; 266: 20062–9.

38. Colletti LM, Remick DG, Burtch GD, Kunkel SL, Strieter RM, Campbell DA. The role of tumor necrosis factor alpha in the pathophysiologic alterations following hepatic ischemia/reperfusion injury. J Clin Invest 1990; 85: 1936–43.

39. Goto M, Takei Y, Kawano S, Tsuji S, Fukui H, Fushimi H, Nishimura Y, Kashiwagi T, Fusamoto H, Kamada T. Tumor necrosis factor and endotoxin in the pathogenesis of liver and pulmonary injuries after orthotopic liver transplantation in the rat. Hepatology 1992; 16: 487–93.

40. Currin RT, Reinstein LJ, Lichtman SN, Thurman RG, Lemasters JJ. Inhibition of tumor necrosis factor release from cultured rat Kupffer cells by agents that reduce graft failure from storage injury. Transplant Proc 1993; 25: 1631–2.

41. Henley KS, Lucey MR, Normolle DP, Merion RM, McLaren ID, Crider BA, Mackie DS, Shieck VL, Nostrant TT, Brown KA, Campbell DA, Ham JM, Appelman HD, Turcotte JG. A double-blind, randomized, placebo-controlled trial of prostaglandin E_1 in liver transplantation. Hepatology 1995; 21: 366–72.

42. Cywes R, Brendan J, Mullen M, Stratis MS, Greig PD, Levy GA, Harvey PR, Strasberg SM. Prediction of the outcome of transplantation in man by platelet adherence in donor liver allografts. Transplantation 1993; 56: 316–23.

43. Jaeschke H, Farhood A. Neutrophil and Kupffer cell-induced oxidant stress and ischemia–reperfusion injury in rat liver. Am J Physiol 1991; 260: G355–62.

44. Marzi I, Knee J, Buhren V, Menger M, Trentz O. Reduction by superoxide dismutase of leukocyte-endothelial adherence after liver transplantation. Surgery 1992; 111: 90–7.

45. Koo A, Komatsu H, Tao G, Inoue M, Guth PH, Kaplowitz N. Contribution of no-reflow phenomenon to hepatic injury after ischemia–reperfusion: evidence for a role for superoxide anion. Hepatology 1992; 15: 507–14.

46. Essani NA, Fisher MA, Manning AM, Farhood A, Jaeschke H. Tumor necrosis factor-α and interleukin-1 induce hepatic intercellular adhesion molecule-1 (ICAM-1) mRNA expression in a murine endotoxin shock model. In: Wisse E, Knook DL, Wake K (eds), Cells of the Hepatic Sinusoid, Vol. 5, The Kupffer Cell Foundation, Leiden 1995; 177–9.

47. Nishimura Y, Takei Y, Goto M, Nagai H, Kawano S, Fusamoto H, Kamada T. Expression of ICAM-1 is involved in the mechanism of liver injury after orthotopic liver transplantation In: Wisse E, Knook DL, Wake K (eds), Cells of the Hepatic Sinusoid, Vol. 5. The Kupffer Cell Foundation, Leiden 1995; 231–3.

48. Peng X-X, Currin RT, Musshafen TL, Thurman RG, Lemasters JJ. Lipopolysaccharide treatment of donor rats causes graft failure after orthotopic rat liver transplantation. In: Wisse E, Knook DL, Wake K (eds), Cells of the Hepatic Sinusoid, Vol. 5. The Kupffer Cell Foundation, Leiden 1995; 234–5.

49. van Goor H, Rosman C, Grond J, Kooi K, Wübbels GH, Bleichrodt RP. Translocation of bacteria and endotoxin in organ donors. Arch Surg 1994; 129: 1063–6.

50. Todo S, Demetris AJ, Makowa L, Teperman L, Podesta L, Shaver T, Tzakis A, Starzl TE. Primary nonfunction of hepatic allografts with preexisting fatty infiltration. Transplantation 1989; 47: 903–5.

51. Teramoto K, Bowers JL, Kruskal JB, Clouse ME. Hepatic microcirculatory changes after reperfusion in fatty and normal liver transplantation in the rat. Transplantation 1993; 56: 1076–82.

52. Hayashi M, Tokunaga Y, Fujita T, Tanaka K, Yamaoka Y, Ozawa K. The effects of cold preservation on steatotic graft viability in rat liver transplantation. Transplantation 1993; 56: 282–7.

53. Gao W, Connor HD, Lemasters JJ, Mason RP, Thurman RG. Primary non-function of fatty livers produced by alcohol is associated with a new antioxidant-insensitive free radical species. Transplantation 1995; 59: 674–9.

54. Lemasters JJ, Gao W, Currin RT, Thurman RG. Ultrastructure of livers from alcohol-treated rats following orthotopic liver transplantation. Toxicologist 1994; 14: 284.

55. Currin RT, Toole JG, Thurman RG, Lemasters JJ. Evidence that Carolina rinse solution protects sinusoidal endothelial cells against reperfusion injury after cold ischemic storage of rat liver. Transplantation 1990; 50: 1076–8.

56. Gao W, Takei Y, Marzi I, Lindert KA, Caldwell-Kenkel JC, Currin RT, Tanaka Y, Lemasters JJ, Thurman RG. Carolina rinse solution – a new strategy to increase survival time after orthotopic liver transplantation in the rat. Transplantation 1991; 52: 417–24.

57. Post S, Rentsch M, Gonzalez AP, Palma P, Otto G, Menger MD. Effects of Carolina rinse and adenosine rinse on microvascular perfusion and intrahepatic leukocyte-endothelium interaction after liver transplantation in the rat. Transplantation 1993; 55: 972–7.

58. Bachmann S, Caldwell-Kenkel JC, Oleksy I, Steffen R, Thurman RG Lemasters JJ. Warm Carolina rinse solution prevents graft failure from storage injury after orthotopic rat liver transplantation with arterialization. Transplant Int 1992; 5: 108–14.

59. Gao W, Currin RT, Lemasters JJ, Connor HD, Mason RP, Thurman RG. Reperfusion rather than storage injury predominates following long-term (48 h) cold storage of grafts in UW solution: studies with Carolina rinse in transplanted rat liver. Transplant Int 1992; 5 (Suppl. 1): S329–35.

60. Sanchez-Urdazpal L, Gores GJ, Lemasters JJ, Thurman RG, Steers JL, Wahlstrom HE, Hay EI, Porayko MK, Wiesner RH, Krom RAF. Carolina rinse solution decreases liver injury during clinical liver transplantation. Transplant Proc 1993; 25: 1574–5.

61. Gao W, Hijioka T, Lindert KA, Caldwell-Kenkel JC, Lemasters JJ, Thurman RG. Evidence that adenosine is a key component in Carolina rinse responsible for reducing graft failure after orthotopic liver transplantation in the rat. Transplantation 1991; 52: 992–8.

62. Bachmann S, Caldwell-Kenkel JC, Currin RT, Lichtman SN, Steffen R, Thurman RG, Lemasters JJ. Protection by pentoxifylline against graft failure from storage injury after orthotopic rat liver transplantation with arterialization. Transplant Int 1992; 5 (Suppl. 1): S345–50.

63. Reinstein LJ, Lichtman SN, Currin RT, Wang J, Thurman RG, Lemasters JJ. Suppression of lipopolysaccharide-stimulated release of tumor necrosis factor by adenosine: evidence for A_2 receptors on rat Kupffer cells. Hepatology 1994; 19: 1445–52.

64. Bachmann S, Caldwell-Kenkel JC, Currin RT, Tanaka Y, Takei Y, Marzi, I Thurman RG, Lemasters JJ. Ultrastructural correlates of liver graft failure from storage injury: studies of graft protection by Carolina rinse solution and pentoxifylline. Transplant Proc 1993; 25: 1620–4.

65. Weinberg JM, Davis JA, Abarzua M, Rajan T. J Clin Invest 1987; 80: 1446–54.

66. Dickson RC, Bronk SF, Gores GJ. Glycine cytoprotection during lethal hepatocellular injury from adenosine triphosphate depletion. Gastroenterology 1992; 102: 2098–107.

67. Marsh DC, Vreugdenhil PK, Mack VE, Belzer FO, Southard JH. Glycine protects hepatocytes from injury caused by anoxia, cold ischemia and mitochondrial inhibitors, but not injury caused by calcium. Hepatology 1993; 17: 91–8.

68. Currin RT, Caldwell-Kenkel JC, Lichtman SN, Bachmann S, Takei Y, Kawano S, Thurman RG, Lemasters JJ. Protection by Carolina rinse solution, acidotic pH and glycine against lethal reperfusion injury to sinusoidal endothelial cells of rat livers stored for transplantation. Transplantation 1996, in press.

69. Bachmann S, Peng X-X, Currin RT, Thurman RG, Lemasters JJ. Glycine in Carolina rinse solution reduces reperfusion injury, improves graft function and increases graft survival after rat liver transplantation. Transplant Proc, 1995; 27: 741–2..

70. den Butter G, Lindell SL, Sumimoto R, Schilling MK, Southard JH, Belzer FO. Effect of glycine in cog and rat liver transplantation. Transplantation 1993; 56: 817–22.

71. Marzi I, Zhong Z, Lemasters JJ, Thurman RG. Evidence that graft survival is not related to parenchymal cell viability in rat liver transplantation: the importance of nonparenchymal cells. Transplantation 1989; 48: 463–8.

72. Marotto ME, Thurman RG, Lemasters JJ. Early midzonal cell death during low-flow hypoxia in the isolated, perfused rat liver: protection by allopurinol. Hepatology 1988; 8: 585–90.

73. Currin RT, Thurman RG, Lemasters JJ. Carolina Rinse solution protects adenosine triphosphate-depleted hepatocytes against lethal cell injury. Transplant Proc 1991; 23: 645–7.

16 | Pharmacological agents in organ preservation

DAVID ANAISE

1. Introduction

Pharmacological agents have played only a minor role in clinical organ preservation. Several decades of intensive research on the pathophysiology of hypothermic ischaemia led to the introduction of numerous pharmacological agents that were shown to ameliorate this condition, but few of these promising agents are currently used in clinical organ procurement. Research efforts have been directed primarily toward the development of flush solutions. The primary research effort was to overcome cellular swelling. Both Collins' solution [1] and the University of Wisconsin solution [2] contain impermeant sugars and specific electrolytes designed to combat tissue swelling noted during cold storage. Most flush solutions also contain a mixture of additives designed to interfere with various ischaemic processes. The use of these agents remains empirical and the significance of each component has not been ascertained.

For organ retrieval from stable donors, and for organ preservation up to 36 h, these solutions offer adequate protection. The need to expand the donor pool by increased use of organs from marginal donors and from non-heart beating cadaver donors will, however, require new approaches and new solutions must be found. The additives and cocktails need to be replaced with specifically targeted pharmaceutical agents capable of blocking multiple ischaemic processes. Rather than discussing each drug studied, it is more useful to review the prime processes that lead to cell death as a result of ischaemia and point to the usefulness of selected metabolic blockers and inhibitors.

2. Calcium inhibitors

Advances in cellular biology have recently led to the recognition of calcium as a prime mediator of many key enzymes and cellular processes [3] (Fig. 1). Calcium activates several enzymatic systems, including glycogenolysis, lipases, and phospholipases and inhibits other enzymatic systems, such as pyruvate kinase and phospholipid synthesis. Calcium is also intimately involved in hormonal regulation, including the release of insulin, steroids, vasopressin and catecholamine and the binding of prostaglandin to membranes. Calcium also may react with cells by activating

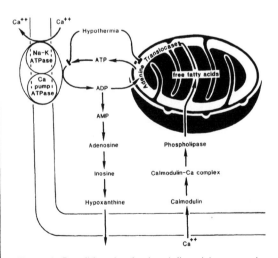

Figure 1. Possible role of calmodulin calcium complex on mitochondrial respiration and phosphorylation during hypothermic ischaemia.

G.M. Collins, J.M. Dubernard, W. Land and G.G. Persijn (eds). Procurement, Preservation and Allocation of Vascularized Organs 145–151
© 1997 Kluwer Academic Publishers.

and deactivating another intracellular messenger cyclic AMP, through its regulatory effects on both adenyl-cyclase and phosphodiesterase [4].

In the cytosol, calcium is bound to calmodulin [5], a protein known to be a prime mediator of important cellular functions. Activated calmodulin is known to regulate membrane phosphorylation, microtubule dis-assembly, activation of phosphorylase A2 and B kinase and the release of neurotransmitters. The precision with which this protein regulates these enzymes may be due to conformational changes of its α-helical structure. Such conformation is caused by the successive binding of calcium to its four molecular calcium-binding sites [6]. The binding of calcium to one site was shown to activate phosphodiesterase, while the binding of calcium to all four sites resulted in activation of myosin light chain kinase [7].

The fine tuning of cellular reactions mediated by calcium may require calcium in the cytosol to be kept at a very low level of activity. Cytosolic calcium level can then fluctuate widely and rapidly around this low level, to alternately switch intracellular targets on and off [8]. During hypothermic ischaemia the enzymatic systems responsible for the efflux of calcium across plasma membranes are deactivated [9,10]. The result-ing massive influx of calcium into the cytosol leads to relentless deterioration of cellular functions and, ultimately, to cell death [11,12].

The precise mechanism by which calcium induces cellular necrosis is not clear. Recent findings suggest that cell death is caused by damage to the mito-chondrial and cell membrane phospholipid moiety [13,14]. Phospholipids not only form the backbone of the membrane bilayer, but also provide sites of attach-ment and an optimal environment for energy trans-ducing units. Trump et al. [15] have shown that during ischaemia the calmodulin–calcium complex activates phospholipase A. Phospholipase A in turn fuses the inner and outer membranes of the mitochondria to form a pentalammelar structure. Such fusion results in a decrease in inner membrane function [16]. Pro-longation of the ischaemic insult produces swelling of the inner membrane compartments that leads to rupture of the outer membrane [15].

In detailed metabolic studies of the hypothermic kidney, Southard et al. [17] have shown that mito-chondrial dysfunction is a principal limitation to cold storage. The adenine translocase system is a rate-limiting step in the transfer of ADP from the cytosol to the mitochondria. During hypothermia this system is deactivated. Therefore, despite adequate supply of oxygen and substrate, energy stores cannot be restored by phosphorylation, and cellular deterioration ensues.

In further studies, Southard et al. [18] showed that mitochondria obtained from kidneys preserved for 72 h contained high levels of free fatty acids. The accu-mulation of these acids in the mitochondria resulted in the uncoupling of respiration from phosphorylation [19]. Mittnacht [20] has shown that activation of phospholipase A by calcium releases free fatty acids. The accumulation of fatty acids leads to uncoupling, by suppression of the adenine translocase system. The inability to phosphorylate ADP results in dephosphory-lation of ADP to AMP and then to further degradation of AMP to hypoxanthine. The latter is freely diffusible, and thus provides a mechanism for loss of adenine nuclide from the cell [21].

Damage to cellular membranes during hypothermic ischaemia is also mediated by the action of calmodulin on the cytoskeleton [22]. Calmodulin mediates the calcium-dependent assembly and disassembly of microtubules [23]. Studies of renal tubular cells sub-jected to anoxia have shown that damage to cyto-skeletal structures is associated with increased membrane permeability, impairment of receptor sites and formation of exotropic blebs. This damage leads to formation of obstructive casts in the distal tubules [24]. Cell separation may be another important mechanism underlying organ failure after ischaemic damage [25]. Endothelial cell separation due to cyto-skeletal damage may result in exposure of collagen which can lead to platelet aggregation and intra-vascular coagulation. This may be the mechanism underlying the 'no reflow phenomenon' reported in kidneys damaged by prolonged hypothermic ischaemia [26].

Taken together (Fig. 2), these data suggest that cellular necrosis following hypothermic ischaemia may be a consequence of a rapid influx of calcium into the cytosol. Activation of the calmodulin calcium complex causes phospholipase activation, with membrane breakdown, cytoskeletal damage and adverse effects on mitochondrial respiration. If allowed to progress, these events will result in irreversible cell damage. This deleterious calcium cascade may potentially be interrupted at three points (Fig. 2): reducing the influx of calcium, inhibition of the calmodulin calcium complex and by inhibition of some target cellular reaction like activation of phospholipase A.

Dawidson et al. [27] have shown that administration of verapamil intra-arterially after revascularization and orally after transplantation reduces acute tubular necro-sis in humans. They noted improved haemodynamics and graft survival in patients receiving verapamil. Sobh et al. [28] administered the calcium channel blocker verapamil to the donors as well as the recipi-

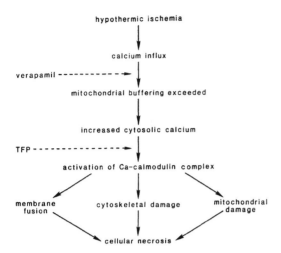

Figure 2. Possible role of calcium calmodulin complex in cellular deterioration during hypothermic ischaemia, and potential blocking sites of trifluoperazine and verapamil.

ents of living related kidney transplants. Delayed graft function (as defined by presence of oliguria and lag in a drop in the serum creatine) was noted in 33% of the control group. Only 7% of the patients treated with verapamil suffered delayed graft function. Elkadi *et al.* [29] administered the calcium channel blockers verapamil and nicardipine to dogs before renal ischaemia. Administration of these calcium antagonists improved animal survival and renal haemodynamics, protected cellular adenine nucleotides and reduced the structural damage associated with ischaemia.

Wagner *et al.* administered the calcium channel blocker Diltiazam to the donor and the recipient and observed a reduction in delayed graft function [30]. Similar observations were noted by Puig *et al.* [31] and Alcaraz *et al.* [32]. No beneficial effects of calcium channel blockers were noted by other investigators [33,34]. Calcium channels are not the only mechanism by which calcium can enter the cytosol: it can also gain entry through leaks in the cell membrane or may be released from internal organelles [35]. As calcium exerts its effect by saturating the calmodulin calcium-binding sites, blocking calmodulin may, therefore, ameliorate ischaemia even when the cytosol is flooded by calcium.

Several classes of pharmacological agents have been shown to have a high binding constant for calmodulin and thus may inhibit its function. The most potent agents include phenothiazine diphenyl-butyropiperidine, thioxathenes and butyrophenones [36]. The phenothiazines trifluoperazine (Stelazine) and chlor-

promazine (Thorazine) bind to the calcium-activated form of calmodulin [37,38] and inhibit its interaction with cellular target proteins. The binding of calcium to calmodulin exposes a hydrophobic domain which seems to be essential for interaction with its receptor protein [39]. Phenothiazine binds to this domain and prevents this receptor activation. In this regard phenothiazine may block the activation of the final pathway of the calcium cascade even without lowering cytosolic calcium concentration. This capacity may have a specific application in attenuating organ ischaemia.

Studies in dogs have shown that addition of Stelazine to EuroCollins' flush solutions permitted cold storage of kidneys for up to 72 h [40]. While only 33% of the kidneys stored in EuroCollins' solutions alone could sustain life after transplantation, addition of Stelazine increased graft viability to 75%. Further studies, using radiolabelled microspheres [41] have shown progressive deterioration in the integrity of the renal cortical microcirculation over time. In contrast, the microcirculation of Stelazine-flushed kidneys was well preserved.

McAnulty *et al.* [42] have shown that calcium plays an important role in the maintenance of kidney viability during perfusion preservation. Both mitochondrial function and post-transplant viability were improved when the perfusate contained 0.5 mM calcium. Without added calcium or with 1.5 mM calcium the mitochondria had reduced function and transplants failed. Donor pretreatment with Chlorpromazine improved the survival of kidneys preserved with a higher calcium content for 5 days. Quinacrine, a phospholipase A inhibitor, improved mitochondrial function and allowed successful preservation of dog kidneys for 7 days [43]. Collins has shown [44] that the addition of Chlorpromazine or Stelazine to his sodium lactobionate sucrose solution resulted in dramatic improvement in rat liver graft survival. He has recently reported superior results of this solution in a clinical trial comparing this solution with Viaspan [45].

3. Reperfusion injury and free oxygen radicals

Recent studies indicate that reperfusion, rather than marking the end-point of ischaemic damage, actually exacerbates the consequences of ischaemic damage [46]. It has been suggested that the mechanism of reperfusion injury may be related to the release of oxygen-free radicals [42].

A free radical is a molecule containing an open bond or a half-bond rendering it chemically reactive. The reaction of a radical with a non-radical (notably an unsaturated lipid bond) results in a formation of yet another free radical, thus leading to destructive chain reactions. The major pathway for oxygen free radical release in post-ischaemic tissues appears to be the enzyme xanthine oxidase [48]. This enzyme is synthesized as xanthine dehydrogenase, but undergoes conversion to xanthine oxidase under ischaemic conditions. Xanthine dehydrogenase catalyses the interaction of xanthine and NAD, to form uric acid and NADH; xanthine oxidase catalyses this same reaction, but can use molecular oxygen instead of NAD and thus may produce superoxide, hydrogen peroxide, or both. The conversion of xanthine dehydrogenase to xanthine oxidase during ischaemia is thus the chief cause of formation of free radicals [49]. Ischaemia also results in depletion of energy stores and the accumulation of hypoxanthine. During reperfusion oxygen and xanthine oxidase oxidize hypoxanthine to produce oxygen free radicals. This reaction leads to lipid peroxidation, membrane damage and cellular necrosis.

Oxygen free radicals are extremely short lived. The evidence that the generation of oxygen free radicals contribute measurably to ischaemic injury is largely based on the ability of superoxide antagonists to ameliorate ischaemic damage. Free radical scavengers such as superoxide dismutase, catalase, and allopurinol offer some protection against the deleterious effect of ischaemia in a variety of models [50–53]. Their protective effect, however, seems to be limited. Leahy and Wait [54] showed only a minimal protective effect of superoxide dismutase or catalase on rat kidneys subjected to 45 min ischaemia. In contrast, the administration of verapamil resulted in improved survival and function of such treated kidneys. No beneficial effect was noted when superoxide dismutase was added to the verapamil regimen. Koyama [55] evaluated the protective effect of superoxide dismutase on cold stored pig kidneys. Infusion of 20 mg superoxide dismutase into the renal artery during reperfusion significantly ameliorated 24 h of cold storage damage. Blocking the generation of superoxide radicals with allopurinol (a known inhibitor of xanthine oxidase) offered similar protection. The combination of superoxide dismutase with catalase and allopurinol did not improve upon these results. The beneficial effect of free radical scavengers were limited however to optimal kidney procurement.

Allopurinol was effective in ameliorating ischaemia in the canine model but not in humans [56]. Hoshino et al. [57] observed improved renal function after the administration of either superoxide dismutase or allopurinol to ischaemic porcine kidneys. Human data did not support this observation. In a double-blind randomized study [58] intra-arterial injection of superoxide dismutase failed to improve allograft function.

Amelioration of ischaemic damage by free radical scavengers in rats [59,60] may be the result of the heightened sensitivity of the rodent kidney to free radical release. Southard et al. [60] measured xanthine oxidase activity in rat, canine and human kidneys: the activity of xanthine oxidase in the rat kidney was 30 times greater than that observed in the dog kidney and 60 times greater than that in the human kidney. The authors found low activity levels of xanthine oxidase in dog kidneys preserved for 3 and 5 days. They concluded that oxygen free radicals are probably not important in the damage occurring during preservation of dog and human tissues. The high level of xanthine oxidase in the rat kidney may signify a heightened susceptibility of the rodent species to reperfusion injury mediated by free radical release. Oxygen free radicals may be of little significance in human liver and kidney preservation because endogenous xanthine oxidase has a relatively low activity, compared with a high endogenous activity of superoxide dismutase which scavenges superoxide anions [62]. In contrast, injury caused by oxygen free radicals may be of great importance in the lung and the intestine, which are sensitive to such damage.

Free radical release may become important in prolonged machine preservation. Bennett et al. [61] evaluated the effect of specific scavengers of oxygen-derived free radicals on the immediate function rate of rabbit kidneys preserved for 24 h by hypothermic perfusion. Improvement in creatinine clearance was seen when the perfusate was treated with superoxide dismutase and catalase. This effect was enhanced if a long lasting polyethylene glycol-linked form of superoxide dismutase was used. In contrast, no effect of free radical scavengers could be demonstrated in kidneys which were cold stored whether the agents were added to the flush solution, given to the recipient, or both.

Loss of glutathione from the kidney can increase sensitivity to oxygen free radical-induced injury. Boudjema et al. [62] demonstrated that during 5 days of continuous machine perfusion of the kidney there was a loss of glutathione from the renal cortex. Perfusion with reduced glutathione suppressed this loss. The addition of the three amino acids that make up glutathione (glycine, glutamic acid, and cysteine) stimulated the synthesis of glutathione in the kidney during hypothermic perfusion. These data suggest that the no-reflow phenomenon often seen in cold stored

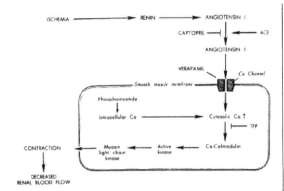

Figure 3. The effect of angiotensin II on vascular smooth muscle during reperfusion. Note the potential blocking effects of captopril, verapamil, and trifluoperazine (TFP) on angiotensin-mediated vasoconstriction.

kidneys is not necessarily caused by free oxygen radicals. Other events that occur during reperfusion, including the release of angiotensin [65] may have a more significant role in the pathogenesis of the no-reflow phenomenon (Fig. 3). Freer [63], Peach [66] and Hoff [35] have shown that the activation of angiotensin receptors on smooth muscle membranes involves receptor-linked channels which allow influx of extracellular calcium, as well as the release of calcium from intracellular pools. Activated calmodulin in turn activates myosin light chain kinase, which then phosphorylates light chain myosin, to initiate smooth muscle contraction [67]. Angiotensin-induced vasoconstriction deprives the preserved organ of oxygen at the time that it needs it most. Blocking angiotensin release or smooth cell myosin phosphorylation immediately after completion of the vascular anastomosis are attractive strategies to ameliorate reperfusion injury [68].

4. Prostaglandins

Prostanoids (leukotrienes, thromboxane and prostaglandins) are synthesized from arachidonic acid as the result of phospholipid hydrolysis. Prostacyclin, PGI_2 and PGE_2 are potent vasodilators, decrease platelet aggregation and, when given to the ischaemic kidney, have a protective effect [69,70]. In contrast, thromboxane, is a potent vasoconstrictor that induces platelet aggregation and contributes to the release of oxygen free radicals and proteases [71].

Mangino *et al.* [72] have shown heightened thromboxane production in the renal cortex following reper-

fusion of kidneys subjected to 48 h of cold storage. PGE_2 and 6-keto PGE_1 production were not, however, affected significantly by ischaemia and reperfusion. Enhanced thromboxane production was not seen with ischaemia alone (without reperfusion) or after reperfusion with an oxygen saturated buffer. It was noted only after reperfusion with blood.

Aspirin is a cyclooxygenase inhibitor that suppresses the formation of prostaglandins and thromboxane. Furegrelate is an inhibitor thromboxane synthetase but allows production of prostaglandins. Schilling *et al.* [73] perfused canine kidneys for 5–7 days with furegrelate added to the perfusate and with aspirin given to the recipient before transplantation. Aspirin was beneficial for up to 5 days of preservation, but not after 7 days of preservation. Furegrelate allowed 7 days' canine kidney preservation.

Anderson *et al.* [74] have shown that thromboxane caused endothelial injury during machine preservation. Schilling *et al.* [73] have noted that furegrelate was beneficial in machine but not cold storage preservation. These observations suggest a different mechanism of injury in perfused kidneys and cold stored kidneys. It is possible that the availability of oxygen in a perfused model allows conversion of arachidonic acid to thromboxane. Other prostaglandin agonist and antagonists have shown promise in organ preservation. Kin *et al.* [75] added the thromboxane inhibitor OKY046 to the University of Wisconsin solution and successfully preserved segmental canine pancreata for 96 h.

Prostacyclin is a potent vasodilator and probably the most potent inhibitor of platelet aggregation yet discovered. Mundy *et al.* [76] administered prostacyclin to dogs before 45 min of ischaemia and documented excellent protection of renal function in the treated subjects.

5. Conclusion

This chapter outlines three major pathways leading to cellular destruction as a consequence of hypothermic ischaemia. Clearly, these pathways are not the only ones involved in ischaemia, nor are the agents identified the most promising agents. Since cell death is the result of multiple insults, a combination of agents is needed to enable successful long term preservation. Combinations of pharmacological agents may result in either additive or synergistic, but often antagonistic, responses. Careful studies are thus needed to identify the combination of drugs that will best protect the preserved organs from ischaemia.

In 1993, 9698 kidneys were recovered from 4849 cadaver donors. Only 7503 of these were actually transplanted [77] – 22.6% of the recovered kidneys were discarded. Improved methods of preservation may have allowed the transplantation of many of those kidneys. In 1993 many transplant centres began to explore the potential of non-heart beating cadaver donors. Utilization of this donor source will require further development of organ preservation sciences.

Acknowledgement

I wish to thank Jimmy Light M.D. and Ann Kowalski R.N for their help in preparing this manuscript.

References

1. Collins GM, Bravo-Sugerman MB, Terasaki P. Kidney preservation for transportation. Lancet 1969; 2: 1219.
2. Kalayoglu M, Stratta RJ, Sollinger HW et al. Clinical results liver transplantation using UW solution for extended preservation. Transplant Proc. 1989; 21: 1342.
3. Carafoli E. Membrane transport and the regulation of the cell calcium levels. In: Cowley PA, Trump BF (eds) Pathophysiology of Shock, Anoxia, and Ischemia. Williams and Wilkins, Baltimore 1982. pp. 95.
4. Cheung WY. Cyclic 3′5′-nucleotide phosphodiesterase: pronounced stimulation by snake venom. Biochem Biophys Res Commun 1967; 29: 478.
5. Cheung WY. Calmodulin plays a pivotal role in cellular regulation. Science 1980; 207: 19.
6. Richman PG, Klee CB. Specific perturbation by Ca^{2+} of tyrosyl residue 138 of calmodulin. J Biol Chem 1979; 254: 5372.
7. Anderson JM, Gimbrone MA Jr, Alexander RW. Angiotensin II stimulates phosphorylation of the myosin light chain in cultured vascular smooth muscle cells. J Biol Chem 1981; 256: 4693.
8. Carafoli E, Crompton M. The regulation of intracellular calcium. Curr Topics Membrane Transplant 1978; 10: 151.
9. Schatzmann HJ. Dependence on calcium concentration and stoichiometry of the calcium pump in human red cells. J Physiol 1973; 235: 551.
10. Gmaj P, Murer H, Kinne R. Calcium ion transport across plasma membranes isolated from rat kidney cortex. Biochem J 1979; 178: 549.
11. Judah JD, Ahmed K, McLean AEM. Possible role of ion shifts in liver injury. In: de Renck AVS, Knight J (eds), Ciba Foundation Symposium on Cellular Injury. Little, Brown & Co., Boston, 1964; pp. 187–205.
12. Trump BF, Mergner WJ, Kahng MW, Saladino AJ. Studies on the subcellular pathophysiology of ischemia. Circulation 1976; 53 (suppl. 1): 17.
13. Osornior AR, Berezesky IK, Mergner WJ, Trump BF. Mitochondrial membrane fusions in experimental myocardial infarction. Fed Proc 1980; 39: 634.
14. Sun ST, Day EP, Ho JT. Temperature dependence of calcium-induced fusion of sonicated phosphatidylserine vesicles. Proc Natl Acad Sci USA 1978; 75: 4325.
15. Trump BF, Berezesky IK, Cowley RA. The cellular and subcellular characteristics of acute and chronic injury with emphasis on the role of calcium. In: Cowley RA, Trump BF (eds), Pathophysiology of Shock, Anoxia, and Ischemia. Williams & Wilkins Co., Baltimore 1982; p. 6.
16. Wakabayashi T, Green DE. Membrane fusion in mitochondria. I. Ultrastructural basis for fusion. J Electron Microsc 1977; 26: 305.
17. Southard JH, Hoffmann RM, Belzer FO. Mechanism of loss of mitochondrial functions during hypothermic storage of kidneys. In: Pegg DE, Jacobsen IA, Hala NA (eds), Organ Preservation: Basic and Applied Aspects. MTP Press, Boston 1982; pp. 127.
18. Southard JH, Senzig KA, Hoffmann RM, Belzer FO. Toxicity of oxygen to mitochondrial respiratory activity in hypothermically perfused canine kidneys. Transplantation 1980; 29: 459.
19. Shug AL, Shrago E, Bittar N, Folts JD, Koke JR. Acyl-CoA inhibition of adenine nucleotide translocation in ischemic myocardium. Am. J Physiol 1975; 228: 689.
20. Mittnacht S, Jr, Sherman SC, Farber JL. Reversal of ischemic mitochondrial dysfunction. J Biol Chem 1979; 254: 9871.
21. Feinberg H. Energetics and mitochondria. in: Pegg DE, Jacobsen IA, Halasz NA (eds), Organ Preservation: Basic and Applied Aspects. MTP Press Boston, 1982; p. 3.
22. Welsh MJ, Dedman JR, Brinkley BR, Means AR. Tubulin and calmodulin. Effects of microtubule and microfilament inhibitors on localization in the mitotic apparatus. J Cel Biol 1979; 81: 624
23. Marcum JM, Dedman JR, Brinkley BR, Means AR. Control of microtubule assembly-disassembly by calcium-dependent regulator protein. Proc Natl Acad Sci USA 1978; 75: 3771.
24. Donohoe JF, Venkatachalam MA, Bernard DB, Levinsky NG. Tubular leakage and obstruction after renal ischemia: Structural-functional correlations. Kidney Int 1978, 13: 208.
25. Loewenstein WR, Rose B. Calcium in (junctional) intracellular communication and a thought on its behavior in intracellular communication. Ann NY Acad Sci 1978; 307: 285.
26. Diethelm AG, Devries BS, Hartley MW, Phillips SJ. The no-reflow phenomenon after canine renal preservation with medium 199. J Surg Res 1975; 19: 55.
27. Dawidson I, Rooth P, Lu C, Sagalowsky A et al. Verapamil improves the outcome after cadaver renal transplantation. J Am Soc Nephrol 1991; 2: 983–90.
28. Sobh MA, Shehab el-Din AB, Moustafa FE, el-Far MA et al. A prospective randomized study of the protective effect of verapamil on ischemic renal injury in renal allotransplants. Transplant Proc 1989; 21: 1230–2.
29. Elkadi HK, Mardan AH, Nghiem DD, Southard JH. The role of calcium antagonists in the management of renal warm ischemia. J Urol 1989; 141: 974–80.
30. Wagner K, Albrecht S, Neumayer HH. Prevention of post-transplant acute tubular necrosis by the calcium antagonist diltiazem: a prospective randomized study. Am J Nephrol 1987; 7: 287–91.
31. Puig JM, Lloveras J, Oliveras A, Costa C, Aubia J Masramon J. Usefulness of diltiazem in reducing the incidence of acute tubular necrosis in Euro-Collins-preserved cadaveric renal grafts. Transpl Proc 1991; 23: 2368–9.
32. Alcaraz A, Oppenheimer F, Talbot-Wright R, Fernandez-Cruz L, Manalich M, Garcia-Pages E, Cetina A, Vendrell JR, Carretero P. Effect of diltiazem in the prevention of acute tubular necrosis, acute rejection, and cyclosporine levels. Transpl Proc 1991; 23: 2383–4.
33. Pirsch JD, D'Alessandro AM, Roecker EB, Knechtle SJ et al. A controlled, double-blind, randomized trial of verapamil and cyclosporine in cadaver renal transplant patients. Am J Kidney Dis 1993; 21: 189–95.
34. Koller J, Wieser C, Kornberger R, Furtwangler W et al. Does systemic pretreatment with verapamil prevent acute tubular necrosis after renal transplantation? Transplant Proc 1988: 20: 905–6.
35. Hoff RP, Vuorela HJ, Neumann P. PY 108–068, a new, potent, and selective inhibitor of calcium-induced contraction of rabbit aortic rings. J Cardiovasc Pharmacol 1982; 4: 344.

36. Weiss B, Prozialeck W, Cimino M, *et al.* Pharmacological regulation of calmodulin. Ann NY Acad Sci 1980; 356: 319.

37. Levin R, Weiss B. Specificity of binding of trifluoperazine to the calcium dependent activator of phosphodiesterase and to a series of other calcium binding proteins. Biochim Biophys Acta 1981; 540: 197.

38. Osborn M, Weber K. Damage of cellular functions by trifluoperazine, a calmodulin specific drug. Exp Cell Res 1981; 130: 484.

39. LaPorte DE, Weirman BM, Strom DR. Calcium induced exposure of a hydrophobic surface on almodulin. Biochemistry 1980; 19: 3814.

40. Asari H, Anaise D, Bachvaroff RJ *et al.* Preservation techniques for organ transplantation: I. Protective effects of calmodulin inhibitors in cold-preserved kidneys. Transplantation 1984; 37: 113.

41. Anaise D, Sato K, Atkins H *et al.* Scintigraphic evaluation of the viability of cold-preserved kidneys before transplantation. J Nucl Med 1984; 25: 1304.

42. McAnulty JF, Ploeg RJ, Southard JH, Belzer FO. Successful five day perfusion preservation of the canine kidney. Transplantation 1989; 47: 37–41.

43. McAnulty JF, Vreugdenhil PK, Southard JH, Belzer FO. Improved survival of kidneys preserved for seven days with a phospholipase inhibitor.

44. Tokunaga Y, Wicomb WN, Concepcion W. Nakazato P, Cox K, Esquivel CO, Collins GM. Improved rat liver preservation using chlorpromazine in a new sodium lactobionate sucrose solution. Transpl Proc 1991; 23: 660–1.

45. Collins GM, Wicomb WN, Warren R. Wong L, Bry WI, Feduska NJ, Salvatierra O. Canine and cadaver kidney preservation with sodium lactobionate sucrose solution. Transpl Proc 1993; 25: 1588–90.

46. Ames A, Wright RL, Kowada M, Thurston JM, Majno G. Cerebral ischemia II, the no reflow phenomenon. Am J Pathol 1968; 52: 437.

47. McCord JM. Oxygen-derived free radicals in post-ischemic tissue injury. N Engl J Med 1985; 312: 159.

48. Roy RS, McCord JM. Superoxide and ischemia: conversion of xanthine dehydrogenase to xanthine oxidase. In: Greenwald R, Cohen G (eds), Oxy Radicals and Their Scavenger Systems. Vol. 2. Cellular and Molecular Aspects. Elsevier, New York 1983; pp. 145–53.

49. Della Corte E, Stirpe F. The regulation of rat liver xanthine oxidase. Involvement of thiol groups in the conversion of the enzyme activity from dehydrogenase (Type D) into oxidase (Type O) and purification of the enzyme. Biochem J 1972; pp. 126: 739.

50. Hansson R, Gustavsson B, Jonsson O *et al.* Effect of xanthine oxidase inhibition on renal circulation after ischemia. Transplant Proc 1982; 14: 51.

51. Ouriel K, Smedira NG, Ricotta JJ. Protection of the kidney after temporary ischemia: free radical scavengers. J Vasc Surg 1985; 2: 49.

52. Paller MS, Hoidal JR, Ferris TF. Oxygen free radicals in ischemic acute renal failure in the rat. J Clin Invest 1984; 74: 1156.

53. Stuart RS, Baumgartner WA. Borkon AM *et al.* Five hour hypothermic lung preservation with oxygen free-radical scavengers. Transplant Proc 1985; 17: 1454.

54. Leahy AL, Wait RB. Verapamil, superoxide dismutase, and catalase in post-ischemia renal failure. Surg Forum 1984; 35: 24.

55. Koyama I, Bulkley GB, Williams GM. Im MJ. The role of oxygen free radicals in mediating the reperfusion injury of cold-preserved ischemic kidneys. Transplantation 1985; 40: 590.

56. Toledo-Pereyra LH, Simmons RL, Olson LC, Najarian JS. Clinical effect of allopurinol on preserved kidneys: a randomized double-blind study. Ann Surg 1977: 185: 128–31.

57. Hoshino T, Maley WR, Bulkley GB, Williams GM. Ablation of free radical-mediated reperfusion injury for the salvage of kidneys taken from non-heartbeating donors. A quantitative evaluation of the proportion of injury caused by reperfusion following periods of warm, cold, and combined warm and cold ischemia. Transplantation 1988; 45: 284–9.

58. Bry WI, Collins GM, Halasz NA. Jelliner M. Improved function of perfused rabbit kidneys by prevention of oxidative injury. Transplantation 1984; 38: 579.

59. Green CJ, Healing G, Lunec J, Fuller BJ, Simpkin S. Evidence of free-radical-induced damage in rabbit kidneys after simple hypothermic preservation and autotransplantation. Transplantation 1986; 41: 161.

60. Southard JH, Marsh DC, McAnulty JF, Belzer FO. Oxygen free radical damage in organ preservation: activity of superoxide dismutase and xanthine oxidase. Transplant Proc 1987; In Press.

61. Bennett JF, Bry WI, Collins GM, Halasz NA. The effects of oxygen free radicals on the preserved kidney. Cryobiology 1987; 24: 264–9.

62. Boudjema K, Southard JH, Belzer FO, Jaeck D, Cinqualbre J. Changes in glutathione levels in the renal cortex of dogs during preservation by continuous hypothermic pulsatile perfusion. Chirurgie 1991; 117: 575–82.

63. Freer RJ. Calcium and angiotensin tachyphylaxis in rate uterine smooth muscle. Am J Physiol 1975; 228: 1423.

64. Peach MJ. Molecular actions of angiotensin. Biochem Pharmacol 1981; 30: 2745.

65. Adelstein RS. Calmodulin and the regulation of the actin–myosin interaction in smooth muscle and non-muscle cells. Cell 1982; 30: 349.

17 | Kidney preservation

GEOFFREY M. COLLINS

1. Introduction

The evolution of clinical organ transplantation over the past 25 years has had a major influence on the methods used for kidney preservation. The work of Belzer and his colleagues [1] and that of Collins *et al.* [2] provided the foundation for the two alternative methods of continuous hypothermic perfusion or initial flushing followed by ice storage. For some years the processes of cadaver donor maintenance, organ procurement, and preservation were focused solely on the needs of the kidney. Donors were vigorously fluid-loaded, usually without regard for the effect on the heart, lungs or other abdominal organs. Kidneys were often dissected and removed individually, and in most cases were flushed with Collins' solution and stored on ice until transplanted. A minority of centres used continuous hypothermic perfusion. Those using perfusion claimed better immediate function, while advocates of simple flushing justified their choice in terms of lower cost, greater simplicity and essentially equivalent results [3]. The discovery of cyclosporine, and its introduction into general clinical use in 1984 changed the picture substantially. While in earlier years it was the exception to procure thoracic and extrarenal abdominal organs along with the kidneys, this is now the rule. As a result, the emphasis in donor management, organ procurement and preservation methods has shifted to the needs of the heart, lungs and the extrarenal abdominal organs. Donor hydration is now practised conservatively to avoid inducing pulmonary or visceral oedema. The abdominal organs are usually procured *en bloc*, and preservation methods are chosen with the liver and pancreas primarily in mind.

The principles of donor preparation, the surgical techniques of organ procurement, and the basic physiology and biochemistry of hypothermic organ preservation are discussed elsewhere, and this discussion will be confined to the practical issues of kidney preservation by ice storage or by continuous hypothermic perfusion.

2. Ice storage

The benefit of hypothermia to kidney preservation derives from metabolic suppression. The decay of total adenine nucleotide in the renal cortex after 24 h at 4°C is roughly equivalent to that seen following 30 min of normothermic ischaemia – a 50-fold improvement in biochemical tolerance is produced by cooling [4]. Since surface cooling alone is too slow to effectively cool the relatively large human kidney [5], early work on kidney preservation concentrated on the development of suitable flush solutions to produce rapid core cooling. Collins' solution was the first of these to preserve kidneys better than a simple electrolyte solution. It was formulated to resemble intracellular fluid (see Table 1) in the belief that it would control ionic and fluid exchanges across the cell membrane during hypothermic storage [2]. It originally contained 30 mM magnesium sulphate, which led to a tendency for magnesium phosphate crystals to precipitate over time. To avoid this, Eurotransplant modified the solution by removing the magnesium and increasing the glucose content to compensate for the reduced osmolarity. This new solution known as EuroCollins' (EC) and the original composition remain in limited use today for living donors and for kidney-only cadaveric donors.

G.M. Collins, J.M. Dubernard, W. Land and G.G. Persijn (eds). Procurement, Preservation and Allocation of Vascularized Organs 153–157
© 1997 Kluwer Academic Publishers.

Table 1. Flush solution composition (mM).

Component	Collins'	Sacks 2	Ross and Marshall	PBS[(A)]	UW[(B)]
Sodium	10	14	80	120	35
Potassium	115	126	80		125
Magnesium	30	8	35		5
Citrate			55		
Sulphate	30		35		5
Phosphate	50	60		60	25
Chloride	15	16			
Bicarbonate	10	20			
Lactobionate					100
Glucose	140				
Sucrose				140	
Raffinose					30
Mannitol		208	190		
Glutathione					3
Adenosine					5
Allopurinol					1
Hydroxyethyl starch					50 g/l
Dexamethasone					16 mg/l
Insulin					40 U/l
Penicillin					2×10^5 U/l

Since there is both experimental and clinical evidence to show that the magnesium in Collins' solution is beneficial [6–8], we use the original composition for flushing, and EC for immersion to avoid any possibility of magnesium phosphate 'frosting' on the kidney surface.

Once it had been established that flush cooling and ice storage was an effective method for kidney preservation, the basic questions became how these flush solutions worked and whether their composition could be improved. The major component of modern kidney storage solutions is an impermeant solute such as phosphate, lactobionate, glucose, sucrose or raffinose which is used to control hypothermic swelling. There is less agreement about the need for some of the other minor components, including buffers to control acidosis, reducing agents to minimize oxidative reperfusion injury, adenine nucleotide precursors for high-energy phosphate regeneration after revascularization, and both potassium and magnesium to prevent loss of intracellular cations.

Among the best known of these flush solutions are Sacks [9], Ross and Marshall [10] and phosphate buffered sucrose (PBS) [11] (see Table 1). Kidney preservation for 3 days has been achieved experimentally with each of these solutions, and all have been used successfully for cadaver kidney preservation. However, in recent years they have been superseded by the University of Wisconsin (UW) solution. Currently, UW is the preferred method for liver preservation and it has been quite natural, therefore, to use it simultaneously for the kidneys in the usual multi-organ donor. In experimental studies UW was found to be superior to both EC and PBS solutions [12], and in a multicentre clinical trial UW solution was associated with a significantly higher incidence of immediate kidney function (77%) compared with EC preservation (67%) [13]. However, other trials failed to show a difference between UW and Collins' when the latter was made up with magnesium [8,14]. If Collins' solution is to be used as a less expensive alternative to UW for kidney-only donors, it would seem wise to include the magnesium sulphate.

Although UW is the accepted standard for kidney preservation, there is evidence to suggest that its composition might be further improved, or at least simplified. Of its many constituents there is general agreement only on the value of lactobionate. HES and adenosine may not be necessary, and other sugars can often be substituted for raffinose without loss of efficacy [15–17]. There is evidence that a high-sodium composition may be superior to the standard high-potassium composition [18,19]. In a clinical trial of one such high sodium variant (SLS), we found significantly better kidney function compared with UW when storage times exceeded 30 h (82.7% for SLS versus 65.5% for UW) [19]. Avoidance of delayed graft function by using improved flush solutions can appreciably improve the prospects for kidney transplantation by reducing the length of hospital stay, as well as the costs, and improving 1-year graft survival [20,21]. However, as pointed out above, new flush solutions are unlikely to find a place in kidney preservation unless they are also shown to be superior to UW for liver and pancreas.

3. Perfusion preservation

Continuous hypothermic perfusion with cryoprecipitated plasma was the first technique to be used in clinical practice for extended renal preservation, although its popularity waned somewhat with the introduction of effective ice storage methods. However, there seems to be a resurgence of interest in kidney perfusion as cost containment policies stress the need for immediate graft function, and the increasing use of imported kidneys fuels concerns about the quality of their procurement and preservation. The basic physiological parameters for hypothermic kidney perfusion were established by Belzer and his colleagues in 1967 [1], and have not been superseded. These include pulsatile flow at a pressure of 30–60 torr, a pulse rate of around 60 ppm, and a temperature of 4–10°C. Their original perfusate was cryoprecipitated plasma, in which the freezing and filtration steps were designed to remove lipoprotein aggregates which might otherwise have led to rising vascular resistance. In an attempt to simplify perfusate preparation, other perfusates have been based on plasma albumin [22–24]. This avoided the cryoprecipitation step, but the solutions still needed to be prepared freshly from the basic ingredients prior to each kidney perfusion, and were subject to the variability inherent in biological products. To overcome these disadvantages, the Belzer group developed an entirely synthetic solution using 5% hydroxyethyl starch (HES) as the colloid. This proved to be superior to a similar solution containing albumin [25] and had the major advantage of being stable on storage.

The composition of the Belzer gluconate solution is shown in Table 2. It contains, in addition to HES, a number of ingredients designed to reduce cell swelling and to support metabolism. Although 3-day kidney preservation is readily achievable with this solution, quite sufficient for clinical practice, Belzer and his colleagues have continued to work towards extending preservation times further. Their approach has been to study hypothermic metabolism as a guide to optimiz-

Table 2. Perfusion solution composition (Belzer gluconate solution, mM).

Component	Concentration
Sodium gluconate	80
Potassium phosphate	25
Glucose	10
Magnesium gluconate	5
HEPES	10
Adenine	5
Ribose	5
Mannitol	30
Penicillin	2×10^5 units
Dexamethasone	12 mg
Phenol red	12 mg
Insulin	100 units
Calcium chloride	1.5

ing the constituents. McAnulty et al. reported successful 5-day preservation by setting the calcium content of the perfusate at 0.5 mM [26], and 7-day storage by the addition of a phospholipase inhibitor, quinacrine, to the perfusate [27]. They also reported that adenine plus ribose was more effective than the parent adenosine for maintaining adenine nucleotide levels on perfusion [28]. The composition of the UW lactobionate solution is similar to that of the gluconate solution. However, the Wisconsin group has shown that the lactobionate anion is less effective than gluconate for kidney perfusion, but better than the latter for cold storage [17,29].

4. Choice of preservation method

The obvious advantages to transplanting well-preserved cadaveric kidneys are a greater likelihood of immediate function, a reduced need for dialysis and a lower cost of hospitalization. Delayed graft function also appears to lead to poorer long term outcome [21], although in some cases this may be explained by an unrecognized rejection process. Indeed, poor preservation may itself promote the onset of rejection [30]. The fact that a well preserved kidney may be treated 'kindly' by the immune system is exemplified by the outcome of living unrelated kidney transplantation. Within this group, spouse transplants do as well as two haplotype-matched related donors, and all living unrelated transplants fair considerably better than equally mismatched cadaveric donor transplants [31].

Other issues which must be considered by each transplant program when selecting a method for cadaveric kidney preservation include (1) any influence their choice might have on long term outcome, apart from any direct effect on early graft function, (2) suitability of the method for regional exchange of kidneys on the basis of established organ sharing arrangements, (3) the cost of solutions, equipment and staff required to implement the chosen method, and (4) the average duration of preservation required. This will be determined by logistical considerations, such as where the patients and kidneys typically come from, time taken to complete the necessary arrangements such as histocompatibility typing, and availability of the operating room. A recent study by Koyama et al. bears on the first of these issues [8]. They summarized the effects of preservation methods on the outcome of more than 15 000 first cadaver kidney transplants reported to the UNOS registry. Perfusion preservation yielded the highest rate of immediate graft function (83% at 1 week), 10% better than that obtained with cold-stored kidneys. However, the 1 year graft survival of perfused kidneys was significantly lower (78%) than with the use of Collins' (81%) or UW (83%) solutions. Our own experience comparing ice storage and machine perfusion appears to generally support the findings of the pooled data (see Table 3). The rate of immediate function for pumped (actually mixed perfusion preservation, since perfusion on average accounted for only 50% of preservation time) was 91%, 10% better than with cold storage. As with the pooled data the higher immediate function rate did not translate into a higher incidence of 1-year graft function. However, ice storage, particularly with UW, failed progressively beyond 30 h of storage whereas machine perfusion still maintained a 91% immediate function rate. Furthermore, with long preservation times machine-perfused kidneys appeared to have a better 1-year graft survival than ice-stored organs. On the basis of these data we have adopted a policy of placing all kidneys on the pump whether procured locally or at a distance when the preservation time is likely to exceed 30 h. We have been able thereby to increase the rate of early function even when kidneys have been ice stored for most of the preservation period. Our policy appears to have reduced length of hospital stay by several days in this group of recipients without prejudicing long term function. The resulting cost savings more than offset any expenses incurred in running the perfusion machine.

References

1. Belzer FO, Ashby BS, Dunphy JE. Twenty-four-hour and 72-hour preservation of canine kidneys. Lancet 1967; 2: 536–9.
2. Collins GM, Bravo-Shugarman M, Terasaki Pl. Kidney transportation. 3. Initial perfusion and 30 hour storage. Lancet 1969; 2: 1219.
3. Opelz G, Terasaki Pl. Advantage of cold storage over machine perfusion for preservation of cadaver kidneys. Transplantation 1982; 33: 64–8.
4. Buhl MR, Jorgensen S. Breakdown of 5′adenine estimated by oxypurine excretion during perfusion. Scand J Clin Lab Invest 1975; 35: 211–17.
5. Kerr WK, Kyle VN, Keresteci AA, Smythe CA. Renal hypothermia. J Urol 1960; 81: 236–42.
6. Collins GM, Halasz NA. Forty-eight hour ice storage of kidneys: importance of cation content. Surgery 1976; 79: 432.
7. Collins GM, Barry JM, Maxwell JG, Sampson D, VanderWerf BA. The value of magnesium in flush solutions for human cadaveric kidney preservation. J Urol 1984; 131: 220–2.
8. Koyama H, Cecka JM, Terasaki Pl. A comparison of cadaver donor kidney storage methods: pump perfusion and cold storage solutions. Clin Transplant 1993; 7: 199–205.
9. Sacks SA, Petritsch PH, Leong CH, Kaufman JJ. Experiments in renal preservation: 48 and 72-hour canine kidney preservation by initial perfusion and hypothermic storage. J Urol 1974; 111: 434–8.
10. Jablonski P, Howden B, Marshall V, Scott D. Evaluation of citrate flushing solution using the isolated perfused rat kidney. Transplantation 1980; 30: 239–43.
11. Lam FT, Mavor AID, Potts DJ, Giles GR. Improved 72-hour renal preservation with phosphate-buffered sucrose. Transplantation 1989; 47: 767–71.
12. Ploeg RJ, Goosens D, McAnulty JF, Southard JH, Belzer FO. Successful 72-hour cold storage of dog kidneys with UW solution. Transplantation 1988; 46: 191–6.
13. Ploeg RJ, Van Bockel JH, Langendijk PTH, Groenewegen M, Van Der Woude P, Persijn GG, Thorogood J, Hermans J. Effect of preservation solution on results of cadaveric kidney transplantation. Lancet 1992; 340: 129–36.
14. Collins GM, Bry WI, Warren R, Mollenkopf F, Feduska NJ. Clinical comparison of UW with Collins' solution for cadaveric kidney preservation. Transplant Proc 1991; 23: 1305–6.

Table 3. Ice storage versus machine perfusion (primary cadaveric transplants).

Function	All storage times			> 30 h storage		
	n	1 week	1 year	n	1 week	1 year
Machine perfusion	46	91.3%	81.4%	33	90.9%	80.1%
Ice storage	596	78.9%	83.9%	312	74.4%	76.6%

15. Jamieson NV, Lindell S, Sundberg GS, Southard JH, Belzer FO. An analysis of the components in UW solution using isolated perfused rabbit liver. Transplantation 1988; 46: 512–16.

16. Yu W, Coddington D, Bitter-Suermann H. Rat liver preservation. I. The components of UW solution that are essential to its success. Transplantation 1990; 49: 1060–6.

17. Sumimoto R, Jamieson NV, Kamada N. Examination of the role of the impermeants lactobionate and raffinose in a modified UW solution. Transplantation 1990; 50: 573–6.

18. Moen J, Claeson K, Pienaar H, Lindell S, Ploeg RJ, McAnulty JF, Vreugdenhil P, Southard JH, Belzer FO. Preservation of dog liver, kidney, and pancreas using the Belzer-UW solution with a high-sodium and low-potassium content. Transplantation 1989; 47: 940–5.

19. Collins GM, Wicomb WN, Warren R, Wong L, Bry Wl, Feduska NJ, Salvatierra O. Canine and cadaver kidney preservation with sodium lactobionate sucrose solution (SLS). Transplant Proc 1993; 25: 1588–1590.

20. Almond PS, Troppmann C, Escobar F, Frey DJ, Matas AJ. Economic impact of delayed graft function. Transplant Proc 1991; 23: 1304.

21. Rosenthal JT, Danovitch GM, Wilkinson A, Ettenger RB. The high cost of delayed graft function in cadaveric renal transplantation. Transplantation 1991; 51: 1115–17.

22. Johnson RWG, Anderson M, Flear CTG. Evaluation of a new perfusion solution for kidney preservation. Transplantation 1972; 13: 270–5.

23. Halasz NA, Collins GM. Simplification of perfusion preservation methods: colloid and buffer studies. Transplantation 1974; 17: 534–6.

24. Toledo-Pereyra LH, Condie RM, Malmberg R, Simmons RL, Najarian JS. A fibrinogen-free plasma perfusate for preservation of kidneys for 120 hours. Surg Gynecol Obstet 1974; 38: 901–5.

25. Hoffman RM, Southard JH, Lutz M, Mackety A, Belzer FO. Synthetic perfusate for kidney preservation. Its use in 72-hour preservation of dog kidneys. Arch Surg 1983; 118: 919–21.

26. McAnulty JF, Ploeg RJ, Southard JH, Belzer FO. Successful five day perfusion preservation of the canine kidney Transplantation 1989; 47: 37–41.

27. McAnulty JF, Vreugdenhil PK, Southard JH, Belzer FO. Improved survival of kidneys preserved for seven days with a phospholipase inhibitor. Transplant Proc 1991; 23: 1991; 691–2.

28. McAnulty JF, Southard JH, Belzer FO. Improved maintenance of adenosine triphosphate in five-day perfused kidneys with adenine and ribose. Transplant Proc 1987; 19: 1376–9.

29. McAnulty JF, Vreugdenhil PK, Southard JH, Belzer FO. Use of UW cold storage solution for machine perfusion of kidneys. Transplant Proc 1990; 22: 458–9.

30. Howard TK, Klintmalm GBG, Cofer JB, Husberg BS, Goldstein RM, Gonwa TA. The influence of preservation injury on rejection in the hepatic transplant recipient. Transplantation 1990; 49: 103–7.

31. Terasaki PI, Cecka JM, Lim E. Takemoto S, Cho Y Gjertson D, Ogura K, Koyama H, Mitsuishi Y, Yuga J, Cohn M. Overview. Clin Transplants 1991; 409–30.

18 | Liver preservation: historical review of preservation techniques

N.V. Jamieson

1. Introduction

In his early transplant work Carrel (1908) used Locke's solution at room temperature to flush organs prior to transplantation and used the same solution chilled to preserve an artery for several days [1]. Locke's solution was used as a physiologically balanced solution and reference is made to the 'poisonous effects of the pure sodium salt'. He later worked with Charles Lindbergh (the same Lindbergh who had piloted the *Spirit of St. Louis* across the Atlantic) and together they studied perfusion preservation of organs at normothermia using large volumes of oxygenated plasma to keep tissues viable for many days, but then did not go on to test their results in a transplant model [2]. Carrel thus pioneered not only organ transplantation but also the techniques of simple cold storage and of machine perfusion which were to re-emerge in the 1960s for clinical organ preservation. In his work he quotes Le Gallois (1770–1814) as predicting 'If one could substitute for the heart a kind of injection … of arterial blood, either natural or artificially made … one would succeed easily in maintaining alive indefinitely any part of the body'. This apparently simple prediction has proved remarkably difficult to achieve in practice.

In the experimental development of liver grafting Moore and his colleagues [3] noted the success of previous workers in extending the tolerance of the liver to hypoxia using hypothermia (< 28°C). Cold isotonic salt solution was placed in the peritoneal cavity to render the donor animal hypothermic and surface cooling continued until the temperature of the liver was around 28°C. Starzl and his co-workers used a similar technique but contributed the refinement of the

concept of 'core cooling' [4]. They cooled the donor in an ice bath to a temperature of 25–30°C before opening the abdomen and then used an *in situ* flush of 1 l of chilled Ringer's lactate via the portal vein to provide rapid cooling of the interior of the liver. During perfusion the core temperature of the liver fell to 10–20°C, but preservation times were still limited to 2 h. This experimental observation is illustrated in Fig. 1, with the addition of the subsequent cooling seen when the organ is packed and stored in melting ice, as in current clinical practice.

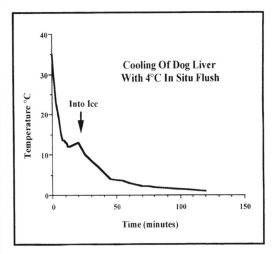

Figure 1. The rate of cooling of a dog liver during an in situ flush with 1500 ml of a chilled (4°C) preservation solution followed by immersion in melted ice for storage. Core temperature measured using a thermistor probe.

G.M. Collins, J.M. Dubernard, W. Land and G.G. Persijn (eds), Procurement, Preservation and Allocation of Vascularized Organs 159–167
© 1997 Kluwer Academic Publishers.

In 1963, the same year as the first attempted human liver transplant, Marchioro investigated the use of a femoro-femoral extracorporeal perfusion system to preserve organs in a canine model [5], maintaining the organ temperature at 12–15°C. The results in the dog were disappointing: the satisfactory upper limit for this technique proving to be 6 h for the kidney and less than 2 h for the liver. A short human trial proved unsuccessful since technical problems were encountered in establishing and maintaining the perfusion, and the technique was abandoned. Kestens enjoyed greater success in his model with a similar technique using perfusion with oxygenated blood at 10–18°C [6]. Livers were maintained in this fashion in donor dogs for periods of 90–325 min and then transplanted orthotopically, with nine of 12 dogs surviving for more than 5 days. Despite these successes the technique was not developed further.

Asanguinous perfusion as pioneered by Carrel attracted considerable interest at this time, representing a logical and appealing technique for organ preservation and offering a means of providing nutrients and removing waste products to permit maintenance of metabolism, albeit at a reduced rate under hypothermic conditions. In 1967 Slapak reported the first application of this technique to the liver [7]. Puppy livers perfused with a cold balanced salt solution at 4°C under hyperbaric conditions for 24 h were transplanted into the necks of adult dogs. Eight of 19 livers produced bile after grafting and were still functioning at the time of elective sacrifice at 48 h, with reasonable histological appearances. The same year saw one of the landmark papers in preservation from Belzer et al. [8]. They described machine perfusion of canine kidneys with consistent success after 72 h preservation. Brettschneider and his co-workers devised a complex but effective perfusion technique for the liver which they applied both experimentally in dogs and clinically in man. The grafts were placed inside a refrigerated (4°C) hyperbaric chamber and perfused via the artery and the portal vein with a perfusate consisting of 50% blood and 50% balanced salt solution with the addition of low molecular weight dextran, dextrose, magnesium sulphate and procaine. In the dog this gave good preservation at 8–9 h with minimal biochemical disturbances in liver function, similar to control animals. A preservation period of 24 h gave less satisfactory results but nonetheless three of five animals survived for over 7 days [9]. The technique was subsequently used in seven human recipients with preservation times of 242–427 min and all survived the first week with adequate immediate function, their subsequent course being determined by the effects of rejection, immuno-suppression and infection. The technique was thus effective but complex and expensive and was soon superseded by simpler and cheaper alternatives [10].

In 1969 Collins reported a new simple flush solution for cold storage of kidneys [11]. Collins based his solution on the concept of using a modified intracellular solution rich in potassium and magnesium to minimize the ionic shifts known to occur in anoxic kidney slices stored in the cold. Kidneys were simply flushed with the new solution and then stored on ice at 0–4°C. Collins noted prophetically 'There is no reason to presume that the concentration of ions in the new perfusate is the best that can be achieved for dogs or man'. Many groups preferred the simplicity and cheapness of the system, adopting it in preference to Belzer's machine perfusion, and thus marked the beginning of a controversy over the relative merits of the two techniques which has continued to this day.

In 1969 Schalm and his co-workers [12] published a flush cooling technique for the liver which had been the basis of a thesis the previous year and which had been used in four orthotopic human liver transplants in 1968 [13]. The technique used an initial vascular flush with a dextran-based solution followed by storage in a plasma solution with added glucose, procaine, bicarbonate hydrocortisone and penicillin.

Belzer had by now turned his attention to the liver and used his cryoprecipitated plasma solution in a series of experiments on the application of machine perfusion preservation in a pig orthotopic transplant model [14]. This was carried out at 8–10°C, continuous flow being used for the portal vein and pulsatile flow via the hepatic artery. The technique was successful for 8–10 h but attempts to extend this preservation period to 24 h were disappointing. At longer preservation times uncontrollable bleeding was encountered, attributed to vascular endothelial damage and a consumptive coagulopathy [15].

Meanwhile similar results had been obtained for simple cold storage in the pig, using Schalm's technique with slight modification following 5–8 h preservation [16,17]. Longer preservation times were not successful in this model, although in the baboon Mieny and Myburgh [18] achieved survival after 19–20 h preservation using a dextran-electolyte-sorbitol solution, but once again no animals survived following 24 h preservation.

Addition of chlorpromazine, phenoxybenzamine and hydrocortisone to Schalm's solution and the use of hyperbaric oxygen permitted 12 h preservation [19]. Calne reported good results in porcine liver grafting after preservation for 12–18 h at 4°C using an intermittent squirt perfusion technique [20]. The perfusate used was once again derived from Schalm's solution, being based in this instance on human plasma protein fraction. This combination of simple cold storage with some of the features of machine perfusion represented the best preservation reported in this more difficult model.

Rather belated attention was now turned to Collins' solution and its possible use in the liver. Lambotte and his colleagues, using an isolated perfused canine liver model and reperfusion with oxygenated blood at 20°C, demonstrated an advantage for Collins' C4 over Ringer's lactate [21]. They went on to orthotopic transplantation in the dog. In a control group which received livers preserved at 4°C in Ringer's lactate there were no survivors when storage times were > 3.5 h. Satisfactory preservation was achieved for 6 h using Collins', and 13–19 h preservation was possible, although the postoperative course was difficult with a bleeding diathesis requiring fresh blood transfusions and treatment with ε-amino caproic acid. Increasing the magnesium sulphate concentration in the Collins solution resulted in some survivors after 24–26 h preservation of the graft.

By now a modification of Schalm's technique was in regular clinical use in Cambridge, initial perfusion using Hartmann's solution and plasma protein fraction (PPF) forming the basis of the preservation medium used subsequently for graft storage [22]. This allowed distant organ procurement, but preservation times were still kept down to 3–4 h. In 1977 Benichou published a comparison of Ringer's lactate, the Cambridge PPF solution and Collins' solution in a dog orthotopic transplant model [23]. After 9 h of preservation the survival of dogs receiving livers preserved with the three solutions was similar but peak postoperative transaminase release was less in the Collins' group. Following 18 h of preservation there were no survivors in the Ringer's lactate group but comparable survival in the other two groups, with a probable advantage in favour of Collins solution with respect to SGPT release. Encouraged by these results Starzl changed his clinical organ preservation to Collins' solution and reported in the same paper seven human liver grafts removed from donors in Los Angeles and transferred by air to Denver.

Numerous studies performed during the 1970s [24,25] and early 1980s [26] aimed at elucidating the mechanisms of action of the existing storage solutions and methods, and the significance of the various components in the often complex solutions being devised. Isolated organ perfusion, tissue slice studies and whole organ transplantation in many different species were all used by various authors in addressing these issues. These studies often raised more questions than they answered. Collins and Halasz [27] showed that the

inclusion of procaine in the original C_3 solution was actually detrimental and that the high potassium 'intracellular' formulation could be changed to a high sodium variant with only a slight decrease in effectiveness. Similarly it appeared that phosphate could be replaced with sulphate without detrimental effect and, indeed, possibly a slight benefit [28]. A committee set up by the Eurotransplant organization devised the simplified variant known as EuroCollins in 1976, which omitted amongst other things magnesium sulphate from the solution. This avoided the problem of the formation of crystals of magnesium phosphate (for which the original solution is supersaturated) during storage. Despite these changes from Collins' original formulation this solution proved effective both in clinical practice and in the laboratory [29] and became the standard preservation solution for both kidney and liver preservation in continental Europe and the USA during the early 1980s.

Nonetheless a picture was developing of the underlying principles of successful organ preservation. The situation for machine perfusion was at least readily understandable where an attempt was being made to replace the natural circulation and supply appropriate substrates to maintain normal, albeit reduced, cell metabolism but the principles of simple cold storage were rather more difficult to grasp. These centred around the beneficial effects of hypothermia in reducing metabolic activity and thus the cells' requirements for oxygen and other nutrients, together with a reduction in catabolic processes and the production of potentially toxic waste products. Homeostatic as well as damaging processes are reduced under hypothermic conditions but in simple cold storage, unlike machine perfusion, there is not the facility to continue aerobic metabolism to maintain the internal milieu. It is, therefore, necessary to rely on manipulation of the physicochemical nature of the extracellular environment to minimize the adverse effects of hypothermia on these homeostatic processes. Additional benefits may be obtained by pharmacological manipulation in order to improve initial washout, prevent release of lysosomal enzymes, mitigate their effects or to minimize the effects of free radicals generated at the time of reperfusion. Similarly any naturally occurring protective substances such as glutathione which are known to be lost or consumed during storage can be supplemented [30].

Cell swelling has been identified as a major damaging event in hypothermia. The normal mechanisms by which cell volume is maintained are still poorly understood, representing a balance between active and passive molecular and ionic movements across the cell membrane. Much has been made of the role of the sodium pump in this regard by MacKnight and Leaf

[31]. They believe that the colloid osmotic pressure of the intracellular macromolecules is offset by the exclusion of sodium from the cells; this is undoubtedly a valuable concept, although many inconsistencies remain to be resolved. Na+, K+-ATPase is largely inactive at the temperatures (0–4°C) used in simple cold storage in all tissues [32] and thus cell swelling would be expected in the absence of any preservation solution effect to prevent it. It is interesting to note that all of the effective cold storage solutions described so far include in their constituents impermeant substances which remain in the extracellular space and help to provide this property [24,28]. Glucose is the principal impermeant in Collins' solution: although this is an impermeant in the kidney the hepatocyte cell membrane is freely permeable to glucose [33], and this may be a crucial factor in the difference between the longer preservation times achieved with this solution for the kidney but not the liver.

Clinical liver transplantation underwent substantial expansion during this period following the 1983 NIH Consensus Conference report. Safe preservation limits of 6–8 h were established using either EuroCollins' or the Cambridge PPF-based solution. These time limits allowed practical use of donors from a wide area but required close coordination of donor and recipient procedures. The recipient operation commenced as soon as the donor team confirmed that the graft appeared satisfactory, the aim being to allow the recipient team to reimplant the liver as soon as it arrived in the operating theatre. Donor procedures usually take place in the evening, at a time convenient to the donor hospital at the end of their routine operating day, with the result that the donor team are usually travelling during the hours of darkness, often by air due to the time constraints involved. This resulted in most transplant operations being carried out during the night, increasing the organizational difficulties of arranging support staff for the procedure and adding the complication of darkness and possible poor weather conditions to the transport of the donor organ. Unforeseen problems with transport arrangements or unexpected time consuming difficulty in the recipient hepatectomy could result in the ischaemic time of the graft being prolonged towards or beyond the limits of safe preservation. Starzl described the procedure as 'an exercise in urgency and administrative inconvenience'.

2. The introduction of UW solution

The interests of the University of Wisconsin preservation laboratory had continued to be directed primarily towards machine perfusion, but examination of the properties of lactobionate and raffinose in preventing hypothermic cell swelling led to the description of a new cold storage solution for pancreas preservation by Wahlberg and his co-workers who achieved successful experimental preservation times of 48 and 72 h [34]. Lactobionic acid (mol. wt 358 kDa) is derived from lactose. The lactobionate anion is used in UW solution to replace chloride and raffinose (mol. wt 504 KDa) is a trisaccharide included as an impermeant.

Jamieson and his co-workers from the same department applied this solution and some simpler variants to liver preservation using first an isolated perfusion model and later an orthotopic canine transplant model, achieving 24 and 48 h preservation [35,36]. Some of this work included simplified variants on the initial solution and dog livers were successfully preserved for 48 h despite the omission of hydroxyethyl starch, adenosine and dexamethasone from the initial formulation [36]. Further analysis of the components essential for liver preservation carried out in an isolated perfused rabbit liver model confirmed the importance of lactobionate, raffinose and glutathione in the solution, but suggested that the other components could be omitted without serious adverse effects [37]. This initial experimental work was soon followed by clinical application of the solution with preservation times up to 24 h at the University of Wisconsin [38], University of Pittsburgh [39] and University of Cambridge where simplified versions of the new UW solution were also used successfully [40].

The introduction of UW solution has permitted substantial changes in clinical practice and is now in routine use throughout the world. The more prolonged safe preservation period has allowed safer distant procurement and permitted the transplant procedure to be booked as a 'semi-elective' procedure. When difficulty in donor hepatectomy is encountered slow careful dissection can proceed without undue concern about the deleterious effects of a longer preservation time. For standard transplantation procedures preservation times of up to 12–16 h are more than adequate. The longer preservation times of 24, 30 and even 48 h which can be achieved experimentally [36] represent the limits of what can be achieved under ideal procurement conditions with a healthy donor and recipient animal, and do not represent times which should be routinely utilized in clinical practice. These long preservation times represent the limits of what can be achieved under perfect laboratory conditions; the AST release observed in the initial 24 and 48 h preservation groups of 2092 ± 960 IU/l and 4875 ± 1904 IU/l, respectively, represent substantial but recoverable hepatocellular injury.

Our own initial experience with UW solution and two simplified derivatives involved mean preservation times of 10–11 h, permitting the organ to be harvested late in the evening at the convenience of the donor hospital and reimplanted next morning [41]. We used clinically not only the standard UW solution but also the simplified solution used in some of the initial dog experiments [36], omitting adenosine, insulin, dexamethasone and hydroxyethyl starch, and the Cambridge II solution which is similar but with a reversed Na^+/K^+ ratio, and which had been previously tested in a rat model [42] (Table 1). Results with all three solutions were good with no significant difference in ALT release (Table 2) blood requirement or graft survival between the three groups [40,41]. Mean

transaminase release in all groups was well below 1000 IU/l, compared with higher values observed in the long preservation experimental studies.

More recent clinical studies have further addressed this issue of increasing degrees of organ damage with prolonged storage. The most worrying reports have related to the occurrence of biliary strictures following long cold ischaemic times [43–45]. Ninety-one patients receiving liver transplants at the Mayo clinic, and without any of the accepted risk factors for biliary strictures (ABO incompatibility, arterial thrombosis and chronic rejection), surviving for at least 3 months, have been analysed and a strong correlation between cold ischaemic time and non-anastomotic biliary strictures noted. Thirty-five percent of grafts preserved for over 11.5 h developed such strictures and reduction of mean ischaemic times to 9 h reduced the occurrence of

Table 1. The composition of the three lactobionate based solutions which have been used in clinical practice in Cambridge.

	Commercial UW solution	Simplified solution	Cambridge II solution
K lactobionate (mM)	100	100	–
Na lactobionate (mM)	–	–	100
NaKH$_2$PO$_4$ (mM)	25	25	25
MgSO$_4$ (mM)	5	5	5
Glutathione (mM)	3	3	3
Raffinose (mM)	30	30	30
Allopurinol (mM)	1	1	1
Adenosine (mM)	5	–	–
Penicillin (U)	200 000	200 000	–
Insulin (U)	40	–	–
Dexamethasone (mg)	16	–	–
Hydroxyethyl starch (g%)	5	–	–
Gentamicin (mg)	–	–	8
Ampicillin (g)	–	–	1
Na (mM)	30	30	120
K (mM)	120	120	30
pH	7.4	7.4	7.4
Osmolality (mOsm/l)	320–330	305–315	305–315

Table 2. Clinical use of lactobionate solutions – ALT release.

	Commercial UW solution	Simplified solution	Cambridge II solution
Preservation time (h)	11 ± 4.4	10.1 ± 4	10.5 ± 4.5
Number of cases	89	93	24
Mean ± S.D. (IU/l)	501 ± 475	528 ± 559	284 ± 151
Median (IU/l)	354	317	281
Range	44–3465	28–2863	25–564

The ALT levels are those measured on the day after operation.

this complication to 1.7% [44]. Other centres, including our own, have not noted such a marked cut-off point [46–48] and have emphasized the known injurious effects of bile on the biliary epithelium and highlighted the importance of careful irrigation of the biliary tree [49]. Work in our own department by Saxena, using corrosion casting techniques, has demonstrated that the vascular pattern around the bile duct is surprisingly sparse in the region of the major bifurcations, explaining the increased vulnerability of these regions to ischaemic injury and 'non-anastomotic' stricture formation.

Nonetheless it is increasingly accepted that preservation times in excess of 12–16 h are achieved only at the price of increased risk of impaired early graft function with a concomitant increase in graft failure [50,51]. The effects of long preservation will exacerbate any pre-existing liver impairment and the presence of known risk factors such as fatty infiltration, long donor ICU stay, heavy inotrope dependence of the donor and the added injurious effect of liver reduction procedures. A number of attempts have been made to improve assessment of donor organs but in this area and that of donor manipulation to improve graft quality much work remains to be done. The MEGX test is the system which has been most extensively applied in donor organ assessment, using the liver's ability to metabolize lignocaine as an index of hepatic function [52]. Early enthusiasm for this technique [52,53] using set cut-off points to indicate which donor organs should be used for transplantation and which discarded has been dampened by a realization that even organs with low MEGX values in the donor can be transplanted successfully [54–56]. The arterial ketone body ratio (AKBR) has been used in a similar manner in both living related and cadaveric transplantation [57] with initial promising results. Both AKBR and MEGX have also been applied as post-operative liver function tests [58–60] to predict early graft outcome. Studies of donor manipulation to improve graft quality have been sparse and in some cases contradictory. Preservation in fasted rats has been shown to be superior [61] but increased glycogen content has been shown to be beneficial in man and hyperalimentation of donors suggested [62]. Hormonal manipulation in donors has not yet been shown to be effective.

To date the renewed experimental activity stimulated by the introduction of UW solution has not resulted in the production of any solution which is clinically superior. Trials of the existing Bretschneider HTK solution have progressed from an initial pilot study [63] with short ischaemic times to 20 h preservation [64] and subsequently to a comparison of UW and HTK in 60 patients. There was similar survival of grafts in both groups with preservation times up to 15 h, but with higher levels of enzyme release in the HTK group, suggesting poorer preservation quality with this fluid. This is in keeping with a comparison in the dog showing that longer preservation was possible using UW solution but that 24 h preservation could be achieved with both HTK and UW [65].

The advantages of using a single solution for preservation of all of intra-abdominal organs is obvious, but there has been considerable discussion on the issue of the initial washout solution to be used prior to the storage of the organs in the UW solution. The initial experimental work in the liver used UW solution throughout [36] and the Wisconsin group have advocated this as correct practice in the clinical setting [66]. This viewpoint is supported by experimental work in both the isolated perfused liver [67] and the rat liver transplant model [68]. Nonetheless the high cost of UW has encouraged some groups to use cheaper solutions as the initial washout solution, UW being reserved for the final flush to reduce costs. One clinical study has addressed this issue in a randomized fashion and showed no difference in graft function or outcome when EuroCollins' was used in place of UW solution for the initial flush [69].

3. Experimental developments

Initial work concentrated on assessing the role of the various components in UW solution to determine which were essential to its effectiveness. The isolated perfused liver model was used initially and demonstrated the importance of lactobionate, raffinose and glutathione [37], the place of the former being attributed to their impermeant properties and that of glutathione to its central antioxidant role [30]. Subsequent studies have used this type of isolated perfusion system, isolated hepatocytes [70] and rat liver transplant models [42,71,72]. The overall conclusions of these studies are similar and emphasize the importance of the key components, but also serve to illustrate the difficulty and complexity of this form of analysis by omission of single or multiple components from an existing solution. The ability to change from a high potassium to a high sodium content has been successfully demonstrated by several groups [37,42,71] and extended to the dog [73] and to man [41,74].

Attempts to produce more effective solutions have met with mixed results. A combined histidine-lactobionate solution (HL) was shown to be superior to other solutions, including UW, in rat liver preservation

[75,76] as well as in the heart and pancreas [77,78]. However, when this solution was tested in the dog model there was no significant difference between HL and UW after 48 h preservation [79]. The gluconate-based UW machine perfusion solution has also been applied to the liver with perfusion via the portal vein for 72 h. Seven of eight dogs survived for 7 days after transplantation with such livers, although bilirubin rose progressively [80].

The importance of the oxidation state of glutathione in preservation solutions was first suggested in a paper on heart preservation when it was noted that freshly made UW solution was superior to stored solutions, and it was speculated that the glutathione became oxidized during storage [81]. This was subsequently tested in a dog liver transplant model, and addition of fresh reduced glutathione to UW solution immediately prior to use clearly improved survival of recipient animals after 48 h storage, but not after 24 h storage [82]. A similar limited human trial demonstrated a small difference, but results did not reach statistical significance [83]. N-Acetylcysteine is a glutathione precursor and its use has been advocated to maintain or restore glutathione levels following reperfusion [90].

The effects of pharmacological additives have also been examined. Using a high sodium lactobionate and sucrose based solution it has proved possible to obtain superior rat liver preservation than that achieved with UW solution, and this was improved still further by addition of chlorpromazine [84]. A later study showed similar benefits from addition of trifluoperazine or nisoldipine [85].

Washing the liver with a 'rinse' solution immediately prior to reperfusion has also been advocated to reduce the damage occurring at this time. The initial work simply used nitrogen-bubbled ice-cold Ringer's lactate and showed an advantage for this approach attributed to the removal of toxic metabolites or toxic precursors in an oxygen-free environment. This observation was combined with studies on mechanisms of graft injury at the time of reperfusion related to endothelial cell damage, Kupffer cell activation, leucocyte adherence and microcirculatory disturbance, and led to the development of the Carolina rinse (CR) solution [86]. The formula for Carolina rinse solution is given in Table 3. It is slightly acidic and contains anti-oxidants, iron chelators, free radical scavengers and calcium channel blockers, together with fructose, glucose and insulin, which have been suggested to improve post-ischaemic energy status.

CR has been tested in the rat liver transplant model, where significant benefits were demonstrated after 12 h storage in UW and rinsing in either Ringer's lactate,

Table 3. The composition of Carolina rinse solution.

KCl	5 mM
NaCl	115 mM
CaCl$_2$	1.3 mM
KH$_2$PO$_4$	1 mM
MgSO$_4$	1.2 mM
Glutathione	3 mM
Desferrioxamine	1 mM
Allopurinol	1 mM
Nicardipine	2 μM
Adenosine	1 mM
Fructose	10 mM
Glucose	10 mM
Insulin	100 U/l
Dexamethasone	–
Hydroxyethyl starch	5 g%
MOPS	20 mM
Na (mM)	115
K (mM)	6
pH	6.5
Osmolality (mOsm/l)	290–305

fresh UW or CR [87]. Microvascular perfusion has been shown to be improved in a similar model, and leucocyte adherence was decreased [88]. A preliminary trial in human transplantation has suggested a small advantage for the Carolina rinse solution in terms of reduced postoperative bilirubin, alkaline phosphatase and lower early transaminase levels [89].

4. Conclusions

The major advances which have occurred in organ preservation have allowed the development of a practical system for sharing of liver grafts, transportation over long distances and subsequent transplantation. Nevertheless there remains considerable room for further improvement to allow increased safe storage times, improve the quality of organs from borderline donors and minimize organ wastage. Simple cold storage offers many practical advantages but perfusion systems are a more logical route if truly long term preservation is to be achieved. Nonetheless Le Gallois's prediction that 'one would succeed easily in maintaining alive indefinitely any part of the body' has proved impossible to achieve.

Preservation research remains a major challenge with many studies raising as many questions as they answer. Further progress in this complex field will involve a synthesis of techniques, information and expertise from many fields including cellular physiology, molecular biology, biophysics, pathology, pharmacology, cryobiology and perfusion technology.

References

1. Carrel A. Results of the transplantation of blood vessels, organs and limbs JAMA 1908; 51: 1662.
2. Carrel A, Lindbergh CA. The culture of whole organs. Science 1935; 81: 621.
3. Moore FD, Smith LL, Burnap TK et al. One stage homotransplantation of the liver following total hepatectomy in dogs. Transplant Bull 1959; 6: 103.
4. Starzl TE, Kaupp HAJ, Brock DR, Lazarus RE, Johnson RV. Reconstructive problems in canine liver homotransplantation with special reference to the postoperative role of hepatic venous flow. Surg Gynecol Obstet 1960; 111: 733.
5. Marchioro TL, Huntley RT, Waddell WR, Starzl TE. Extracorporeal perfusion for obtaining postmortem homografts. Surgery 1963; 54: 900.
6. Kestens PJ, Mikaeloff P, Haxhe JJ et al. Homotransplantation of the canine liver after hypothermic perfusion of long duration. Bull Soc Chir 1966; 6: 647.
7. Slapak M, Wigmore RA, Maclean LD. Twenty-four hour preservation by the use of continuous pulsatile preservation and hyperbaric oxygen. Transplantation 1967; 5: 1154.
8. Belzer FO, Ashby BS, Dunphy JE. 24-hour and 72-hour preservation of canine kidneys. Lancet 1967; ii: 536.
9. Brettschneider L, Daloze PM, Huguet C et al. The use of combined preservation techniques for extended storage of orthotopic liver homografts. Surg Gynecol Obstet 1968; 126: 263.
10. Brettschneider L, Groth CG, Starzl TE. Experimental and clinical preservation of orthotopic liver homografts. In: Starzl TE, Putnam CW (eds), Experience in Hepatic Transplantation. Saunders and Co, Philadelphia 1969:
11. Collins GM, Bravo-Sugarman M, Terasaki PI. Kidney preservation for transportation. Lancet 1969; i: 1219.
12. Schalm SW, Terpstra JL, Drayer B, van den Berg C, Vectkamp JJ. Simple method for short term preservation of a liver homograft. Transplantation 1969; 8: 877.
13. Calne RY, Williams R. Liver transplantation in man. I. Observations on technique and organisation in five cases. Br Med J 1968; 4: 535.
14. Belzer FO, May R, Berry MN, Lee JC. Short term preservation of porcine livers. J Surg Res 1970; 10: 55.
15. Perkins HA, May RA, Belzer FO. Cause of abnormal bleeding after transplantation of pig liver stored by a perfusion technique. Arch Surg 1970; 101: 62.
16. Hadjiyannakis EJ, Calne RY, Marshall VC, D.R. D. Supply and preservation of kidneys. Br J Surg 1971; 58: 835.
17. Spilg H, Uys CJ, Hickman R, Saunders SJ, Terblanche J. Successful liver transplantation after storage for 6–8 hours, using a simple hypothermic immersion technique. Transplantation 1971; 11: 457.
18. Mieny CJ, Myburgh JA. Successful 20 hr preservation of the primate liver by simple cooling. Transplantation 1971; 11: 495.
19. Spilg H, Uys CJ, Hickman R, Saunders SJ, Terblanche J. Twelve-hour liver preservation in the pig using hypothermia and hyperbaric oxygen. Br J Surg 1972; 59: 273.
20. Calne RY, Dunn DC, Herbertson BM et al. Liver preservation by single passage hypothermic 'squirt' perfusion. Br Med J 1972; 4: 142.
21. Lambotte L, Pontegnie-Istace S, Otte JB, Kestens PJ. The effect of Isoproterenol and Collins' solution on the preservation of canine livers with simple cooling. Transplant Proc 1974; 6: 301.
22. Wall WJ, Calne RY, Herbertson BM et al. Simple hypothermic preservation for transporting human livers long distances for transplantation. Transplantation 1977; 23: 210.
23. Benichou J, Halgrimson CG, Weil R, Koep LJ, Starzl TE. Canine and human liver preservation for 6 to 18 hours by cold infusion. Transplantation 1977; 24: 407.
24. Downes G, Hoffman R, Huang J, Belzer FO. Mechanism of action of washout solutions. Transplantation 1973; 16: 46.
25. Bishop MC, Ross BD. Evaluation of hypertonic citrate flushing solution for kidney preservation using the isolated perfused rat kidney. Transplantation 1978; 25: 235.
26. Jablonski P, Howden B, Marshall V, Scott D. Evaluation of citrate flushing solution using the isolated perfused rat kidney. Transplantation 1980; 30: 239.
27. Collins GM, Halasz NA. Forty-eight hour ice storage of kidneys: importance of cation content. Surgery 1976; 79: 432.
28. Collins GM, Green RD, Halasz NA. Importance of anion content and osmolarity in flush solutions for 48 to 72 hr hypothermic kidney storage. Cryobiology 1979; 16: 217.
29. Dreikorn K, Horsch R, Rohl L. 48- to 96-hour preservation of canine kidneys by initial perfusion and hypothermic storage using the EuroCollins solution. Eur Urol 1980; 6 221.
30. Kosower NS, Kosower EM. The glutathione status of cells. Int Rev Cytol 1978; 54: 109.
31. MacKnight ADC, Leaf A. Regulation of cellular volume. Physiol Rev 1977; 57: 510.
32. Martin DR, Scott DF, Downes GL, Belzer FO. Primary cause of unsuccessful liver and heart preservation: cold sensitivity of the ATPase system. Ann Surg 1972; 175: 111.
33. Cahill GF, Ashmore J, Scott Earle A, Zottu S. Glucose penetration into liver. Am J Physiol 1960; 192: 491.
34. Wahlberg JA, Love R, Landegaard L, Southard JH, Belzer FO. Successful 72 hours' preservation of the canine pancreas. Transplant Proc 1987;.
35. Jamieson NV, Sundberg R, Lindell S, Southard JH, Belzer FO. A comparison of cold storage solutions for hepatic preservation using the isolated perfused rabbit liver. Cryobiology 1988; 25: 300–10.
36. Jamieson NV, Sundberg R, Lindell S et al. Preservation of the canine liver for 24–48 hours using simple cold storage with UW solution. Transplantation 1988; 46: 517–22.
37. Jamieson NV, Lindell S, Sundberg R, Southard JH, Belzer FO. An analysis of the components in UW solution using the isolated perfused rabbit liver. Transplantation 1988; 46: 512–16.
38. Kalayoglu M, Sollinger HW, Stratta RJ et al. Extended preservation of the liver for clinical transplantation. Lancet 1988; 1: 617–19.
39. Todo S, Nery S, Yanaga K, Podesta L, Gordon R, Starzl TE. Extended preservation of human liver grafts with UW solution. JAMA 1989; 261: 711–14.
40. Jamieson NV, Johnston PS, O'Grady JG et al. Clinical use of UW solution or a simplified liver preservation solution prior to transplantation in 179 human livers, December 1987–July 1989. Transplant Proc 1990; 22: 2189–90.
41. Jamieson NV. Review article: improved preservation of the liver for transplantation. Aliment Pharmacol Ther 1991; 5: 91–104.
42. Sumimoto R, Jamieson NV, Wake K, Kamada N. 24-hour rat liver preservation using UW solution and some simplified variants. Transplantation 1989; 48: 1–5.
43. Sanchez-Urdazpal L, Gores GJ, Ward EM et al. Ischemic-type biliary complications after orthotopic liver transplantation. Hepatology 1992; 16: 49–53.
44. Krom RA, Sanchez-Urdazpal L. The biliary tree – the Achilles tendon of liver preservation? Transplantation 1992; 53: 1167
45. Li S, Stratta RJ, Langnas AN, Wood RP, Marujo W. Shaw BJ. Diffuse biliary tract injury after orthotopic liver transplantation. Am J Surg 1992; 164: 536–40.
46. Colonna JOI, Shaked A, Gomes AS et al. Biliary strictures complicating liver transplantation. Ann Surg 1992; 216: 344–52.
47. Belzer FO, D'Alessandro AM, Hoffmann RM et al. The use of UW solution in clinical transplantation. Ann Surg 1992; 215: 579–85.
48. Belzer FO, Southard JH, D'Alessandro AM, Knechtle SJ. Sollinger HW, Kalayoglu M. Update on preservation of liver grafts. Transplant Proc 1993; 25: 2010–11.
49. Belzer FO, D'Alessandro A, Hoffmann R, Kalayoglu M, Sollinger H. Management of the common duct in extended

preservation of the liver. Transplantation 1992; 53(5): 1166–68.

50. Ploeg RJ, D'Alessandro AM, Knechtle SJ et al. Malfunction of the liver after transplantation: an analysis of potential risk factors. Transplant Proc 1993; 25: 1659–61.

51. Adam R, Bismuth H, Diamond T et al. Effect of extended cold ischaemia with UW solution on graft function after liver transplantation. Lancet 1992; 340: 1373–6.

52. Oellerich M, Burdelski M, Ringe B et al. Lignocaine metabolite formation as a measure of pre transplant liver function. Lancet 1989; 1: 640.

53. Adam R, Azoulay D, Astarcioglu I et al. Reliability of the MEGX test in the selection of liver grafts. Transplant Proc 1991; 2: 2470–1.

54. Reding R, Wallemacq P, de Ville de Goyet J et al. The unreliability of the lidocaine/monoethylglycinexylidide test for assessment of liver donors. Transplantation 1993; 56: 323–6.

55. Adam R, Azoulay D, Astarcioglu I et al. Limits of the MEGX test in the selection of liver grafts for transplantation. Transplant Proc 1993; 25: 1653–4.

56. Tesi RJ, Elkhammas EA, Davies EA et al. Safe use of liver donors with MEGX values less than 90 ng/ml. Transplant Proc 1993; 2: 1655–6.

57. Yamaoka Y, Washida M, Manaka D et al. Arterial ketone body ratio as a predictor of donor liver viability in human liver transplantation. Transplantation 1993; 55: 92–5.

58. Potter JM, Hickman PE, Lynch SV et al. Use of monoethylglycinexylidide as a liver function test in the liver transplant recipient. Transplantation 1993; 56: 1385–8.

59. Asonuma K, Takaya S, Selby R et al. The clinical significance of the arterial ketone body ratio as an early indicator of graft viability in human liver transplantation. Transplantation 1991; 51: 164.

60. Egawa H, Shaked A, Konishi Y et al. Arterial ketone body ratio in paediatric liver transplantation. Transplantation 1993; 55: 522–66.

61. Sumimoto R, Southard JH, Belzer FO. Livers from fasted rats acquire resistance to warm and cold ischemia injury. Transplantation 1993; 55: 728–32.

62. Adam R, Reynes M, Bao YM et al. Impact of glycogen content of the donor liver in clinical liver transplantation. Transplant Proc 1993; 25: 1536–7.

63. Gubernatis G, Pichlmayr R, Lamesch P et al. HTK-solution (Bretschneider) for human liver transplantation. First clinical experiences. Langenbecks Arch Chir 1990; 375: 66–70.

64. Gubernatis G, Dietl KH, Kemnitz J et al. Extended cold preservation time (20 hours 20 minutes) of a human liver graft by using cardioplegic HTK solution. Transplant Proc 1991; 23: 2408–9.

65. van Gulik TM, Reinders ME, Nio R, Fredericks WM, Bosma A, Klopper PJ. Preservation of canine liver grafts using HTK solution. Transplantation 1994; 57: 167–71.

66. Belzer FO. Clinical organ preservation with UW solution Transplantation 1989; 47: 1097–8.

67. Sundberg R, Ar'Rajab A, Ahren B. Evaluation of initial cooling solutions for liver preservation using isolated perfused rabbit liver. Transplant Proc 1990; 22: 509–10.

68. Yu W, Coddington D, Bitter SH. Rat liver preservation. II. Combining UW solution with EuroCollins solution or Ringer's lactate abrogates its protective effect. Transplant Int 1990; 3: 238–40.

69. Cofer JB, Klintmalm GB, Morris CV et al. A prospective randomized trial between Euro-Collins and University of Wisconsin solutions as the initial flush in hepatic allograft procurement. Transplantation 1992; 53: 995–8.

70. Southard JH, van GT, Ametani MS et al. Important components of the UW solution. Transplantation 1990; 49: 251–7.

71. Marshall VC, Howden BO, Jablonski P et al. Analysis of UW solution in a rat liver transplant model. Transplant Proc 1990; 22: 503–5.

72. Yu W, Coddington D, Bitter-Suermann H. Rat liver preservation. I. The components of UW solution that are essential to its success. Transplantation 1990; 49: 1060–6.

73. Moen J, Claesson K, Pienaar H et al. Preservation of dog liver, kidney, and pancreas using the Belzer-UW solution with a high-sodium and low-potassium content. Transplantation 1989; 47: 940–5.

74. Kurzawinski TR, Hardy SC, Appleby J et al. A prospective randomised double blind clinical trial of high sodium versus high potassium liver preservation solution. ESOT 6th Congress 1993;.

75. Sumimoto R, Kamada N, Jamieson NV, Fukuda Y, Dohi K. A comparison of a new solution combining histidine and lactobionate with UW solution and Eurocollins for rat liver preservation. Transplantation 1991; 51: 589–93.

76. Sumimoto R, Jamieson NV, Kobayashi T, Fukuda Y, Dohi K, Kamada N. The need for glutathione and allopurinol in HL solution. Transplantation 1991; 52: 565–7.

77. Sumimoto R, Dohi K, Urushihara T et al. An examination of the effects of solutions containing histidine and lactobionate for heart, pancreas, and liver preservation in the rat. Transplantation 1992; 53: 1206–10.

78. Urushihara T, Sumimoto R, Sumimoto K et al. Prolonged rat pancreas preservation using a solution with the combination of histidine and lactobionate. Transplant Int 1992; 5(Suppl 1): 336–9.

79. Sumimoto R, Lindell SL, Southard JH, Belzer FO. A comparison of histidine-lactobionate and UW solution in 48-hour liver preservation. Transplantation 1992; 54: 610–14.

80. Pienaar BH, Lindell SL, Van GT, Southard JH, Belzer FO. Seventy-two-hour preservation of the canine liver by machine perfusion. Transplantation 1990; 49: 258–60.

81. Wicomb WN, Collins GM. 24-hour rabbit heart storage with UW solution – effects of low-flow perfusion, colloid and shelf storage. Transplantation 1989; 48: 6–9.

82. Boudjema K, Van Gulik TM, Lindell SL, Vreugdenhil PS, Southard JH, Belzer FO. Effect of oxidised and reduced glutathione in liver preservation. Transplantation 1990; 50: 948–51.

83. Boudjema K, Ellero B, Barguil Y et al. Addition of reduced glutathione to UW solution: clinical impact in liver transplantation. Transplant Proc 1991; 23: 2341–3.

84. Tokunaga Y, Wicomb WN, Concepcion W, Nakazato P, Collins GM, Esquivel CO. Successful 20-hour rat liver preservation with chlorpromazine in sodium lactobionate sucrose solution. Surgery 1991; 110: 80–6.

85. Tokunaga Y, Collins GM, Esquivel CO, Wicomb WN. Calcium antagonists in sodium lactobionate sucrose solution for rat liver preservation. Transplantation 1992; 53: 726–30.

86. Currin RT, Toole JG, Thurman RG, Lemasters JJ. Evidence that Carolina rinse solution protects sinusoidal endothelial cells against reperfusion injury after cold ischemic storage of rat liver. Transplantation 1990; 50: 1076–8.

87. Gao W, Tskei Y, Marzi I et al. Carolina rinse solution – a new strategy to increase survival time after orthotopic liver transplantation in the rat. Transplantation 1991; 52: 417–24.

88. Post S, Rentsch M, Gonzalez AP, Palma P, Otto G, Menger MD. Effects of Carolina rinse and adenosine rinse on microvascular perfusion and intrahepatic leukocyte-endothelium interaction after liver transplantation in the rat. Transplantation 1993; 55: 972–7.

89. Sanchez-Urdazpal L, Gores GJ, Lemasters JJ et al. Carolina rinse solution decreases liver injury during clinical liver transplantation. Transplant Proc 1993; 25: 1574–5.

90. Vivot C, Stump DD, Schwartz ME, Theise ND, Miller CM. N-aetylcysteine attenuates cold ischaemia/reperfuson injury in the isolated perfused rat liver. Transplant Proc 1993; 25: 1983–4.

19 | Heart and lung preservation

Winston N. Wicomb

1. Introduction

Preservation of the heart and lung has lagged behind that of the intra-abdominal organs. Although the first heart transplant was performed close to three decades ago, the maximum safe preservation period for both heart and lung remains at approximately 6 h [1,2]. This slow progress in the case of the heart is due to the difficulty in countering the effects of loss of the Ca^{2+} regulatory mechanisms produced by ischaemia, and in the case of the lung it results from the fragility of the alveolar structure [3,4]. In the heart this damage usually manifests itself as low cardiac output and in the lung as postoperative deterioration in circulatory oxygen tension, decreased compliance and increased pulmonary vascular resistance [5,6]. For heart preservation the general consensus favours the use of extracellular solutions (St Thomas II), whereas an intracellular formulation is preferred for the storage of lungs [7,8]. Many modifications of these solutions have been tried, including the addition, replacement or removal of colloids, pharmacological agents, biological and synthetic antioxidants, antiplatelet activating factor, calcium antagonists and vasodilators such as prostaglandins PGE_1 and PGI_2 [9–11]. Critical comparisons among these solutions is complicated by the numerous methods used for testing. The ultimate test, of course, remains orthotopic transplantation for hearts and unilateral, double, or heart–lung transplantation for lungs.

2. Heart preservation

For many years, cardiac surgeons have preserved donor hearts with the same cardioplegic solutions as those used for arresting the heart in open-heart operations. These solutions generally resemble extracellular fluid with a somewhat higher potassium content (15–40 meq/l) to induce rapid arrest. Although high-potassium solutions such as Collins' and UW have been accepted for some time as being optimal for abdominal organ preservation [12], there has been a reluctance to use them for the heart since Melrose reported that high levels of potassium in flush solutions damaged the myocardium [13]. Subsequently, Kohno et al. [14] explained this effect as activation of the slow calcium channels causing an influx of calcium. This calcium flux is also responsible for the transient vasospasm noted in most organs when flushed with hyperkalaemic solutions [15].

The success of UW in abdominal organ preservation has prompted a recent re-evaluation of this high-potassium solution for storage of the thoracic organs [16,17]. In a randomized blinded prospective clinical trial, Jeevanandam et al. compared UW with a crystalloid cardioplegic solution. Hearts preserved in UW were subjectively more vigorous and rhythmic on reperfusion. However, there was no evidence of ischaemic injury or conduction abnormalities on ECG in either group [18]. Using an in vitro model, Stringham et al. tested UW for its efficacy in maintaining high-energy phosphates during preservation. At 12 and 24 h of preservation heart function had fallen to 73% and 42% of control function respectively, and ischaemic contracture was evident in the latter group [19]. This 12 h limit for UW in heart preservation is far short of what has been achieved with this solution in abdominal organ preservation. The explanation may lie in the special problem of intracellular control of calcium in a muscular organ [19], and Southard recently reported improved results by adding BDM, a

G.M. Collins, J.M. Dubernard, W. Land and G.G. Persijn (eds). Procurement, Preservation and Allocation of Vascularized Organs 169–172
© 1997 Kluwer Academic Publishers.

potent Ca^{2+} antagonist, to UW [20]. It is also possible that some of the components of UW may be harmful to the heart. For example, the glutathione in commercial UW rapidly oxidizes, resulting in loss of myocardial collagen [21]. By adding reduced glutathione immediately before use these detrimental effects can be avoided [22]. In a study comparing UW with St Thomas's solution, Tian et al. demonstated that UW produced an increased rate of phosphocreatine, nucleotide and ATP depletion and poorer functional recovery of pig hearts stored at 12°C. No difference was evident between the two groups when hearts were stored at 4°C [23]. These effects may explain why in the early clinical trials the advantages of UW over standard cardioplegic solutions have been small [24,25].

At the present time, heart transplant surgeons remain unwilling to risk clinical storage times beyond 4–8 h [26,27]. Present research, therefore, is directed towards attempting to extend the time limits for the heart storage to 24 h or more, as is possible with the liver and kidney [28]. If this could be achieved, the potential donor pool would be substantially increased, with consequent improved prospects for recipients for whom local donors are difficult to find, given the present restraints.

Promising lines of investigation include two new concepts that have made it possible to preserve rabbit hearts for 24 h with residual function comparable to that of controls. The first is the use of a very low flow perfusion technique called microperfusion [29]. This appears to work by control of acidosis, and requires the perfusate to contain a colloid to ensure adequate distribution within the heart at low perfusion pressures. UW solution made up freshly (with reduced glutathione) provided good 24 h preservation with this technique. However, significantly better results were obtained by substitution of 5% polyethylene glycol (PEG) for hydroxyethyl starch in a modified UW [30] yielding a new solution called 'Cardiosol'. In combination with microperfusion, Cardiosol resulted in rabbit hearts stored for 24 h performing at the same level as fresh, control hearts. This new solution has been used clinically in a limited trial with good results [31]. All 20 recipients of primary heart transplants originally preserved with Cardiosol are alive more than 6 years later. The benefits can undoubtedly be ascribed to the PEG, which probably acts as a free-radical scavenger [32,33]. Its primary action may be to ameliorate the reperfusion injury since a PEG solution has been found to improve kidney preservation when used only as a terminal rinse after 48 h ice storage [34]. Recent studies in our laboratory have shown that a 10% PEG

20 linear is superior to the 5% solution used previously in Cardiosol, making 24 h ice storage possible even without microperfusion. The value of PEG in heart preservation is further supported by recent experiments by Malhotra et al. [35]. They stored rat hearts in Collins' solution containing 8% PEG and demonstrated superior myocardial protection in this group. These new techniques, perhaps in conjunction with the use of calcium antagonists such as BDM, offer the possibility of making heart transplantation a less emergent procedure.

3. Lung preservation

The selection of donors and the procedures for excision of the lungs or the heart–lung block are reviewed in detail elsewhere [36]. The lung, because of its delicate structural alveolar and capillary network, is especially susceptible to injury from infection, brain death, and ischaemic and operative trauma. As a result, less than 20% of the available donors are suitable for heart–lung or lung transplantation [37] and technical failures related to poor preservation contribute towards more than 40% of the early deaths following lung transplantation [38]. Furthermore the results of transplantation have been disappointing and inconsistent when compared with the experimental data reported in dogs and primates [39].

The first experimental model for lung preservation was the normothermic autoperfusion system developed by Robicsek in the late 1950s [40]. The technique of donor core-cooling without pulmonary artery flush has also been used for distant organ procurement [41]. An advantage of this technique is that it allows uniform cooling of donor organs while blood flow is maintained. The major drawback of this method is the need to transport bypass equipment to the donor centre. This method of preservation was simplified by Bando et al., who used core cooling, non-recirculating retrograde heart perfusion and hypothermic lung immersion in a solution containing human superoxide dismutase [42]. Although they achieved 8 h of preservation the results were only marginally better than those achieved with total donor core cooling [43]. Recently, Chien et al. achieved successful 24 h preservation using a modified multi-organ autoperfusion preparation [44]. The disadvantage of these systems is their complexity, which renders them too cumbersome for clinical use.

Ice storage in the inflated state [45,46] is the preferred method of lung preservation for clinical transplantation. Collins' solution was first used for lung storage by the Stanford group in 1984 [47] and became accepted as the standard method, supported by numerous experimental studies. Using Collins' as the flush solution, Puskas et al. reported 18 h of lung preservation following PGE_1 pretreatment, and 30 h heart–lung preservation by donor lung hyperinflation [48,49]. However, in a clinical trial Keenan et al. showed increased perioperative lung preservation injury in lungs procured in Collins' solution [50]. Kawahara et al. compared UW with the Collins' solution for 24-h lung preservation, measuring changes in airway pressure, static lung compliance and pulmonary vascular resistance [51]. They found most parameters significantly improved in the UW group, including less pronounced oedema formation. On the other hand, Hardesty demonstrated no significant difference in graft function between lungs stored in UW or Collins', although the ischaemic time was somewhat longer in the UW group [8]. Aeba et al. compared these solutions in the rat left lung transplant model, and found better preservation with UW at 6 h, but not at 12 h, at which time graft injury was similar in the two groups. Only the lipid peroxides were higher in the Collins' group after 12 h of cold ischaemia [52]. They attributed the improved function at 6 h to the higher viscosity of UW, which they postulated might provide a more even distribution of the solution into constricted vessels. Defects in experimental design make it difficult to evaluate some other studies in which UW appeared to be better than Collins solution for lung preservation. In one study, for example, the period of functional evaluation after transplantation was too short to draw valid conclusions [53]. In another, a significant proportion of animals died early from progressive cardiac failure or ionic imbalance [37]. In a rabbit heart–lung transplant experiment, Miyoshi et al. used a low K^+ UW and obtained superior preservation compared with the standard solution [54]. In baboons, Human et al. evaluated UW and the Bretschneider solution (HTK) after 16 h of ice storage. Although the heart performed better in the UW group, the lungs were better protected in the HTK solution. The UW group also exhibited a more notable increase in pulmonary oedema [55]. These conflicting findings make it difficult to determine which composition is best for lung preservation.

At the present time, study of the use of UW solution is the most rewarding line of investigation in thoracic organ preservation. However, the precise molecular and cellular mechanism of protection offered by UW and its PEG-containing variant is incompletely understood. Our own focus of attention is on the action of these solutions on the vascular endothelium and their potential for protecting against oxygen free radical attack. These reactive species are not only a consequence of hypothermia and reperfusion, but may also result from oxidants generated by chemical changes in the organic components of preservation solutions. At the present time PEG appears to be the most promising UW additive that can protect the heart and successfully extend the cold ischaemic period beyond 12 h of preservation.

References

1. Haverich A, Wahlers T, Schafers HJ et al. Distant organ procurement in clinical lung and heart-lung transplantation. Eur J Cardiothorac Surg 1990; 4: 245–9.
2. Yacoub MH, Khagahani A, Banner N, Takarimi S, Fitzgerald M. Consistent organ procurement for heart and lung transplantation. Transplant Proc 1989; 21: 2548–50.
3. Modry DL, Walpoth BW, Cohen RG et al. Heart–Lung Preservation in the dog followed by lung transplantation. A new model for the assessment of lung preservation. Heart Transplant 1983; 2: 287–98.
4. Hunter DN, Morgan CJ, Yacoub M, Evans TW. Pulmonary endothelial permeability following lung transplantation. Chest 1992; 102: 417–21.
5. Kao RL, Magovern GJ. Prevention of reperfusional damage from ischemic myocardium. J Thorac Cardiovasc Surg. 1986; 91: 106–11.
6. Unruh HW. Vascular and interstitial effect of University of Wisconsin solution on canine lung. Ann Thorac Surg 1992; 54: 1168–71.
7. Hearse DJ, O'Brien K, Braimbridge MV. Protection of the myocardium during ischemic arrest. J Thorac Cardiovasc Surg 1981; 81: 873–79.
8. Hardesty RL, Aeba R, Armitage JM, Kormos RL, Griffith BP. A clinical trial of University of Wisconsin solution for pulmonary preservation. J Thorac Cardiovasc Surg 1993; 105: 660–66.
9. Wicomb WN, Cooper DKC. Storage of the donor heart. In: Cooper DKC, Novitzky D (eds). The Transplantation and Replacement of Thoracic Organs. Kluwer Academic Publishers, Dordrecht 1990; pp. 51–61.
10. Pillai R, Bando K, Schueler S, Zebley M, Reitz BA, Baumgartner WA. Leucocyte depletion results in excellent heart lung function after 12 hours of storage. Ann Thorac Surg 1990; 50: 211–14.
11. Wahlers TH, Hirt SW, Haverich A, Fieguth HG, Jurmann M, Borst HG. Future horizons of lung preservation by application of a platelet-activating factor antagonist compared with current clinical standards. J Thorac Cardiovasc Surg 1992; 103: 200–5.
12. Southard JH, Belzer FO. The University of Wisconsin organ preservation solution: components, comparisons, and modifications. Transplant Rev 1993; 7: 176–90.
13. Melrose DG, Dreyer B, Dentall HH, Baker BE. Elective cardiac arrest. Lancet 1955; 2: 21–3.
14. Kohno H, Shiki FK, Ueno Y, Tokunaga K. Cold storage of the rat heart for transplantation: two types of solutions required for optimal preservation. J Thorac Cardiovasc Surg 1987; 93: 86–94.
15. Keshavjee S, Yamazaki F, Cardoso PF, McRitchie DL, Patterson GA, Cooper JD. A method for safe twelve-hour pulmonary preservation. J Thorac Cardiovasc Surg 1989; 89: 529–34.
16. Jeevanandam V, Barr ML, Auteri JS et al. University of Wisconsin solution for human donor heart preservation: initial clinical experience. Ann Thorac Surg 1991; 50: 1213–16.

17. Hirt SW, Wahlers T, Jurmann MJ et al. University of Wisconsin versus modified Euro-Collins' solution for lung preservation. Ann Thorac Surg 1992; 53: 74–9.

18. Jeevanandam V, Barr L, Auteri JS et al. University of Wisconsin solution versus crystalloid cardioplegia for human donor heart preservation. J Thorac Cardiovasc Surg 1992; 103: 194–9.

19. Stringham JC, Southard JH, Hegge J, Triemstra L, Fields BL, Belzer FO. Limitations of heart preservation by cold storage. Transplantation 1992; 53: 287–94.

20. Stringham JC, Southard JH, Fields BL et al. Improved myocardial preservation with 2,3 Butanedione monoxime, calcium and the UW solution. Transplant Proc 1993; 25: 1625–6.

21. Wolowicz PE, Caulfield JB. Cardioplegia with aged UW solution induces loss of cardiac collagen. Transplantation 1991; 51: 898–901.

22. Wicomb WN, Perey R, Portnoy V, Collins GM. The role of reduced glutathione in heart preservation using a polyethylene glycol solution, Cardiosol. Transplantation 1992; 54: 181–2.

23. Tian G, Smith KE, Smith KE et al. A comparison of UW cold storage solution and St Thomas' solution II: A P^{31} NMR and function study of isolated porcine hearts. J Heart Lung Transplant 1991; 10: 975–85.

24. Jeevanandam V, Auteri JS, Sanchez JA, Hsu D, Marboe C, Smith CR, Rose EA. Cardiac transplantation after prolonged graft preservation with the University of Wisconsin solution. J Thorac Cardiovasc Surg 1992; 104: 224–8.

25. Demertzis S, Wippermann J, Schaper J, Wahlers T, Schafers HJ, Wagenbreth I, Hausen B, Haverich A. University of Wisconsin versus St. Thomas' Hospital solution for human donor heart preservation. Ann Thorac Surg 1993; 55: 1131–7.

26. Novitzky D, Wicomb WN, Rose AG, Cooper DKC, Reichart B. Pathophysiology of pulmonary edema following experimental brain death in the Chacma baboon. Ann Thorac Surg 1987; 43: 288–94.

27. Wicomb WN, Hill DJ, Avery JG, Collins GM. Donor heart preservation – limitations of cardioplegia and warm ischemia. Transplantation 1992; 53: 947–9.

28. Sumimoto R, Jamieson MV, Kamada N. Examination of the role of the impermeants lactobionate and raffinose in a modified UW solution. Transplantation 1990; 50: 573–6.

29. Wicomb WN, Collins GM. 24-Hour Rabbit heart storage with UW solution: Effects of low flow perfusion, colloid, and shelf storage. Transplantation 1989; 48: 6.

30. Wicomb WN, Hill JD, Avery J, Collins GM. Optimal cardioplegia and 24-hour heart storage with simplified UW solution containing polyethylene glycol. Transplantation 1990; 49: 261–4.

31. Collins GM, Wicomb WN, Levin BS, Verma S, Avery J, Hill JD. A heart preservation solution containing polyethylene glycol: an immunosuppressive effect? Lancet 1991; 338: 890–91.

32. Mack JE, Kerr JA, Vreugdenhil PK, Belzer FO, Southard JH. Effect of polyethylene glycol on lipid peroxidation in cold-stored rat hepatocytes. Cryobiology 1991; 28: 1–7.

33. Marsh DC, Lindell SL, Fox LE, Belzer FO, Southard JH. Hypothermic preservation of hepatocyte. Role of cell swelling. Cryobiology 1989; 26: 524–34.

34. Collins GM, Wicomb WN. New organ preservation solutions. Kidney Int 1992; 42: s197–s202.

35. Malhotra D, Zhou HZ, Kong YL, Shapiro JI, Cahan L. Improvement in experimental cardiac preservation based on metabolic considerations. Transplantation 1991; 52: 1004–8.

35. Haverich A, Novitzky D, Cooper DKC. Selection of the donor; excision and storage of donor organs. In: Cooper DKC, Novitzky D (eds), The transplantation and replacement of thoracic organs. Kluwer Academic Publishers, Dordrecht 1990; pp. 273–81.

36. Jamieson SW, Baldwin J, Stinson EB et al. Clinical heart–lung transplantation. Transplantation 1984; 37: 81–4.

37. Hirt SW, Wahlers T, Jurmann M, Fieguth HG, Dammenhayn L, Haverich A. Improvement of currently used methods for lung preservation with prostacyclin and University of Wisconsin solution. J Heart Lung Transplant 1992; 11: 656–64.

38. Haverich A, Scott WC, Jamieson SW. Twenty years of lung preservation: a Review. Heart Transplantation 1985; 4: 234–40.

39. Robicsek F, Sanger PW, Taylor FH. Simple method at keeping the heart 'alive' and functioning outside of the body for prolonged periods. Surgery 1963; 53: 525–30.

40. Kontos GJ, Adachi H, Borkon AM et al. A no-flush, core-cooling technique for successful cardiopulmonary preservation in heart–lung transplantation. J Thorac Cardiovasc Surg 1987; 94: 836–42.

41. Bando K, Teramoto S, Tago M et al. Successful extended hypothermic cardiopulmonary preservation for heart–lung transplantation. J Thorac Cardiovasc Surg 1989; 98: 137–46.

42. Hammerschmidt DE, Stroncek DF, Bowers TK et al. Complement activation and neutropenia occurring during cardiopulmonary bypass. J Thorac Cardiovasc Surg 1981; 81: 370–7.

43. Chien S, Deltgen PR, Diana JN, Shi X, Nilekani SF, Salley R. Two-day preservation of major organs with autoperfusion multiorgan preparation and hibernation induction trigger. A preliminary report. J Thorac Cardiovasc Surg 1991; 102: 224–34.

44. Aeba R, Killinger WA, Keenan RJ et al. Lazaroid U74500A as an additive to University of Wisconsin solution for pulmonary grafts in the rat transplant model. J Thorac Cardiovasc Surg 1992; 104: 1333–9.

45. Nicholas TE, Barr HA. Control and release of surfactant phospholipids in the isolated perfused rat lung. J Appl Physiol 1981; 51: 90–8.

46. Jamieson SW, Stinson EB, Oyer PE, Baldwin JC, Shumway NE. Operative technique for heart–lung transplantation. J Thorac Cardiovasc Surg 1984; 87: 930–5.

47. Hardesty RLl, Aeba R, Armitage JM, Lormos RL, Griffith BP. A clinical trial of University of Wisconsin solution for pulmonary preservation. J Thorac Cardiovasc Surg 1993; 105: 660–6.

48. Puskas JD, Cardoso FG, Mayer E, Shi S, Slutsky AS, Patterson GA. Equivalent eighteen-hour lung preservation with low-potassium dextran or Euro-Collins' solution after prostaglandin E_1 infusion. J Thorac Cardiovasc Surg 1992; 104: 83–9.

49. Puskas JD, Hirai T, Christie N, Mayer E, Stutsky AS, Patterson GA. Reliable thirty-hour lung preservation by donor lung hyperinflation. J Thorac Cardiovasc Surg 1992; 104: 1075–83.

50. Keenan RJ, Griffith BP, Kormos RL, Armitage JM, Hardesty RL. Increased perioperative lung preservation injury with lung procurement by Euro-Collins' solution flush. J Heart–Lung Transplant 1991; 10: 50–5.

51. Kawahara K, Ikari H, Hisano H et al. Twenty-four-hour canine lung preservation using UW solution. Transplantation 1991; 51: 584–7.

52. Aeba R, Keenan RJ, Hardesty RL, Yousem SA, Hamamoto I, Griffith BP. University of Wisconsin solution for pulmonary preservation in a rat transplant model. Ann Thorac Surg 1992; 53: 240–6.

53. Naka Y, Shirakura R, Matsuda H et al. Canine heart–lung transplantation after twenty-four-hour hypothermic preservation with Belzer-UW solution. J Heart Lung Transplant 1991; 10: 296–303.

54. Miyoshi S, Shimokawa S, Schreinemakers H. Comparison of the University of Wisconsin preservation solution and other crystalloid perfusates in a 30-hour rabbit lung preservation model. J Thorac Cardiovasc Surg 1992; 103: 27–32.

55. Human PA, Holl J, Vosloo S. Extended cardiopulmonary preservation: University of Wisconsin solution versus Bretschneider's cardioplegic solution. Ann Thorac Surg 1993; 55: 1123–30.

20 | Small bowel preservation

FRANCISCO J. RODRÍGUEZ-QUILANTÁN AND LUIS H. TOLEDO-PEREYRA

1. Introduction

Despite early developments in transplantation techniques and preservation of the small bowel, few significant changes have occurred in the last two decades [1–22]. In recent years, however, transplantation of the small bowel has been reintroduced as a potential treatment for acute or chronic irreversible intestinal failure, more often indicated for short small bowel syndrome [23]. Most of the experience with preservation and transplantation of the small bowel has been experimental [1–6,10,13–14,17–22,24]. In the clinical arena, the longest survivor for small bowel transplantation has lived more than 3 years, with satisfactory results, after receiving bowel with liver and other organs in a cluster operation [25]. As better results of small bowel transplantation (SBTx) are obtained, a comparative analysis with established techniques of ambulatory parenteral nutrition (APN) will have to be attained in order to offer the best perspective for patients with end stage small bowel disease (ESSBD) [23].

With regard to the preservation of the small bowel, multiple solutions and methods have been used with variable results. Here, we will review the historical background, organ procurement and preservation of the small bowel for transplantation.

2. Historical background

2.1. Preservation methods

2.1.1. *Early stages*
Attention has been oriented towards the development of methods for cold storage and transplantation of the small bowel since the early work of Lillehei and associates in 1959 [1]. They transplanted autografts in dogs after several hours of cold ischaemia, achieving satisfactory nutritional support and several years' survival in some of these animals. Years later, the same group reported their results of small bowel auto- and allo-transplantation in dogs [2], and in 1967 extended these techniques to their clinical use in patients with ESSBD [3].

Cohen and associates [4] focused on the absorptive properties of jejunal canine auto and homografts after transplantation. In 1973 Toledo-Pereyra and Najarian [5] began to compare perfusion and non-perfusion systems for preservation of the small bowel, assuming that pulsatile perfusion was the most satisfactory method for preservation of intestinal grafts, and in the mid 1970s [6] they achieved better results using cryo-precipitated plasma and human plasma as intestinal preservation solutions in dogs.

G.M. Collins, J.M. Dubernard, W. Land and G.G. Persijn (eds). Procurement, Preservation and Allocation of Vascularized Organs 173–179
© 1997 Kluwer Academic Publishers.

Based on the fact that control of preservation injury might be an important element in the protection of small bowel allografts, and that associated immunological factors are important, during the mid- and late 1970s, drugs such as allopurinol, chlorpromazine, methylprednisolone and antilymphoblast globulin were used to improve small bowel preservation [7].

2.1.2. *Middle stages*

The 1980s was characterized by its emphasis in the prevention and amelioration of ischaemia–reperfusion injury (IRI). Several groups extensively studied the role of oxygen free radicals (OFR), leukotriene B_4 (LTB$_4$), platelet-activating factor (PAF), prostacyclin (PGI$_2$), thromboxane A$_2$ (TxA$_2$) and complement warm and cold ischaemic damage. Administration of superoxide dismutase, catalase, dimethyl sulphoxide, allopurinol, mannitol, desferroxamine and other oxygen free radical scavengers, or various antagonists (against PAF, LTB$_4$, TxA$_2$) administered to the recipient during or immediately before the reperfusion considerably decreased the tissue damage seen after IRI [8–11]. The high concentrations of xanthine dehydrogenase and xanthine oxidase in the small bowel of small animals

have made this organ particularly suitable for the study of free radical injury.

2.1.3. *Late stages*

Notwithstanding the importance of OFR scavengers, the discovery of new immunosuppressive drugs such as Cyclosporine A changed the immunological response of transplantation [12]. Several publications discussed the results of small bowel transplants, particularly in large animals, combined with treatment with Cyclosporine alone or associated with methylprednisolone [13,14]. In the late 1980s, researchers at the University of Wisconsin designed their preservation solution (UW), originally developed for pancreas preservation, and later demonstrated to show protective function for kidney and liver [15,16]. This solution was also utilized for short term preservation of heart and lung with preliminary acceptable results [24]. For small bowel preservation, the UW solution has not produced the level of protection observed for preservation of the pancreas; it has shown experimentally moderately good results [17–22], and clinically it has not attained the consistent results obtained in the preservation of other organs [23,25] (Fig. 1).

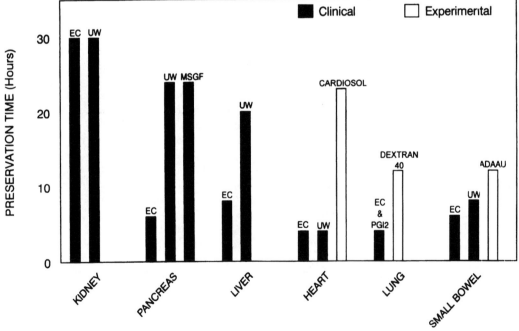

Figure 1. Comparative results of the different times and solutions for preservation of various transplantable organs. Note the shorter times of successful preservation obtained for the small bowel when compared to other organs. EC: EuroCollins' solution; UW: University of Wisconsin preservation solution; MSGF: modified silica gel fraction; PGI$_2$: prostacyclin; ADAAV: albumin, Dextran 40, adenosine, allopurinol and verapamil. (Reproduced with permission from reference [24].)

2.1.4. *Current status*

Of significant relevance is the beneficial role of donor depletion of neutrophils on cell function and morphology after small bowel revascularization [26]. In the 1990s, special attention was paid to cytokines (interleukin-1, interleukin-6 and tumour necrosis factor) and their role in reperfusion injury has been emphasized, particularly, in models of liver transplantation [27]. Endothelium-derived relaxing factor (later identified as nitric oxide; NO), has also been found to be important in small bowel preservation [28,29].

The production of a potent vasoconstrictor, endothelin, and the expression of adhesion molecules (integrins, selectins and the immunoglobulin superfamily) in preservation–reperfusion models have been proposed as the main factors in the injury associated with ischaemia during and after reperfusion [30]. In this decade, the global mechanism of the complex preservation – reperfusion injury has been conceptualized as a conjunction of phenomena in which the adhesion molecules, neutrophils, cytokines and OFR play an important role (Fig. 2). Regarding new immunosuppressive drugs, FK-506, along with Rapamycin and substances such as free radicals scavengers and antioxidants, have been recently utilized with promising results [31–35].

2.2. Harvesting and transplantation techniques

2.2.1. *Experimental*

Lillehei and his group introduced the techniques of auto and homo intestinal transplantation in large animals. In 1971 Monchik and Russell [36] emphasized the immunological response of the host and graft after transplantation, using inbred and hybrid Lewis rats, without cold storage, and described the technique of heterotopic intestinal transplantation (Fig. 3). Kort and his associates, in 1973, described the technique of orthotopic intestinal transplantation in the rat, created for physiological, nutritional and mechanical purposes as well as immunological reasons (Fig. 4) [37]. Years later, Deltz and Thiede, modified Kort's technique in a two-stage procedure [38]. Recently, the revascularization of the intestine in the recipient rat has been improved by utilizing the non-suture cuff technique using the left renal artery and vein of the recipient and the donor's superior mesenteric artery and portal vein, and left nephrectomy [39]. Although some authors propose venous drainage directly to the portal vein in the recipient, most experiments use portal vein drainage of the donor to the inferior vena cava or, with modification of the technique, to the left renal vein [40].

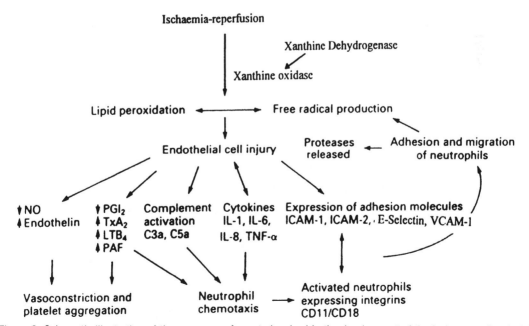

Figure 2. Schematic illustration of the sequence of events involved in the development of the lesion associated with ischaemia–reperfusion. (Modified from reference [9].)

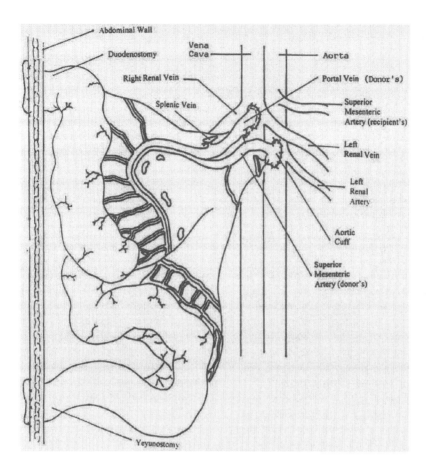

Figure 3. Technique of heterotopic small bowel transplantation in the rat. (Reproduced with permission from reference [18].)

2.2.2. *Clinical*

In 1967, Lillehei and his group described the first two published human small bowel transplants (with pancreas and duodenum, and small bowel plus right colon respectively). Few cases were performed for several years, until the late 1980s when European surgeons published their initial cases, some of which were associated with liver transplantation. They utilized the UW preservation solution, with a longest preservation time and survival of 10.5 h and 17 months respectively [41,42]. No longer clinical preservation time has been achieved.

In 1984 Starzl and his group [43] described the multiple organ procurement technique, including the small bowel, subsequently modified in 1987 by the same group [44] to receive less operating time. Currently, this is the conventional technique for procurement and transplantation *en bloc* of abdominal organs, including the small bowel, flushed and preserved with UW solution [45] (Fig. 5A–C). When the isolated small bowel is transplanted, the vascular pedicle is dissected out directly from the major abdominal vessels, with an aortic cuff in cases of cadaveric donors.

3. Conclusions

Transplantation of the human small bowel is not now a rare event. It is being performed more frequently, in spite of the fact that current preservation solutions do not offer consistent protection for periods of time similar to those attained with other transplantable abdominal organs. Improvements to the present preservation solutions, e.g. UW solution, and protection of the donor graft from IRI, will be needed to obtain

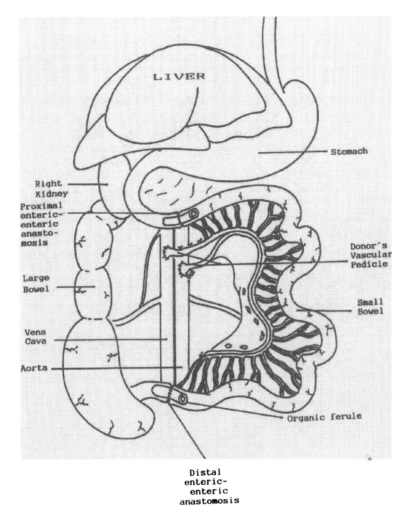

Figure 4. Technique of orthotopic small bowel transplantation in the rat. (Reproduced with permission from reference [18].)

better results and improve the logistics of small bowel preservation for transplantation.

References

1. Lillehei RC, Gott B, Miller FA. The physiologic response of the small bowel of the dog to ischemia, including *in vitro* preservation of bowel with successful replacement and survival. Ann Surg 1959; 150: 543–560.
2. Lillehei RC, Goldberg S, Gott B and Longerbeam JK. The present status of small bowel transplantation. Am J Surg 1963; 105: 58–72.
3. Lillehei RC, Idezuki Y, Feemster JA, Dietzman RH *et al.* Transplantation of stomach, intestine and pancreas: experimental and clinical observations. Surgery, 1967; 62: 721–41.
4. Cohen WB, Hardy MA, Quint J and State D. Absorptive function in canine jejunal autografts and allografts. Surgery 1969; 65: 440–6.
5. Toledo-Pereyra LH, Najarian JS. Small bowel preservation: Comparison of perfusion and non-perfusion systems. Arch Surg 1973; 107: 875–7.
6. Toledo-Pereyra LH. Small bowel preservation. In: Toledo-Pereyra LH (ed.), Basic concepts of organ procurement, perfusion and preservation for transplantation. Academic Press, New York 1982; pp. 317–331.
7. Toledo-Pereyra LH. Small bowel preservation: evolution of methods and ideas and current concepts. Transplant Proc 1992; 24: 1083–4.
8. Southard JH, Marsh DC, McAnulty JF and Belzer FO. Oxygen-derived free radical damage in organ preservation: Activity of superoxide dismutase and xanthine oxidase. Surgery 1987; 101: 566–70.
9. Grace PA. Ischaemia–Reperfusion injury. Br J Surg 1994; 81: 637–47.

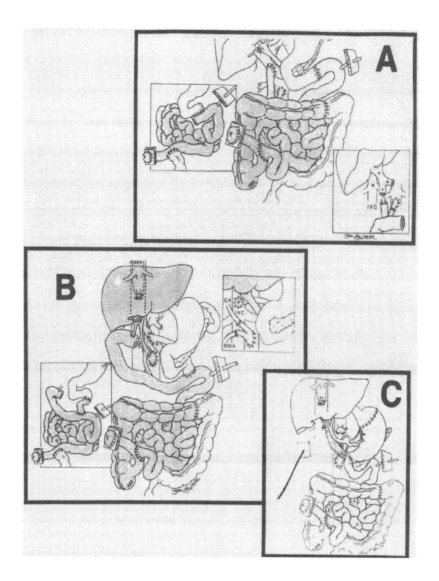

Figure 5. Artistic depiction of the various possibilities of small bowel transplantation in humans, along with other abdominal organs. (A) Isolated intestinal transplantation including one half of the colon or the small intestine only. (B) Hepatic and intestinal transplantation with and without part of the colon. (C) Multivisceral operation. (Reproduced with permission from reference [45].)

10. Toledo-Pereyra LH, Granger DN. Small bowel ischemic and reperfusion injury: Pathophysiological mechanisms. In: Das DK (ed.). Pathophysiology of reperfusion injury. CRC Press, Boca Raton, 1993; pp. 137–47.

11. Parks DA, Bulkley GB and Granger DN. Role of oxygen free radicals in shock, ischemia and organ preservation. Surgery 1983; 94: 428–34.

12. Calne RY, White DJG. The use of cyclosporin A in clinical organ grafting. Ann Surg 1982; 196: 330–7.

13. Raju S, Didlake RH, Cayirli M *et al.* Experimental small bowel transplantation utilizing cyclosporine. Transplantation 1984; 38: 561–6.

14. Diliz-Perez HS, McClure J, Bedetti C *et al.* Successful small bowel transplantation in dogs with cyclosporine and prednisone. Transplantation 1984; 37: 127–32.

15. Whalberg JA, Southard JH, and Belzer FO. Development of a cold storage solution for pancreas preservation. Cryobiology 1986; 23: 477–81.

16. Belzer FO, D'Alessandro AM, Hoffmann RM *et al.* The use of UW in clinical transplantation. Ann Surg 1992; 215: 579–85.

17. Schweizer E, Gassel AM, Deltz E and Schroecer P. A comparison of preservation solutions for small bowel transplantation in the rat. Transplantation 1994; 57: 1406–8.

18. Rodríguez-Quilantán FJ, Toledo-Pereyra LH, Suzuki S. Total heterotopic small bowel transplantation in the rat: Technical considerations in the procurement, preservation and transplantation of the graft. Gac Med Mex 1993; 129: 131–7.

19. Rodríguez-Quilantán FJ, Toledo-Pereyra LH, Suzuki S. Role of neutrophils following small bowel transplantation in the rat. Transplant Proc 1993; 25: 3209.

20. Fabian MA, Bollinger RR, Wyble CW et al. Evaluation of Solution for small intestinal preservation. Biochemical changes as a function of storage time. Transplantation 1991; 52: 794–9.

21. Rodríguez-Quilantán FJ, Toledo-Pereyra LH, Suzuki S. Twenty-four-hour total small bowel hypothermic storage preservation and transplantation in the rat: A study of various preservation solutions. J Invest Surg 1994; 7: 439–51.

22. Taguchi T, Zorychta E, Guttman. Evaluation of UW solution for preservation of small intestinal transplants in the rat. Transplantation 1992; 53: 1202–5.

23. Shanbhogue LKR and Molenaar JC. Short bowel syndrome: metabolic and surgical management. Br J Surg 1994; 81: 486–99.

24. Toledo-Pereyra LH, Rodríguez-Quilantán FJ. Scientific basis and current status of organ preservation. Transplant Proc 1994; 26: 309–11.

25. Abu-Elmagd K, Todo S, Tzakis A, Reyes J, Nour B et al. Three years' clinical experience with intestinal transplantation. J Am Coll Surg 1994; 179: 385–400.

26. Sisley MC, Desai T, Harig JM, Gewertz BL. Neutrophil depletion attenuates human intestinal reperfusion injury. J Surg Res 1994; 57: 192–6.

27. Toledo-Pereyra LH, Suzuki S. Neutrophils, cytokines and adhesion molecules in hepatic ischemic and reperfusion injury. J Am Coll Surg 1994; 174: 758–62.

28. Mueller AR, Platz KP, Langrehr et al. The effects of administration of nitric oxide inhibitors during small bowel preservation and reperfusion. Transplantation 1994; 58: 1309–16.

29. Villareal D, Grisham MB, Granger DN. Nitric oxide donors improve gut function after prolonged hypothermic ischemia. Transplantation 1995; 59: 685–9.

30. Heemann UW, Tullius SG, Azuma H, Kupiec-Weglinsky J, Tilney NL. Adhesion molecules and transplantation. Ann Surg 1994; 219: 4–12.

31. Murase N, Demetris AJ, Woo J et al. Graft-Versus-Host disease after Brown Norway-to-Lewis and Lewis-to-Brown Norway Rat Intestinal Transplantation Under FK-506. Transplantation 1993; 55: 1–7.

32. Stepkowski SM, Chen HF, Wang ME et al. Inhibition of host-versus-graft and graft-versus-host responses after small bowel transplantation in rats by rapamycin. Transplantation 1992; 53: 258–64.

33. Harward TRS, Coe G, Souba WW et al. Glutamine preserves gut glutathione levels during intestinal ischemia/reperfusion. J Surg Res 1994; 56: 351–5.

34. Katz SM, Sun S, Schechner RS et al. Improved small intestinal preservation after lazaroid u74389g treatment and cold storage in University of Wisconsin preservation solution. Transplantation 1995; 59: 694–8.

35. Sun SC, Greenstein SM, Schechner RS et al. Superoxide dismutase: enhanced small intestinal preservation. J Surg Res 1992; 52: 583–90.

36. Monchik GJ, Russell PS. Transplantation of small bowel in the rat: technical and immunological considerations. Surgery 1971; 70: 693–702.

37. Kort WJ, Westbroeck DL, MacDicken J, Lameijer LDF. Orthotopic total small bowel transplantation in the rat. Eur Surg Res 1973; 5: 81–9.

38. Deltz E, Thiede A. Microsurgical Technique for small intestinal transplantation. In: Thiede A, Deltz E, Engemann R (ed.), Microsurgical models in rat for transplantation research. Springer-Verlag, Berlin 1985; pp. 51–5.

39. Wallander J, Holtz A, Larsson E et al. Small-bowel transplantation in the rat with a nonsuture cuff technique. Transplant Int 1988; 1: 135–9.

40. Schraut WF, Abraham VS, Lee KKW. Portal Versus Caval drainage of small bowel allografts: technical and metabolic consequences.

41. Grant D, Wall W, Mimeault R, Zhong R et al. Successful small-bowel/liver transplantation. Lancet 1990; 335: 181–4.

42. Schroeder P, Goulet O and Lear PA. Small-bowel transplantation: European experience. Lancet 1990; 336: 110–11.

43. Starzl TE, Hakala TR, Shaw BW Jr. Hardesty RL et al. A flexible procedure for multiple cadaveric organ procurement. Surg Gynecol Obstet 1984; 158: 223–30.

44. Starzl TE, Miller C, Broznick B, Makowka L. An improved technique for multiple organ harvesting. Surg Gynecol Obstet 1987; 165: 343–8.

45. Todo S, Tzakis A, Abu-Elmagd K, Reyes J, Furukawa H et al. Abdominal multivisceral transplantation. Transplantation 1995; 59: 234–40.

21 | Pancreas preservation

David E.R. Sutherland, Kay Moudry-Munns and Angelika Gruessner

1. Introduction

Organ preservation is essential for transplantation to be logistically practical. The principles of solid organ preservation by either simple cold storage or machine perfusion have been well described [1]. Numerous experiments on pancreas preservation with both techniques have been published since the 1960s [2–5]. By the mid-1980s, it was generally conceded that cold storage was superior for the pancreas [6]. Hyperosmolar plasma-based solutions were found to be superior to the simple intracellular electrolyte solutions (Collins' or Collins'-like) that were widely used for kidney preservation [7]. Plasma-based solutions were able to preserve canine pancreas grafts for 48–72 h, while Collins' solution was effective for no more than 24 h [8,9]. Clinically, through most of the 1980s, most centres that used Collins' or Collins'-like solutions limited human pancreas preservation to < 12 h [10]. At the University of Minnesota, silica-gel filtered (SGF) plasma solution made hyperosmolar with mannitol was used to successfully preserve human pancreas grafts for up to 30 h [11–14].

The drawback of plasma-based solutions was, of course, the risk of transmission of human viruses. In 1987 Wahlberg published an article on the use of a new synthetic intracellular electrolyte solution in which lactobinate (a cellular impermanent) replaced chloride as the dominant anion and raffinose was used as the osmotic agent [15]. This solution was capable of preserving canine pancreases for up to 72 h. Termed Belzer solution or University of Wisconsin (UW) solution, it was introduced clinically for all organs shortly thereafter [16].

A comparison at the University of Minnesota showed no difference in clinical outcome for human pancreases preserved in either UW or SGF [14]. Both were able to preserve pancreas grafts for at least up to 30 h; UW, however, eliminated the possibility of disease transmission and was made commercially available [16]. It has virtually replaced all other solutions for pancreas preservation. This occurred more rapidly in the USA than in Europe or other locations, but since 1990 UW solution has been used to preserve 95–100% of pancreas transplants annually world-wide (Fig. 1).

2. Methods

The purpose of this chapter is to relate pancreas graft survival rates to preservation solution and preservation time, as documented in the International Pancreas Transplant Registry (IPTR) database. More than 5500 pancreas transplants were reported to the IPTR between 1966 and 1993 [17], and several overall analyses have been published [10,18].

The data analysed in this chapter have accumulated since October 1987 [17]. More than 90% of pancreas grafts have been transplanted simultaneously with a kidney. The best results are achieved with bladder

G.M. Collins, J.M. Dubernard, W. Land and G.G. Persijn (eds). Procurement, Preservation and Allocation of Vascularized Organs 181–191
© 1997 Kluwer Academic Publishers.

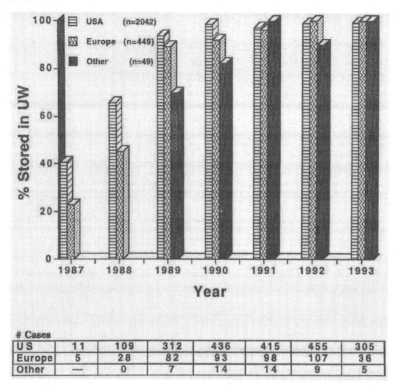

# Cases							
US	11	109	312	436	415	455	305
Europe	5	28	82	93	98	107	36
Other	—	0	7	14	14	9	5

Figure 1. Percentage of pancreas grafts preserved in University of Wisconsin (UW) solution by location and year. During the late 1980s, UW solution was used for a higher proportion of pancreases transplanted in the USA than in Europe or other locations, but in the 1990s UW solution has been used nearly exclusively.

drainage [17]. Since this is the technique most commonly used, the analysis on preservation was restricted to 2754 cadaver bladder-drained (BD) pancreas transplants performed simultaneously with a kidney (SPK). World-wide graft outcome according to preservation solution was analysed for all cases since 1987. However, since UW has emerged as the dominant solution used, a separate analysis was undertaken for grafts stored in UW solution since 1989 in order to reflect results according to current practice. Since variables other than preservation time or solution may affect results, Cox regression analyses were also performed according to multiple variables, including location (USA or non-USA), and transplant year.

The univariate and multivariate statistical analyses were performed using the SAS program. Pancreas grafts were considered functioning for as long as the recipients were insulin-independent. Death with a functioning graft was counted as a graft failure. Graft survival rates were calculated actuarially using the Kaplan–Meier method. For the univariate analyses, the probability values were calculated by the Wilcoxon

(WC) and log-rank (L-R) tests, and refer to the significance of differences among the overall survival curves. The WC test is primarily used to calculate the probability that early differences are significant, while the L-R test is used to calculate the probability for late differences; actual p values are given for those < 0.2. For the multivariate analysis (Cox regression), exact p values are given for all comparisons.

3. Demographics

The duration of preservation times according to solutions used for cases from October 1987 to November 1993 are shown in Table 1. Only UW or plasma-based solutions were used for preservation times exceeding 24 h (3% and 8% of the grafts, respectively). Over 50% of grafts preserved in UW solution were preserved for > 12 h, while only 11% and 15%, of those preserved in Collins' or other solutions, respectively, exceeded 12 h.

Table 1. Number of pancreas transplants world-wide according to preservation solution and preservation time October 1987–November 1993.

Preservation solution	< 12 h	12–23 h	24–29 h	≥ 30 h
UW (n = 2393)	45% (1082)	51% (1227)	3% (80)	< 1% (4)
Collins (n = 131)	88% (116)	11% (15)	0 (0)	0 (0)
Other (n = 11)	82% (9)	18% (2)	0 (0)	0 (0)
Plasma (n = 59)	49% (29)	36% (21)	14% (8)	2% (1)

UW was used for an ever-increasing proportion of cases beginning in the late 1980s, but was accepted more readily in the USA than elsewhere (Fig. 1). However, by the 1990s UW was virtually the only solution used at all centres, and this has continued to the present (Fig. 1). Even with the UW solution, preservation for ≥ 24 h is exclusively performed in the USA. No non-USA grafts were reported to be stored for longer than 24 h, and nearly two-thirds of non-USA grafts were stored for less than 12 hours. In contrast, in the USA approximately two-thirds were stored for longer than this.

4. Results

4.1. Results by solution and multiple variables

When outcomes for all SPK BD cases from 1987 to 1993 were analysed according to the various preservation solutions, there were no differences (Fig. 2). Graft functional survival rates at 1 year were 76% for UW (n = 2425), 74% for those stored in plasma-based solutions (n = 58) and 69% for those stored in Collins' solution (n = 137). However, the mean duration of

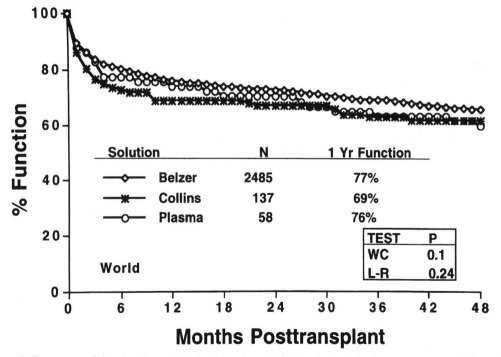

Figure 2. Pancreas graft functional survival rates for cadaveric bladder-drained simultaneous pancreas/ kidney (SPK) transplants performed world-wide from 1987 to 1993 according to preservation solution.

preservation was different between the three groups, being significantly shorter ($p = 0.0001$) with Collins' (6.4 ± 4.2 h) than with UW (12.4 ± 5.5 h) or plasma-based solutions (13.6 ± 8.3 h).

Cox regression analysis of the risk of graft loss for technical reasons (thrombosis, pancreatitis, primary non-function, etc.) showed that solution and preservation time had no influence, but year of transplant did (Table 2). The risk for technical failure has decreased annually. In a second Cox analysis of overall risk for graft loss from all causes (rejection included), preservation solution again emerged as being non-significant (Table 3), while year of transplant remained significant. Unexpectedly, the relative risk for graft loss was actually lower with increasing preservation time. Because this finding seemed aberrant, separate univariate analyses were performed for grafts preserved in UW solution, and other variables were included in the Cox model to account for a possible centre effect (see below).

4.2. Results by preservation time in UW solution

Since pancreas grafts are almost exclusively preserved in UW solution, the analysis of outcome according to storage times was performed only for these cases. The graft functional survival rates of cadaver bladder-drained pancreas transplants in recipients of simultaneous kidney transplants according to the preservation time in UW solution overall (world-wide) since 1989 are shown in Fig. 3. The differences were minimal, with 1 year graft functional survival rates of 77% for those stored for < 12 h ($n = 775$), 78% for those stored for 12–23 h ($n = 1005$), and 80% for those stored for 24–29 h ($n = 60$). Separate analyses were carried out for European (Fig. 4) and American (Fig. 5) cases. In Europe more than two-thirds of grafts were stored < 12 h and none was stored for ≥ 24 h. Graft functional survival rates were virtually identical for pancreas stored for < 12 h ($n = 197$) and 12–23 h ($n = 89$) – 85% and 86%, respectively at 1 year.

In the USA, 4% of pancreas grafts were stored for 24–30 h. On simple univariate analyses, no penalty for extending preservation time could be discerned (Fig. 5). The 1 year function rates were 75% for those stored for < 12 h ($n = 556$), 77% for those stored for 12–23 h ($n = 847$) and 81% for those stored for 24–30 h ($n = 65$). The higher graft survival rates with increasing storage times was unexpected, and could reflect a centre effect since those with the most experience and the best results might be more liberal in accepting longer storage times.

It could be that the most experienced or larger centres with the best overall results are more likely to use pancreases under circumstances requiring extended preservation. If the results obtained at the centres that used grafts stored for > 24 h were compared with the outcome of those stored for a shorter time, a benefit of extended preservation time might not be seen. A review of the database showed that all but three of the centres reporting grafts stored for ≥ 24 h had performed more than 50 transplants. Thus, separate analyses were done within two groups of centres; those reporting ≥ 50 total pancreas grafts (nine centres) and those reporting fewer transplants (96 centres). The results of these analyses are shown in Figs. 6 and 7, respectively.

Table 2. Relative risk (RR) for pancreas graft loss due to technical failures according to Cox regression analysis of cadaver bladder-drained simultaneous pancreas/kidney transplants for USA and European cases 1987–1993.

Variable	p	RR
Transplant Year*	0.0650	0.921
USA versus Europe	0.4414	0.991
Collins' versus UW	0.2598	1.322
Plasma versus UW	0.6545	0.837
Preservation Time	0.5983	1.088

* Risk for technical failure is progressively decreasing. Preservation factors and continent of transplant had no influence in this analysis but did when centre size was taken into account (see Table 4).

Table 3. Relative risk (RR) for pancreas graft loss according to Cox regression analysis of cadaver bladder-drained simultaneous pancreas/kidney transplants for USA and European cases 1987–1993.

Variable*	p	RR
Transplant Year	0.0002	0.891
USA versus Europe	0.0105	1.332
Collins' versus UW	0.7281	1.061
Plasma versus UW	0.8214	0.951
Preservation Time	0.0603	0.986

* Preservation time up to 30 h at least does not increase risks for graft loss. The appearance in the univariate analysis that risk is less with increasing preservation time is explained by a centre effect (see Table 5).

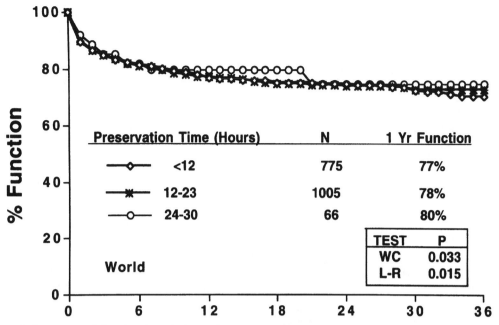

Figure 3. Pancreas graft functional survival rates for bladder-drained simultaneous pancreas/kidney transplants performed world-wide in 1990–1993 according to preservation time in UW solution.

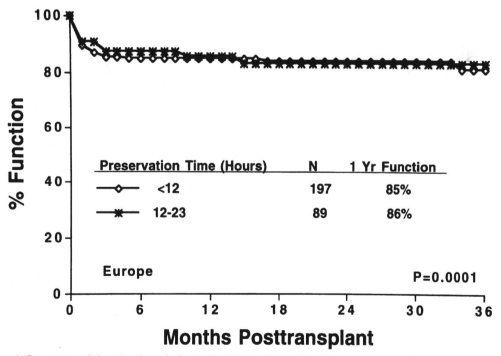

Figure 4. Pancreas graft functional survival rates for bladder-drained simultaneous pancreas/kidney transplants performed in Europe in 1990–1993 according to preservation time in UW solution.

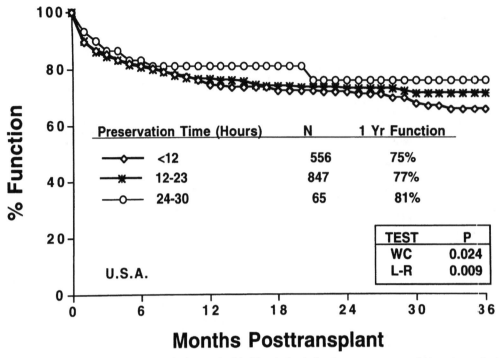

Figure 5. Pancreas graft functional survival rates for bladder-drained simultaneous pancreas/kidney transplants performed in the USA in 1990–1993 according to preservation time in UW solution.

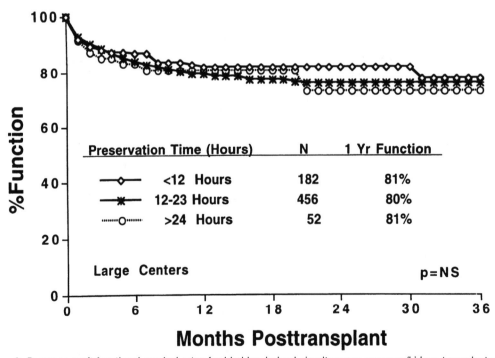

Figure 6. Pancreas graft functional survival rates for bladder-drained simultaneous pancreas/kidney transplants performed in 1990–1993 at large (≥ 50 cases) institutions (*n* = 9) according to preservation time in UW solution.

In the centres reporting > 50 cases, graft survival rates were highest with the shortest (< 12 h) preservation time (Fig. 6). Of the 96 centres with ≤ 49 cases each, the graft survival rate curves were not significantly different no matter what the preservation time, but only 14 grafts were stored for > 24 h (Fig. 7). At each preservation time, the graft survival rate curves tended to be higher in the analysis for larger centres than for smaller centres (~ 4–5% difference at 1 year). Since about 80% of grafts stored for > 24 h were performed at the large centres, in the overall analysis the survival rate at this storage time was higher than for shorter preservation times, since most of the latter were performed at the small centres. That the centre effect is real was shown in a Cox regression analysis (Tables 4, 5).

The relative risk for technical failure was 50% less (p = 0.002) at large centres than at small centres (Table 4). Independently, the risk of technical loss increased when preservation time was lengthened, an effect that was seen even when centre size was included in the model. The risk for technical failure increases approximately 3% for each hour by which preservation is extended. In a comparison Cox analysis of overall risk for pancreas graft loss from all causes (rejection included), preservation time had no effect on outcome

Table 4. Relative risk (RR) for pancreas graft loss due to technical failure according to Cox regression analysis of cadaver bladder-drained simultaneous pancreas/kidney transplants preserved in UW solution for USA and European cases with centre size* as variable 1990–1993.		
Variable*	p	RR
Transplant Year	0.4626	0.946
USA versus Europe	0.4533	1.175
Centre Large versus Small*	0.0002	0.513
Preservation Time	0.0356	1.032

* Large ≥ 50 Cases
Small ≤ 49 Cases
When centre size is taken into account there is a detrimental effect of increasing preservation time. The risk for technical failure at large centres is 50% less than at small centres, but the overall risk increased as preservation time increased.

(Table 5). However, the centre effect persisted, the risk for graft loss being 35% less at large than at small centres.

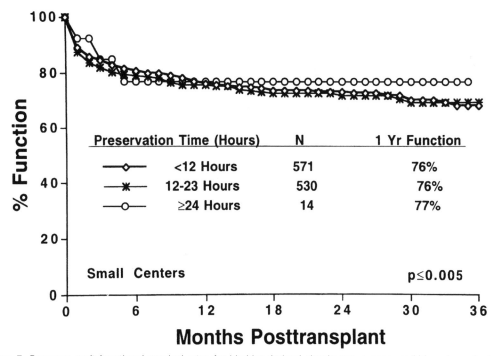

Figure 7. Pancreas graft functional survival rates for bladder-drained simultaneous pancreas/kidney transplants performed in 1990–1993 at small (≤ 49 cases) institutions (n = 96) according to preservation time in UW solution.

Table 5. Relative risk (RR) for pancreas graft loss according to Cox regression analysis of cadaver bladder-drained simultaneous pancreas/kidney transplants preserved in UW solution for USA and European cases with centre size* as variable 1990–1993.

Variable*	p	RR
Transplant Year	0.0046	0.855
USA versus Europe	0.0002	1.867
Centre Large versus Small*	0.0003	0.658
Preservation Time	0.6056	1.005

*Large ≥ 50 Cases
Small ≤ 49 Cases
When centre size is taken into account there is no beneficial effect of increasing preservation time. The overall risk for graft loss is significantly less at large centres.

Thus, we conclude that extending preservation time slightly increased the risk of graft failure. The higher graft survival rates seen at > 24 h in the univariate analysis was an artefact. Large centres have better results at long preservation times than those obtained by small centres using grafts with short preservation times. Nevertheless, at all centres, regardless of size, preservation up to 30 h had only a minimal effect on the overall probability of success.

4.3. Effect of preservation time on pancreas graft endocrine function

Whether there is an effect of longer preservation time on the degree of graft endocrine function is also uncertain. Only one study has addressed this problem. Morel *et al.* [14] analysed the metabolic profiles and glucose tolerance test results in recipients of pancreas grafts performed at the University of Minnesota according to the duration of graft preservation. Metabolic profiles (Fig. 8) and intravenous (Fig. 9) and oral (Fig. 10) glucose tolerance test results were similar in recipients of grafts stored for < 6, 6–12, 12–24 or > 24 h. Thus, graft functional survival rates in terms of insulin-independence of the recipients are similar, and the degree of endocrine function is similar for pancreas preservations times up to 30 h.

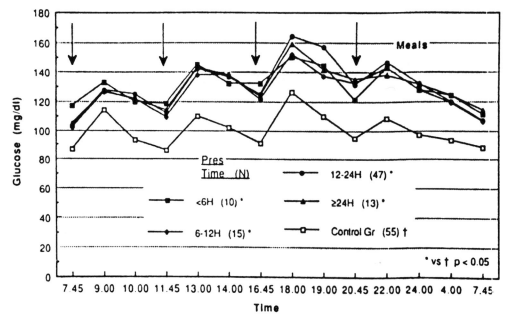

Figure 8. Plasma glucose levels during 24 h metabolic profiles 2–6 weeks' post-transplant according to duration of graft preservation in cases performed at the University of Minnesota from 1984 to 1989. There were no significant differences between the four preservation times, but the glucose values in the normal controls are significantly lower at each time point. (Reproduced from reference [14].)

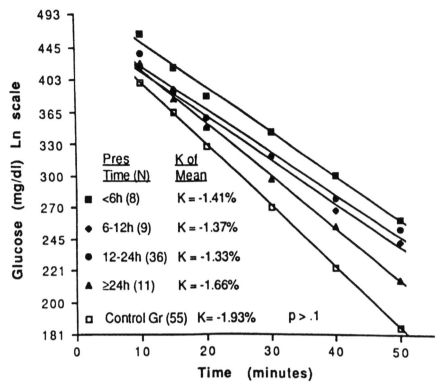

Figure 9. Mean glucose levels 10–50 min after injection during i.v. glucose tolerance tests 2–6 weeks' post-transplant according to duration of pancreas graft preservation in cases performed at the University of Minnesota from 1984 to 1989. There were no significant differences between the groups. (Reproduced from reference [14]).

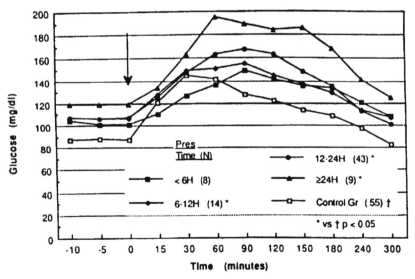

Figure 10. Mean glucose levels during oral glucose tolerance tests 2–6 weeks' post-transplant according to duration of pancreas graft preservation in cases performed at the University of Minnesota from 1984 to 1989. There was no statistically significant difference in the mean glucose rise at any time between the four preservation time groups, but after 90 minutes the mean glucose values are significantly lower in the control group than in any of the four preservation groups. (Reproduced from reference [14].)

5. Discussion

The upper limits of storage time for a human pancreas in UW solution or other solutions is not known. Canine pancreas grafts can be stored for up to 72 h in either a plasma-based [9] or UW solution [15] prior to transplantation. In humans, storage times for > 30 h have rarely been tested [14]. Of nine grafts reported to the Registry stored for more than 30 h [17], four were technical failures but another four remained functioning for more than 1 year.

However, 30 h is sufficient to complete the logistical manoeuvres usually required to accomplish transplantation, even when the donor and recipient are at long distances from the transplant centre. No one would want to test a hypothesis that might have detrimental effects by trying > 30 h preservation, unless there were extenuating circumstances. For example, if an individual with a high proportion of antibodies to the panel has a negative cross-match graft available under conditions that would require > 30 h preservation to accomplish the transplant, the hypothesis could justifiably be tested. If cases accumulate and show consistently successful results at > 30 h preservation, then the type of patients for whom extended preservation would be acceptable could be expanded, e.g. exceptionally good HLA matches, even if the candidate does not have high panel reactivity. Ultimately, longer times could be used in order to ease the burden of having to perform some transplants at night.

The preservation times tolerated are sufficient such that all pancreases procured should be utilized. There are approximately 4500 cadaver donors in the USA annually, but in 1993 only approximately 800 pancreases were transplanted [17]. Now that storage times of up 30 h are known to be possible, the number of transplants should be able to be expanded with routine sharing from organ procurement organizations or centres that cannot utilize a pancreas to those that can, as has been the practice at the University of Minnesota for several years [19].

6. Summary and conclusion

Pancreas grafts can be preserved for up to 30 h in UW or plasma-based solutions with no difference in outcome. UW is now routinely used by nearly all centres for pancreas preservation, since it is totally synthetic and eliminates the risk of disease transmission, and it is commercially available. For bladder-crained pancreas grafts transplanted simultaneously with a kidney, functional survival rate for those stored in UW solution for < 12 h was 77%, with survival of 78% for those stored for 12–23 h and 80% for those stored for 24–30 h. Preservation is not a limiting factor in the application of pancreas transplants, and efforts should be made to increase the utilization rate so the maximum number of diabetic patients can benefit from cure of their disease.

References

1. Belzer FO, Southard JH. Principles of solid-organ preservation by cold storage. Transplantation 1988; 45: 673–6.
2. Idezuki Y, Feemster JA, Dietzman RH, Lillehei KC. Experimental pancreaticoduodenal preservation and transplantation. Surg Gynecol Obstet 1002; 126: 1002–14.
3. Brynger H. Twenty-four-hour preservation of the duct-ligated canine pancreatic allograft. Eur Surg Res 1975; 7: 341–54.
4. Baumgartner D, Sutherland DER, Najarian JS. Studies on segmental pancreas autotransplants in dogs: technique and preservation. Transplant Proc 1980; 12 (Suppl. 2): 163–71.
5. Florack G, Sutherland DER, Heil JE, Zweber BA, Najarian JS. Long term preservation of segmental pancreas autogratts. Surgery 1982; 92: 260–9.
6. Florack G, Sutherland DER, Heil JE, Squifflet JP, Najarian JS. Preservation of canine segmental pancreatic autog·afts: Cold storage versus pulsatile machine perfusion. J Surg Res 1983; 34: 493–504.
7. Sutherland DER, Morrow CE, Florack G et al. Cold storage preservation of islet and pancreas grafts as assessed by *in vivo* function after transplantation to diabetic hosts. Cryobiology 1983; 20: 138–50.
8. Abouna GM, Heil JE, Sutherland DER, Najarian JS. Factors necessary for successful 48-hour preservation of pancreas grafts. Transplantation 1988; 45: 270–4.
9. Heise JW, Sutherland DER, Heil JE, Najarian JS. 72-hours' preservation of pancreatic autotransplants in dogs using a urinary drainage technique. Transplant Proc 1988; 20: 1029–30.
10. Sutherland DER, Moudry KC, Dunn DL, Goetz FC. Najarian JS. Pancreas-transplant outcome in relation to presence or absence of end-stage renal disease, timing of transplant, surgical technique, and donor source. Diabetes 1989; 38 (Suppl 1): 10–12.
11. Abouna GM, Sutherland DER, Florack G, Najarian JS. Function of transplanted human pancreatic allografts after preservation in cold storage for 6 to 26 hours. Transplantation 1987; 43: 630–6.
12. Florack G, Sutherland DER, Heise JW, Najarian JS. Successful preservation of human pancreas grafts for 28 hours. Transplant Proc 1987; 19: 3882–5.
13. Florack G. Sutherland DER, Morel P. Condie RM, Najarian JS. Effective preservation of human pancreas grafts. Transplant Proc 1989; 21: 1369–71.
14. Morel P. Moudry-Munns KC. Najarian JS, Gruessner RWG. Dunn DL, Sutherland DER. Influence of preservation time on outcome and metabolic function of bladder-drained pancreas transplants. Transplantation 1990; 49: 294–303.
15. Wahlberg J. Southard JH. Belzer FO. Development of a cold storage solution for pancreas preservation. Cryobiology 1986; 23: 77–82.
16. Belzer FO. Clinical organ preservation with UW solution. Transplantation 1989; 47: 1097–8.
17. Sutherland DER. Moudry-Munns KC. Gruessner A. Pancreas transplant results in United Network for Organ Sharing United States of America Registry with a comparison to non-USA data in the International Registry. In: Terasaki PI (ed.), Clinical

Transplants 1993. UCLA Tissue Typing Laboratory, Los Angeles 1994; pp. 47–69.

18. Sutherland DER, Gruessner A, Moudry-Munns KC. International pancreas transplant registry report. Transplant Proc 1994; 26: 407–11.

19. Dunn DL, Schlumpf RB. Gruessner RWG *et al.* Maximal use of liver and pancreas from cadaveric organ donors. Transplant Proc 1990; 22: 423–4.

Section III
Allocation and Logistics

22 | Principles of kidney allocation

J. De Meester and G.G. Persijn

1. Allocation principles

It is generally accepted that a model for kidney allocation should be equitable. The two principles of primary importance for policy decisions concerning allocation of donor organs in organ transplantations are medical utility and justice [1,2]. These allocation principles are usually explained with regard to the individual transplant candidate. Patient selection based upon medical utility points towards the predictably best outcome of a donor organ in a transplantation, i.e. the maximum number of patient–years of graft function. Selection based upon justice is related to giving an organ to those who are worst off, either at the particular moment that an organ is to be allocated or from the 'over-a-lifetime' perspective, so that their condition will be improved. Strictly speaking, these two principles are mutually conflicting.

In any allocation model, the decision of whether to use an allocated organ remains the privilege of the transplant surgeon and/or physician responsible for the care of the patient, who must evaluate both the donor organ quality and the transplant circumstances of the patient. The patient also has the right to decline the offered transplant.

2. Allocation factors

Factors, used in the different organ allocation models, can be divided into medical and non-medical. Examples of medical factors are ABO blood group, HLA-typing (and thus HLA-matching between donor and recipient), cross-match result, body size parameters, virological results, recipient and/or donor age, cold ischaemia time, medical urgency of a transplant and HLA-sensitization. Time on the waiting list, donor organ exchange balance, geographical areas, logistical issues and centre transplant activity are categorized as non-medical factors. In addition, the factors themselves, and their ultimate use, are related to either or both allocation principles and to the type of organ to be allocated. The use of HLA-typing, cross-match results, ABO blood group, medical transplantability and body size parameters are supported by the medical utility principle, whereas medical urgency, waiting time, HLA-sensitization, likelihood of finding a suitable organ in future and geographical aspects reside under the justice principle. Factors such as HLA-typing and HLA-sensitization are almost exclusively used in kidney allocation models; body size parameters are only a factor in thoracic organ and liver allocation

G.M. Collins, J.M. Dubernard, W. Land and G.G. Persijn (eds), Procurement, Preservation and Allocation of Vascularized Organs 195–199
© 1997 Kluwer Academic Publishers.

models. Furthermore, each individual allocation factor ought not to be applied in the same manner by different organ exchange organizations. Schemes often depend upon the results of the scientific analyses and/or on general consensus within the transplant community.

This is illustrated by the application of HLA-matching in kidney allocation models. The Euro-transplant (ET) organ exchange organization (which covers Austria, Belgium, Germany, Luxemburg, and the Netherlands) fully prioritizes patients without an HLA-antigen mismatch between donor and recipient on the HLA-A,B,DR loci. Thereafter, HLA-A,B,DR mismatch classes are ranked by increasing number of mismatches. Highest priority is given to a zero HLA-DR antigen mis-match (scale 0-2), followed by a zero HLA-B antigen mismatch (scale 0-2), which, in turn, has more weight than an HLA-A antigen mismatch (scale 0-2). In con-trast, the United Kingdom Transplant Support Service Special Health Authority (UKTSSA), which covers England and Scotland, regards zero HLA-A,B,DR mis-match recipients as well as those which have only a single HLA-A or HLA-B antigen mismatch (called 'beneficial matching') as priorities. The United Network for Organ Sharing (UNOS; US) recently changed its policy regarding the factor HLA-typing: the first right for a kidney, formerly assigned only to the recipients who exactly shared all HLA-A,B,DR antigens of the donor, currently also concerns patients with no HLA-A,B,DR mismatch. Thereafter, both in UKTSSA and in UNOS, several HLA-A,B,DR mismatch classes are grouped together and, subsequently, ranked or weighted.

The definition of (highly) sensitized recipients also varies [3,4]. In ET, UKTSSA, France and Scandiatransplant, a high degree of immunization of a recipient means incompatibility with $\geq 85\%$ of a stan-dard donor lymphocyte panel (%PRA). In UNOS, $\geq 80\%$ positive reactions are sufficient for the status of 'highly sensitized',whereas Swiss Transplant defines patients with $\geq 50\%$ positive reactions as being highly immunized. Even more variation is seen in the definition of sensitization, which ranges from 1%PRA (UKTSSA), through 5%PRA (ET, Swiss Transplant), up to 20%PRA (UNOS).

Concerning the geographical areas, the justice principle is often quoted in order to assign, in the event of locally available donor organs, priority to 'local' recipients listed at the local transplant programme associated with the donor hospital over 'non-local' recipients. The local programme should have some reward for the efforts involved in effecting organ donation in its local donor area. Sometimes, local priority is also defended by the medical utility prin-ciple: reduction of cold ischaemia times will benefit the outcome of the transplant. Last but not least, financial expenses associated with organ exchange and budgetary constraints, oblige geographical features to be taken into account more often. Many allocation pro-tocols therefore include geographical aspects: donor organs are first to be allocated locally, then regionally, then nationally and then internationally (UNOS, France, UKTSSA).

Some allocation models incorporate the so-called organ export:import balance of a transplant pro-gramme. This is the difference between the organs pro-cured and the organs transplanted (ET); following the principle of justice, neutral organ export : import balances should be achieved. An alternative method to meet the loss of potential local transplants is the so-called organ pay-back. i.e. transplant centre A should return an organ to centre B that offered an organ for a patient listed at centre A (UNOS).

3. Allocation modes

As a first allocation mode, the direction of the organ offer should be assessed: patient-oriented or centre-oriented. In the first category, the organ offer is made to a specific patient, while, in the latter, the offer is made to a transplant centre which subsequently selects the best suitable recipient. The two types are often combined. The ultimate example of a patient-oriented offer is the widely applied concept of mandatory ex-change. Whenever transplant candidates for a particu-lar organ appear in this category the offer and/or exchange of an organ is obligatory. The definition of mandatory exchange is different according to the donor organ and between the different organ exchange organ-izations. In ET, with regard to kidney transplantation, zero HLA-A,B,DR mismatched recipients, current and non-currently sensitized recipients selected by the acceptable mismatch programme [5] and eligible recipients in the highly immunized trial (HIT) protocol are included in the 'mandatory exchange' category. Mandatory exchange of zero HLA-A,B,DR mis-matched recipients is not performed in France, however.

An allocation model should also use a specific mode to generate the allocation lists, whether a points system, a (stepwise) hierarchical system or a strictly rotational system. In a points system several factors are weighted simultaneously, either per patient or per centre, and the sum is used for ranking the patients or the centres, e.g. kidney allocation in UNOS (patients). In the stepwise hierarchical system (most often patient-oriented), the factors are sequentially used: one factor after the other is sorted according to a predetermined pattern in order to generate the final recipient allocation list, e.g. kidney allocation in ET.

4. HLA-allo-sensitization and crossmatch

Sensitized patients have a high chance of a positive cross-match with a particular donor. In order to minimize inappropriate offers to these recipients, some organ exchange organizations demand the regular shipment of sera of (highly) sensitized patients on the kidney waiting list to all tissue typing laboratories within the organ exchange organization. A kidney is only offered to (highly) sensitized patients who have a negative preliminary cross-match at the donor centre. At the recipient centre, the cross-match must be repeated before transplantation (ET). In Australia, however, sera shipment involves all kidney patients on the waiting list, regardless of the level of sensitization. The cross-match performed at the donor centre is not repeated at the recipient centre in order to reduce the cold ischaemia time.

Efforts made to transplant immunized kidney patients have led to the development of special programmes by reference tissue typing laboratories of the organ exchange organization [5,6]. In ET, the acceptable mismatch programme allows the incorporation of HLA-A and HLA-B mismatched antigens, which are expected not to result in a positive cross-match, in the HLA-typing of the kidney transplant candidate. The chance of finding a suitable donor kidney without a positive cross-match will, therefore, be greater. If selected by the programme, the recipient has the first priority for the kidney on offer.

5. Life of (kidney) allocation systems

Allocation systems are not fixed over time. Scientific advances in immunology and clinical transplant medicine, socio-economic and political climates, and societal and ethical standards influence allocation systems repeatedly: minor and/or major changes in the selection of allocation factors and mode(s), of the short and long term goals, and concerning the degree to which each of the principles of justice and medical utility are considered are unavoidable. In practice, an allocation system is redesigned upon compromise solutions which ultimately satisfy the vast majority of the transplant programmes.

As an illustration, the kidney allocation systems, operational in the ET foundation from 1981 to 1996 are described. In March 1996, a totally new kidney allocation system was implemented.

5.1. ET Kidney allocation system 1981–1995

5.1.1. *Basic hierarchic structure*
First, there was a system of mandatory exchange, whose impact on the allocation varied a lot over time. Since 1990, the impact of such an exchange for a kidney is about 15–20%. The offer was always patient-specific and was made by the central allocation office of Eurotransplant. Second, the transplant programmes which were associated with the donor hospital decided whether a local transplantation was possible. If this was so, the programme selected the best suitable recipient, in compliance with a minimum set of rules. For kidneys, this followed ABO blood group matching and, additionally, minimum HLA-antigen sharing criteria. The third level consisted of the allocation of donor organs which could not be used locally. These donor organs had to be offered to the Eurotransplant pool and were placed by the 24 h duty office of Eurotransplant, following specific allocation rules.

5.1.2. *Kidney allocation rules*
At the first level, donor kidney exchange was mandatory for patients with zero HLA-mismatches, patients selected by the acceptable mismatch programme and patients selected by the HIT procedure. With the exception of the two latter programmes, blood group type O kidneys were allocated only to blood group type O and/or B recipients and there was no priority for ABO identical versus ABO compatible blood groups in matching the donor. Zero HLA-mismatched recipients were sorted first according to current allo-sensitization and then according to time on the waiting list.

At the second level, the local transplant programme selected the best suitable recipient(s) on the waiting list, respecting the above-mentioned ABO blood group and minimum HLA-antigen sharing rules. The HLA-antigen sharing for a kidney transplant had to be a minimum of either 2 HLA-DR antigens (as of 1993) or one HLA-B antigen plus one HLA-DR antigen common between the donor and the recipient (as of 1987).

At the third level, if donor kidneys were offered to the Eurotransplant pool, potential recipients were sequentially sorted using different allocation factors: first according to the medical urgency, second by HLA-mismatch class, third by sensitization and finally on the basis of waiting time. With regard to medical urgency, priority was given to patients, with severe physical and/or psychological problems. The HLA-mismatch classes concerned the HLA-A, HLA-B and HLA-DR loci: HLA-DR mismatches were weighted more than HLA-B mismatches, which in turn had more impact than HLA-A mismatches, e.g. HLA-A-B-DR mismatch class order: 1-0-0, 2-0-0, 0-1-0, 1-1-0, 2-1-0, 0-0-1, 1-0-1, 2-0-1, 0-2-0, 1-2-0, 2-2-0, 0-1-1, 1-1-1 and 2-1-1. With regard to sensitization, priority was given first to highly immunized patients (85–100% PRA), then to immunized patients (6–84% PRA) and then to the non-immunized patients (0–5% PRA).

No offer was made to sensitized patients with a positive crossmatch at the donor centre, to patients below the minimal degree of HLA-antigen sharing and, since April 1994, to patients belonging to a transplant programme with a net kidney import excess of five or more.

5.2. ET Kidney allocation system 1996

5.2.1. Introduction

Three major points of criticism about the ET kidney allocation model used since 1981 were voiced during 1995: (1) a constantly high proportion of patients was on the renal transplant waiting list for more than 5 years ($\pm 10\%$); (2) there was little chance of a transplant for recipients with a relatively rare HLA-phenotype or with homozygous HLA-loci, probably as a result of an allocation system too much focused on HLA-matching; and (3) there were increasing imbalances at the centre and country level between kidney procurement and kidney transplantation.

Two studies addressed these problems [7,8]; an allocation technique, totally different from that in use at ET, had been designed via simulation studies, and was said to be able to correct for many of the comments raised, while guaranteeing a favourable HLA-match distribution and an overall transplant success rate near the theoretically possible optimum.

The possibility of introducing the proposed allocation model was thoroughly examined by experts chosen from the Eurotransplant transplant community. Simulation analyses were performed over the period 1989–1995, using a ET tailor-made model. As shown in Table 1, the results showed that a markedly better waiting list structure and national procurement/transplantation balance could be realized. The decision for definitive implementation of the model was made, supported by the Board of Eurotransplant and the renal transplant programmes.

Table 1. Comparison between two allocation systems (real data versus data from simulation).

	1989–1995 Old system Real	1989–1995 New model Simulation
HLA-mismatch		
0 (%)	22	24
1–2 (%)	40	44
3 (%)	29	25
> 3 (%)	9	7
Waiting time		
Average (years)	2.1	1.6
Maximum (years)	20.0	13.0
> 3 years (%)	28	17
> 5 years (%)	11	3
Balance		
Centre		
Average	± 13	± 13
Maximum	± 65	± 80
Country		
Austria	– 9	– 2
Belgium	– 31	– 11
Germany	+ 47	+ 7
Netherlands	– 5	+ 6
Distance		
Local (%)	46	52
+ Regional (%)	54	65
+ National (%)	71	82

5.2.2. Basic structure

In the allocation structure, the 'local centre' allocation level has been eliminated, leading to the creation of a one-pool system. Nevertheless, the idea of mandatory exchange is kept. New allocation factors have been entered: an HLA-mismatch probability factor assessing the frequency of the HLA-phenotype of a transplant candidate, the national kidney balance, and a factor related to the distance between the donor-reporting transplant centre and the transplant programme where the potential recipient is listed. The greatest change is the process by which recipients on the allocation list are ranked, upon the availability of a donor. Instead of the previously applied method of sequential sorting, all eligibile recipients are given points on five allocation factors, the sum of which determines their position on the list. These five allocation parameters are shown in Table 2.

The HLA-mismatch factor has been simplified, by using only seven mismatch grades (0–6). The more HLA-mismatches on the HLA-A, HLA-B and HLA-

Table 2. Allocation factors.

	Points	Weight	Max. Points	Formula
HLA-A,B,DR mismatch	100	4	400	$400 \times (1 - \text{HLA MM} / 6)$
Mismatch probability	100	1	100	$100 \times (1 - [\text{ABO} \times \{1 - (\% \text{ PRA}/100)\} \times (\text{MMP0} + \text{MMP1})])^{1000}$
Waiting time	100	2	200	$200 \times [(\text{WT} + \text{bonus})/\text{max WT}]$
Distance donor > transplant programme	100	2,6	260	Local = 260; Regional = 208; National = 104; Other ET countries = 0
National import/export balance	100	2	200	$200 \times [(\text{highest balance} - \text{balance country recipient}) / (\text{highest balance} - \text{lowest balance})]$

DR loci, the fewer points allocated. The mismatch probability factor assesses the chance of 0 and 1 HLA-mismatch in 1000 kidney offers. This chance is adjusted for the ABO blood group match possibilities and for the level of HLA-allosensitization (% PRA screening), to protect the ABO blood group recipients and to compensate for the higher chance of a positive crossmatch respectively. The lower the overall chance, the more points are allocated.

The time waiting factor uses, as determinator, the waiting time of the longest waiting transplant candidate, being transplantable and having the identical ABO blood group as the donor. A bonus waiting time is assigned to paediatric recipients, following the agreement to give some priority to their transplantation. The distance between donor centre and transplant programmes compensates for the elimination of the local centre allocation level. Recipients at the local transplant programme receive more points than those at the other transplant programmes in the donor country. No points are given to those on waiting lists in the other Eurotransplant countries. The national kidney balance relates to the difference between kidney transplantation and kidney procurement, both calculated at the national level and over a period of 365 days. Patients listed at a transplant programme in a country with the highest net balance (more transplants than procurements) will have zero points.

5.2.3. *Results*
An audit committee will monitor whether the new allocation model fulfils its goals, and whether discrepancy will occur between the simulated and real-life results.

6. Epilogue

Allocation models are constructed by consensus among the participating transplant programmes, balancing between the principles of medical utility and justice. As a tool to create and/or adapt allocation procedures, increasing numbers of experiments will be performed with simulation techniques (e.g. liver allocation simulation analyses in UNOS; personal communication from W. Graham). Despite the fact that assumptions are inevitable with this technique, it seems to be possible to compare reliably different allocation models and variants of numerous outcome parameters, medical (survival, mortality on the waiting list) as well as non-medical (exchange, transport, cost profile of health care).

References

1. Milford EL. The end-stage renal disease transplant program: an experiment in participatory democracy and national health care. Semin Dialysis 1994; 1: 69–74.
2. 1991 UNOS Ethics Committee. General principles for allocating human organs and tissues. Transplant Proc 1992; 24: 2227–35.
3. Matesanz R, Hors J, Persijn G et al. (eds). Council of Europe Transplant Volume 04; 1992.
4. Matesanz R, Hors J, Persijn G et al. (eds). Council of Europe Transplant Volume 05; 1993.
5. Claas FHJ, De Waal LP, Beelen J et al. Transplantation of highly sensitized patients on the basis of acceptable HLA-A and HLA-B mismatches. Clin Transplant 1989; 20: 185–90.
6. Special schemes for transplanting highly sensitized patients. In: Gore SM, Bradley BA (eds). Renal transplantation: sense and sensitization. Kluwer Academic Publishers, Dordrecht: 1988: 268–81.
7. Wujciak T, Opelz G. Computer analysis of cadaver kidney allocation procedures. Transplantation 1993; 55: 516–21.
8. Wujciak T, Opelz G. A proposal for improved cadaver kidney allocation. Transplantation 1993; 56: 1513–17.

23 | Principles of liver allocation in Eurotransplant

Uwe Jost and Burkhard Ringe

1. Introduction

Transplantation of organs has made enormous progress over the last 30 years. Technical developments in organ transplantations gave rise to questions of more moral and ethical nature [1], with the need for discussions about the determination of brain death, donor and recipient selection and allocation of these scarce resources. Immunological research contributed significantly to the successes of transplantation [2,3]. As already repeatedly reported during recent years, a growing need for liver transplantations exists now that this has become standard therapy for patients with end stage liver disease. Considering the fact that many patients die on the waiting list, it is of great importance that an efficient and rapid procedure for organ allocation is established [4,5].

For many years Eurotransplant based the allocation of donor livers on blood group compatibility, size, clinical urgency and waiting time. Many offers were needed before a liver graft was finally accepted, and the most critical patients could often not be transplanted on time. As the number of liver transplantations increased, moral pressure was exerted for the development of an efficient, transparent and rapid organ allocation system to reduce the number of the organizationally lost organs. A new liver allocation system (ELAS) was developed within Eurotransplant in 1990 and implemented in April 1991.

2. History

The first allocation system used within the Eurotransplant area was developed in the early 1980s. All potential liver recipients were classified according to their clinical urgency (high urgency, urgent, transplantable, not transplantable). In addition to restricted blood group compatibility (blood group A to A or AB, B to B or AB, O to O or B; and AB to AB), waiting time (all recipients on one central waiting list with the longest-waiting recipient on top) played an important role. Height and weight were considered with different weighting. However, the clinical status and medical urgency of potential liver recipients was not always clearly defined, and showed significant variations among different transplant centres. Acceptance and refusal of a liver graft was influenced by many factors. After a few years' urgency categories of potential recipients changed. In addition 'no capacity' in the transplant centre because of lack of ICU beds, operating facilities or surgeons became an important factor. Many potential available donor livers (up to 15%) were not transplanted for organizational reasons (response time, organization of the explantation team, arrival). In the summer of 1990 renewed discussion of organ allocation was started. Neuhaus (Berlin) proposed a rotating allocation system [6]. After further discussions during the 'Liver Club' meeting in

G.M. Collins, J.M. Dubernard, W. Land and G.G. Persijn (eds). Procurement, Preservation and Allocation of Vascularized Organs 201–207
© 1997 Kluwer Academic Publishers.

Cambridge in September 1990 the liver group from Hannover presented a new proposal [7] for a liver allocation system. This concept was accepted at the Eurotransplant meeting in September 1990. A Eurotransplant Liver Allocation Committee (ELAC) was established to develop allocation and a practicible program (ELAS). The ELAS was implemented April 8, 1991 for a 2-year study period with a specially developed PC program.

3. Theoretical principles of the new system

The goal of ELAS was the establishment of an effective, fast and transparent liver allocation system which would reduce the number of livers not used for organizational reasons. The responsible physicians at the respective transplant centre should judge the individual transplantation necessity of potential recipients and select the most urgent patient.

The important advantages of the new concept are summed up in the following. First, the system is fundamentally patient (recipient) oriented, final judgment of the physician responsible for patient care giving the priority for transplantation to the most urgent recipient (not always the longest waiting). Second, the waiting time for an individual recipient can be estimated more exactly, which allows application of specific pretreatment protocols. Third, allocation of donor organs is more objective, since it is based on realistic transplantation numbers which reflect the need of each single centre. Fourth, there would be equal benefit for all transplant centres: those with high activity have a more frequent supply of donor organs; smaller centres which occasionally have no suitable recipient on their own waiting list, would obtain a bonus for altering a locally recovered donor to the pool, resulting in a better position on the 'rank list'. Finally, organ allocation via Eurotransplant should take less time in purchase.

4. Practical principles

ELAS allocates organs according to a centre-adapted procedure, taking into account transplantation activity of the individual centre in relation to the activity of all centres [7]. Offers are made only to centres with a suitable recipient on their waiting list (blood group identical, weight compatible, transplantable status) and with transplantation capacity (ICU, surgeon, etc.). The activity of the centres was calculated from the transplantations performed in the previous 6-month period

(e.g. 1.1.94 to 30.6.94). Each transplant centre thus acquires a 'STEP'-factor. For example, the total number of all transplantations from all centres over a certain period is 500. The activity of centre X is 100 in this period. The resulting 'STEP' is 500/100 = 5 for the following 6 months. Smaller transplant centres with fewer transplantation activity receive a larger 'STEP': those performing 20 transplants are calculated as 500/20 = 25. In this way each centre receives an individual 'STEP' for a limited period, which influences the number of further offers to the centres.

The basis for liver allocation is a so-called 'rank list' constructed on a points system and including all active liver transplant centres in Eurotransplant. Offers are always made to the highest ranked centre on this list, under observance of the above listed conditions. At the start of ELAS all rank points were equal to the calculated 'STEP' (Table 1). Every transplant performed influences the rank points and thus the position in the rank list as follows.

4.1. Liver offer accepted and transplantation effect

A donor liver is initially offered via Eurotransplant to the centre with the highest rank position and accepted. The new rank position of the centre is calculated by addition of the centre's STEP (Table 2). For example;

Table 1. Example of rank listing at the start of the system (April 1991).

Position	Centre	Rank points	STEP
1	A	1	5
2	B	1	10
3	C	1	20
4	D	1	50
5	E	1	100

Table 2. Example of rank listing after a transplantation has been performed and points recalculated: position is changed compared with Table 1.

Position	Centre	Rank points	STEP
1	B	1	10
2	C	1	20
3	D	1	50
4	E	1	100
5	A	6	5

centre A has the highest rank. According to its STEP of 5 the rank point of this centre increases from 1 to 6. This results in a change of the rank position of the centre A and centre B has now the pole position. A change in the rank position of a centre following transplantation allows equitable organ distribution.

If the second, third or fourth offer is accepted and transplantation is effected, the 'rank points' increase by only a half STEP. If acceptance is made of the fifth offer or after, the rank points are not increased. If a liver is offered via Eurotransplant from outside the organization and is transplanted no STEP is added to the rank points.

4.2. Liver offer refused

A donor liver offered via Eurotransplant can be refused by a centre for various reasons. When this happens more than three times in a row and the livers are transplanted elsewhere, the rank points of the refusing centre increase by one STEP. The major objective of this rule is to avoid a selection or accumulation of so-called 'optimal' donor organs by single centres. Analyses of the 2-year trial period during which these guidelines were applied showed that this rule had to be

utilized only in very rare cases. Usually the larger centres were affected.

4.3. Local donor organ retrieved and transplantation performed in the same centre

A donor liver procured locally can be used prefentially in the same transplant programme, independently of the actual position on the rank list, except if a potential recipient is registered as highly urgent elsewhere. Following transplantation the new rank position of this particular centre is calculated by addition of only half a STEP. This is an indirect advantage for a donor centre.

4.4. Local donor organ retrieved and offered to Eurotransplant

If a donor liver procured by a liver transplant programme and no local transplantation is possible, the graft is offered to Eurotransplant and will be distributed according to the general guidelines, i.e. to the centre with the highest rank position. For this offer the donor centre will be given a bonus of 50% of the dif-

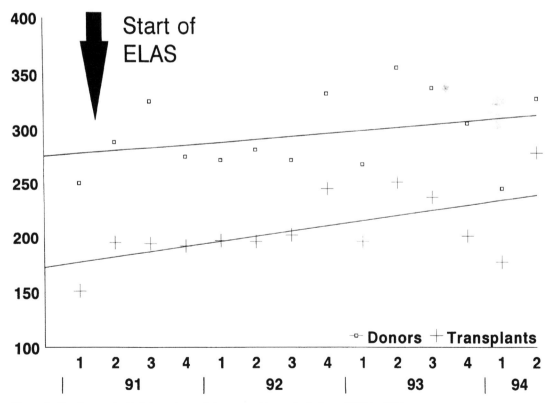

Figure 1. Development of total numbers of donors and transplants from 1991 to 1994.

ference between its own rank points and the rank points of the centre in the top rank. If the organ has to be offered obligatorily for a high urgency recipient in another centre, the bonus increases to 75% of the above mentioned difference.

4.5. High urgency registration

A patient suffering from acute graft failure and fulminant hepatic failure has to be transplanted within 3 days and has the highest priority for any suitable liver available within Eurotransplant. Every centre with a high urgency request will obtain the next liver available, irrespective of the actual position on the rank list. For this registration request special data have to be faxed to ET. After transplantation has been performed the rank points change with addition of one STEP.

4.6. Temporary cancellation and special donor requirements

A transplant centre may temporarily withdraw its registration on the rank list completely or selectively for single blood groups, e.g. for capacity problems. At registration special donor requirements, such as upper and lower weights limits, can also be incorporated. There is no penalty if a centre cancels their registration, since the actual rank points will be kept, and it will move relatively upwards on the list. Upon renewal of the registration this centre will be taken into distribution as before. Unnecessary offers to transplant programmes are thereby reduced and time is saved when making the offers. The centre can reactivate itself any time completely.

5. Results

Since the introduction of ELAS in April 1991 the number of organ donors has become stable, although slowly from 1140 in 1991 to over 1200 donors reported in 1993 [8–11]. As shown in Figure 1, the proportion of livers used increased significantly in relation to donor numbers. Table 3 shows the current numbers from 1990 to 1994. One of the most important goals of ELAS was reached: the proportion of livers not used fell from 46% in 1990 to 30% in 1993.

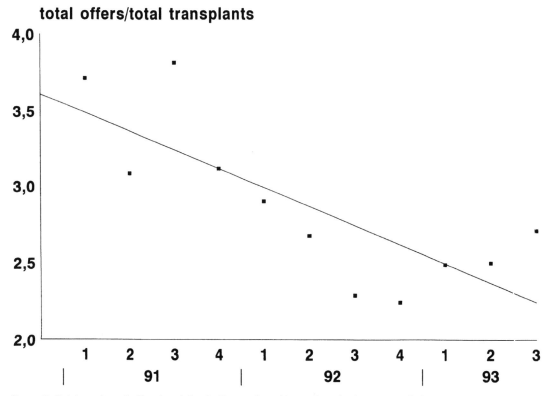

Figure 2. Total number of offers in relation to the number of transplants in the same period.

Table 3. Total number of transplants, proportion of livers not used, and reasons for refusal of a liver graft.

	1990	1991	1992	1993
Transplants (n)	599	768	765	859
Not used (%)	46	38	33	30
Reasons				
Medical	327	363	322	318
Organizational	169	79	42	33
No recipient	23	23	15	18

that the proportion of 'high urgency' requests remained stable at around 20%. The improved effectiveness of the system also shows itself in the required number of offers made before final allocation of the organ. In 1990 an average of 3.8 offers were necessary to achieve a successful transplantation or to receive a definitive refusal of a potential donor liver. Figure 2 shows the development over the last 3 years. In 1993 an average of 2.8 offers was necessary before final placement of a liver. This resulted in a reduction of two futile offers daily, allowing 700–800 transplantations per year to be performed. This clearly means less efforts in the allocation and less burden for the transplant centres. Faster allocation also improves organization in the donor hospitals. Critics of the new system, especially smaller centres, supposed that so-called 'big centres' would become dominant and others would have no possibility for expansion. In a separate evaluation the active transplant centres were divided into three groups according to the number of transplants performed in 1990. Figure 3 shows the development of these three groups with lower, medium and high activity. It is obvious that the groups with lower and medium activity were particularly able to raise

Initial numbers for 1994 confirm this trend, and the long term utilization rate is expected to reach 80%. Considering the reasons for this improvement shows that, first of all, there was a clear improvement in organization. Although 15% of donor livers were not used in 1990 with the old system, still for organizational reasons, this decreased to 3% in 1993. The percentage of medical rejection reasons remained constant. Investigations of Eurotransplant have also shown

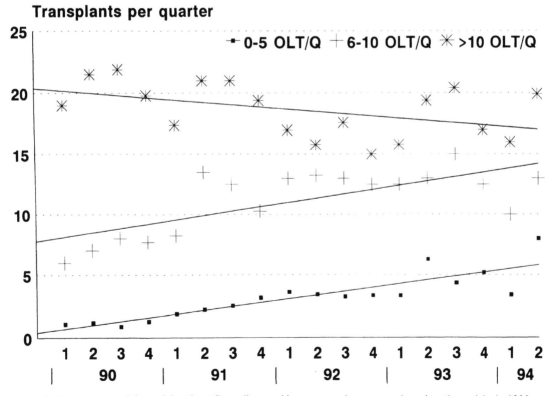

Figure 3. Development of the activity of small, medium and larger transplant centres based on the activity in 1990.

their transplant numbers. The few 'big centres' barely maintained their old level of activity. These figures also relate, however, to individual problems in some centres as well as to the increase in the total number of liver transplant centres from 19 to 27 over the last 5 years.

6. Other countries, other customs?

If one considers the development of organ transplantation in other European countries or in the USA, it becomes obvious that countries with a low number of transplant centres have no problems with allocation of organs. The Mediterranean [12] countries and Britain pursue a simple rotation system: donor livers are transplanted locally if possible, or are transferred, according to the generally valid rules, and following telephone agreement, to another centre. This principle can function, however, only with few centres and homogeneous donor and transplant activity. In France a variant of the ELAS has been used since 1992. Here, liver grafts are distributed according to similar rules; in addition a local and a regional rank list exist as well as national rank list. First, organs can be transplanted on the lowest plane; if no local transplantation is possible, the graft is distributed to the regional and later to the national list. A 'high urgency' message requires the imperative delivery of a donor liver. The donor centre is set immediately on the supreme rank position and soon receives a liver offer. The transparency is guaranteed over a PC-video-telephone-system (Minitel, BTX). Each centre is able to retrieve all allocation data.

A more complicated system underlies the allocation mode of UNOS (United Network of Organ Sharing) [12–14], and its modified variant used in Japan [15]. Here a points system has been established for many years, based mainly on the clinical status and the waiting time. The transportation of donors, transplant centre and recipients throughout the country play a larger role, as in Europe. The large number of potential recipients has, however, led to the situation that only patients with top priority can be transplanted (hospital stay, ICU).

7. Discussion

An analysis of the new liver allocation system over the last three years shows that most of the stated goals of the program were reached. The proportion of unused livers was reduced due to improvement in the organ-

ization of organ allocation. Organs were offered only to centres with a suitable recipient, taking into account the capacity (ICU, surgeons, etc.). The reasons for rejection of an offer therefore almost always only related to medical events. The slightly increased number of organ donors and transplantations, the reduction of fruitless offers, as well as the increased activity in smaller and medium centres clearly show the advantages of the new system. Persistent criticism improved the system by the subsequent integration of many 'sub-rules', which resulted in organ allocation and calculations being performed mysteriously for transplant centres. Improvement in the transparency of the organization was demanded repeatedly. Eurotransplant has accommodated many of these demands, and much of the important data relating to each centre are now available via Pioneer or the transplantation information system (TIS). These include the rank list, the blood group preview and an activity list for each centre. ELAS presents the optimal system for efficient and rapid organ allocation. The fact that each centre has the freedom to select the most urgent recipient themselves, makes possible patient-oriented organ allocation. Controversy still exists over the different indications for liver transplantation [16–18]; these cannot be solved by an allocation programme.

References

1. Bondolfi A. Allocation and fairness problems in current medicine exemplified by transplantation medicine. Z Arztl Fortbildung Jena, 1993; 87: 547–51.
2. Rhodes R. A review of ethical issues in transplantation. Mt Sinai J Med 1994; 61: 77–82.
3. Edwards BJ. Ethical considerations in organ transplantation. Semin Periop Nurs 1992; 1: 33–6.
4. Toledo-Pereyra LH. Global organ sharing: dreams and realities. Transplant Prod 1991; 23: 2697.
5. Burdick JF, Diethelm A, Thompson JS, van Buren CT, Williams GM. Organ sharing – present realities and future possibilities. Transplantation 1991; 51: 287–92.
6. Neuhaus P. A new rotary allocation system. Eurotransplant Newsl 8/90.
7. Jost U, Ringe B. Proposal for liver allocation in Eurotransplant. Eurotransplant News 2/91, 8–14.
8. Jost U, Ringe B, de Boer J, Mühlbacher F, Neuhaus P, Otter JB, Slooff M, Persijn G. Preliminary experience with a new Liver Allocation System within Eurotransplant. XIVth International Congress of the Transplantation Society, Paris 16–21 Aug. 1992 (Abstract 355) Transplant Proc 1993.
9. Jost U, Ringe B, de Boer J, Slooff M, Persijn G. Two years' critical analysis of the new Eurotransplant liver allocation system; 6th Congress of the European Society of Organ Transplantation, Rhodos, 25–28 Oct. 1993.
11. De Boer J, Slooff M, Jost U, Persijn G. Eurotransplant Liver Allocation System (ELAS): State of the Art. Eurotransplant Newsl 10/94, 119, 19–21.
12. Scheaffer MJ, Alexander DC. U.S. system for organ procurement and transplantation. Am J Hosp Pharm 1992; 49: 1733–40.

13. Ferree DM. Cadaveric organ sharing: the organ center. In: Phillips MG, (ed.) UNOS – Organ Procurement, Preservation and Distribution in Transplantation. William Byrd Press, Richmond 1991; pp. 129–44.

14. Wolf JS. The role of the United Network of Organ Sharing and designated organ procurement organizations in organ retrieval for transplantation. Arch Pathol Lab Med 1991; 115: 246–9.

15. Shimada M, Akazawa K, Morigychi S, Odaka T, Nose Y. A personal computer network system for equitable allocation of cadaver organs. Med Inform Lond 1991; 16: 199–305.

16. Sanfilippo F. Organ allocation: current problems and future issues. Transplant Proc 1993; 25: 2467.

17. Thomas DJ. Organ transplantation in people with unhealthy lifestyles. AACN Clin Issues Crit Care Nurs 1993; 4: 665–8.

18. Muto P, Freeman RB, Haug CE, Lu A, Rohrer RJ. Liver transplant candidate stratification systems. Implications for third-party payors and organ allocation. Transplantation 1994; 57: 306–8.

24 | Principles of heart allocation

AXEL HAVERICH

1. Introduction and historical background

Cardiac transplantation has emerged as an accepted mode of therapy for end stage heart failure. Patients whose life expectancy would otherwise be measured in weeks or months can be offered a form of surgical intervention that is very likely to significantly extend their life, with an exellent prospect of rehabilitation. The importance of cardiac transplantation can be seen from the rate of approximately 3000 transplants performed world-wide per year, with a total of over 27 000 such interventions being performed during the past 20 years (Fig. 1). This achievement represents the culmination of a long series of surgical experiences and innovations, a steadily increasing understanding of myocardial physiology and preservation and co-

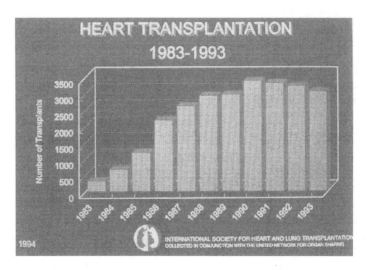

Figure 1. Annual number of heart transplantations reported to the registry of the International Society of Heart and Lung Transplantation.

G.M. Collins, J.M. Dubernard, W. Land and G.G. Persijn (eds). Procurement, Preservation and Allocation of Vascularized Organs 209–216
© 1997 Kluwer Academic Publishers.

operative progress in the fields of post-operative graft surveillance and patient care. A major impediment to the further increase of this therapeutic option has been the limitation of sufficient numbers of donor hearts world-wide and in Europe.

1.1. Historical background

The idea of cardiac replacement is very old, but the first reported cardiac transplantation occurred in 1905 when Carrel and Guthrie described a cervical hetero-topic transplant in a dog [1]. In the 1950s, the speed of advancement in cardiac surgery increased dramatic-ally, and the field of cardiac transplantation paralleled this trend. In Russia during the 1950s, Demikhov per-formed canine thoracic heterotopic transplantation and demonstrated the ability of the donor heart to sustain the animal's circulation independently [2]. The development of a reliable cardiopulmonary bypass technique in 1953 by Gibbon in Philadelphia set the stage for successful cardiac transplantation and cardio-vascular surgery in general [3,4].

In 1960, Shumway and Lower, using the technique of topical hypothermic myocardial preservation, suc-cessfully carried out orthotopic cardiac transplantation in dogs [5–7]. These studies clearly demonstrated that a denervated heart could support the recipient's cir-culation and that some anatomic reinnervation returned months after transplantation [8,9]. Other important information gained from these experiments included the recognition of hypothermia as a protective adjunct to the preservation of the donor organ. Experimentally, the donor heart could be placed in hypothermic storage for hours and still be transplanted successfully with good graft function. This observation led the way to the present system of long-range donor organ pro-curement using hypothermic transfer of the donor heart between hospitals.

The first human cardiac transplantation was carried out in 1964, when James Hardy and associates trans-planted a heart of chimpanzee into a 68-year-old man who was dying of left ventricular failure [10]. The patient succumbed, but the attempt served to focus interest on the possibility of clinical implementation and on the area of xenograft utilization, an area of regained interest today.

In December 1967, C.N. Barnard performed the first human orthotopic cardiac allograft at the Groote Schuur Hospital in Capetown, South Africa [11]. This operation attracted considerable interest, and despite the fact that the patient lived less than 3 weeks, enthus-iasm for the procedure burgeoned. During the fol-lowing year more than 100 cardiac transplantation procedures were performed at more than 60 centres, with generally poor survival results because of rejec-tion despite heavy immunosuppression. The clinical cardiac transplantation programme at Stanford Uni-versity, based on a long laboratory experience, com-menced in January 1968. This programme has been active continuously since that time, with steadily improving results. By 1985 more than 350 cardiac transplantation procedures had been performed and the 1 year survival rate exceeded 80%. Many North American and European centres have since started individual heart transplant programmes: more than 30 cardiac surgical units had embarked on this treatment within the Eurotransplant Community by 1994.

2. Selection of donor hearts

The importance of a well-functioning donor heart cannot be over-emphasized. It is clearly crucial to the success of the heart transplant procedure, particularly if orthotopic transplantation is to be performed. Early donor heart failure accounts for approximately 25% of the deaths of heart transplant patients and is, therefore, an area where significant improvements can still be made (Fig. 2). Careful selection and meticulous management of a potential donor therefore remains essential.

2.1. Donor age

As the incidence of coronary artery disease in men increases markedly after the age of 50, it has until recently been our policy to exclude men above this age from donation of hearts. For similar reasons, women over the age of 55 were also excluded. The shortage of donor hearts has become so acute, however, that we now consider hearts of both men and women up to the age of 65 years as long as echiocardiography, and basic pressure measurements, as well as inspection of the donor heart at the time of retrieval, reveal no significant disease. Many centres use donor hearts of brain-dead patients older than 55 years only in recipi-ents of approximately the same age. However, these hearts can be safely used in younger patients in an emergency, as shown by various groups [12,13]

2.2. Donor size

It is generally accepted that hearts taken from donors whose body mass is within approximately 25% of that of the potential recipient will support the circulation after orthotopic transplantation. The relative heights

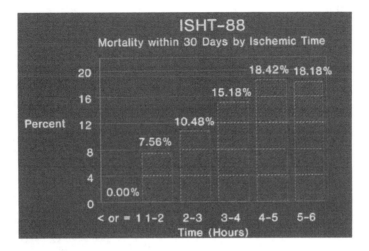

Figure 2. Perioperative mortality (30 days) after heart transplantation in relation to the ischaemic time of donor hearts.

are the measurements most easily obtained over a long distance, other measures are usually rough estimates. The muscle masses of the two subjects should also be taken into consideration in assessing the suitability of a donor heart for a specific recipient. In general, all male donors would be able to fullfil the demands of the circulation of another male subject, irrespective of his height (Fig. 3). The same holds true for female to female transplantation. Only in female to male cardiac replacement or with paediatric donors does donor size become critical in our experience. In the rare instance when a donor heart is more than 30% smaller than the recipient, heterotopic heart transplantation may be considered. The value of implanting larger donor hearts in

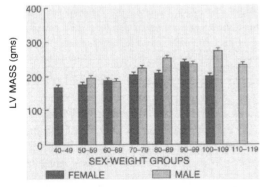

Figure 3. Left ventricular (LV) mass in relation to weight (kg) in normal male and female subjects. Except for females < 49 kg and both sexes > 100 kg, there is no significant difference in LV mass *per se* when looked at in 10 kg increments (Reproduced from reference [14].)

recipients with pulmonary hypertension has been advocated but has not been addressed by specifically designed clinical trials.

2.3. Donor blood group

ABO blood group compatibility between donor and recipient is essential. There is an estimated approximately 60% risk of early hyperacute or accelerated acute rejection in the presence of ABO incompatibility. A recent report has suggested that a recipient who receives a heart from an ABO-identical donor (e.g. O to O or A to A) will survive longer than one who receives a heart from an ABO non-identical, yet compatible, donor (e.g. O to A), though this has not been confirmed by a multicentre trial [15]. The shortage of donors is such, however, that most groups will transplant if there is ABO compatibility. Rhesus compatibility is not thought to be of importance.

2.4. Presence of lymphocytotoxic antibodies in the recipient

Whenever lymphocytotoxic (LCT) antibodies are demonstrated to be present in the recipient serum (by prior screening against a panel of lymphocytes), the result of a donor lymphocyte–recipient serum crossmatch should be obtained. In the presence of a positive crossmatch (demonstrating antibodies to be present in the recipient serum against the donor cells), the risk of hyperacute rejection of the transplanted heart is high, and that donor should not be used for that specific recipient.

2.5. Exclusion of cardiac disease

Patients with pre-existing cardiac disease are obviously unsuitable for heart donation. Severe or long-standing diabetes mellitus and hypertension may also preclude donation. The presence of a cardiac disorder can be excluded by taking, whenever possible, a clinical history from the patient's relatives or his/her own medical practitioner, by clinical examination, by study of a chest radiograph, transthoracic echiocardiography, and a 12-lead ECG. Intracranial damage itself may cause ST and T wave changes on the ECG [16,17]. Hypothermia leads to bradycardia and/or the presence of J waves, which are of no pathological significance, but which can be confused with electrocardiographic changes suggestive of ischaemia. Brain death is associated with many cardiac and haemodynamic disturbances which have recently been investigated experimentally (Sebening). Nevertheless, cardiac catheterization and angiography are rarely indicated to exclude suspected cardiac disease.

Echocardiography should be used to determine ventricular wall shortening fraction in questionable situations to give some indication of the quality of myocardial contractility. Septal motion is often paradoxical in brain-dead subjects, though the cause of this is unclear; in our experience its presence does not appear to be associated with impaired ventricular function in the post-transplant period.

Ideally, there should be no history of severe hypotension or cardiac arrest at any time. Recovery from such episodes, however, with return of an adequate blood pressure and diuresis, suggests that myocardial function remains satisfactory. Our group recently showed that previous resuscitation of the organ donor does not affect short or long term prognosis of the recipient [18].

Many cardiac surgeons believe that the most reliable means of assessing donor heart function is by direct inspection of the organ at the time of procurement, and we concur that this is a most important part of donor selection. It is therefore essential that an experienced surgeon should assess each donor heart on an individual basis. Donor heart assessment and retrieval is not a procedure that can be left to an unsupervised junior member of the surgical team.

2.6. Transferable disease

Hearts should not be transplanted from donors with transferable disease, such as a malignant lesion (other than a primary tumour of the central nervous system) or certain serious infections. The presence of pyrexia in the hours or days before death may be related to the brain injury itself, and does not necessarily indicate serious infection, although every effort must be made to exclude this possibility. Once brain death has occurred, body temperature usually falls to sub-normal levels over the course of a few hours. The length of time that the patient has been ventilated mechanically is equated with an unavoidable degree of infection, overt or otherwise; not more than 5 days is desirable, and longer than 10 days is usually unacceptable.

The presence of acute pulmonary infection certainly precludes donation of the lungs, but does not rule out heart donation. Infection in the renal tract of the donor is also not a contraindication to use of the heart. Many hearts have been transplanted successfully from donors with positive blood cultures; the decision to use a heart from such a donor is a difficult one, and not without risk but, if the infected organism is known, the recipient can be given the appropriate antibiotics. Our own policy is liberal in regard to the chance finding of a positive blood culture; if the patient has overwhelming sepsis, however, then organs should not be excised for transplantation. In any case, inspection of the donor heart valve should exclude bacterial endocarditis prior to implantation.

Positive human immunodeficiency virus (HIV) antibody serology should preclude transplantation, and whenever possible, this test should be performed before donor heart excision. A positive test should be repeated as false-positive results can occur. If the donor is believed to be at high risk for HIV positivity (e.g. homosexuals, i.v. drug abusers, haemophiliacs), but is HIV-negative, the decision on whether to use the organ must be based on the urgency of the recipient's condition, after full discussion with the patient and/or his or her family. When making such a decision, the possible risks to operating room, intensive care unit and laboratory staff must also be taken into consideration. HIV transmission by heart and kidney transplantation has been reported and the present evidence is that organs from high risk donors should not be used electively [19–22].

Blood specimens are taken for bacterial culture and serological tests for syphilis, cytomegalovirus, and hepatitis B and C surface antigens. Although the results may not be available before the organ is transplanted, they may, if positive, be of considerable importance in the subsequent care of the recipient. The presence of a positive test for venereal disease in the donor need not preclude donation, but it would seem wise to give the recipient a course of antibiotic therapy to prevent transfer of the disease. An IgM level suggestive of recent cytomegalovirus infection would not preclude use of the heart for transplantation, though many groups would not use such a donor for a heart–lung transplantation in a cytomegalovirus-negative recipient. When the presence of hepatitis B or C antigen is strongly suspected, the result of the serological investigation must be awaited; it remains our policy not to transplant organs from patients in whom a positive result is obtained. When the need of the recipient is urgent, however, a strongly positive hepatitis antibody reaction possibly should not prevent donation as long as the recipient is covered by a course of gamma globulin.

3. Preservation of donor hearts

The goal of organ preservation is to maintain the viability of an organ *ex vivo* for a period of time that will accomplish the following objectives: (1) allow transportation of the cadaveric organ to the transplant centre; (2) provide time for donor–recipient tissue matching; (3) yield good initial function following transplantation. Additionally, preservation time should be sufficient to make the surgery semi-elective, to preserve organs injured by warm ischaemia or a period of hypotension, to provide time for organ sharing between transplant centres, and in general to allow the use of all available cadaveric organs. The exact period necessary to accomplish this objective, is ideally, 48 h or more. These objectives have yet to be attained for cardiac or pulmonary transplants, and myocardial preservation research continues to hold widespread interest.

3.1. Methods of preservation

Three methods are used to preserve organ and tissues, and each is dependent upon hypothermia. These are simple cold storage after vascular flushout, continuous hypothermic perfusion and cryopreservation below 0°C. Hypothermia is only one of the essential components of successful preservation (albeit perhaps the most important); the composition of the preservation medium is also a critical determinant of preservation quality, as outlined below.

The heart has little time to regain function after preservation and transplantation and little preservation-induced damage can be tolerated. Two forms of damage can affect the viability of the heart: that due to preservation and damage that occurs during the initial period of reperfusion. Reperfusion injury may limit the viability of the heart more than preservation-induced damage. The kidney and liver may be capable of

regaining function in hours following transplantation by the resynthesis of depleted energy stores, the correction of tissue oedema, re-establishment of a normal electrolyte content in the cell and other processes of cellular repair. However, the heart requires an immediate and continuous supply of high-energy compounds, as well as an intact cell membrane to regulate the flux of calcium (Ca) that regulates myocardial contraction. Without the time necessary to repair tissue damage, the reperfused heart may continue to lose viability and fail.

Heart transplantation is a demanding process and difficult for many experimental laboratories to perform routinely and successfully. Consequently, methods to evaluate the efficacy of a preservation protocol are often judged on the basis of metabolic studies performed on isolated perfused hearts or by analysing tissue metabolism and morphological features. Although these tests are useful in evaluating the outcome of the preservation procedure, unless orthotopic transplantation is performed the succes of the preservation is questionable.

3.1.1. *Cold storage*
The method used to preserve the heart clinically is simple cold storage following cardioplegic arrest, and Baumgartner's group demonstrated in 1979 that 5–7 h of preservation by cold saline flush-out could be successful [23]. Even with the use of modern cardioplegic solutions this is still the limit of the clinical application of preservation techniques. Experimentally, hearts have been preserved in a variety of cold storage fluids, most of which are similar to Collins' solution. The cause of failure of the heart to support the circulation of the recipient is not known. In general, left ventricular function is depressed after preservation, and the heart often becomes haemorrhagic and oedematous on reperfusion. Functionally, the right ventricle appears to be much more susceptible to preservation injury than the left. This damage is characteristic of that seen after releasing the clamps from a heart that has been made ischaemic. It appears to be partially due to the limited resynthesis of ATP, influx of extracellular calcium and the inability of the reperfused heart to re-establish volume control of the heart cells.

3.1.2. *Continuous perfusion*
Many attempts have been made to obtain successful perfusion preservation of the heart. Perfusates tested include CPP, a Krebs' type of solution containing dextran, modified blood, an amino acid-containing perfusate, and a perfusate devoid of colloids but containing 130 mM glycerol. In some cases, 24 h of

successful preservation has been reported using both the orthotopic and heterotopic transplant models [24–31]. However, none of the methods evaluated experimentally is currently used clinically. Today, the vast majority of donor hearts is preserved by cardioplegic arrest followed by cold storage.

3.1.3. *Novel techniques*
In Europe, either St. Thomas's Hospital solution or Bretschneider solution are most commonly used for initial cardioplegic arrest. In recent years some groups have changed their technique and now use of the University of Wisconsin (UW) solution with equally good success. However, no clear advantages of UW solution were seen in a prospective randomized study [32]. Free oxygen radical scavengers, such as superoxide dismutase and catalase, as well as chelate ion binding substances have been evaluated in animal experiments on long-term preservation of donor hearts [33–35]. At present, these techniques have not been applied to the clinical setting of cardiac transplantation, since results have not been very convincing.

The method of 'controlled reperfusion', often used in routine cardiac operations involving either acutely ischaemic or chronically damaged myocardium, is not widely used in cardiac transplantation. There are a few reports of improved early donor heart function using this technique [36], but there does not appear to be a general acceptance of this technique.

4. Allocation of donor hearts in Europe

Historically, organ allocation (for renal transplantation) within Eurotransplant was performed according to ABO blood group compatibility, HLA matching and waiting time, in this order of preference. HLA compatibility never played a role in heart transplantation since the logistics of procurement donor hearts did not allow for matching procedures due to the time constraints. In principle, organ allocation for heart transplantation can be organized locally, within a certain

region, or on a national or international level. In addition to these geographic criteria, individual patient characteristics such as waiting time and urgency of the potential recipient are used by many allocation systems. A centre-specific (but not patient-related) rotational allocation system can also be successfully used, as demonstrated by the liver allocation system within the Eurotransplant Foundation and the current allocation procedure for cardiac allografts within UK Transplant. Thus, four basic characteristics are used for heart allocation (Table 1).

The current practice of heart allocation within the Eurotransplant Foundation takes into consideration three of the four principle characteristics: geographic criteria, patient criteria and immunologic criteria. Centre criteria are currently of no importance.

If a donor heart is offered from a hospital which is not co-operating with a heart transplant centre, it is allocated to the patient within Eurotransplant with the longest waiting time. This is done within the ABO compatibility criteria (Fig. 4). If a potential recipient is listed under an increased urgency, he will be transplanted first. Currently, three levels of urgency are pro-

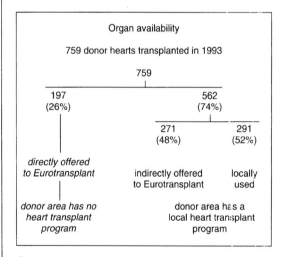

Figure 4. Availability of donor hearts and mode of allocation of organs reported to Eurotransplant in 1993.

Table 1. Principles of organ allocation.			
Geographical criteria (donor origin)	Patient criteria	Centre criteria	Immunological criteria
Local Regional National International	Waiting time Urgency Size	Size (activity)	ABO compatibility HLA matching

vided within the waiting list of Eurotransplant, along with a fourth category of not transplantable:

Transplantable
High urgency
Special urgency request

Transplantable means that the patient can be operated on according to normal criteria. High urgency is only allowed in situations of acute retransplantation, within 7 days after the initial operation. This level of urgency is under dispute, since results after acute retransplantation are definitely inferior to those following first transplant procedures. Nevertheless, the allocation committee sticks to this rule for the time being. Special urgency requests can be made by heart transplant centres on behalf of individual recipients whose cardiac function deteriorates while they are on the waiting list. To avoid abuse of this system, the total number of special urgency requests allowed for a specific centre is limited to 15% of the number of transplants performed in the previous year. New centres have allowance of two special urgency requests within their first year of activity (Fig. 5). Usually, high urgency requests and special urgency requests both result in allocation of a donor heart within 3–4 days within the Eurotransplant community. ABO blood group compatibility is still respected in this situation. A not transplantable status can be indicated temporarily (< 6 month), if transplantation is impossible due to intercurrent complications.

In order to increase donor procurement in local areas, the heart transplant committee gives the local recipient centre priority for the use of locally available donor hearts, unless there is a recipient within the Eurotransplant waiting lists at a higher degree of urgency. Currently, about 50% of donor hearts are used locally, the other 50% being allocated within the rules of Eurotransplant (Fig. 4).

This apparently complicated allocation system is felt to provide a balanced service to both the transplant centres and the individual recipients on the waiting list. Local use of donor hearts increases the transplantation activity of centres with many organ donors. Any higher urgency requirements, however, break this rule and hearts are allocated on an international basis. In future, it may be necessary to reduce local donor heart usage again, in order to maintain the number of hearts available to Eurotransplant for international allocation. With this current system in use it does not appear to be necessary to introduce a rotating system with centre criteria rather than patient criteria as the basic principle of allocation.

In summary, world-wide figures for heart transplantation are stagnating despite the increasing use of borderline organs with respect to age and size matching, functional performance and ischaemic times. Matching criteria beyond ABO blood group compatibility, such as HLA typing, have still not been introduced into the clinical practice of heart transplantation due to the time constraints of organ retrieval and long distance procurement.

In central Europe, donor hearts are allocated through Eurotransplant using three different urgency levels, transplantable, high urgency, and special urgency request. Recipient criteria such as waiting time and size still are major allocation principles, and local organ procurement is supported by the system to encourage for regional promotion of organ donation. In the future, every effort must be made to increase the number of donor hearts and to further decrease the number of potential donor hearts not transplanted for various reasons. This is thought to be achieved best by legislation indicating organ donation to be an act of humanity, but also through further information to the public as to the beneficial effects of organ transplantation as a means of prolonging life and increasing quality of life in the recipients.

Requirements for a 'SU' request

- availability of 'SU' grants
- only 1 'SU' on the list at any time (per TX type)
- registration forms
- in accordance with the eligibility criteria

HEART	HEART and LUNG
permanent hospitalization and/or stay on ICU	permanent hospitalization and/or stay on ICU
severe cardiac insufficiency despite therapy and need for inotropic support and/or IABP/ECMO	severe cardiopulmonary insufficiency despite therapy and need for permanent O_2 support and/or for mechanical ventilation
patients with a VAD are not eligible unless device-related complications	

Figure 5. Requirements for a special urgency request within Eurotransplant including current criteria in heart and heart–lung transplantation.

References

1. Carrel A, Guthrie CC. The transplantation of veins and organs. Am J Med 1905; 10: 1101.

2. Demikhov VP. Experimental transplantation of vital organs. Transl Basil Haigh (New York Consultants' Bureau) p. 126, 1962.
3. Gibbon JH Jr. Application of a mechanical heart and lung apparatus to cardiac surgery. Minn Med 1954; 37: 171.
4. Cass MH, Brock R. Heart excision and replacement. Guys Hosp Rep 1959; 108: 285.
5. Lower RR, Shumway NE. Studies on orthotopic transplantation of the canine heart. Surg Forum 1960; 11: 18.
6. Lower RR, Dong E, Shumway E. Long-term survival of cardiac homografts. Surgery 1965; 58: 110.
7. Lower RR, Dong E, Shumway E. Suppression of rejection crisis in the cardiac homograft. Ann Thorac Surg 1965; 1: 45.
8. Dong E, Hurely EJ, Lower RR, et al. Performance of the heart two years after autotransplantation. Surgery 1964; 56: 270.
9. Baumgartner WA, Reitz BA, Oyer PE et al. Cardiac transplantation. Curr Prob Surg 1979; 16: 6.
10. Hardy JD, Chavez CM, Kurrus FD et al. Heart transplantation in man: developmental studies and report of a case. JAMA 1964; 188: 1132.
11. Barnard CN. The operation S Afr Med J. 1967; 41: 1271.
12. Schüler S, Warnecke H, Loebe M, Fleck E, Hetzer R. Extended donor age in cardiac transplantation. Circulation 1989; 80 (Suppl 3): 133–9.
13. Mulvagh SL, Thorton B, Frazier HH et al. The older cardiac tranplant donor. Relation to graft function and recipient survival longer that 6 years. Circulation 1989; 80 (Suppl 3): 126–32.
14. Chan B, Fleischer K, Bergin J et al. Weight is not an accurate criterion for adult cardiac transplant size matching. Ann Thorac Surg 1991; 52: 1230–6.
15. Nakatani T, Aida H, Mearis MP, Frazier OH. Effect of ABO blood type on survival of CSA treated cardiac transplant patients. J Heart Transplant 1988; 7: 81.
16. Fentz V, Gormsen J. Electrocardiographic patterns in patients with cerebrovascular accidents. Circulation 1962; 25: 22.
17. Cooper DKC. The donor heart: present position with regard to resuscitation, storage, and assessment of viability. J Surg Res 21: 363.
18. Brandt M, Hirt S, Harringer W, Kanngiesser M, Robien N, Haverich A. Transplantation von Spenderherzen nach Reanimation – frühpostoperativer Verlauf und Ergebnisse. Transplantationsmedizin Suppl 6, 1994.
19. L'Age-Stehr J, Schwarz A, Offermann G, Langmaack H, Bennhold L, Niedrig M, Koch MA. HTLV-III infection in kidney transplant recipients. Lancet 1985; 2: 1361.
20. Prompt CA, Reis MM, Grillo FM, Kopstein J, Kreamer B, Manfro RC, Maia MH, Comiran JB. Transmission of AIDS virus at renal transplantation. Lancet 1985; 2: 672.

21. Schwarz A, Hoffmann F, L'Age-Stehr J, Tegzess AM, Offermann G. Human immunodeficiency virus transmission by organ donation. Transplantation 1987; 44: 21.
22. Rubin RH, Jenkins RL, Shaw BW, Shaffer D, Pearl RH, Erb S, Monaco AP, Van Thiel DH. The acquired immunodeficiency syndrome and transplantation. Transplantation 1987; 44: 1.
23. Baumgartner WA, Reitz BA, Oyer PE et al. Cardiac homotransplantation. Curr Probl Surg 1979; 16: 61.
24. Proctor E, Matthews G, Archibald J. Acute orthotopic transplantation of hearts stored for 72 hours. Thorax 1971; 26: 99.
25. Copeland J, Jones M, Spragg R et al. In vitro preservation of canine hearts for 24–28 hours followed by successful orthotopic transplantation. Ann Surg 1973; 178: 687.
26. Suadeau J, Kolobow T. Isolated sheep heart hypothermic (5–13°) perfusion with fresh blood. Successful preservation for 24–72 hours with continuous strong ventricular activity. Cryobiology 1977; 14: 337.
27. Suros J, Wood JE. Twenty-four hour preservation of the canine heart. J Surg Res 1974; 16: 672.
28. Toledo-Pereyra LH, Chee M, Lillehei RC. Effect of temperature upon heart preservation. Cryobiology 1978; 15: 551.
29. Watson DC. Consistent survival after prolonged donor heart preservation. Transplant Proc 1977; 9: 297.
30. Pausescu E, Mendler N, Gebhardt K et al. Exceptional performance in heart preservation with an amino acid-containing perfusion fluid. World J Surg 1978; 2: 109.
31. Cooper DYC, Wicomb WN, Rose AG et al. Orthotopic allotransplant and autotransplantation of the baboon heart following 24 hours' storage by a portable hypothermic perfusion system. Cryobiology 1983; 20: 385.
32. Demertzis S, Schäfers H-J, Wahlers T, Wippermann J, Jurmann M, Cremer J, Haverich A. Clinical myocardial preservation with the UW solution. First results in cardiac transplantation. Transplant Int 1992; 5 (Suppl. 1): 343–4.
33. Karck M, Appelbaum Y, Schwalb H, Haverich A, Chevion M, Uretzky G. TPEN, a transition metal chelator, improves myocardial protection during prolonged ischema. J Heart Lung Transplant 1992; 11: 979–85.
34. Jurmann M, Schäfers H-J, Dammenhayn L, Haverich A. Oxygen free radical scavengers for amelioration of reperfusion damage in heart transplantation. J. Thorac Cardiovasc Surg 1987; 95: 368–77.
35. Jurmann M, Dammenhayn L, Schäfers H-J, Haverich A. Pulmonary reperfusion injury: evidence for oxygen-derived free radical mediated damage and effects of different free radical scavengers. Eur J Cardiothorac Surg 1990; 4: 665–70.
36. Haverich A, Dammenhayn L, Jurmann M, Laas J, Hoppe R. The effect of controlled reperfusion in porcine hearts submitted to three hours of cold global ischemia. Transplant Int 1989; 2: 78–83.

25 | Kidney allocation in highly sensitized patients

FRANS H.J. CLAAS

1. Introduction

Among the kidney transplantation candidates highly sensitized patients form a special subgroup which is extremely difficult to transplant [1]. Highly sensitized patients have formed HLA alloantibodies against many foreign HLA antigens in response to previous pregnancies, blood transfusions or failed transplants. These antibodies are the main cause of their accumulation on the waiting lists of the different organ exchange organizations: cross-matches with almost all potential donors will be positive, and a positive cross-match is generally considered to be a contraindication to transplantation [2].

A second reason why those patients are considered to be a difficult group is the fact that graft survival in highly sensitized patients is generally inferior compared to that of non-immunized patients [3]. Many of these patients return to the waiting list after rejection of a graft which is generally associated with the formation of even more antibodies. We first provide some background information on the reasons why patients become highly sensitized, followed by a more exact definition of those highly sensitized patients, which are the most difficult to transplant. Finally, different approaches to the selection of suitable (i.e. cross-match negative) kidney donors for these patients will be discussed.

2. The hyperimmunized patient

In contrast to sensitization against the ABO blood groups, natural antibodies do not play a role in sensitization against the HLA alloantigens. Renal transplant candidates with alloantibodies will have been confronted previously with foreign HLA antigens in one way or another. The three factors which lead to sensitization of patients waiting for a renal allograft are pregnancy, blood transfusion and failed transplants [1]: it is therefore not surprising that females are predominant amongst the (highly) sensitized patients. This higher incidence of sensitization is not only a result of antibody formation against the paternal HLA antigens of the foetus during pregnancy, but multiparous women are also more likely to develop broadly reactive antibodies after blood transfusions [4,5]. Patients, who are homozygous for one of the supertypic HLA antigens (i.e. Bw4 and Bw6) are also at risk for the development of broadly reactive antibodies.

Although transplanted patients receive several immunosuppressive drugs, antibody formation is regularly observed after transplantation – especially, but not exclusively, during rejection episodes [6,7]. Indeed, patients reappearing on the waiting list for a retransplantation show a higher level of alloantibodies than those waiting for a first graft.

Although the risk factors described above can easily be determined, not every patient is equally likely to become sensitized by such contacts with HLA alloantigens [8]. This may relate either to the immunogenicity of the alloantigens or to the immune response genes in the patients, predisposing to antibody formation against foreign HLA antigens.

Several factors may contribute to the immunogenicity of blood used for transfusions, including the amount of blood given per transfusion and the number of transfusions. A very important factor is the amount of viable leucocytes in the transfusate. A systematic study on the immunogenicity of platelets both in man

G.M. Collins, J.M. Dubernard, W. Land and G.G. Persijn (eds). Procurement, Preservation and Allocation of Vascularized Organs 217–222
© 1997 Kluwer Academic Publishers.

[9] and in the mouse [10] showed that the presence of viable leucocytes in the platelet suspension is a prerequisite for the induction of alloantibodies against MHC antigens. Foreign MHC class II antigens are necessary for the activation of T-helper (TH2) cells in the recipient, which, in turn, activate B-cells which then develop into alloantibody producing plasma cells. The probability of sensitization in renal transplant patients increases with an increasing number of viable leucocytes in the transfused blood [11]. Several recent studies suggest that the immunogenicity of blood transfusions is critically dependent on the number of HLA-DR antigens shared between blood donor and recipient [12,13].

When donor and recipient differ for both HLA-DR antigens, antibodies are induced significantly more often than when donor and recipient share at least one HLA-DR antigen. Furthermore, when antibodies are formed in the latter case these are mainly of the IgM type, whereas HLA-DR-mismatched transfusions induce IgG antibodies (De Waal et al., personal communication). As the switch from IgM to IgG antibodies depends on the interaction between T-helper cells and B-cells (plasma cells), these data suggest that DR-mismatched transfusions lead to activation of T-helper cells whereas DR-matched transfusions do not. This is in line with the differential effect of blood transfusions on the cytotoxic T-cell repertoire. HLA-DR matched transfusions lead to down-regulation of the donor-specific cytotoxic T-cell repertoire [12], whereas HLA-DR-mismatched transfusions lead to priming of donor specific cytotoxic T-cells [14].

Next to the HLA class II antigens, the number of HLA class I mismatches between donor and recipient plays a determining role in whether a patient becomes sensitized. However, even when challenged with very immunogenic products, only a minority of the patients become highly sensitized. For instance HLA-DRw6-positive patients are more likely to reject an HLA-DR-mismatched graft and to develop antibodies reactive against B-cells and monocytes after graft rejection than are patients positive for other HLA-DR antigens [15]. On the other hand the HLA-DR1 antigen has been associated with low sensitization and a high degree of kidney transplant survival [16]. These data suggest that genetic factors in the recipient also play a role with respect to the level of sensitization.

2.1. What is a hyperimmunized patient?

Generally, immunization of renal transplant recipients is determined by an antibody screening against a panel of HLA-typed blood donors. The most commonly used

assay is the complement-dependent lymphocytotoxicity test. Positive reactions are observed when antibodies in the serum of the recipient are able to bind to donor cells, followed by complement activation and lysis of the target cells. Such tests for leukocyte antibodies were initiated by the observation that the presence of donor-specific leukocyte antibodies in the serum of the recipient is associated with hyperacute graft rejection [17,18]. A hyperimmunized patient is defined by the presence of serum antibodies reacting with the majority of the panel donors (i.e. within Eurotransplant with > 85% of the donors). The problem, however, is that positive reactions may be based on different antibody specificities. It is well known that antibodies directed against donor HLA class I antigens will probably result in graft rejection. However, leukocytes express many more possible target structures for antibodies, some of which are shared by kidney cells and may indeed be transplantation antigens. Others, however, are only expressed on leukocytes and antibodies against these antigens do not harm the graft. A classical example of these irrelevant antibodies are autoantibodies, which in contrast to the classical HLA antibodies, are not generally of the IgG type but of IgM type [19]. It is, therefore, helpful to distinguish a high panel reactivity due to HLA alloantibodies from a high panel reactivity due to autoantibodies.

The situation with regard to antibodies to HLA class II is less clear. Generally, these antibodies are considered to be harmless, although hyperacute rejections have been reported in individual cases, mainly involving patients with high titres of such antibodies [20]. Another aspect, and one which should be taken into consideration, is whether only antibodies present in the most recent serum of the patient are relevant or whether antibodies in historical sera should also be considered as harmful for graft survival. In the early days of cross-matching both historical and current sera were used for cross-matching. Later studies showed, however, that patients with a positive cross-match using historical sera, but with a negative cross-match using the current serum, had a similar graft survival to patients who never had donor specific antibodies [21,22]. The problem with these studies is that no information was given on the specificity and antibody class of the antibodies causing the positive historical cross-match. A few small studies looked in more detail at the relevance of positive historical sera.

The presence of IgG antibodies directed against HLA class I mismatches of the donor was associated with poor graft survival [23,24]. When HLA class I antibodies were of the IgM type, graft survival was acceptable. As mentioned above, the absence of a switch from IgM to IgG antibodies suggests that no T cell activation took place, which is probably the reason why these positive historical cross-matches are not harmful. Recent experiments support the reasoning that it is not the antibodies themselves, but the fact that the formation of IgG antibodies is associated with priming of donor-specific helper and cytotoxic T-lymphocytes that explains why graft survival is poor in patients with a positive historical cross-match due to IgG antibodies [25]. When the historical antibodies are autoantibodies or are directed against HLA class II, generally a good graft survival is observed.

Taking all these facts into consideration, a hypersensitized patient should preferentially be defined as a patient with IgG antibodies directed against the HLA class I antigens of more than 85% of the panel donors. These antibodies may be present in current and/or historical sera. Therefore it is essential to determine beforehand, the specificity and immunoglobulin class of the antibodies causing the high panel reactivity. In patients with autoantibodies a crossmatch in the absence and presence of the reducing agent DTT (dithiothreitol) should be performed. If the crossmatch is positive without DTT but becomes negative in the presence of DTT, transplantation can be performed without any need for further special allocation strategies [26]. Only patients, who are hyperimmunized and have a high panel reactivity due to HLA alloantibodies of IgG type, are dependent on special treatments and/or allocation systems in order to be transplanted within a reasonable time with a crossmatch negative donor.

3. Strategies to increase the chance of finding a suitable donor for highly sensitized patients

The main problem for highly sensitized patients is the fact that they have made antibodies against almost all foreign HLA antigens. The serological cross-match with almost all donors will be positive, which excludes them from transplantation. In principle, two different kinds of strategies can be applied. Either one accepts that the patient has so many antibodies and tries to develop sophisticated ways to find a cross-match-negative donor, or one aims to remove the harmful antibodies. With respect to the latter, cyclophosphamide treatment in combination with plasma exchange has been effective in a number of highly sensitized patients [27]. However, this treatment is

rather aggressive, often resulting in infectious complications and even death in some patients.

A more common approach to remove the HLA antibodies is the use of extracorporeal immunoadsorption (IA) by *Staphylococcus* protein A columns [28–30]. Although these columns are effective in removal of antibodies, the treatment is often followed by high levels of *de novo* resynthesis of anti-HLA antibodies. IA is, therefore, usually performed in combination with immunosuppressive treatment in order to prevent resynthesis of antibodies. Nevertheless, variable effects of IA on antibody removal are obtained. Resynthesis of antibodies is not always prevented by this treatment [30,31] and some HLA antibodies, especially of the IgG3 class, are poorly absorbed by protein A. The use of protein G for IA is suggested to be more effective in removing all anti-HLA IgG antibodies [32]. Once the antibodies have been successfully removed, variable results are also reported with respect to graft survival. Several groups show that this approach is useful to remove the antibodies and successfully transplant the patients [28,29,33]. On the other hand, and particularly when transplants are performed in the presence of positive historical cross-matches, a large number of failures have been reported [30,31]. This may be due to the fact that antibody formation is accompanied by the activation of cytotoxic T-cells against the same HLA mismatches [25]. When only the antibodies are removed, the remaining primed cytotoxic T-cells may be responsible for the high incidence of rejection. Prophylactic treatment with anti-T-cell reagents (i.e. ATG, OKT3) may be helpful in mitigating this detrimental effect of these primed T-cells.

If one accepts that a patient is highly sensitized, the only way to transplant the patient is to find a cross-match-negative donor. The obvious solution is, of course, transplantation with an HLA-identical or compatible donor but the chance of finding such a donor is often very low due to the extensive polymorphism of the HLA system. Other schemes involve the distribution of the sera from these patients to many different tissue typing laboratories. The cells of every ABO-compatible donor are tested in a serological cross-match and donor–recipient combinations with negative cross-matches are identified by trial and error [34,35]. Originally HLA class II matching was not involved in these schemes. Currently, HLA-DR matched combinations are preferentially transplanted as matching for HLA-DR was found to improve graft survival significantly in these highly sensitized patients [36,37]. The introduction of these schemes has indeed contributed to a shorter waiting time and acceptable graft survival in hyperimmunized patients.

Another approach, which is based on extensive anti-body specificity analysis, is the determination of acceptable mismatches. Patient sera are routinely screened in complement-dependent cytotoxicity against panels of HLA-typed blood donors. If these panels are large enough, one can determine the specificities of HLA alloantigens toward which the patient did not form antibodies by looking carefully at the HLA typings of the cross-match-negative panel donors. Knowledge of these acceptable HLA antigens (or epitopes shared amongst different antigens) can be used for the selection of future organ donors [38,39].

The acceptable mismatch programme, which is used within the Eurotransplant area, is based on this principle. The protocol is based on earlier data obtained within Eurotransplant which show that, in the case of a negative cross-match with both current and historical sera, HLA-A and -B mismatches are less important for graft survival in highly sensitized patients, whereas matching for HLA-DR has a significant influence, especially in retransplantation [40]. The aim of the acceptable mismatch programme is an exact definition of those HLA-A and -B incompatibilities which will not result in a positive cross-match. Therefore, the sera from highly immunized patients are screened against a panel of lymphocyte donors, who are selected on the basis of having only one HLA-A or -B mismatch with the specific patient (Table 1).

Using this approach HLA-A and/or -B antigens towards which the patient has not developed antibodies can be detected. Kidney donor selection takes place by inputting the HLA-A, -B and -DR antigens of every potential donor into the central computer, which then selects cross-match-negative recipients on the basis of the patients' own HLA-A, -B and -DR antigens in combination with the acceptable HLA-A and -B mismatches [41]. In this way the donor is always matched for HLA-DR (either identical or compatible) but may have several HLA-A and -B mismatches. The sera from more than 300 highly sensitized patients have been tested so far for the absence of specific allo-

antibodies against HLA-A and -B antigens using such patient-specific panels. All these patients showed anti-body reactivity against > 85% of the panel donors in complement-dependent lymphocytotoxicity. This anti-body reactivity was due to multispecific alloantibodies to HLA class I antigens; autoantibodies were excluded. In patients with < 100% panel reactivity a first indica-tion concerning these acceptable HLA-A and -B mis-matches was deduced from the HLA antigens of the negative panel donors in the screening. Nevertheless, patients with 100% panel reactivity were also found to have acceptable mismatches, which, due to the com-position of the panel, were not detectable in the standard screening. A panel of lymphocyte donors with only one HLA-A or -B mismatch with the specific patient, however, will reveal these 'holes' in the antibody reper-toire of the highly immunized patient. In 90% of the patients it was possible to define such acceptable mismatches using such patient-specific panels.

Even HLA antigens with a high phenotype fre-quency, such as HLA-A1 and HLA-A3, were found to be acceptable in some patients. Addition of the accept-able HLA-A and -B antigens to the patient's own HLA-A, -B and -DR antigens with respect to kidney donor selection will increase the chance of finding a cross-match-negative donor significantly (Table 2). Over 200 of these patients have been transplanted fol-lowing this scheme with a 1 year graft survival of > 80%. Some of these patients had been waiting for 10 years for an HLA-compatible graft. Of the patients transplanted the mean waiting time between inclusion in the acceptable mismatch programme and transplantation was about 6 months [42].

We conclude that the determination of acceptable HLA-A and -B mismatches contributes to a significant

Table 2. Consequences of acceptable mismatches for kidney donor selection.

Patient: A1 A2 B7 B8 DR2 DR3   100% panel reactivity

Acceptable mismatches: A3 B35

DR compatible donors, who will be selected on the basis of their acceptable mismatches

A1 A3 B7 B8	A2 A2 B35 B35	A3 A3 B35 B35
A2 A3 B7 B8	A2 A3 B7 B35	A3 A3 B7 B7
A3 A3 B7 B8	A2 A3 B8 B35	A3 A3 B8 B8
A1 A2 B7 B35	A1 A3 B7 B35	A1 A3 B35 B35
A1 A2 B8 B35	A1 A3 B8 B35	A1 A3 B7 B7
A1 A2 B35 B35	A3 A3 B7 B35	A1 A3 B8 B8
A1 A1 B35 B35	A3 A3 B8 B35	A2 A3 B35 B35
A2 A3 B8 B8	A2 A3 B7 B7	

Table 1. Principle of detection of acceptable HLA-A and/or -B mismatches in highly sensitized patients.

HLA-type of the patient: A1 A2 B7 B8

Selected panel donors	Cross-match with patient sera
A1 A2 B7 B44	+
A1 A2 B2 B35	–
A1 A2 B7 B60	+
A1 A3 B7 B8	–

Acceptable mismatches: A3 and B35

increase of the potential donor pool for highly immunized patients. Based on laboratory work, which is performed beforehand in the recipient centre, a central organ-sharing office can select all HLA-DR-compatible kidney donors who will give a negative cross-match with all sera from a given a highly immunized patient.

This approach has several advantages compared with other schemes to select cross-match negative donors for highly sensitized patients. First, there is no need for distribution of patient sera to other tissue typing centres; second, instead of performing cross-matches with all donors, most of which will be positive, selection is based on a predictable negative cross-match; finally, selection of potential donors is based on data of the recipient centre, which has all information concerning the immunological background (transfusion, specific alloantibodies, autoantibodies etc.) of the patient and not on a negative cross-match in another tissue typing centre. A disadvantage of the scheme might be that the amount of laboratory work is considerable.

The finding that in about 50% of the highly immunized patients the acceptable mismatches include HLA-A and/or -B antigens of the mother of the patient, which have not been inherited by the patient, is certainly helpful in the search for acceptable HLA-A and -B antigens [43].

The good survival of patients transplanted with the help of the acceptable mismatch programme is in line with observations of Maruya et al. [44], who demonstrated that in the total patient population (sensitized and non-sensitized) certain HLA mismatches seem not to be recognized by the immune system of the recipient. Mismatches for these so-called 'permissible mismatches' lead to a significantly better graft survival than other (non-permissible) mismatches. Future studies should reveal whether acceptable mismatches (non-responsiveness on the level of antibody formation) are related to permissible mismatches (non-responsiveness on the level of graft survival). Once we know the rules and mechanisms underlying why some HLA mismatches (or HLA epitopes) lead to immune reactivity and others do not, organ allocation programmes for both sensitized and non-sensitized patients will have the possibility of finding an optimal donor for far more recipients than is presently the case.

References

1. Gore SM, Bradley BA (eds). Renal Transplantation: Sense and Sensitization. Kluwer Academic Publishers, Dordrecht, 1988.
2. Scornik SC, Brunson ME, Howard RS, Pfaff WK. Alloimmunization, memory, and the interpretation of crossmatch results for renal transplantation. Transplantation 1992; 54: 389–96.
3. Opelz G. Kidney transplantation in sensitized patients. Transplant Proc 1987; 19: 3737–41.
4. Sirchia G, Scalamogna M, Mercurial F. Evaluation of the blood transfusion policy of the North Italy Transplant Programme. Transplantation 1981; 31: 388–94.
5. Opelz G, Graver B, Mickey MR. Lymphocytotoxic antibody responses to transfusions in potential kidney recipients. Transplantation 1981; 32: 177–82.
6. Suciu Foca N, Reed E, D'agati V, Ho E, Cohen DJ, Benenisty AI, MacCabe R, Brensilver JM, King DW, Hardy MA. Soluble HLA antigens, anti-HLA antibodies and anti-idiotypic antibodies in the circulation of renal transplant recipients. Transplantation 1991; 51: 593–601.
7. Park MS, Terasaki PI, Lau M, Iwaki Y. Sensitization after transplantation. Clin Transplant 1987: 393–7.
8. Sanfilippo F, Vaughn WK, Bollinger RR, Spees EK. Comparative effects of pregnancy, transfusion and prior graft rejection on sensitization and renal transplant results. Transplantation 1982; 34: 360–7.
9. Eernisse JG, Brand A. Prevention of platelet refractoriness due to HLA-antibodies by administration of leukocyte poor blood components. Exp Haematol 1981; 9: 77–83.
10. Claas FHJ, Smeenk RJT, Smidt R, Eernisse JG. Alloimmunization against the MHC antigens after platelet transfusions is due to contaminating leucocytes in the platelet suspension. Exp Haematol 1981; 9: 84–9.
11. Martin SM, Dyer PA, Harris R. Successful renal transplantation of patients sensitized following deliberate unrelated blood transfusions. Transplantation 1985; 39: 256–61.
12. Van Twuyver E, Mooijaart RJD, Ten Berge RJM, Van der Horst AR, Wilmink JM, Kast WM, Melief CJM, De Waal LP. Pretransplant blood transfusion revisited. N Engl J Med 1991; 325: 1210–13.
13. Lagaaij EL, Henneman IPH, Ruigrok MB, De Haan MW, Persijn GG, Termijtelen A, Hendriks GFJ, Weimar W, Claas FHJ, Van Rood JJ. Effect of one HLA-DR antigen matched and completely HLA-DR mismatched blood transfusions on survival of heart and kidney allografts. N Engl J Med 1989; 321: 701–5.
14. Van Twuyver E, Mooijaart RJD, Ten Berge RJM, Van der Horst AR, Wilmink JR, Claas FHJ, De Waal LP. High affinity cytotoxic T lymphocytes after non-HLA sharing blood transfusion, the other side of the coin. Transplantation 1994; 57: 1246–51.
15. Hendriks GFJ, Schreuder GMTh, Claas FHJ, D'Amaro J, Persijn GG, Cohen B, Van Rood JJ. HLA-DRw6 and renal allograft rejection. Br Med J 1983; 286: 85–7.
16. Cooke DJ, Cecka M, Terasaki PI. HLA-DR1 recipient have the highest kidney transplant survival. Transplant Proc 1987; 19: 675–7.
17. Kissmeyer-Nielsen F, Olsen S, Peterson BP, Fjedborg O. Hyperacute rejection of kidney allografts associated with pre-existing humoral antibodies against donor cells. Lancet 1966; 2: 662–5.
18. Patel R, Terasaki PI. Significance of the positive crossmatch test in kidney transplantation. New Engl J Med 1969; 280: 735–9.
19. Chapman JR, Taylor CJ, Ting A, Morris PJ. Immunoglobulin class and specificity of antibodies causing positive T cell crossmatches. Relationship to renal transplant outcome. Transplantation 1986; 42: 608–13.
20. Scornik JC, LeFor WM, Ciciarelli JC et al. Hyperacute and acute kidney graft rejection due to antibodies against B cells. Transplantation 1992; 54: 61–6.
21. Cardella CJ, Falk JA, Nicholson MJ, Harding MJ, Cook GT. Successful renal transplantation in patients with T cell reactivity to donor. Lancet 1982; 2: 1240–2.
22. Norman DJ, Barry JM, Wetzsteon PJ. Successful cadaver kidney transplantation in patients highly sensitized by blood transfusions. Unimportance of the most reactive serum in the pretransplant crossmatch. Transplantation 1985; 39: 253–5.

23. Taylor CJ, Chapman JR, Ting A, Morris PJ. Characterization of lymphocytotoxic antibodies causing a positive crossmatch in renal transplantation. Transplantation 1989; 48: 953–8.

24. Ten Hoor GM, Coopmans M, Allebes WA. Specificity and Ig class of preformed alloantibodies causing a positive crossmatch in renal transplantation. Transplantation 1993; 56: 298–305.

25. Roelen DL, Van Bree FPMJ, Ten Hoor GM, Hoitsma A, Van Rood JJ, Allebes WA, Claas FHJ. Activated HLA class I reactive T lymphocytes associated with a positive historical crossmatch predict early graft rejection. In: Thesis DL. Roelen (University of Leiden): 1994; 99–110.

26. Vaidya S, Ruth J. Contributions and clinical significance of IgM and autoantibodies in highly sensitized renal allograft recipients. Transplantation 1989; 47: 956–8.

27. Taube DH, Williams DG, Cameron JS, Bewick M, Ogg CS, Rudge CJ, Welsh KI, Kennedy LA, Thick MG. Renal transplantation after removal and prevention of resynthesis of HLA antibodies. Lancet 1984; 1: 824–8.

28. Palmer A, Taube D, Welsh K, Bewick M, Gjorstrup P, Thick M. Removal of anti-HLA antibodies by extracorporeal immunoadsorption to enable renal transplantation. Lancet 1989; 1: 10–20.

29. Hakim RM, Milford E, Himmelfarb J, Wingard R, Lazarus JM, Watt RM. Extracorporeal removal of anti-HLA antibodies in transplant candidates. American J Kidney Dis 1990; 16: 423–31.

30. Kupin WL, Venkat KK, Hayashi H, Mozes MF, Oh HK, Watt R. Removal of lymphocytotoxic antibodies by pretransplant immunoadsorption therapy in highly sensitized renal transplant recipients. Transplantation 1991; 51: 324–9.

31. Hiesse C, Kriaa F, Rousseau P, Farahmand H, Bismuth A, Fries D, Charpentier B. Immunoadsorption of anti-HLA antibodies for highly sensitized patients awaiting renal transplantation. Transplantation 1992; 7: 944–51.

32. Barocci S, Nocera A. In vitro removal of anti-HLA IgG antibodies from highly sensitized transplant recipients by immunoadsorption with protein A and protein G sepharose columns: a comparison. Transplant Int 1993; 6: 29–33.

33. Ross CN, Gaskin G, Gregor-Macgregor S, Patel AA, Davey NJ, Lechler RI, Williams G, Rees AJ, Pusey CD. Renal transplantation following immunoadsorption in highly sensitized recipients. Transplantation 1993; 55: 785–9.

34. Schäfer AJ, Hasert K, Opelz G. Collaborative transplant study crossmatch and antibody project. Transplant Proc 1985; 17: 2469–71.

35. Bradley BA, Klouda PT, Ray TC, Gore SM. Negative crossmatch selection of kidneys for highly sensitized patients. Transplant Proc 1985; 17: 2465–6.

36. Klouda PT, Corbin SA, Ray TC, Rogers CA, Bradley BA. Renal transplantation in highly sensitized patients: five years of the SOS scheme. Clin Transplant 1990; 69–73.

37. Opelz G. Collaborative transplant study kidney exchange trial for highly sensitized recipients. Clin Transplant 1991; 61–4.

38. Oldfather JW, Anderson CB, Phelan DL, Cross DE, Luger AM, Rodey GE. Prediction of crossmatch outcome in highly sensitized dialysis patients based on the identification of serum HLA antibodies. Transplantation 1986; 42: 267–70.

39. Duquesnoy RJ, White LT, Fierst JW, Vanek M, Banner BF, Iwaki Y, Starzl TE. Multiscreen serum analysis of highly sensitized renal dialysis patients for antibodies toward public and private class I HLA determinants. Implications for computer-predicted acceptable and unacceptable donor mismatches in kidney transplantation. Transplantation 1990; 50: 427–37.

40. Hendriks GFJ, De Lange P, D'Amaro J, Schreuder GMTh, Claas FHJ, Persijn GG, Cohen B, Van Rood JJ. Eurotransplant experience with highly immunized patients. Scand J Urol Nephrol 1985; 92: 81–6.

41. Claas FH, Gijbels Y, Van Veen A, De Waal LP, D'Amaro J, Persijn GG, Van Rood JJ. Selection of cross-match negative HLA-A and/or -B mismatched donors for highly sensitized patients. Transplant Proc 1989; 21: 665–6.

42. Claas FH, De Waal LP, Beelen J, Reekers P, Berg-Loonen PV, De Gast E, D'Amaro J, Persijn GG, Zantvoort F, Van Rood JJ. Transplantation of highly sensitized patients on the basis of acceptable HLA-A and -B mismatches. Clin Transplant 1989; 185–90.

43. Claas FHJ, Gijbels Y, Van der Velde-de Munck J, Van Rood JJ. Induction of B cell unresponsiveness to noninherited maternal HLA antigens during fetal life. Science 1988; 241: 1815–17.

44. Maruya E, Takemoto S, Terasaki PI. HLA matching: identification of permissible mismatches. Clin Transplant 1993; 511–20.

26 | Principles of lung allocation

KEITH MCNEIL AND JOHN WALLWORK

1. Introduction

Lung transplantation is now an established therapeutic option for patients with a variety of advanced cardiopulmonary disorders, with resulting improvements in survival and quality of life. Currently the number of transplants performed is limited by the availability of donor organs. The United Kingdom Transplant Support Service Authority figures for 1995 showed a total of 171 heart–lung and lung transplants performed, with 253 patients still awaiting transplantation at that time. Thus the number of potential recipients far exceeds the number of organs which become available, and an active donor organ allocation process must therefore occur.

The allocation of a donor lung block is based first on the selection of a recipient with a disease process and stage appropriately treated by a lung transplant, and second on the matching of donor and recipient on the basis of total lung capacities, ABO blood group and cytomegalovirus infection status. If two or more potential recipients satisfy these criteria, allocation will necessarily depend on largely subjective answers to questions such as whether the sickest patients are transplanted first, or whether patients with the best chance of a successful outcome are preferred? Should younger patients take priority over older patients or should those who have been waiting longest have preference? These questions raise complex social, moral and ethical issues which must be addressed if donated organs are to be allocated fairly, consistently and equitably while still ensuring that the maximum benefits are achieved.

2. General recipient criteria

Lung transplantation is generally considered for patients with limited survival prospects. There are exceptions to this general rule, with some patients considered on the basis of their symptoms, as it has been shown that an early and sustained improvement in their quality of life can be expected following lung transplantation [1]. Most patients, however, are considered when their life expectancy is less than 2 years. It is important to consider potential recipients before their disease is so advanced that malnutrition and other organ dysfunction results, with a consequent increase in the incidence of post-operative morbidity and mortality.

The diseases amenable to treatment with a lung transplant are now well established. Table 1 lists the indications for lung transplants performed at Papworth Hospital from 1984 to 1996. Although some debate continues over the place of single lung transplantation in bullous emphysema and pulmonary hypertension, in general, agreement exists over the major indications. Contraindications are likewise well established [2,3] but with increasing experience most are now relative rather than absolute.

G.M. Collins, J.M. Dubernard, W. Land and G.G. Persijn (eds). Procurement, Preservation and Allocation of Vascularized Organs 223–226
© 1997 Kluwer Academic Publishers.

Table 1. Major indications for lung transplantation, Papworth Hospital 1984–1996.

Heart–lung transplantation

Cystic fibrosis	138
Eisenmenger's syndrome	58
Primary pulmonary hypertension	43
Emphysema	27
Bronchiectasis	31
Fibrosing alveolitis/pulmonary fibrosis	20
Sarcoidosis	5
Thromboembolic pulmonary hypertension	6
Other	23
Total	351

Double lung transplantation

Bronchiectasis	9
Emphysema	7
Cystic fibrosis	6
Total	22

Single lung transplantation

Emphysema	71
Fibrosing alveolitis/pulmonary fibrosis	33
Sarcoidosis	5
Other	14
Total	123

3. Allocation of the donated lung

When a donor organ becomes available a recipient is selected from the waiting list constructed according to the above principles. The initial allocation of the donor lungs involves a matching of donor/recipient total lung capacity, ABO blood group and cytomegalovirus infection status (as determined by serology).

3.1. Total lung capacity (TLC)

All potential recipients have their TLC measured at assessment by body plethysmography. The donor's TLC is predicted according to the following equations:

males: $TLC = (7.8 \times \text{height in metres}) - 7.3$
females: $TLC = (7.46 \times \text{height in metres}) - (0.013 \times \text{age}) - 6.42$

The predicted donor TLC will usually be matched to a recipient with either the same or a slightly larger (up to 10%) measured TLC. Allocating donor lungs to recipients with a smaller TLC is avoided because of the potential for developing post-operative atelectasis.

3.2. ABO blood group

Donors and recipients are matched according to their ABO blood group status. Rhesus factor and minor blood group matching is not required. Potential recipients are also screened for preformed antibodies against a random panel of 'donor' lymphocytes. On the basis of this result, a prospective donor-specific lymphocyte cross-match may be necessary prior to the final allocation of the donor lungs.

3.3. Cytomegalovirus (CMV) infection status

All donors and recipients are tested serologically to determine their CMV status. Mismatching (allocating organs from a CMV-positive donor to a CMV-negative recipient) is avoided because of the significant morbidity and mortality associated with primary post-transplant CMV pneumonitis. The role of CMV prophylaxis (ganciclovir or hyperimmune globulin) has not been established in respect of lung transplantation but is currently under trial. The results from other solid organ transplant programs should not be extrapolated to lungs at this stage.

After matching these three criteria, one or more potential recipients may be deemed suitable to be allocated a particular set of donor lungs. If only one recipient fulfils the matching criteria, allocation of the donor lungs is straightforward. However, where two or more potential recipients are suitable, allocation will depend on less objective criteria which include:

(1) need for a transplant in terms of survival – should the sickest patients be transplanted first even though they are at higher risk of significant morbidity and mortality?
(2) prediction of the likely outcome – should patients with the best chance of a good outcome be preferred to those at higher risk of morbidity and mortality?
(3) status of the donor organs – should the 'best' organs be allocated to the patients with the best chance of a good outcome, thus maximizing the likely benefits of this scarce resource?
(4) maximizing the number of recipients transplanted from each donor – a heart–lung block can be potentially used for one heart–lung recipient or split to provide two single lungs and one heart for transplantation, thus benefiting 3 recipients.

Other questions to be considered include: whether younger patients have priority over older patients, and whether the length of time spent on the waiting list is a factor to be considered?

3.4. Allocation according to need

A recent study of survival after acceptance for heart–lung transplantation showed the underlying diagnosis to be the only factor significantly associated with survival on the waiting list [4]. Patients with Eisenmenger's syndrome had a significantly longer survival than all other diagnostic groups. Patients with fibrosing alveolitis had a slightly shorter survival, although this was only a small group. Patients with Eisenmenger's syndrome – who are often transplanted on the basis of quality of life rather than survival – were transplanted at a slower rate, reflecting the need of the other diagnostic groups for transplantation, to improve their survival.

Although there exists the general principle that sicker patients are given priority in respect of the provision of medical care, they may not always be the best candidates for transplantation because of factors such as malnutrition, cachexia and other organ dysfunction [3,5]. Such patients are ill-equipped to cope with the physical stress of a lung transplant and are at greater risk of significant morbidity and mortality arising from factors such as poor wound healing, impaired ventilation and cough secondary to respiratory muscle weakness, and an increased susceptibility to infection.

3.5. Allocation according to likely outcome

Consideration of the likely short and long term outcomes following transplantation is based on the principle of maximizing the benefits from organ donation. The principle of sicker patients being given priority assumes that eventually every patient will receive treatment. This is, however, not the case with lung transplantation: a significant number of patients die on the waiting list as a direct result of the shortage of donor lungs [4]. In effect, a triage decision may be necessary when allocating a donor lung, with patients clearly at higher risk of significant morbidity and mortality passed over in favour of those likely to have a more favourable outcome.

Successful transplantation depends not only on favourable physical factors but also on stable psychosocial, behavioural and economic circumstances [5,6]. Once transplanted, the patient must be willing and able to comply with a complicated medication regimen, and attend for frequent follow-up often involving repeated invasive procedures. It is difficult to find objective parameters when assessing such factors; however, they must be considered and evaluated not only at the initial assessment but also prior to the definitive allocation of the donor lungs.

3.6. Allocation according to the status of the donor organs

For a number of reasons, some donor organs will be 'better' than others. This judgement will reflect factors such as the prior health and fitness of the donor, the quality of the donor's care prior to organ procurement, donor organ ischaemic time and preservation techniques. Although the logistics of the transplant procedure dictate that the latter factors are unlikely to figure in any decision regarding allocation, the first factor certainly may. Should the 'best' organs be allocated to those recipients likely to use them to their maximum capacity? There can be no dogmatic answer, but this question may need to be considered during the allocation process.

3.7. Maximizing the use of available donors

A heart–lung transplant is the least efficient use of a thoracic organ donor as only one recipient will benefit. Potentially however, one heart–lung block could provide two single lungs and one heart for transplantation, thus benefiting three recipients. There will always be patients who require replacement of both the heart and lungs, but in some cases additional strategies may be available to improve donor organ supply. The domino heart transplant utilizes the heart from a heart–lung transplant recipient for a patient requiring heart transplantation. In this case two recipients benefit from a heart–lung transplant procedure. In some cases of Eisenmenger's syndrome it may be possible to surgically correct the heart defect and treat the associated pulmonary hypertension with a single lung transplant. Finally, the issue of living-related lobe transplantation is currently being explored, again as a means of expanding the donor pool. These alternatives should be considered for suitable patients on the waiting list to ensure that available donor organs are used in the most efficient manner.

3.8. Allocation according to age

Lung transplantation has been successfully extended to older patients, with a consequent increase in the size of the potential recipient pool and most units set an age limit for considering patients for a lung transplant. Increasingly, however, older patients are competing with younger patients for donor organs. The long term outcome in terms of functional recovery in the older age groups is not clear [3]. Co-existing disorders associated with advancing age, such as osteoporosis, renal impairment, atherosclerosis, not only prolong postoperative recovery and hospitalization but are likely to limit the benefits of transplantation, and as stated previously, maximizing benefits is a prime objective determining the allocation of donor lungs. As life expectancy following a lung transplant is limited, it may be that the older more mature patient can utilize the benefits conferred equally or even more effectively than an adolescent patient. In this respect we may mitigate against older patients because of our own emotions and expectations rather than evaluating each situation on an individual basis.

3.9. Time on the waiting list

This factor is unlikely to figure significantly in allocating donor lungs, as in general the previous arguments will take precedence. If however all other factors are equal, then waiting time may influence the final decision.

In the final analysis, the allocation of donor lungs involves a combination of science and economics, sociology and psychology, and common sense. We cannot separate the arguments for need or projected outcome from a consideration of the complex psychosocial issues involved. Any allocation process must therefore take into account not only the needs of individual patients but must also recognize the attendant responsibility of ensuring that each set of donor organs is allocated with the expectation that the maximum benefit will result from the final decision.

References

1. Caine N, Sharples LD, Smyth R, Scott J, Hathaway T, Higenbottam TW, Wallwork J. Survival and quality of life of cystic fibrosis patients before and after heart–lung Transplantation. Transplant Proc 1991; 23: 1203–4.
2. Wallwork J. Indications for operation, patient selection and assessment. In: Wallwork J (ed.), Heart and Heart–lung Transplantation. WB Saunders Co. Philadelphia 1989; pp. 449–62.
3. Mitchell AG. Indications, selection and management of the recipient. In: Cooper DKC, Novitsky D (eds), The Transplantation and Replacement of Thoracic Organs. Kluwer Academic Publishers, Lancaster 1990; pp. 267–72.
4. Sharples LD, Belcher C, Dennis CM, Higenbottam T Wallwork J. Who waits longest for heart and lung transplantation? J Heart Lung Transplant 1994; 13: 282–91.
5. Vagelos R, Fowler MB. Selection of patients for cardiac Transplantation. Cardiol Clin 1990; 8: 23–38.
6. Higenbottam T, Otulana BA, Wallwork J. Transplantation of the lung. Eur Respir J 1990; 3: 594–605.

27 | Organization and logistics in organ exchange

B. Haase-Kromwijk, J.M.J. De Meester and G.G. Persijn

1. Introduction

Organ transplantation is considered as the logical treatment for patients with end stage organ failure. Organs for transplantation may be obtained either from living or post-mortem donors. The organization of these two types of donation is quite different, mainly due to the fact that living donation is restricted to the narrow circle of recipient, donor and physician, in contrast to post-mortem organ donation which has rapidly evolved to a much broader environment with intense international cooperation.

This chapter outlines the infrastructure required to coordinate, beyond the local donor hospitals and transplant programmes, post-mortem organ donation, allocation and transplantation: the so-called organ exchange organization.

2. Organizational aspects

The need to organize post-mortem donation and organ allocation on a large scale is directly proportional to the number and/or the organ type of transplant programmes located in a particular geographical area.

National public health structures and services should be able to establish and maintain post-mortem organ transplant programmes, and hospitals should be equipped with intensive care facilities and be able to cooperate as sources of cadaveric donor organs with nearby transplant programmes. The inability to achieve this type of system explains the rarity of post-mortem organ transplant programmes in many countries in Latin America, Africa, South-East Asia and South-West Asia. If transplantation is to be performed in these areas, more interest is shown in the use of living related and unrelated (kidney) donors, for which screening for suitable donors, time point of explanation and transplantation, etc. can be organized more easily in a single hospital.

The legal acceptance of the 'brain death' concept, i.e. the total and irreversible loss of brain functions, to determine the death of a person, as an alternative to the more classical concept of 'absence of cardiac activity and cessation of respiration', is crucial to the development of transplant programmes. This concerns, in particular, the non-renal organs: successful transplantation

G.M. Collins, J.M. Dubernard, W. Land and G.G. Persijn (eds). Procurement, Preservation and Allocation of Vascularized Organs 227–232
© 1997 Kluwer Academic Publishers.

of heart, lung, liver and pancreas is simply not possible following circulatory arrest. This factor hampered the establishment of non-renal transplant programmes in Denmark up to 1990, the year in which the 'brain death' concept was accepted by parliament [1]. As at the beginning of 1995, no official approval by the Japanese Congress has yet been declared to the adoption of the 'brain death' concept. Therefore, in addition to their living donor kidney transplant activity, some Japanese centres have started a living related liver transplant programme.

3. Organ exchange organizations in a restricted sense

An organ exchange organization is, in the restricted sense, an alliance of donor hospitals and transplant programmes, together with their accompanying tissue typing laboratories, all of which follow the same set of general policies, standard operating procedures and organ allocation rules. Currently, such organ exchange organizations are found in Europe [2–7], North-America [8,9] and Australia [10].

The concept of such a supra-local cooperation already dates from the early days of kidney transplantation [11] and was based upon two requirements, which were also relevant upon the definitive emergence of the non-renal transplant programmes.

3.1. Reduction of the waste of organs by maximum possible transplantation of all donated organs

The maximum possible usage of donated organs depends on the size of the area and/or the pool of transplant candidates to be served. Characteristics of donors show large variations, accentuated by the current liberation of several donor criteria (age, size); the definition of appropriate donor organ quality is not constant among transplant programmes. The larger an organ exchange organization, the greater and the more diverse the waiting list of transplant candidates and the more mansplant programmes, the higher the chance of ultimately using organs suitable for a transplant within the service area, and thus, the lower the wastage of useful conor organs.

Although the reasoning behind recipient pooling could be a plea for wide international, or even worldwide, agreements, limited service areas of organ exchange organizations are demanded because of the restricted ischaemic tolerance of the donor organs and

modes of organ transplant, and due to financial considerations.

3.2. Optimal usage and transparent allocation of donor organs

Organ allocation within the area of an organ exchange organization should primarily aim at the transplantation of two categories of patients: those with the best transplant outcome, achievable by 'matching' donor and recipient as well as possible, and those who are in the most urgent need of a transplant. Subsequently, the benefit of a cooperation was also seen in the approval of a uniform and justifiable organ allocation policy. Transparent execution of these organ allocation policies, with the inevitable necessity of compliance monitoring, would eliminate doubts, voiced by government, general public and patients, about the fairness of selection and the possible existence of special interests that take inappropriate advantage of donated organs for single transplant programmes or patients [9].

In order to realize maximum usage, achieve optimal usage and maintain allocation transparency, compliance from donor hospitals and transplant programmes is essential. The transplant programmes should prospectively list all transplant candidates on the composite waiting list of the organ exchange organization, together with data which are required to enable them to be matched with donors; the donor centres should report every post-mortem donor to the organ exchange organization, in order to match the donor against the waiting list before an organ is offered and used for transplantation.

4. Organ exchange organizations in a broader sense

Most organ exchange organizations have adopted one or more of the following activities.

4.1. Scientific research

Scientific research is performed in order to assess the importance of donor- and/or recipient-related factors which could affect recipient selection and transplant outcome, and to monitor characteristics of used and non-used donors and donor organs. Results are subsequently used to improve the existing organ allocation algorithms, to re-define the guidelines for donor organ eligibility, and to formulate recommendations for donor management. In addition, the individual transplant programmes are given the opportunity to sound out their local policies. Therefore, the transplant programmes should provide regularly all relevant donor, recipient, transplant and transplant follow-up data to the organ exchange organization [6,12].

4.2. Reference tissue typing laboratory

Through the establishment of a central tissue typing laboratory, standardized procedures of the tissue typing involved in organ donation and transplantation can be implemented. This is realized by organizing training courses and bench workshops, and by the distribution of standard reagents and material. A second goal is quality assurance and control, accomplished by post-hoc donor re-typing at the central laboratory and/or by the establishment of regular specific proficiency testing schemes [4]. Uniform as well as reliable donor and recipient HLA typing, recipient anti-HLA antibody screenings and cross-match results are the aim. In the case of odd HLA-typing and/or cross-match results, the central laboratory can provide a second opinion service.

4.3. Education programmes for medical professionals, public and/or patients

Organ exchange organizations support all kind of informative and instructive projects to increase the number of organs and tissues donated. These initiatives, e.g. European Donor Hospital Educational Programme (EDHEP), Eurotransplant International Foundation, the organ exchange organization in which Austria, Belgium, Germany, Luxemburg and The Netherlands are cooperating (ET), and Vital Connections (United Network for Organ Sharing (UNOS), the organ exchange organization of the USA), are mostly directed towards health care professionals. Communication strategies are developed to enable clinicians to feel confident and effective in dealing with bereaved relatives and in making an organ and tissue donation request. Sometimes, broad-scale donor awareness campaigns are directed towards health care providers and the general public. Transplant centres themselves most often initiate patient education programmes. Some organizations have established a telephone help-line, to answer any question about donors, organ procurement and transplantation (Spain, UNOS). This service is available for the general public, health professionals and journalists.

4.4. Role in tissue banking and/or bone marrow donor registries

Several organ exchange organizations, such as United Kingdom Transplant Support Service Special Health

Authority (UKTSSA), the organ exchange organization serving the UK and the Republic of Ireland, and Etablissement Français de Greffes (EFG), the organ exchange organization serving France, also concentrate on post-mortem tissues, such as cornea, bone, skin and hearts for valves [2,3]. The main tasks are tissue recovery, coordination of tissue processing for transplantation purposes and tissue allocation. In some cases the tissue banking programme has evolved to a separate organization, maintaining a close working relationship with the founding organ exchange organization, as is the case for Bio Implant Services, which was founded in 1989 by Eurotransplant and which coordinates internationally several tissue banking programmes [7].

Registries of unrelated living bone marrow donors are also being established (Swiss Transplant, France).

5. Structure of an organ exchange organization

The structure of the current organ exchange organizations is a product of evolution rather than design [10]. Historical bonds, national culture and character, geographical and demographic characteristics, medical and immunological progress, changes in political and governmental control, and developments in managerial approach, telecommunication and computer networks have led to a diverse spectrum of possible structures [2,3,5–7,13,14].

5.1. Development and infrastructure

Although most organ exchange organizations operate on a national base, either directly since its foundation (France, 1969) or gradually over time (USA, 1986), for others, cooperation immediately had an international character (ET, 1967: Austria, Belgium, Germany, Luxemburg and The Netherlands; UKTS, 1972: UK and Republic of Ireland; Scandiatransplant, 1969: Denmark, Finland, Iceland, Norway and Sweden). International collaboration for kidney and liver transplants exists between Australia and New Zealand [10]. In contrast, several regional groups continue to work independently in Italy.

It is clear that service areas vary widely: UNOS, 9.4×10^6 km^2 with a population of 253×10^6; Eurotransplant, 5.2×10^6 km^2 with a population of 113×10^6; Spain, 1.5×10^6 km^2 with a population of 38×10^6; north Italy, 0.4×10^6 km^2 with a population of 1.8×10^6.

The organ exchange organizations usually started as a private initiative, founded on the recognition of the special benefits that widespread professional collaboration could attain in the field of transplant surgery. The voluntary cooperating transplant programmes were comparable to the members of a club who agree to abide by the rules set by their profession. The organ exchange organization, as the official of the club, was the custodian and operator of those rules and had to strike a delicate balance in satisfying the demands of the individual transplant programmes while maintaining the integrity of the consensual framework representing all the members.

During the last decade, however, donation systems, transplant programmes and organ exchange organizations have received attention by governments and, in particular, Ministries of Public Health. The motives were the increasing demand made by types of organ transplantation on the organization of the health care system, the constitutional right of equal access to medical care, the shortfall of post-mortem donors, and also the allegations of organ trading, medical tourism and non-compliance with the allocation rules. Some existing organ exchange organizations became attached to the Department of Health (UKTSSA, France), while others were contracted by the government but still remained a private corporation (UNOS). In other countries, the opportunity was taken by the government to create a formal national organ exchange organization, closely linked to the government (Spain, Saudi Arabia). Legislative measures on brain death, organ procurement and transplantation (Austria, Belgium, Sweden, Denmark) and/or decrees concerning authorization of programmes to perform transplants (The Netherlands) were also formulated.

The international organ exchange organization, Eurotransplant, continues to operate on free will and consensus amongst the participants, achieving true international collaboration.

5.2. Policy development

In general, organ exchange organizations have a hierarchical decision-making process [15,16]. Advisory committees are most often related to the different organ types of transplantation, and/or specific specialisms such as ethical or financial committees. An equal representation of the diverse regions and/or programmes in each committee is safeguarded. It is through these committees that recommendations for change of existing policies and for implementation of new regulations are formulated for approval by the Board of the organ exchange organization and/or gov-

ernment. In this policy development process, the transplant community is actively involved. In addition, all policies are regularly monitored and evaluated on request by an individual transplant programme, on the initiative of an advisory committee or upon demand by the Board.

With respect to policy making, it should be said that, in general, all regulations are developed and/or sounded out by medical professionals, actively involved in the field of transplantation. Increasingly, however, appeals are made for participation in decision-making by the general public: e.g. UNOS has on the Board a representative of health organizations serving the interests of patients and of donor families as well as ethicists and economists [12]. Anticipating this trend of non-medical interest, several exchange organizations have standing committees such as Patient Affairs and Ethics.

5.3. Operational structure

5.3.1. *Central office*
Many administrative and some operational tasks of an organ exchange organization are governed by a central office, the tasks of which vary widely. The central office usually runs the system of match and to allocating organs 24 hours a day; sometimes, a central allocation office is established which participates, to a varying extent, in the organ allocation process within the territory of the organ exchange organization (see section 5.3.4). If suitable recipients for an organ are lacking, the central office offers the organs to other organ exchange organizations.

In order to facilitate listing of transplant candidates, reporting of donors, registration of transplants and entry of transplant follow-up, a telecommunications or computer network is operated; the central office collects and handles the requests for statistical analysis. The central office conducts meetings of the advisory committees and the Board; it informs the transplant centres about new decisions and changes; and it acts as the vocal point for the general public and/or to the government.

5.3.2. *Donation side*
The organization of the donor organ reporting and of procurement are managed differently. In UNOS, organ procurement and transplantation are separated due to the establishment of 'organ procurement organizations' (OPO), which are frequently not hospital-based. Within an assigned geographical area, the OPOs promote donation in the hospitals, whether or not these are engaged in transplantation; upon donor report, they

also inform the central office of UNOS about the donor and assist in donor management and subsequent organ allocation. In contrast, in Europe, the transplant centres themselves act as the donor-reporting agency. The procurement area of a transplant centre consists either of a clearly defined geographical area (Austria, The Netherlands, Spain, France) or of a conglomerate of affiliated donor hospitals (Belgium, Germany).

The contact person between the donor/transplant centre and the central office has changed from an interested surgeon or physician who was willing to coordinate the donor procedure or who wished to be informed by the central office upon an organ offer for one of his patients, to persons, who are specially trained for these activities. Introduction of those so-called transplant coordinators has led to a more professional approach towards the organization of donation and transplantation in the designated areas of transplant programmes.

5.3.3. *Transplantation side*
Authorization of transplant programmes is a matter for the Ministry of Health rather than the organ exchange organizations. Some organ exchange organizations have adopted corporate by-laws governing membership standards for establishment of transplant unit and/or for programme continuity (e.g. UNOS, Saudi Arabia). Most often, computer networks between transplant programmes enable the 24 h listing of transplant candidates on the composite waiting list of any organ transplant type. Similar facilities are also made available for transplant registration and the entry of transplant follow-up data.

5.3.4. *Organ matching/allocation*
The differences in the achievement of organ matching and allocation between the organ exchange organizations can be roughly reduced to the presence or absence of a central organ allocation office. Some organ exchange organizations have chosen an organ matching and allocation procedure fully initiated and executed by the donor centre (Scandiatransplant, Australia). Thus, no central allocation office is present. The participation of a central organ allocation office in organ allocation depends on the allocation protocol upon which the transplant community has agreed for the different post-mortem donor organs. On the one hand, the central allocation office is the only one which fully coordinates the matching and allocation ('top-down' approach) [4], on the other, it only assists with the organ placement when needed ('bottom-up' approach) [8]. The former option is more or less in use in Eurotransplant, while the latter exists in UNOS and

France. The central office also often arranges shipment of donor organs from donor centre to transplantation centre and/or transport of explantation teams.

5.4. Financial aspects
The financial structure of an organ exchange organization is dependent on the legal entity of the organization and on the characteristics of the national health care system(s). With regard to the legal entity, a distinction needs to be made between a private non-profit foundation (e.g. ET), a governmental institution as a part of the Ministry of Health (e.g. UKTSSA), and a private non-profit corporation, contracted by the government (e.g. UNOS). Eurotransplant is financed by the health insurance authorities in the participating countries, by means of the payment of a fee for every patient registered on the waiting list. The fee is annually adjusted to meet the Board approved budget. In addition, ET functions as a clearing house: the donor centre is reimbursed by ET as soon as possible for the costs related to donor management, donor explantation and donor organ transport. Later on, ET charges these expenses to the transplant recipients or centres.

The Department of Health is responsible for the operational maintenance of UKTSSA. Adequate funding in the form of a cash limited budget is provided and comes out of public funds raised through general taxation [6].

The UNOS contract is a cost-sharing arrangement in which the government pays only a portion of the costs accrued through contract performance. UNOS pays the remaining costs from patient registration fees [12].

6. Summary
The organization of post-mortem organ donation and allocation differs world-wide due to governmental participation, financial support, historical bonds and socioeconomic factors. Organ exchange and acceptance of the 'brain death' concept are essential to the establishment of renal and non-renal post-mortem organ transplant programmes. In order to avoid wastage of donor organs, to optimize the use of a donor organ in a transplant and to effect equitable and transparent organ allocation, (inter)national alliances of donor hospitals and transplant programmes, all applying the same set of organ allocation rules, or the so-called organ exchange organizations were founded. Many differences exist between the organ exchange organizations with regard to infrastructure and development, financial

support, internal operational structure and decision making about organ allocation protocols.

References

1. World Health Organization Legislative Responses to Organ Transplantation. Martinus Nijhoff Publishers, Dordrecht: 1994.
2. Council of Europe (Matesanz R, Hors J, Persijn G. *et al.* eds.), Transplant, July 92, Volume 04.
3. Council of Europe (Matesanz R, Hors J, Persijn G. *et al.* eds.), Transplant, September 93, Volume 05.
4. Persijn GG, Cohen B. Eurotransplant part I, organizational aspects.Clin Transplant 1986; 35–46.
5. Balderson R. UKTSSA – the support service for transplant units nationwide. Transplant Soc Newsl 1993; 1: 7.
6. Pudlo P. European transplant programs – what can the U.S. learn? J Transplant Coordination 1993; 3: 138–40.
7. Cohen B, Haase-Kromwijk B. Eurotransplant 1990 – progress report. J Transplant Coordination 1991; 1: 5–10.
8. Ferree DM. Post-mortem organ sharing: the organ centre. In: Philips MG, (ed). UNOS: Organ procurement, preservation and distribution in transplantation. William Byrd Press, Richmond 1991, 129–44.
9. Barnes BA. Experience of the New England organ bank. Clin Transplant 1986; 53–60.
10. Armstrong G. Organ donation in Australia – an overview. ETCO Newsl 1994; 2: 3–8.
11. Van Rood JJ. A proposal for international cooperation in organ transplantation: Eurotransplant. Histocompatibility Testing 1967; 451–52.
12. UNOS. New OPTN, Scientific Registry contracts foretell increased responsibilities. UNOS Update 1993; 9: 2–12.
13. Saudi Centre for Organ Transplantation. Regulations of organ transplantation in the Kingdom of Saudi Arabia. Saudi J Kidney Dis Transplant 1994; 5: 37–98.
14. Milford EL. The end-stage renal disease transplant program: an-experiment in participatory democracy and national health care. Semin Dialysis 1994; 1: 69–74.
15. Eurotransplant Newsl 1994; 120: 2–6.
16. Eurotransplant Newsl 1994; 120: 11–21.

28 | Costs of transplantation

F. TH. DE CHARRO, A. DE WIT

1. Introduction

Transplantation is considered by the general public to be a spectacular achievement of modern medicine. Transplantation can be seen as a representation of the power of medicine to prolong life. Nature appears defeated if parts of the body which no longer function properly can be replaced. The idea that substitute organs are derived from the remains of a person who has lost his/her life may increase the perception of transplantation as a victory over death. Mankind recreates itself by performing transplants. The capacity of the human body to reject tissue from outside the body is controlled. The implanted organ, which is normally attacked by the immunosuppressive system, survives because the destructive and deadly process of rejection is disrupted by immunosuppressive agents. There is then a second victory over death when organ failure is prohibited and the implanted organ is permitted to survive, enabling the transplanted patient to live.

Transplantation medicine is also spectacular because of its high cost. Reports of cardiac surgeons flying around the world as part of the jet set contribute to that image. Kidney racers speed along the roads and through the sky. Television broadcasts transplantation as a treatment involving many physicians and attention focuses on expensive stays in hospital to treat the complications. Some even fear that high cost treatments such as transplantation concentrate health care resources on the lives of a few happy patients. Less expensive health care which might help many people could be in danger if high technology medicine, supported by media attention, attracts more and more resources.

Transplantations have been front page news for approximately four decades: somehow there always seems to be an amazing breakthrough within this field of medicine. New and expensive immunosuppressive drugs substitute for relatively cheap ones. The pharmaceutical industry is investing heavily in these new drugs: health economists expect them to be introduced at a price level which equals their marginal benefits to society. These marginal benefits are, in fact, determined by the willingness of decision makers to accept new treatments and drugs, sometimes under considerable public pressure.

Transplantation is an intermediate product: it has no value in itself, but derives its value from the benefits to the patient. Ultimately, every transplantation should be motivated by the consequences for the health of the recipient. The counterpart to this statement is that the costs of transplantation cannot be assessed in themselves. Basically, medical effectiveness manifests itself in improvements in quality of life and increased life span of graft recipients. Costs should be related to medical effectiveness and so enable decision makers to act according to rationality. In The Netherlands, assessment studies have been performed for kidney, heart and liver transplantation. A study on lung transplantation has also been completed, but as yet the results have not been published. An overview of cost-effectiveness of transplant programmes will be presented here based on the available evidence.

A cost-effectiveness analysis is one where the consequences of a project or programme are evaluated using microeconomic concepts of costs and benefits and where output is expressed in an appropriate physical unit [1,2]. Life years gained, sometimes adjusted

G.M. Collins, J.M. Dubernard, W. Land and G.G. Persijn (eds). Procurement, Preservation and Allocation of Vascularized Organs 233–240
© 1997 Kluwer Academic Publishers.

for differences in quality of life, has been used as the output measurement unit in the studies described here. The resulting picture differs substantially for each. These assessments were performed at different times so the cost estimates refer to different time periods and should be used prudently: while prices and wages have increased, skills and experience have also increased, bringing improved productivity. It is not unreasonable to assume that the increase in wage and prices is compensated by increases in productivity. The cost estimates will be presented in British pounds, although the original estimates were in Dutch guilders, using a rate of exchange of 2.5 Dutch guilders to the pound. There is no evidence that this rate of exchange reflects purchasing power parity. On the contrary, a comparative research project on the Dutch and English heart transplant studies resulted in a purchasing power parity of 7 Dutch guilders for one British pound. However the use of an international currency such as the pound is probably more meaningful than the use of a relatively unknown currency such as the Dutch guilder. Kidney transplantation was subjected to an evaluation study in the period 1982–1988 [3]. The heart and liver transplantations were assessed in the period 1985–1988 [4,5].

2. Kidney transplantation

Kidney transplantation is a treatment which substitutes for another life-saving treatment, dialysis. Dialysis is expensive, though some types are more expensive than others, and transplantation is, therefore, a cost saving treatment. Kidney transplantation also improves quality of life. It cannot be proved however that kidney transplantation increases life expectancy in comparison with dialysis.

The first kidney transplantation in The Netherlands was performed in 1966 and the number of transplantations performed each year has increased since, reaching 30 per million in 1995 [6]. The total number of patients living with a functioning graft was 264 per million on 1st January 1996, according to the data of the Dutch End Stage Renal Disease Registry (Renine). The proportion of Dutch ESRD patients living with a functioning graft is about 50.2%.

In the 1980s, the Health Council conducted a study on the cost-effectiveness of ESRD treatments in The Netherlands [7]. Costs to society of transplantation during the first year were estimated at around £28 000 British pounds. These costs included the cost of pre-transplant investigations related to the transplantation, the costs of donor recruitment, explantation, implanta-

tion and the follow-up costs during the year starting on the day of transplantation. Of this amount, slightly more than 60% covered the costs of hospitalization. At that time, average hospital stay for a sample of 70 patients was 50 days. Supplementary services requested around 30%, or £20 000. Included in this figure were the costs of donor recruitment, estimated at £3000. Figure 1 illustrates the distribution of the costs of kidney transplantation.

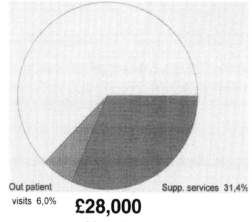

Hospitalization 62,6%

Out patient visits 6,0%   **£28,000**   Supp. services 31,4%

Year 1

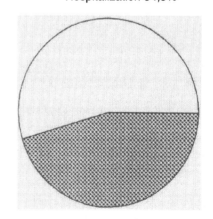

Hospitalization 54,5%

Out patient visits 45,5%

£2,400

Year 2+

Figure 1. Costs of kidney transplantation.

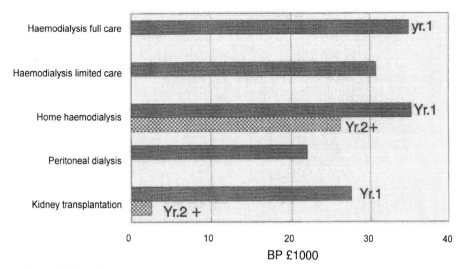

Figure 2. Cost of different treatments for end stage renal disease.

The costs of treatment in the first year of transplantation were approximately the same as the average costs of dialysis. The cost of continuous ambulatory peritoneal dialysis (CAPD) was thought to be somewhat lower, but that for haemodialysis was somewhat higher (Fig. 2).

Since the middle of the 1980s the costs of transplantation have been influenced by the introduction of Cyclosporine (CsA). In a recent study a comparison was made between the costs of transplantation in patients treated with CsA monotherapy or a combination regimen of CsA during the first 3 months and prednisone supplemented by azathioprine (Aza) later on. The cost of CsA monotherapy was higher by an estimated £1250 [8], in the first year. Although the use of CsA is reported to be cost-effective in general, it is difficult to determine the optimal mix of elements in an immunosuppressive regimen. While the use of CsA increases the costs of drugs, the number of hospital days is decreased due to the decreased number of rejection episodes. Improved graft survival also results in avoidance of some dialysis costs.

The quality of life of patients living with kidney grafts is generally perceived to be higher than the quality of life of dialysis patients. Evans *et al.* found that subjective quality of life, summarized in the Index of Life Satisfaction, was even higher than that of the general population [9]. This could partly be attributed to the relief experienced by patients after dialysis treatment ceases. Steroid treatment might also be an influence. However it has also been suggested that the subjective quality of life of dialysis patients is quite

high [10] supposedly due to their capacity to cope. Subjective quality of life may, therefore, have limited value and should be supplemented with information about the objective health status of the patients. According to this measure, the quality of life of transplanted patients is substantially higher, provided the patient is free from rejection [11].

Although treatment during the first year after transplantation is approximately as expensive as dialysis, the following years generate far fewer costs than does dialysis treatment. The exact saving depends to a high degree on the immunosuppressive regimen followed. Without CsA, the costs have been estimated at £2500 (1986 prices). Model calculations using a Markov chain indicated that an increase in the number of transplantations of 1150 (230 per year over a 5-year period), would result in a reduction of the total cost to society of the ESRD programme in The Netherlands of £24 million: a kidney transplantation results in a cost reduction of about £20000 per patient per year. Kidney transplantation is therefore a cost-saving treatment which increases the quality of life of the kidney patients.

In Northern American and Western European countries, it is impossible to perform a substantial number of kidney transplants without also offering a full dialysis programme to treat the majority of patients while they are waiting for a donor kidney. It also enables the patient to fall back on dialysis after an irreversible rejection. It is, therefore, not correct to present figures of the cost per life year gained by kidney transplantation without taking the costs of dialysis into account [12]. The costs of transplantation are inseparable from the costs of dialysis and costs of kidney transplantation should be conceptualized as being negative. Cost per life year gained by the ESRD programme as a whole were estimated at £20 000.

3. Heart transplantation

Heart transplantation makes a substantial demand on resources, but also results in substantial benefits. Heart transplantation has been assessed in the USA by Evans [13] and in the UK by Buxton [14]. In The Netherlands a cost-effectiveness study was performed on the Dutch heart transplant programme in 1985–1988 [15].

The American and English studies showed that survival after transplantation was substantial. Using a number of reasonable assumptions, life expectancy after heart transplantation, was estimated to be about 10 years. However, survival of the patient in the absence of a transplant is not easy to assess, since those who die on the waiting list are probably in relatively poor health. Patients who survive long enough to undergo transplantation are expected to survive for a relatively long period, even in the absence of transplantation. In the Dutch study, the time taken for the screening of patients was used as a proxy for the condition of the patient. The shorter the screening time, the worse the condition of the patient was assumed to be. This information was incorporated into an analysis which resulted in an estimate of expected survival without transplantation of 1.1 year. The

increase in life expectancy of heart transplant patients was thus estimated about 9 years.

That heart transplantation increases quality of life was established in the Dutch study by interviews using a number of quality of life instruments. Some results are described here. The Nottingham Health Profile reflects the degree to which limitations are experienced by the respondents on six dimensions of quality of life: pain, energy, physical mobility, sleep, social isolation and emotional reactions. A score of 0 represents the absence of any limitation in the items relevant for that dimension. A score of 100 indicates that the respondent suffers from all the limitations included in that dimension of the NHP. The scores on the Nottingham Health Profile are presented in Fig. 3. The scores on the dimensions 'sleep' and 'energy' decreased from 53 and 74 before transplantation to 15 and 4.4 months after transplantation, respectively. The Karnofsky score increased from 53 before to 89 4 months after transplantation. The resulting increase in quality of life was again confirmed in interviews with patients 13 months after transplantation. In order to estimate quality-adjusted life years, the observed health states were translated into a single figure quality of life index, summarizing values for health states derived from a sample of the population [16]. The indicator for quality of life was estimated to lie between 0.15 and 0.30 before transplantation and between 0.55 and 0.85 after transplantation. All the measurement instruments used indicated that heart transplantation results in a substantial increase in quality of life. Heart transplan-

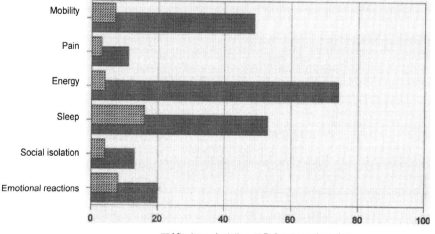

Figure 3. Quality of life before and after heart transplantation.

tation therefore in an increase in both the quantity and quality of life.

Heart transplantation also proved to be an expensive treatment. During the year starting with the operation, the treatment on average cost was £56 000. After this first expensive year, treatment costs went down to £14 000, much of which was due to costs of immuno-suppressive drugs, mainly CsA. Costs related to organ procurement were a minor part of heart transplant costs, amounting to £2000 for registration, laboratory costs, transplant coordinators etc. at the moment a patient was put on the waiting list, and £1800 for the cardiectomy. Ultimately, costs per life year gained were estimated at £23 000. This relatively low figure can be explained by the substantial number of life years gained over which the relatively high costs during the first year after transplantation are spread. These costs include the costs incurred during screening patients for heart transplantation and the costs incurred during the period of time the patients were on the waiting list for a donor organ. Cost has been defined as the extra costs incurred because of the heart transplan-tation: costs of treatment of the original heart disease have not been taken into account, since these costs would have been incurred anyway. The amount in-volved for patients on the waiting list was around £4500. The impact of the costs of screening on the cost per life year gained is dependent on the level of the screening costs, the proportion of patients transplanted and the survival period after transplantation. In the case of heart transplantation, the screening costs are relatively low: 29% of the referred population received a transplant, and the increase in the number of life years gained was long enough to moderate the impact of the screening costs on the costs per life year gained.

Costs per quality-adjusted life year were higher than costs per life year. These costs vary substantially when assumptions are made, based on the single figure quality of life index, after transplantation. If the index assumes that quality of life after heart transplantation is 0.8, and quality of life before heart transplantation is 0.2, the cost per quality adjusted life year is around £23 500. However, if the index shows that after trans-plantation quality of life is lower, e.g. 0.55, cost per quality-adjusted life year goes up to £37 000.

4. Liver transplantation

Liver transplantation differs from heart transplantation in that the survival period without transplantation can be relatively long. In the case of heart transplantation, a model was developed to estimate survival of the patient in the absence of transplantation using the time used for screening as a proxy for the seriousness of the health state of the patient. Survival without a liver transplant is difficult to estimate. Liver transplantation has to be carried out relatively early in the disease, since the probability of success of the operation diminishes with remaining liver function. Survival after transplantation is also less favourable than in the case of heart transplantation. As a result, it is more difficult to provide evidence for a substantial gain in life expectancy due to liver transplantation.

The increase in life expectancy differs according to the primary diagnosis. In a study of patients with primary biliary cirrhosis (PBC), 1 year survival rate with transplantation was estimated at 65%, and 5 year survival was 55%. The estimate of survival without a transplant differed according to the clinical model used. For patients in the Child–Pugh class A, the estimated period of survival without transplantation was close to that observed following transplantation [17]. In those with disease of the more severe Child–Pugh classes B and C there was a significant increase in life expectancy using different clinical prognostic models [18]. The dif-ference between the Child–Pugh classes might be attributed partly to the effect of the timing of the trans-plantation: the longer the waiting time the more severe the disease. As a result of increased experience in The Netherlands, liver transplantations have been carried out later in the patient's history and accordingly the impact of the disease has been more serious.

The increase in the number of life years gained by patients with PBC has been estimated at about 4.5, and in patients with other causes of cirrhosis about 1.5 years [19]. It was impossible to prove an increase in life expectancy for patients with other primary diagnosis.

Liver transplantation increases quality of life. The Karnofsky Performance Index, the State-Trait Anxiety Inventory, Self-rating Depression Scale, The Index of Psychological Affect, the Index of Overall Life Satisfaction and the Nottingham Health Profile all demonstrate an increase if the pretransplantation scores are compared with those 1 year after transplantation. The scores on the Nottingham Health Profile are pre-sented in Figure 4. Quality of life was condensed into a single figure index using the EuroQol instrument [20]. Subjective quality of life after 1 year even exceeds the quality of life of the general population, probably due to relief after the serious deprivation of the period of organ failure.

The costs of liver transplantation are substantial. The costs in the year starting with transplantation was estimated at slightly more than £70 000, 25% of which

Nottingham Health Profile (100 - 0)

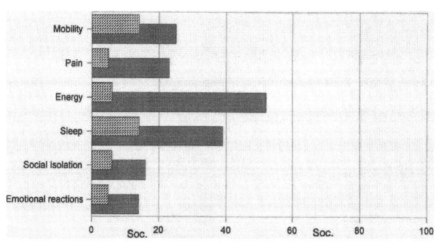

After transplantation ▓Before transplantation

Figure 4. Quality of life before and after liver transplantation.

was spent on the operation itself and 30% on hospital costs. Hospital costs were high due to the rather long stay in intensive care. The costs of screening and treatment during the time on the waiting list were estimated at £7500. Over an 8 year period between 1979 and 1987, 73 transplants were performed in 221 referred patients. In every transplantation programme more patients have to be screened than can be transplanted, and so the burden of the screening activities is proportionally higher. So if for every transplant, three full screening episodes are required, the total costs of the first transplant year and the three screenings would be more than £90 000. The second and consecutive years after transplantation generate considerably lower costs. If CsA is used those costs amount to £11 000 a year, and if not, the costs are approximately £5000. Cost per life year gained will be high if the number of life years gained is low and vice versa. In PBC patients these costs will be low since the number of life years gained is more than 4 and the considerable cost of screening and the transplantation year will be divided over the years gained. However, if the number of life years gained is rather low, an amount of approximately £90 000 can only be divided over this rather low number of life years. Accordingly, costs per life year gained were unacceptably high for patients with diagnoses other than cirrhosis. For PBC patients, costs per life years gained were less, £32 000, which is considered to be acceptable in view of the costs incurred for other patient groups.

5. Lung transplantation

Lung transplantation has been subjected to a recent technology assessment in The Netherlands, but the results are not yet published. Lung transplantations have been performed at the St. Antonius Hospital in Nieuwegein and at the Academic Hospital in Groningen. After some discussion, it was decided to concentrate the experimental lung transplantation programme at the Academic Hospital in Groningen, where 257 patients were screened for lung transplantation in the period 1990–1993. In this group of patients, 35 lung transplantations have been performed. The most common primary diagnosis was pulmonary emphysema, followed by cystic fibrosis, pulmonary hypertension and pulmonary fibrosis. The number of donor organs which have become available during the period 1990–1994 in The Netherlands has been less then 1 per million population. Since the need for lung transplantation is expected to be much higher a discrepancy between the supply and need for donor lungs is anticipated [21]. The 1 year survival period has been reported to be 86%, although this differs substantially according to primary diagnosis: emphysema patients have the highest expectation and pulmonary hypertension the lowest. The cost per life year gained will of course depend on survival, the costs incurred during the first year and the screening/transplantation ratio.

6. Discussion

The state of the art of organ transplantation differs. Kidney transplantation is now an accepted procedure. Although there is still some uncertainty about the optimal immunosuppressive regimen, there is a general consensus that transplantation is a cost-saving procedure and increases quality of life. Kidney transplantation is cost-saving if the health care system has already accepted the high costs of dialysis for those patients, as seems to be the case in all Western European and North American countries.

Heart transplantation is a procedure for which there is no back-up treatment. If the donor heart fails and there is no possibility of retransplantation, the patient dies. Life expectancy after heart transplantation is high enough for costs per life year to be acceptable. Moreover, quality of life improves dramatically as a consequence of the transplantation.

At the moment there is no clear evidence about the number of life years gained by liver transplantation in diagnosis groups other than cirrhosis or in lung transplantation. The medical effectiveness of the intervention differs according to primary diagnosis. Donor availability is a problem in both cases. A figure of around 6 donor livers per million has been mentioned as a first estimate of the donor availability. The number of donor lungs might be dramatically lower. The lower the number of donor organs in relation to the demand, the more difficult it is to avoid an overflow of screening procedures. Since screening costs are not negligible some mechanism is needed to restrict over-screening to a certain extent.

Liver transplantation results in a range of costs per life year gained for a variety of primary diagnoses. For patients suffering from primary biliary cirrhosis and other forms of cirrhosis the costs per life year gained seem to be acceptable and lower than the costs of dialysis treatment, which might serve as a standard of how much society is prepared to pay. In other diagnosis groups, liver transplantation clearly generates very high costs, mostly due to the few life years gained. Policy makers and the medical community might agree that the high costs of transplantation and the suffering of patients who have to undergo the treatments and hospitalization involved do not justify the intervention. Technology assessment in these cases should be diagnosis-specific, and monitoring should continue for those primary diagnoses where results are unsatisfactory until more favourable prospects emerge.

The costs of organ recruitment do not play a substantial role in the decision making process with regard to the acceptability of transplantations. These costs are relatively low in comparison with the total costs during the first transplantation year. These costs involve the resources required to run a registry which enables the identification of an available match between potential recipients and donor organs, laboratory costs, the costs of maintaining an organization which is available at the moment when donor organs become available, the costs of obtaining the donor organ, using either the donor centre or bringing in a team from the transplant centre, and the costs of transporting the donor organ from the donor centre to the transplant centre. Costs of donor recruitment are foremost a problem of distribution, since the costs are incurred in institutions which are not generally performing the transplantation. Donor recruitment costs are high if other treatment costs are high, as will be the case for liver and lung transplantation, and lower if the transplantation has developed into a stage of maturity, as is the case for kidney transplantation. After some time the explantation techniques become routine practice and it is no longer necessary for the surgical team performing the transplant operation to send out a second team to obtain the donor organ.

Ultimately, transplantations are performed to provide benefits to patients. There is, therefore, a strong inclination to use the judgements of patients as a guideline for decision making. It seems, however, that patients' judgements are to a high degree dependent on the circumstances in which they are asked to evaluate their situation. Coping behaviour induces a circumstantial judgement in which dialysis treatment seems to generate an acceptable quality of life for many patients. Their quality of life may sometimes even be high enough to question the desirability of a transplantation. It has been demonstrated that transplantation generates in these patients an experience of life satisfaction which is even higher then that experienced by the general population. It is not known how far this discrepancy between subjective and objective quality of life is due to drugs generating euphoria, but even while neglecting that aspect, it is evident that transplantation is such a major life event that there may be no sound basis for reliable patient judgements. In the end, transplantation for the patients means the difference between life and death and the success of transplantation means the defeat of death.

References

1. Drummond MF, Stoddard GL, Torrance GW. Methods for the Economic Evaluation of Health Care Programmes. Oxford University Press, Oxford 1987.
2. Mishan EJ. Cost-benefit analysis. Unwin Hyman, London.
3. De Charro FT. Kosten-effectiviteitsanalyse van het nierfunktievervangings-programma in Nederland. Eburon, Delft 1988.

4. Van Hout BA, Bonsel G, Habbema D, Van der Maas P, De Charro F. Heart transplantation in the Netherlands; costs, effects and scenarios. J Health Econ 1993; 12: 73–94.

5. Bonsel GJ, Essink-Bot ML, De Charro FT, Van der Maas PJ, Habbema JDF. Orthotopic liver transplantation in the Netherlands. The results and impact of a medical technology assessment. Health Policy 1990; 16: 147–62.

6. Dutch End Stage Renal Disease Registry, Renine: Annual Report. Rotterdam 1995.

7. Health Council. Report on Dialysis and Kidney Transplantation. Report 1986/9. The Hague 1986.

8. Hilbrands LB. Immunosuppressive drug therapy after renal transplantation: balancing the benefits and risks. PhD Thesis, Catholic University of Nijmegen 1996.

9. Evans RW, Manninen DL, Garrison LP et al. The quality of life of patients with end stage renal disease. New Engl J Med 1985; 312: 553–9.

10. de Wit A, Merkus M, de Charro F. Measuring utilities in an end stage renal disease population. In: Badia X, Herdman M, Segura A (eds), Discussion papers of the Plenary Meeting of EuroQol 1995. Catalan Institute of Public Health, Barcelona 1996.

11. Hart LG, Evans RW. The functional status of ESRD patients as measured by the Sickness Impact Profile. J Chronic Dis 1987; 40 (Suppl 1): 1175–130S.

12. Williams A. Economics of coronary artery bypass grafting. Br Med J 1985; 291: 326–9.

13. Evans RW, Manninen DL, Overcast TD et al. The national heart transplantation study; final report. Battelle Human Affairs Research Centres, Seattle 1984.

14. Buxton MR, Acheson R, Caine N. Costs and benefits of the heart transplantation programmes at Harefield and Papworth hospitals. DHSS Research Report No. 12. HMSO, London 1985.

15. Van Hout BA, Bonsel G, Habbema D, Van der Maas P, de Charro F. Heart transplantation in the Netherlands; costs, effects and scenarios. J Health Econ 1993; 12: 73–94.

16. Bonsel GJ., Van Hout BA et al. Utility measurement of health states by the general public using computer assisted interviewing. In: Bonsel GJ (ed.), Methods of Medical Technology Assessment with an Application to Liver Transplantation. Eburon, Delft 1991.

17. Pugh RNH, Marray-Lyon IM, Dawson JL et al. Transection of oesophagus for bleeding oesophageal varices. Br J Surg 1973; 60: 646–9.

18. Bonsel GJ, Klompmaker IJ, Van 't Veer F, Habbema JDF, Slooff MJH. Use of prognostic models for assessment of value of liver transplantation in primary biliary cirrhosis. Lancet 1990; 335: 493–7.

19. Michel BC, Bonsel GJ, Stouthard MEA, Essink-Bot ML, McDonnell J, Habbema D., Liver transplantation: Long term effectiveness. Report no. 92-07. Institute of Public Health, Rotterdam 1992.

20. EuroQol Group. EuroQol, a new facility for the measurement of health related quality of life. Health Policy 1990; 16: 199–208.

21. Mannes GPM, De Boer WJ, Van der Bij W. Ervaringen met 300 patienten verwezen voor longtransplantatie. Ned Tijdschr Geneesk 1996; 140: 228–9.

29 | The role of the transplant coordinator

CELIA WIGHT

1. Introduction

Advances in surgical techniques and improved immunosuppression have led to increasing success in organ grafting. Transplantation is the treatment of choice for most patients in chronic renal failure and the only option for patients with end stage liver, heart and lung disease, and there is an ever-increasing demand for organs and tissue for transplantation. Unlike other surgical procedures, transplantation cannot take place in iso-lation. It requires cooperation between medical colleagues, often working many miles from a transplant centre, and the support of the public [1]. In addition the referral of patients as potential organ donors is an additional labour for intensive care units (ICU) and neurosurgical staff, who see no benefit for their own patients.

The rate of organ procurement differs widely throughout European countries, with a range of 4 donors per million population (PMP) to 25 donors PMP in 1994 (European mean: 14.7 PMP; Fig. 1). The

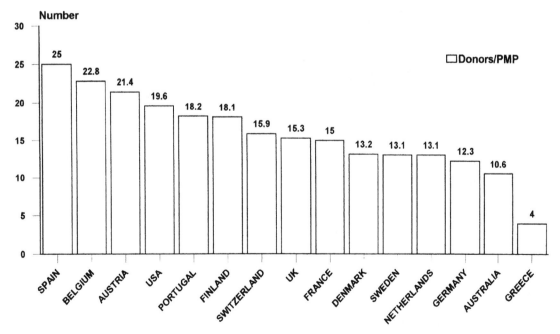

Figure 1. Donors per million population: 1994.

G.M. Collins, J.M. Dubernard, W. Land and G.G. Persijn (eds). Procurement, Preservation and Allocation of Vascularized Organs 241–247
© 1997 Kluwer Academic Publishers.

rate of multi-organ donor procurement also differs throughout Europe, ranging from 28% to 80% of all donors in 1993 (European mean: 64.7%) [2]. In 1994 all countries except Spain experienced a plateau or fall in organ donation, and some saw a rise in relatives' refusals to consent for organ removal. Sensational media coverage can have a very negative impact on the public attitude to organ donation. Transplant coordinators report increasing refusal rates among relatives of potential donors and relatives often state that negative press coverage of organ transplantation has influenced their decision [3]. Presumed consent legislation has been one successful initiative in increasing organ donation. However, comparisons of organ donation figures in different European countries should be undertaken with caution: there are many differences in how these regulations are handled by hospitals and doctors in charge of potential donors [4]. For example, in 1994 the highest number of organs obtained PMP was in Spain, a presumed consent country that chooses not to practice the legislation (Table 1). Presumed consent in countries such as Austria, Belgium and France, however, has not resulted in comparable donation rates. Inefficiencies in the referral process can also cause the loss of potential donor organs; these may arise in both the donating hospital and in the transplant centre (Table 2).

Many factors influence the rate of organ donation and recovery; however, the development of the role of the transplant coordinator (TC), which corresponds with the development of organ exchange organizations (OEO), has done much to make the process easier. This chapter will discuss the role of the TC in Europe and will describe a different model developed in Spain.

2. The role of the transplant coordinator

The main function of transplant coordinators is to help to increase organ donation by providing professional and public education and to organize organ procurement and subsequent transplantation. Following the successful appointment of TCs in the United States in

Table 1. Donor Rates PMP and Donors' Legal Status: 1994.

	Donors PMP	Donors' Legal Status
Spain	25.0	Presumed consent (not practised)
Belgium	22.8	Presumed consent (practised only partially)
Austria	21.4	Presumed consent
Portugal	18.2	Presumed consent (practised only partially)
USA	19.6	Required request
Finland	18.1	Presumed consent
Switzerland (by Canton)	15.0	Presumed consent Informed consent No law
UK and Eire	15.3	Informed consent
France	15.0	Presumed consent (practised only partially)
Denmark	13.2	Informed consent
Sweden	13.1	Informed consent
Netherlands	13.1	No transplant law
Germany	12.3	No transplant law
Australia	10.6	Informed consent
Greece	4.0	Presumed consent (not practised)

the early 1970s, several unofficial posts were created in Europe. However, it was not until 1979, in The Netherlands, that the first full-time TC was appointed. This post was followed by appointments in the UK and Germany. Subsequently, many such posts have been created and currently coordinators provide a nationwide service throughout most of Western Europe. Appointments have been made in Italy and Portugal, although neither of these countries is yet completely provided for. More recently, TCs have been introduced to promote and develop organ donation in Eastern European countries (Fig. 2). However, even in countries with well-established coordination systems, the numbers of TCs PMP remains small (Fig. 3). Most European TCs come from a nursing background, usually dialysis and ICU. Several TCs are medically

Table 2. Inefficiencies in the referral process leading to loss of potential donors.

Problems Arising in Donating Unit	Problems Arising in Tx Centre
Unfamiliar with criteria for organ donation	Uncontactable at time of initial donor referral
Uncertain who to contact in transplant centre	Apparent procrastination, demands and delays
Concerns about burden of extra work	Inappropriate behaviour in operating room

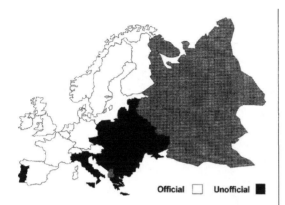

Figure 2. Appointment of transplant coordinators: Europe 1994.

qualified, particularly in The Netherlands, Germany, France and Spain. In some countries a medically qualified TC is in post for only up to 3 years: it can be argued that regular change is disadvantageous to professional relationships between the intensive care and transplant units. On the other hand this arrangement may prevent 'burn out' as is increasingly seen in the USA, where difficulties are experienced in retaining procurement TCs beyond 2 years [5]. Other TCs are appointed from an administrative background and bring important administrative skills to the post.

Traditionally, the European TCs' work base is in the local kidney transplant unit. They are appointed to work within a geographical region that usually corresponds to the catchment area for patients requiring treatment for chronic renal failure and will include several ICUs where potential donors may be identified. Many TCs are involved with both organ procurement and the care of the recipients. However, more recently, in some countries, these tasks have been separated and clinical TCs have been appointed to deal with all matters related to recipients (Fig. 4).

3. Procurement transplant coordinators

All procurement TCs (PTC) work within a designated area and are involved in education and the organization of organ donation.

3.1. Education

At the very least PTCs aim to establish good professional relationships with medical and nursing staff working in the local ICUs. Protocols are provided on the identification and maintenance of potential donors and guidelines are produced on approaching the next of kin. Many PTCs provide formal and informal

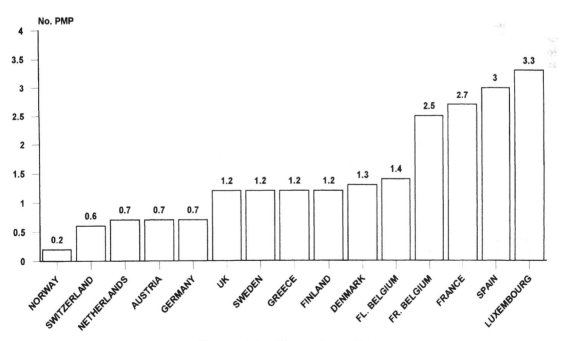

Figure 3. Transplant coordinators per million population: Western Europe 1994.

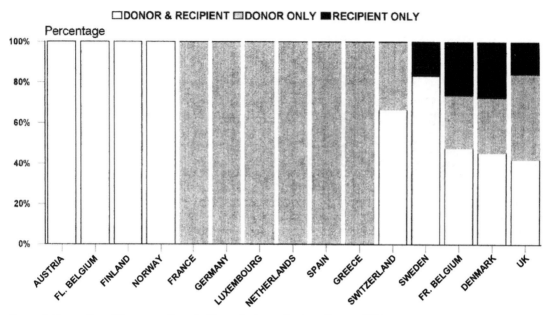

Figure 4. Proportion of time commitment of transplant coordinators: Europe 1994.

lectures to hospital staff on all aspects of organ dona-tion and transplantation. Some PTCs also become in-volved in providing information to the public through interested public groups, schools and the media. However, some TCs feel that public education is not the best use of their time and can be left to others, for example, national kidney foundations and government-led campaigns.

3.2. Organization of organ procurement

PTCs are responsible for the organization and logistics of organ donation. Many will travel to the donating hospital on referral of a potential donor and help the staff with this time-consuming procedure. At this time it is essential that the PTC gains enough information to allow the individual transplant teams the opportunity to determine organ suitability before valuable medical and nursing time has been invested in donor main-tenance and the next of kin have become committed to organ donation. This information requires careful examination of the past medical history and evaluation of the current medical situation; this frequently demands further medical investigations. Only when in possession of this data can the PTC notify the national OEO who will, in turn, offer the organs to the appro-priate transplant units. With a PTC acting as a focus for information it should be possible to inform the

donating hospital which organs are suitable for trans-plantation within 1 hour of the initial referral. These rapid decisions can only be reached with the help of good communication networks within and between the PTC, OEO and the relevant transplant centres and between the PTC and the physician in the donating hospital. Organization of a donor operation can be complex. At the most extreme, in case of multiple organ donation, up to six separate, self-sufficient sur-gical teams (often located many miles apart) can meet in a hospital to remove organs from a donor for several recipients. Telephone calls can run into hundreds and the organization may take many hours (Fig. 5). The PTC will usually attend the donor operation, some as a member of the donor surgical team. Others may use the opportunity to teach operating theatre staff and ensure that the procedure goes smoothly with the least possible inconvenience to the host hospital. The necessity for several surgical teams to participate in organ removal can be expensive, time-consuming and extremely disruptive for any hospital, and may even inhibit future referrals. To improve this part of the do-nation process an initiative has been developed in the UK in which the country has been divided into zones, each with at least one trained surgical team available for organ removal. This has led to a considerable reduction in time wasted in awaiting the arrival of distant surgical teams and in the costs of organ pro-

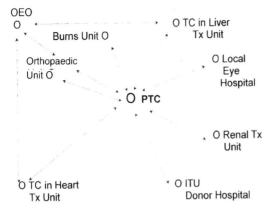

Figure 5. The PTC acts as a focus for information during the time-consuming organization of organ allocation and retrieval.

curement. The surgeons work well together as a team and become well known to the donor hospitals' operating room staff. This arrangement speeds up the procedure and provides a more harmonious atmosphere in the operating room, improvements which are much appreciated by the host hospitals. Once the operation is completed, the PTC is responsible for providing follow up information on the donor and organs removed to the OEO for national statistics. The PTC will also inform the staff in the donating hospital of the results of subsequent transplant operations, and many will also provide the donor's relatives with general information on the outcome of the transplant operations. In some countries, for example, The Netherlands and Great Britain, the PTCs often make follow up home visits to further counsel the relatives.

4. Clinical transplant coordinators

As already described, many PTCs are also involved with some of the care of recipient patients, most usually the organization of the transplant operation. However, where clinical TCs (CTC) have been appointed they are members of the caring medical team, based at a kidney, liver or heart transplant centre. Their main responsibilities are organization of the assessment of patients' suitability for transplantation, entering the names and clinical status on the national OEO waiting list and monitoring and providing support to the patient and his family during the difficult waiting period. When a suitable organ becomes available for a patient, the CTC is contacted by the OEO. Once a decision has been reached to accept the offer, the CTC will organize the transplant operation, the admission to hospital, if necessary, of the chosen patient and support the relatives during this time. As with procurement, recipient information is provided to the OEO for national statistics. The CTC is often involved with patient care during the recovery period and may, with the help of the PTC, help the patient in thanking the family of his donor. Finally, many CTCs will be involved with the out patient and ongoing follow up care of the recipients.

5. The Spanish model

The role of the TC in Spain has developed in a rather different way and is supervised by the national TC based at the national OPO. Seventeen regional TCs work in the 15 regions of Spain: they are all medically qualified and are often based at the regional Depart-

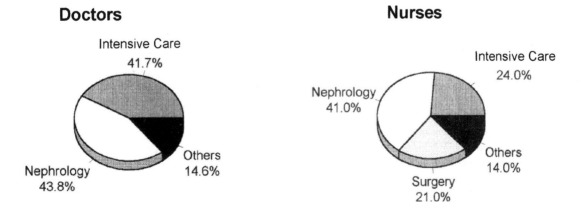

Figure 6. Professional background of medical and nursing members of local TC teams in Spain.

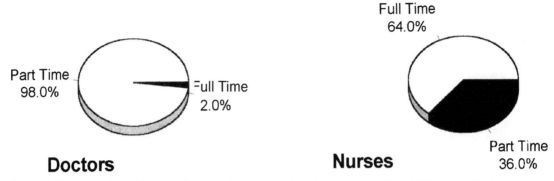

Figure 7. Time commitment to organ donation of medical and nursing members of local TC teams in Spain.

ment of Health. Regional TCs have a mainly managerial function and form the link between the professionals and the local health administrators, and are responsible for all the donation activities affecting the region. The regional TCs meet regularly with the national TC to discuss and evaluate any problems that arise related to organ donation and transplantation. One hundred and eighteen coordinating teams, responsible for the local development of the whole process of organ/tissue procurement and transplantation, have been appointed throughout Spain. The local teams are made up of doctors and nurses from ICU, nephrology, anaesthesiology and surgery (Fig. 6) and are based in all hospitals able to provide donors. Many members of these local TC teams have only a part-time commitment to organ donation (Fig. 7): this takes priority over their other duties on the detection of a patient as a potential organ donor. The part-time medical team members usually return full-time to their original profession after 3 years as a TC. The local TC teams undergo specialist training and are involved in the whole donation process, from donor detection to subsequent organ transplantation.

6. Accountability and training

There are wide differences throughout Europe in the management, accountability, professional status and training of TCs. The PTCs, based in local renal transplant units, tend to be accountable to the local renal transplant team and as a result have individual job descriptions, pay structures, professional standing and working practices. Only in Spain, to a lesser degree in France, Germany, and more recently The Netherlands and Switzerland, has any attempt been made to standardize the role of the TC and establish a national managerial structure and professional recognition. In Spain the local TCs are accountable to the hospital administration and the regional TCs and through the regional TC to the national TC. In France and Germany local TCs are accountable to regional TCs who in their turn are accountable to a recognized individual in the national OEO. In The Netherlands, a much smaller country, the TCs have their own bureau and manage their own affairs with the support of the Board of the national OEO. Only Spain has experienced a consistent increase in organ donation that is largely attributed to the training and support provided to the TCs [6]. In several European countries TCs receive no formal training, while in other countries TCs have provided their own professional support and training, normally managed through a national TC organization. These organizations are also successful in developing professional and public educational material for members. As many TCs do not have their own budget, they are heavily reliant on charities and pharmaceutical companies to provide the resources for this essential educational material. Trying to meet this need the European Donor Hospital Education Programme (EDHEP), a Eurotransplant initiative, was developed in The Netherlands in 1990/1 [7]. Following successful pilot evaluations EDHEP was made available to other interested countries in 1992. This two-part professional education programme aims to increase donation by providing up to date information on all aspects of organ donation and transplantation followed by a communication skills training workshop for all professionals who come in contact with the bereaved. EDHEP has been introduced into most of Europe and in countries in the Middle East, Far East and South America, proving a universal need for more of this type of educational material. All countries report improved professional relationships and increased donor referral following the workshops. The early results of a controlled evaluation of the impact of

EDHEP on the knowledge, self confidence and communication skills of workshop participants in The Netherlands have been most encouraging [8].

The European Transplant Coordinators Organization (ETCO) was founded in the early 1980s to provide a focus for information and standardized training for all European TCs. In addition ETCO aims to encourage European cooperation and to establish its members as professional members of the transplant fraternity. To be a professional, one must have a recognizable qualification. This has been a difficult issue for TCs to address as, nationally, numbers are small and the role has become highly specialized. Again, Spain has taken the lead in this direction by establishing a highly structured training course for TCs with a diploma from the University of Barcelona which is therefore recognized throughout the country.

7. Conclusions

There is no doubt that the role of the TC is now well accepted in Western Europe, where established. TCs have developed a specialized and invaluable role as members of the transplant team. Without the assistance of the TC it is unlikely that any hospital will now consider the referral of a patient as a potential donor. However, because of historically unstructured appointments many TCs, some of whom have been in post for over 10 years, still have no recognized professional status. Some operate in isolation with inadequate or conflicting managerial structures and only through their own organizations is any attempt made to standardize their practice and to improve their professional situation. Some countries have already addressed these issues. It is surely time that other countries followed these examples and looked at the function of TCs and provided the status, structure and tools available to TCs to fulfil their part of the transplant equation.

Acknowledgements

I would like to thank the National Key Members of the European Transplant Coordinators Organization for giving their valuable time to provide national information for inclusion in this chapter.

References

1. Wight C, Calne RY. The Organ Donor: In: Westaby S (ed.), Trauma. Heinemann Medical, London 1988; pp. 382–95.
2. Wight C, Cohen B. Legal and logistic issues in organ transplantation: In: Lindop MJ, Klink JR (eds), Anaesthesia and Intensive Care for Organ Transplantation. Chapman & Hall, London (in press).
3. Cohen B. Finding a Cure to Dramatic fall in organ procurement Rates. Nephrol News/Issues (Europe) 1994; July/August, 21–2.
4. Ripoll J. ETCO Statistics Committee's 1993 Survey on Organ donation and transplantation in Europe. ETCO News. 1994; 12: 3–6.
5. Goldberg R. Kappel D. Organ procurement coordinator success profile: a tool for selection and retention. J Transplant Coordination. 1992; 2: 33–6.
6. Matesanz R, Miranda B, Felipe C. Organ procurement and renal transplants in Spain: the impact of transplant coordination. Clin Transplant 1994; 8: 281–6.
7. Blok GA, Van Dalen J, Jager K, Wight C, Ryan M, Wijnen R. Omgaan met rouw en donatie: een vaardheidsprogramma. In: Metz JCM, Scherpbier AJJA, Houtkoop E (eds), Gezond Onderwijs – 11. Universitair Publikatiebureau. Wageningen 1993; pp. 41–9.
8. Blok GA, van Dalen J, van der Kooy PJ, van Wezel HBN, de Jong IJ, Kranenburg J, Kootstra G. Effect of the European donor hospital education programme. Transplant Proc (in press).

30 | Organ availability in Europe: problems and results

GUIDO G. PERSIJN AND BERNARD COHEN

1. Introduction

The treatment of choice for the majority of patients suffering from end stage organ failure is transplantation. Major progress in the field of 'transplantology' has been achieved during the last decade, resulting in higher survival rates of both grafts and patients. However, the potential impact of these advances is seriously hampered by one persistent problem, the shortage of donor organs. The most successful means of increasing organ donation has been the introduction of so-called presumed consent legislation. The comparison of figures between Eurotransplant countries which appear to have a presumed consent system must, however, be undertaken with caution. There are many differences in how these regulations are handled and practised by hospitals and doctors in charge of potential organ and tissue donors. These might be influenced by cultural and religious aspects but also by social and ethical considerations. Analysing the European data with regard to procurement rates undoubtedly reveals that the number of available organs is the highest in Spain followed by Austria and Belgium (all three have presumed consent). Apparently, presumed consent in countries such as Italy and France has not yet resulted in a similarly high donation rate. In contrast, donation figures in France, Austria and Belgium have recently shown a serious drop, indicating that both public and professionals may not automatically accept presumed consent regulations. What is the Spanish secret? Clearly, a number of major factors contribute to the accomplishments in Spain in recent years. For example,

the appointment of many regional (part-)time transplant coordinators in addition to those in local hospitals, and a relatively high number of fatal road traffic accidents. Such factors may be unique to Spain, but are insufficient to explain this success.

Another barrier to increasing organ donation which is common to all countries no matter which legal system has been adopted is the approach to the next of kin. Refusals to organ donation from the next of kin continue to run between 30 and 40% in all countries, and a significant number of suitable potential donors is, therefore, lost.

One approach to increasing donor awareness may be the introduction of the European Donor Hospital Education Programme (EDHEP). EDHEP is a part of a multifaceted process aimed at closing the increasing gap between available donor organs and the medically indicated demand for organs and tissue for transplantation.

2. European results

Regular European surveys have been conducted to investigate organ donation and transplant activities based on reports of the various national and international organ exchange organizations in Europe [1–4]. Comparison of the figures in European countries will allow us to draw some conclusions which may contribute to the alleviation of the existing donor shortage.

Table 1 shows the 1994 and 1995 results for the major European countries and for Western Europe with

G.M. Collins, J.M. Dubernard, W. Land and G.G. Persijn (eds), Procurement, Preservation and Allocation of Vascularized Organs 249–253
© 1997 Kluwer Academic Publishers.

Table 1. Overview of donation and transplantation activities in the major European countries in 1994 and 1995.

		Euro-transplant[a]	EFG[b]	Scandia-transplant[c]	UK transplant[d]	Spain	Italy	Western Europe total[e]
Non-living donors	1994	1581 (13.9)	878 (15.4)	350 (15.2)	930 (15.2)	960 (25.0)	445 (7.9)	5437 (14.9)
	1995	1620 (14.3)	899 (15.5)	339 (14.7)	964 (15.8)	1037 (27.0)	576 (10.1)	5815 (15.8)
Cadaveric kidney transplants (PMP)	1994	2997 (26.0)	1561 (24.7)	664 (28.8)	1750 (28.8)	1613 (42.0)	830 (14.8)	9969 (27.3)
	1995	3064 (27.0)	1391 (24.0)	604 (26.3)	1765 (28.9)	1765 (46.0)	1042 (18.3)	10157 (27.6)
Heart transplants (PMP)	1994	698 (6.1)	429 (7.5)	119 (5.1)	330 (5.4)	292 (7.6)	304 (5.3)	2230 (6.1)
	1995	732 (6.4)	430 (7.4)	106 (4.6)	337 (5.6)	278 (7.2)	390 (6.8)	2321 (6.3)
Liver transplants (PMP)	1994	916 (8.1)	621 (10.9)	183 (8.0)	644 (10.5)	614 (16.0)	326 (5.8)	3400 (9.3)
	1995	928 (8.2)	645 (11.1)	173 (7.5)	688 (11.3)	698 (18.1)	404 (7.1)	3653 (9.9)
Population in millions	1994	113.4	57.0	23.0	61.1	38.4	56.0	365.7
	1995	113.4	58.0	23.0	61.1	38.4	56.7	367.6

[a] Eurotransplant includes Germany, Austria, Belgium, Luxemburg and The Netherlands.
[b] EFG = Etablissement Français des Greffes, formerly France Transplant.
[c] Scandiatransplant includes Denmark, Finland, Norway and Sweden.
[d] UK Transplant includes UK and Ireland.
[e] Western Europe total also includes Portugal and Switzerland.
PMP, per million population.

regard to kidney, heart and liver transplants. Renal transplant activities in 1995 in Europe varied from 18.3 per million population (PMP) in Italy to 46.0 for Spain (1994: respectively 14.8 and 42.0). However, within the supra-national organ exchange organizations such as Eurotransplant and Scandiatransplant significant differences in the number of cadaveric renal transplants PMP can also be noted. For example, within Eurotransplant in 1995, Austria has the highest number (39.1 PMP) which is one and a half times that of The Netherlands (26.3) and Germany (25.1; Table 2). Nevertheless, Austria previously had even higher renal transplantation rates, namely in 1990, 1991 and 1992 with respectively 51.2, 54.5 and 51.9 transplants PMP. The drop is partly also caused by the high export rate of Austrian-procured kidneys within Eurotransplant. Similar differences can be observed in the Scandinavian countries where, with the exception of Finland, a substantial number of living related renal transplants are also performed.

Interestingly, in 1995 the total number of cadaveric kidney transplants performed dropped somewhat in Scandiatransplant and E.F.G. For Eurotransplant, a

Table 2. Organ transplants in Eurotransplant (PMP).

	Kidney		Heart		Liver	
	1994	1995	1994	1995	1994	1995
Austria	42.2	39.1	11.3	14.4	12.0	14.7
Belgium	37.4	32.2	11.5	9.8	15.9	13.4
Germany	23.7	25.1	5.5	5.8	7.2	7.2
Netherlands	25.8	26.3	3.1	3.2	5.0	6.3

drop was also seen in Austria and Belgium (Table 2), which is certainly partly due to the export of kidneys.

Tables 1 and 2 also give heart transplant figures in Europe. At the top we find in 1995 Austria and Belgium with 14.4 and 9.8 heart transplants PMP. The low figure for The Netherlands, with only 3.2 heart transplants PMP, is surprising. Indeed, there are large differences in the number of hearts procured and transplanted in the different ET countries: The Netherlands is consistently exporting hearts, whereas Germany has consistently been an importing country. Differences in selection policies for transplant candidates might also play an important role. Also in 1995 the number of heart transplants performed dropped in Scandiatransplant and EFG, but also in Spain. For Belgium, this drop was quite substantial – from 11.5 transplants PMP in 1994 to 9.8 in 1995.

With respect to the liver transplant situation in Europe, again Spain, Austria and Belgium had the highest rate in 1995, at 18.1, 14.7 and 13.4 PMP, respectively. Surprisingly, the UK has nearly doubled the number of liver transplants performed, from 5.9 PMP in 1990 to 11.3 in 1995. The low number of 6.3 liver transplants PMP in The Netherlands again does not reflect the procurement rate as many livers are exported each year. The Netherlands apparently has a very small number of patients on the waiting list for liver and heart transplantation. With the exception of Scandiatransplant, the number of liver transplants increased in 1995. However, within ET, Belgium showed again a drop, from 15.9 to 13.4 PMP in 1995.

It has been suggested that the number of transplants realized is related to the number of transplant centres. Table 3 gives an overview of the number of kidney, heart and liver transplant centres in Europe. The low population density in Finland and in Norway may explain the fact that these countries have only one (Norway) or two (Finland) such centre(s). There does indeed appear to be a correlation between the number of kidney, heart and liver transplants performed and the number of active transplant centres per million inhabitants. This is certainly true for Austria, Belgium and France, and maybe also for Switzerland.

Another important factor may be the number of transport coordinators. Table 4 shows the actual number as well as the number of transplant coordinators per million inhabitants in 1995.

No clearcut correlation can be demonstrated between the number of transplant coordinators PMP and the number of post-mortem organ donors PMP, although the countries with the highest procurement rates, i.e. Spain, Austria and Belgium have the highest 'density' of transplant coordinators. Nevertheless, France and Sweden seem to be the exception.

Another important contributing factor may be the number of fatal traffic accidents. Table 5 gives an overview of the 1993 figures for Europe. Although less than half of all suitable organs originate from this category of donors (35–40% in Eurotransplant) this

Table 4. Transplant Coordinators in Europe in 1995 (PMP).

Austria	0.9
Belgium	0.7
Denmark	1.3
France	0.6
Germany	1.8
Netherlands	1.3
Norway	1.0
Spain	0.4
Sweden	0.7
Switzerland	1.0
UK	1.1

Table 3. Inhabitants (in millions) per transplant centre in 1995.

	Kidney	Heart	Liver
Austria	1.5	2.5	2.5
Belgium	1.3	1.7	2.0
Denmark	1.3	5.2	5.2
Finland	2.5	2.5	2.5
France	1.5	1.9	2.4
Germany	2.5	3.2	4.3
Italy	2.8	7.1	6.3
Netherlands	2.1	7.5	5.0
Norway	4.2	4.2	4.2
Portugal	2.0	10.0	5.0
Spain	1.3	7.7	3.0
Sweden	2.1	4.2	2.8
Switzerland	1.2	2.3	1.7
UK	1.7	6.1	6.8

Table 5. Fatal road accidents in 1993 (PMP)[a].

Austria	171
Belgium	166
Denmark	110
Finland	97
France	174
Germany	126
Greece	210
Hungary	153
Ireland	123
Italy	126
Luxemburg	190
Netherlands	84
Spain	168
Sweden	74
Switzerland	111
UK	67

[a] Source: CBS; Central Office for Statistics, Traffic and Transport, The Netherlands. 1994.

Table 6. Transplant laws and practice in Western Europe 1995.

	Legal situation and practice
Austria	Presumed consent (registration possible)
Belgium	Presumed consent but mostly practised as informed consent (registration possible)
Denmark	Informed consent
Finland	Presumed consent
France	Presumed consent but practised as informed consent
Germany	No transplant law but practised as informed consent
Greece	Presumed consent but practised as informed consent
Italy	Presumed consent but practised as informed consent
Luxemburg	Presumed consent but practised as informed consent
The Netherlands	Legislation per May 21, 1996 approved. Informed consent + registration
Norway	Presumed consent
Portugal	Presumed consent but practice varies
Spain	Presumed consent but practised as informed consent
Sweden	Informed consent
Switzerland	Presumed, informed consent or no law, differs per canton
United Kingdom and Ireland	Informed consent

contribution remains significant. The differences in the number of persons killed in traffic accidents in different European countries are striking.

A survey on donation and transplantation activities for so many different countries would not be complete without taking the legal systems into account. Table 6 gives the legal situation in Europe as of June 1995. Germany is now the only country with no legislation on organ donation and transplantation. Most of the countries have so-called 'presumed consent', law which means that every citizen is a donor after death unless he/she has objected during life. However, it should be stressed that the application of this legal system differs from country to country and even within a country. There are many variations, e.g. whether or not the family is approached, whether or not a central registration system exists, and so on. Informed consent means that the deceased has given permission during life by means of a donor card or is registered in a central database as being pro-organ donation. If not, the next of kin of the deceased are approached and asked for permission to remove organs and tissues for transplantation purposes.

3. Discussion

For patients suffering from end stage organ failure, the optimal treatment is organ transplantation. There has been major progress in many fields related to transplant immunology and medicine during the last decade. However, one persistent problem, namely the

shortage of organ donors, is continuously hampering the further development of organ transplantation. Data from European countries show that no solution to this problem has yet been found. Publicity campaigns, distribution of donor cards, appointment of transplant coordinators, implementation of donor protocols in hospitals, reimbursement of donor hospital costs for procurement, educational programmes for hospital personnel and many other initiatives have been introduced. Although these factors may all contribute to a higher donor availability, they have so far failed to increase significantly the donor supply and thus to prevent patients dying while awaiting transplantation. Despite all efforts to increase organ donation results, there has certainly been no substantial growth in Europe during the last 5 years.

The best known factor is the introduction of so-called presumed consent legislation, as used for example in Austria. Analysing the data with regard to procurement rates in Europe undoubtedly reveals that the number of available organs is significantly higher in Spain and Austria than in countries such as The Netherlands and Germany, where no legislative measurements have been taken so far or where the informed consent is practised. Comparing donation figures between countries which seem to have the same legislative system must be undertaken with caution. It should be emphasized that even in countries with presumed consent legislation this important factor is not always a guarantee for optimal procurement rates. In 1995, for unknown reasons, the number of post-mortem donors dropped in Austria and Belgium relative to previous years. There are many differences in how these regulations are handled and practised by the donor hospitals and the doctors in charge of potential donors. There are many different approaches on how to inform donor families. Standardization, uniformity and clarity would be very helpful not only for the doctors in charge but also for the general public.

4. The European Donor Hospital Education Programme[1] – a solution

The European Donor Hospital Education Programme (EDHEP) is a multifaceted programme aimed at closing the gap between available donor organs and tissue and the medically indicated demand [5]. EDHEP is an adaptable training programme that can be adjusted to suit national needs or used to complement existing educational programmes and legislative initiatives which have been adopted in a number of countries in recent years. The programme aims to raise awareness of the donor shortage and to provide some possible solutions, in particular, the perceived need to help doctors and nurses feel effective in dealing with the bereaved and approaching the subject of organ donation. The programme is divided into two parts. EDHEP Part 1, an in-hospital presentation aimed at all hospital personnel, gives a comprehensive briefing on the success of transplantation over the past decade, the shortage of available organs and aims to raise awareness of the key barriers that inhibit a request of the bereaved for organ donation. EDHEP Part 2 is a highly interactive workshop aimed at medical and nursing personnel working in critical care areas of hospitals and addresses some of the common misconceptions about dealing with grief. Health professionals can learn to recognize and respond to different grief reactions and are provided with communication strategies and training for breaking bad news and requesting organ donation.

In 1991, EDHEP was translated from the original English into Dutch and piloted in The Netherlands, where it has become an integral part of hospital in-service training. Since then, the programme has expanded continuously throughout Europe and also in Asia, South Africa, South America, Japan and the Middle East. It is now available in 17 different languages in more than 30 countries worldwide. As countries are at different stages of developing the programme and eager to hear of the experiences of others,

an EDHEP newsletter was introduced in 1992. The newsletter already enjoys a mailing list of more than 700 subscribers. Regular EDHEP demonstration workshops have been held. The young doctors and medical students, who had no previous training in communication skills, were enthusiastic, recognizing their own need for more of this type of training during their medical careers.

Following early evaluation, there can be no doubt that the skills awareness workshop goes some way towards meeting the needs of professionals working in critical care areas of hospitals. Recently, the first evaluation from research conducted in The Netherlands to measure the effectiveness of EDHEP has been obtained. Based on the theoretical notion that behaviour is closely related to knowledge, attitude, mastery of skills and self-appraisal of effectiveness, the EDHEP participants indicated that their behaviour in the context of making an organ donation request is much more confident and, therefore, more effective [6]. It has been demonstrated that EDHEP can lead to a more favourable attitude towards transplantation and that better collaboration and more confident communication on the part of hospital staff confronted with grief and the need to ask for organ donation can result in an increase in organ donation.

Acknowledgements

The authors are indebted to the physicians and their administrative and nursing staffs for providing the Eurotransplant Foundation with the data. Mrs Maya de Beer is gratefully acknowledged for her secretarial assistance.

References

1. Cohen B, Persijn GG and De Meester J. Eurotransplant Annual Report 1994 and 1995.
2. Matesanz R and Miranda B. Transplant Newsl, March 1996, Council of Europe-Conseil de l'Europe
3. Persijn GG, De Meester J, Cohen B. How severe is organ shortage in Eurotransplant? In Touraine JL et al (eds), Organ Shortage: The Solutions Kluwer Academic Publishers, Dordrecht 1995: 3–10.
4. Persijn GG, Cohen B. Self sufficiency in Europe: evaluation of needs. In Englert Y (ed.), Organ and Tissue Transplantation in the European Union. Martinus Nijhoff, Dordrecht 1995; 157–65.
5. Wight C, Jager K, Cohen B, Blok G, van Dalen, J and Wijnen R. The European Donor Hospital Education Programme. In: Englert Y (ed.), Organ and Tissue Transplantation in the European Union. Martinus Nijhoff, Dordrecht 1995; pp. 175–9.
6. EDHEP News, Newsletter nr. 14. Winter 1995 Edit. Writers Inc. Switzerland.

[1] A special contribution by Mrs. Celia Wight, Eurotransplant's EDHEP coordinator.

31 | Donor hospital development in non-university hospitals

Leo Roels

1. Introduction

With the advent of more efficient immunosuppressive drugs such as cyclosporine, growing success rates of solid organ and tissue transplantation have caused a proliferation of transplant centres and an ever-increasing demand for organs that continues to exceed supply in most countries. There is, however, no shortage of potential organ donors and not only is the potential there, but recent surveys indicate an overwhelming support for organ donation amongst the public [1]. Incentives to close the gap between the number of transplants that theoretically may be possible and the number of donations that actually occur include proposals for legislative, financial, educational and organizational measures. With respect to educational and organizational measures, researching, developing and delivering state of the art programmes that focus on intensifying the involvement of health care professionals in the organ recovery process have proven to be most instrumental in solving the organ shortage problem.

Active transplant programmes, although generally concentrated at larger university hospitals, have become increasingly dependent on their cooperation with smaller (e.g. community, private) non-university hospitals to guarantee the uninterrupted supply of cadaveric organs and tissues necessary for a transplant centre to survive. In general, and contrary to the situation in the USA, organ procurement activities in Europe are organized and centralized by university hospitals with transplant activities. Essential to an effective partnership and commitment between these university-based organ procurement organizations (OPOs) and non-university donor hospitals is a sort of systematic process of hospital development with regard to organ and tissue procurement protocols.

This chapter deals with the Leuven experience in establishing and maintaining such an organ and tissue recovery programme with non-university hospitals. Two distinct incentives have contributed to the success of this donor hospital network. The first of these is a donor hospital development programme based on a 'service business' approach, involving motivated nephrologists in referring dialysis centres, supported by their colleagues in surgical and/or anaesthesiological departments. This has recently been combined with a Health Authority supported reimbursement policy of donor management and procurement costs. The second is the implementation of a 'presumed

G.M. Collins, J.M. Dubernard, W. Land and G.G. Persijn (eds), Procurement, Preservation and Allocation of Vascularized Organs 255–262
© 1997 Kluwer Academic Publishers.

consent' legislation that has proven to be flexible enough to combine the individual's rights on self-determination with the greatest respect for the donor relatives' feelings.

2. Donor hospital development

Historically, and until the late 1970s, organ recovery programmes were generally limited to university hospitals with kidney transplant activities, until an ever-advancing medical technology, combined with dramatic improvements in immunosuppressive therapies in the early 1980s, made transplantation of renal (and gradually more non-renal organs) an even more attractive option to both health care professionals and potential recipients.

It became obvious that the resulting growing organ shortage required new strategies to expand the donor pool, e.g. by involving also non-university hospitals in the donor referral process. Health care professionals in smaller community hospitals, however, with no local transplant activity and in the absence of an inherent immediate own benefit, obviously lacked the necessary motivation to participate in more demanding multi-organ donation procedures. Health care budget restrictions further limited the willingness of hospital administrations to be involved in labour-intensive and time-consuming organ and tissue procurement procedures if they are not properly compensated for the employment of their personnel. Any development of an organ and tissue recovery programme in non-university hospitals therefore is deemed to fail if these impediments are not recognized and properly addressed.

2.1. Donor hospital development: the service business approach

For many years several European centres have succeeded in developing organ recovery programmes and donor hospital networks, whereas others failed to obtain satisfactory results. Approaches differ from centre to centre, although analyses of the most successful programmes reveal a remarkably consistent pattern, in many cases developed rather intuitively, mostly as a result of trial and error experiences. Basically, such donor hospital development programmes can be characterized by probably hidden but nevertheless distinct ongoing phases that apply also to marketing: assessment, planning, gaining access and implementation, evaluation and, if necessary, modification of earlier protocols. Since laws of demand and supply are also applicable to organ recovery, it should be no surprise that

these marketing concepts, although not yet widely accepted in Europe, will prove their value in a health care segment that is characterized predominantly by the holy principle of altruism. The only difference is that 'selling' the concept of organ donation should never be confused with selling a commercial product.

The marketing philosophy behind this approach is basically customer oriented and thus aimed at satisfying organizational goals through the identification and satisfaction of customer needs. Customers in this context are both the donor hospital and the transplant centre serviced by the OPO and its procurement transplant coordinator, whether university hospital-based or not. In this concept the OPO acts as a service business whose clients are the donor hospitals, donor relatives, transplant units and the public. That same service business concept implies the existence of different tasks: stimulating demands for services by showing the resulting benefits, removing the obstacles to involvement in an organ recovery programme, and demonstrating the rewards that normally result from such involvement, providing feedback and continual analysis to discover new opportunities in the field of organ and tissue procurement.

2.2. Assessment

A properly conducted 'market segmentation' procedure, avoiding counterproductive trial and error experiences, has been advocated as a prerequisite for a thorough donor hospital development: key groups have to be targeted and, since resources are usually limited, they should preferentially be directed to hospitals with the greatest potential for return. As shown below, some departures from this principle, allowing for further expanding a shrinking donor pool, can be discussed.

Retrospective data analysis should at least encompass review of the total number of hospital deaths versus deaths meeting donor criteria, to determine referral and donation rates that can be expected. In addition to approval for this record review, formal agreement between the donor hospital staff and the OPO representative should include approval for continued contacts with departmental staffs (neurology, neurosurgery, surgery, intensive care, internal medicine, nursing administration, pastoral care, social workers and financial department). It should be recognized that support starting from the 'top' (Hospital Administrator, Medical Director, Medical Council) allows easier contacts with the remaining staff. Assessment of individual departmental needs and concerns about organ donation procedures are essential to create 'customized' answers to local expectations.

2.3. Planning and customization

After most relevant information has been gathered and analysed, one can begin to develop a customized organ recovery protocol, which ideally should include professional in-service education, staff meetings and formation of an in-house organ donation working party. To be efficient, customization should answer the individual needs of key personnel. A systematic evaluation at this stage will reveal key levers affecting future donor recovery rates: each hospital will have key supporters (to be maintained and employed), neutrals (worth investing further efforts) and key opponents (negative impact to be limited).

2.4. Implementation

If applicable, a local organ donation coordinator (liaison officer) can be identified and officialized by his/her hospital staff. Whether or not such a liaison officer will be assigned as a link between the donor hospital and the OPO, this OPO should develop and maintain a high visibility within the donor hospital. This visibility encompasses regular review of protocols, with modifications if necessary, periodic meetings with key persons to assess changing needs, systematic donor and referral follow-up (telephone and written post-recovery evaluation as essential feedback) and initiating and/or assisting with educational activities.

2.5. Evaluation

Quality assurance implies feedback from within the hospital about experiences during donor recovery procedures. A quality service oriented approach also implies a problem solving mindset aimed at satisfying the 'customer': negative procurement experiences and complaints formulated by professionals involved should be considered an opportunity for positive changes.

3. The Leuven Collaborative Group for Transplantation (LCGT): development of a donor hospital network

3.1. Historical background

As a result of efforts to decentralize the routine follow-up of recipients referred for renal transplantation to the Leuven University Hospital by about 20 collaborating non-university dialysis centres, the Leuven Collab-

orative Group for Transplantation (LCGT) was founded in 1978 [2]. This decentralized approach aimed to guarantee optimal and personalized post-transplant recipient care, which should in turn decrease patient non-compliance, and thus further contribute to better survival rates.

As an immediate spin-off of their collaboration with the central transplant centre, associated nephrologists involved were willing to promote organ donation in their local hospital for the benefit of their own dialysis patients on the Leuven waiting list. Most of these nephrologists had graduated at the Leuven University Medical School and now worked all over Flanders (Belgium) to start dialysis centres in smaller, e.g. community, hospitals. Hospitals without dialysis facilities and associated nephrologists, but with surgeons and/or anesthesiologist graduated from the Leuven University Medical School, later joined this group of collaborating donor hospitals (Fig. 1). Since three other university hospitals also developed OPOs in the same Flanders region, an exact recruitment area cannot be defined, but is estimated to service around 3–4 million inhabitants.

3.2. The LCGT donor hospital network: application of the service business approach

In developing the LCGT donor hospital network, the basic rules of assessment, planning, implementation and evaluation were applied almost intuitively, although other favourable conditions also added to the success of the Leuven model.

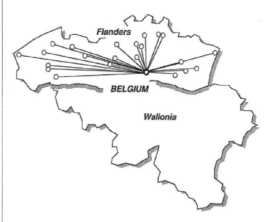

Figure 1. The Leuven Collaborative Group for Transplantation donor hospital network: collaborating hospitals.

3.2.1. *Assessment*

In most instances the 'start at the top and work down' approach to assessing potential resources and gaining access was facilitated by the presence of the above-mentioned motivated local nephrologists, anaesthesiologists or surgeons. They proved to be instrumental in initiating the issue of organ procurement with their hospital administrator, medical director and/or medical council. With the help of these liaison officers, potential local resources could easily be estimated, in most instances without a formal retrospective record review. In many cases, coincident Health Authority-enforced hospital mergers and reforms, which would make such retrospective record reviews rather outdated and thus irrelevant, also restrained us from performing in-depth retrospective record reviews. More accurate assessment of donor potential within cooperating hospitals needs to be performed in the future, once these mergers have resulted in new regional health care tasks divisions.

3.2.2. *Customized planning*

Initial contacts, frequently based on personal relationships, were followed by more formal agreements with hospital, nursing and departmental staff. From the very beginning it was clear that, even at the busiest hospitals, the donation process remains an infrequent event and needs the establishment of a close 'customer-oriented' working relationship with the LCGT procurement coordinator, to answer the sometimes subtle but substantially different expectations experienced during our visits to potential donor hospitals. We meticulously avoided imposing complete procedures, but rather suggested different options of cooperation and service. In general, at least two distinct expectation patterns could be distinguished during this planning phase, and these resulted in the development of two divergent models of hospital development.

Planning the 'fully participating donor hospital staff' model: In hospitals with a motivated abdominal surgery team and the presence of a dedicated local 'liaison officer', local participation was expected to be maximal: local anaesthesiologists, surgeons, ICU and OR personnel were trained in donor management and kidney procurement by the transplant centre's co-ordinator and surgical staff, and felt proud when offered the opportunity to assist visiting teams in multi-organ procurement. By establishing a close and fraternal working relationship, these local surgical teams considered themselves to be active contributors to the university transplant activities. Key to the successful maintenance of this kind of partnership, based mainly on motivation and pride, is a properly con-

ducted feedback system (see below). In this model, and after establishing a detailed referral and procurement procedure, the transplant coordinator's service role could be reduced to a low profile contact function in the background, not even necessarily present during the proper procurement, or limited to assistance in the preservation of the organs.

Obviously, planning and supporting such a 'full participation model' is only possible in hospitals with a high referral potential and/or in cases of 'kidney-only' donors. In cases of multi-organ donation and given the presence of one or more visiting procurement teams, the transplant coordinator should hold a more prominent place in the whole procedure.

Planning an 'all-in' service model for low-profile hospitals: Theoretically, hospitals with a lower donor potential should be serviced in an appropriate but less time-consuming way. Although it seemed inefficient at first glance, a growing organ shortage, and the LCGT's goal to respond to all donor referrals, made us consider the involvement of smaller hospitals. In such hospitals, mostly without neurosurgical facilities, departmental staff usually expected their involvement in organ donation procedures to be restricted as much as possible. Different reasons for this low profile attitude could be identified, but most reflected constraints on medical/nursing staff and finances. In this situation, more complex and time-consuming multi-organ donor management and procurement procedures required a complete 'all-in' service approach from the co-ordinating LCGT transplant centre. This service includes: looking after regulatory medicolegal requirements, assuring appropriate brain death documentation, implementing donor management, organizing appropriate consultations and testing, providing complete documentation of donor information, organizing (multiple) organ/tissue recovery, implementing organ preservation procedures, assuring adequate tissue typing materials and packaging/labelling of organs and tissues, and transporting the organs to the transplant centre.

3.2.3. *Implementation and evaluation*

Both models of cooperation obviously represent extreme situations and intermediate solutions had to be 'tailored' to specific local needs of cooperating hospitals. In both models, however, and because the whole network had to be run by only one procurement coordinator at the transplant centre, the appointment of one or more local liaison officers in collaborating hospitals was considered absolutely essential.

A LCGT donor protocol, including guidelines for brain death diagnosis, legislative guidelines, a donor data collection form and a multi-organ procurement technical guide, was developed to facilitate the task of this local key person(s). With the use of these tools, organizing a complete multi-organ donor referral and procurement in a distant hospital became perfectly feasible with only a few phone calls between the local liaison officer and the LCGT procurement coordinator. Although not absolutely necessary in the first model, the 'visibility' of this coordinator during the proper procurement procedure has been considered beneficial in materializing the link between the local donor team and the transplant centre, whatever the collaboration formula used: the procurement coordinator usually 'finished' the job of the local (kidney) procurement team by taking care of the preservation and packing of the organs. Personal visibility and communication with referral source personnel also allowed further assessment of their attitudes, knowledge base, commitment and educational needs and desires regarding the donation process. In all cases ICU and OR personnel appreciated being informed by the procurement coordinator about the final allocation of the individual organs.

When applying the 'all-in' service formula, the transplant centre's coordinator closely looked after the whole donation process by guiding the ICU staff maximally during identification of donor suitability through meeting individual organ criteria and organizing appropriate consultations, meeting medicolegal requirements, implementing donor management procedures to ensure haemodynamic stability, etc. The involvement of the local OR staff could be limited to an anaesthesiologist and one assisting OR nurse during the proper procurement procedure. The Leuven procurement team, consisting of 2–3 surgeons, one scrub nurse and the procurement coordinator, was always fully equipped to perform the abdominal or/and thoracic organ procurement totally independent of the staff on-site, using its own instruments, cannulas, topical cooling fluid, preservation fluid, sterile ice, even sterile clothing etc.

Earlier problems encountered with foreign, frequently inexperienced, visiting extra-renal teams were avoided as much as possible during recent years by suggesting that the procurement of liver, pancreas and even lungs for other transplant centres should be performed by an own Leuven multiorgan procurement team: in 1993, about 75% of all extra-renal organs from our multi-organ donors were harvested by this abdominal team and transported afterwards to the foreign center. This approach largely facilitated the organization of organ recovery by shortening time delays between referral and procurement; it also reduced team travelling and travel expenses and sub-

stantially facilitated extra-renal organ exchange. Learning from this experience, we were able to promote the concept of a regional multi-organ procurement team and its potential to increase extra-renal organ donation on a larger scale [4].

The implementation phase encompassed professional education, which is not only essential to develop but is even more necessary to continue an effective partnership and commitment between a donor hospital and the transplant centre's OPO. The LCGT transplant coordinator and/or transplant centre's physicians therefore organized or participated in numerous formal in-service presentations in collaborating hospitals to emphasize not only the need for organs and the benefits of transplantation, but also to implement essential donor management principles and to illustrate medicolegal implications, and organizational and reimbursement modalities of cooperation. Frequent informal and personal contacts with key persons in the donor hospital further added to these educational goals. Participating nephrologists were invited to attend workshops or grand round presentations in the transplant centre on a 3-monthly basis. An annual report summarizing recovery and transplant activities within the LCGT was sent to all professionals involved in the donor hospitals. Recently a quarterly LCGT Newsletter has been added to these informative tools.

This feedback on recovery activities and the outcome of the transplanted organs proved to be extremely important in providing quality service to the donor hospital.

3.3. The LCGT donor hospital network: concurrent incentives

3.3.1. *The Belgian law on organ and tissue procurement and transplantation*

The third chapter of the Belgian law on the procurement and transplantation of organs, approved in June 1986 [3], deals with organ and tissue removal after death and has been based on the 'presumed consent' principle: organs or tissues can be removed from every citizen (or foreigner living for more than 6 months in the country) unless it is clear that an objection against removal has been expressed. By-laws have secured an easy and unique system of central registrations of objections: every citizen (parents or legal guardians may do so for minors or incapacitated individuals) can register an objection against post-mortem removal in their local Town Hall. This statement is transmitted immediately to a file of the National Registry in the capital, which is permanently accessible by modem to the transplant centres. Consultation of this database is mandatory before physicians can proceed with any organ or tissue removal. This Belgian law should be considered a 'weakened' presumed consent law: in the absence of any registered decision from the deceased person himself, relatives can use their full right to object against donation. Physicians, however, are no longer obliged to burden the relatives with any decision about donation: relatives are merely consulted and informed about the intentions to remove organs from the deceased, on first sight a subtle but nevertheless substantial difference. Although opinions differ within the professional community about the translation of the opting out principle in practice, one can consider the flexibility of this law as one of its merits: the treating physician keeps his individual responsibility to decide whether or not, or to what extent, he informs the relatives about the intention of organ recovery [5].

3.3.2. *Donor hospital reimbursement*

A subsequent step in maximizing the involvement of non-university hospitals and their medical staff was a fair reimbursement system covering the increasing expenses of adequate donor management and organ removal. Based on calculations of real management and recovery costs by LCGT staff members, a Royal Decree was implemented in January 1990 to reimburse donor management costs to the donor hospital with fixed lump sums per organ procured and consecutively transplanted. Similarly, local surgical teams are reimbursed if they perform organ procurement and preservation themselves, again powerful incentives aimed at further increasing multi-organ donation.

3.4. The LCGT donor hospital network: results

Figure 2 illustrates the organ procurement activities of the LCGT donor hospital network since 1984. During the last 10 years 1742 transplanted organs (1182 kidneys, 254 hearts, 247 livers, 30 lungs and 29 pancreases) originated from this group of collaborating hospitals. Since 1987, primarily as a result of legislative incentives, the number of kidneys procured has almost doubled. It should be noted that lung and pancreas donation has been fully encouraged only since 1992, as a result of starting transplant programme for these organs at the transplant centre. Our policy to consider each referred organ donor as a potential multi-organ donor, unless the contrary can be proved, resulted in a 83.3% and 84.2% multi-organ donation rate in respectively 1992 and 1993; in 1993, 88.6% of 53

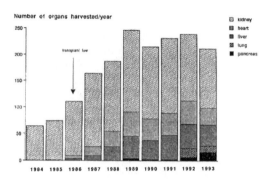

Figure 2. The Leuven Collaborative Group for Transplantation organ procurement activities (1984–1993).

donors less than 55 years old were multi-organ donors with pancreas donation in 57.4% (25.5% whole pancreas and 31.9% islets) and lung donation in 27.6% of these multi-organ donors. In comparison, the overall multi-organ donation rate in the Eurotransplant area in 1992 was 58%, with 72% in Belgium and only 56% and 44% in respectively Germany and The Netherlands [6].

4. Discussion

Several factors have contributed to the excellent results achieved with the LCGT donor hospital network: the implementation of a presumed consent law, incentives to increase awareness and motivation of donor hospital staff, state-of-the-art donor management procedures, a custom-tailored organization, educational tools such as the guidelines for brain death diagnosis, legislative guidelines, a donor data collection form and a multi-organ procurement technical guide, and reimbursement measures.

An adequate Belgian 'presumed consent' legislation should be considered as the cornerstone and necessary framework within which the above organizational incentives could further add to an efficient donor recruitment system. After its first voting in the Belgian Senate in 1985, the contribution of collaborative hospitals in donor referrals to the Leuven transplant centre has increased to 70% during recent years (Fig. 3). Of the legal and other incentives proposed to answer growing organ shortages, probably none will ever ensure completely the individual's right of self-determination, since both opting in and opting out approaches have demonstrated an inherent reluctance of the public to reflect on distant death, not to mention registering an explicit intention to donate organs. The Belgian approach, however, seems to offer a fair com-

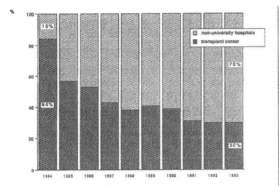

Figure 3. The Leuven Collaborative Group for Transplantation donor hospital network: relative contribution of collaborative donor hospitals in donor referrals compared with the Leuven transplant centre (1984–1993).

promise between collective altruism, rights of self-determination and respect for the next-of-kin's feelings when faced with the sudden death of their beloved.

Although principles of 'market segmentation' focus primarily on servicing hospitals with a reasonable number of potential donors per year, our flexible 'all-in' service approach, with minimal involvement of only a limited number of local staff and the procurement of extra-renal organs by one experienced Leuven team, was quite productive, especially in those hospitals with a lower potential for donation: during the last 5 years, of a total of 414 referrals, 94 donors (23%) originated from 18 hospitals with less than 5 donors/year, which resulted in the procurement of 163 kidneys, 55 hearts and 59 livers that otherwise would not have been available for transplantation.

Frequent organizational and surgical–technical problems encountered by inexperienced visiting procurement teams caused us to promote abdominal organ recovery by one expert local or regional procurement team instead of involving a kidney, a liver and a pancreas team. This approach has greatly facilitated the organization of a multi-organ donation procedure by shortening the time between donor referral and procurement, reducing team travelling time and expenses, and enlarging the exchange rate without jeopardizing the quality of the organs harvested. The Standardization of Eurotransplant Organ Procurement Procedures (SEOPP) Committee is currently studying the feasibility of implementing a certified regional procurement team concept [4]. A similar positive experience with regard to lung recovery by a local thoracic team resulted recently in increased exchange of not locally transplantable lungs, which explains the superior lung recovery rates within the LCGT during

1993 (17 lungs from 47 multi-organ donors younger than 55 years).

Since the implementation of the Belgian transplant law, the LCGT donor recruitment system has been able to answer the need for transplantable organs: contrary to the situation in neighbouring countries, our waiting list for e.g. cadaveric kidney transplantation, representing more than 60% of the patients in the Flanders region, did not increase for about 5 years, and even tended to decrease

4.1. Organ procurement in the future: new challenges, new opportunities

The excellent results obtained so far with this LCGT donor hospital development programme cannot be ignored, yet it would be naive to simply continue this approach without appropriate adaptations in order to answer new challenges. In a small country like Belgium, with a population of only 10 million inhabitants, eight transplant centres are becoming increasingly competitive today in 'claiming' scarce donor resources. This competition will further jeopardize donor recruitment in smaller hospitals: their medical staff, confused by claims from different transplant centres, will decline potential donor referrals, rather than to create local frictions between colleagues graduated from different medical schools.

New strategies obviously need to answer changing needs and concepts. One of these emerging challenges will be to find an answer to the question of who actually 'owns' a donor and will be allocated the organs: should it be the particular transplant centre that coincidentally could secure this donor via an 'old friends' network, or merely the larger regional community served by different transplant centres via an independent procurement organization with one common waiting list, in a system where transplant recipients have the freedom to choose their transplant centre of preference? In a society that is rightly demanding a more fair and transparent organ allocation system, measures need to be taken by governments, regional Health Authorities and/or supranational exchange organizations to protect against unfair preferences in allocating organs that result from an altruistic move by this society. Such developments being the case, it can be expected that in the near future the organization of organ/tissue donor recovery will become more and more independent from the influence of local transplant centres in Europe as a whole.

Whether hospital-based or not, these new recruitment structures can learn from previous experiences with donor hospital development, as realized within the LCGT. This donor hospital development should continue to be founded on basic 'service business' rules: obstacles to involvement should be removed and service demands stimulated. Ongoing analysis to find new opportunities in donor recovery should maximize recovery rates in the setting of a growing scarcity of resources. Regular feedback to the donor hospital should encourage professionals involved and demonstrate the 'rewards' of organ and tissue recovery for the society.

References

1. The Gallup Organization, Inc. 'The American Public's Attitudes Toward Organ Donation and Transplantation', conducted for The Partnership for Organ Donation, Boston, MA, February 1993.
2. Vanrenterghem Y, Waer M, Roels L, *et al.* Shortage of kidneys, a solvable problem? The Leuven Experience. In: Terasaki (ed.), Clinical Transplants 1988, UCLA Tissue Typing Laboratory, Los Angeles; 1988, pp. 91–7.
3. Wet betreffende het wegnemen en transplanteren van organen (13 June, 1986). Belgisch Staatsblad 14 February, 1987, pp. 2129–40.
4. Standardization of Eurotransplant Organ Procurement Procedures (SEOPP) Committee. Minutes of the Fügen 1993 Meeting. Eurotransplant Newsl 1993; 111: 9.
5. Roels L. Donor recruitment in Belgium. In de Charro FTh, Hessing DJ, Akyeld JEM (eds), Erasmus University, Rotterdam 1992, pp. 39–54.
6. de Boer J, De Meester J. Multi organ donor/transplant activities. In: Cohen B, Persijn G (eds), Eurotransplant Annual Report. 1992; pp. 35–48.

32 | Kidney preservation and graft outcome: Eurotransplant experience

J.M.J. DE MEESTER, J.M.A. SMITS, G.G. PERSIJN

1. Introduction

In organ transplantation, preservation techniques are used to counteract loss of functional and structural integrity of the organ during the period starting with its removal from the donor and ending with its implantation into the recipient. Successful preservation would enable maximum utilization of donor organs, and organ allocation schemes to be in compliance with medical and ethical principles. It also would allow surgery to be scheduled as a semi-elective procedure instead of an emergency operation, providing more time for immunological monitoring and recipient preparation. Last but not least, it would secure the immediate and optimal re-functioning of the transplanted organ.

This chapter outlines the principles of organ preservation and its impact on renal graft outcome, as analysed on the Eurotransplant Research Database.

2. Principles of kidney preservation

The basics of renal organ preservation are the use of hypothermia (0–4°C) and a so-called preservation solution. Hypothermia effectively suppresses the rate of cell death by slowing down cell metabolism, but after a couple of hours the organ will cease to be viable. Preservation solutions counteract, albeit to a variable extent and with varying success, the undesirable cellular damaging and metabolic changes such as cell swelling and acidosis, which emerge as result of hypothermia, and upon reperfusion with blood after the implantation of the organ [1].

The process of renal organ preservation can be divided into two phases: organ flush-out and organ storage. Two different methods are used for the second phase, organ storage (Table 1). In simple cold storage, the procured organ is placed in a bag containing the preservation solution (anaerobic) and stored on ice (0–4°C) in a container [2], until implantation. The second method is continuous hypothermic machine perfusion, in which the kidney is gently pulse-perfused, via the cannulated artery, with a cold (5–10°C) solution in a low concentration of oxygen [3] (aerobic); the perfusate allows substrates to be supplied and waste products of the metabolically active kidneys to be removed.

The first phase, organ flush-out, is practically the same for either method of organ storage. Immediately after circulatory arrest the vascular system of the organ is flushed in order to remove all blood from the organ and to cool the organ rapidly. The method of storage determines the type of solution. If simple cold storage is applied, the organ is to be flushed by the same preservation fluid as will be used for its storage. In order to secure optimal equilibration of all organ com-

G.M. Collins, J.M. Dubernard, W. Land and G.G. Persijn (eds). Procurement, Preservation and Allocation of Vascularized Organs 263–270
© 1997 Kluwer Academic Publishers.

Table 1. Organ storage modalities.

Modality	Simple cold storage (CS)	Hypothermic machine perfusion (MP)
Principle	Flush-out with cold storage preservation solution	Flush-out with 0.9% saline or Ringer's lactate
	Organ bagged with preservation solution and put in a box, filled with melting ice	Organ put in a small chamber, artery cannulated, continuously perfused with cold solution
	Anaerobic conditions Hypothermic, 0–4°C	Aerobic conditions Hypothermic, 5–10°C
Solution	EC, UW-CS, HTK Sachs, HOC	UW-MP
Assistance	No particular maintenance Check condition and amount ice	Well-trained technician to supervise pressure, flow rate, pump, etc.
Transport	Easy to arrange Cheap Flight: hands of crew	Difficult Expensive Flight: extra seat
Maximum successful kidney preservation	36–48 h	48–72 h
Delayed graft function	± 25%	± 10%

partments with the solution, an adequate volume should be administered, taking into consideration perfusion flow rate and hydrostatic pressure. When machine perfusion is used as the storage method, the flush solution can be 0.9% saline or Ringer's lactate. It should be noted that the preservation solutions used with the cold storage method are different from those used during machine perfusion, in terms of both components and concentrations (Table 2) [4].

Although machine perfusion produces a better quality of preservation over longer storage periods [3] with, on average, a lower incidence of primary non-function of the grafted kidneys, cold storage preservation has become the method of preference world-wide because of its better practicality for storage and transport.

3. Kidney preservation in Eurotransplant

In the Eurotransplant organization, the collaborating countries, Austria, Belgium, Germany, Luxemburg and The Netherlands, have mainly always used the cold storage method to preserve donor kidneys. In 1976, during the annual Eurotransplant meeting, the Organ Preservation Working Committee decided to introduce the EuroCollins' (EC) solution as the standard solution for donor kidneys in order to replace the existing wide variety in cold storage solutions [5]. As of 1988, the University of Wisconsin (UW) cold

storage solution [6] gradually replaced EC solution as the preservation fluid for abdominal organs obtained from multi-organ donors, because of its superiority in liver and pancreas preservation. Simultaneously, some centres also utilized the histidine-tryptophan-ketoglutarate (HTK) cold storage solution [7] derived from Bretschneider's solution for cardioplegia [8]; this was used mainly in kidney-only donors.

Between August 1988 and August 1989, Eurotransplant was the platform for the European multicentre randomized clinical trial comparing preservation with UW solution and EC solution in liver and pancreas transplantation, in kidney transplantation from multi-organ donors as well as in kidney-only donors [9,10]. Between July 1990 and August 1992, a two-arm randomized trial was performed, comparing HTK versus EC solution and HTK versus UW solution, both in kidney-only donors [11].

4. Characteristics of EC, UW and HTK cold storage solutions

Table 2 shows the different composition of the three cold storage solutions. In brief, the EC solution is rich in glucose, which serves as energy substrate and impermeant, contains a phosphate buffer and has an electrolyte composition which resembles the intracellular milieu. Histidine buffer, a low potassium level and a low viscosity are the main features of the HTK

Table 2. Composition of cold storage preservation solutions (EC, HTK and UW-CS) and the machine perfusion solution UW-MP.

		EC	HTK	UW-CS	UW-MP
Sodium	(mmol/l)	10	15	30	100
Potassium	(mmol/l)	115	10	120	25
Magnesium	(mmol/l)	–	4	5	5
Sulphate	(mmol/l)	–	–	5	–
Calcium	(mmol/l)	–	–	–	05
Bicarbonate	(mmol/l)	10	–	–	–
Chloride	(mmol/l)	15	50	–	20
Phosphate	(mmol/l)	67	–	25	15
Histidine/Histidine-HCl	(mmol/l)	–	180/18	–	–
HEPES	(mmol/l)	–	–	–	10
Glucose	(mmol/l)	194	–	–	10
Lactobionate	(mmol/l)	–	–	100	–
Raffinose	(mmol/l)	–	–	30	–
Hydroxyethyl starch	(g/l)	–	–	50	50
Mannitol	(mmol/l)	–	30	–	30
Gluconate	(mmol/l)	–	–	–	85
Ribose	(mmol/l)	–	–	–	5
Adenosine	(mmol/l)	–	–	5	–
Adenine	(mmol/l)	–	–	–	5
Glutathione	(mmol/l)	–	–	3	3
Allopurinol	(mmol/l)	–	–	1	1
Tryptophan	(mmol/l)	–	2	–	–
Ketoglutarate	(mmol/l)	–	1	–	–
Insulin	(U/l)	–	–	100	40
Dexamethasone	(mg/l)	–	–	8	4
Penicillin G	(U/l)	–	–	200 000	200 000
Osmolarity	(mOsm/l)	355	310	320	320
pH		7.25	7.3	7.4	7.4
Price of 1 l solution ($US)		10	85	300	–

solution. The UW solution, again potassium-rich and containing a phosphate-buffer, uses raffinose and lactobionate to prevent cell swelling and contains many substances which are either stimulators of ATP synthesis or anti-oxidants.

5. Efficacy of EC, UW and HTK

Many publications on the transplantation of kidneys procured from heart-beating donors indicate the superiority of UW over EC, measured by a reduced incidence of delayed graft function [9,12], and/or of vascular complications [13], and/or by an overall improved graft survival [9,14]. The few studies comparing EC and HTK demonstrated the better performance of HTK-preserved kidneys [15]. An interim report on the prospective trial comparing HTK and UW in cadaveric kidney transplant

found no significant difference in delayed graft function and 1-year graft survival [11].

Regarding kidney transplantation from non-heart-beating donors. there is again evidence that UW is superior to EC [16] and also to HTK [17].

6. Renal graft outcome and preservation solutions: Eurotransplant experience

6.1. Materials and methods

All transplantations using kidneys from cadaveric heart-beating donors performed between 1988 and 1994 in the Eurotransplant countries were included ($n = 15011$). Combined kidney and non-renal organ transplants were excluded.

The kidney allocation scheme of Eurotransplant starts with a mandatory exchange for '000' HLA-A, B, DR mismatched donor–recipient combinations; the local transplant programme then selects its best local recipient(s), taking into account a minimal degree of HLA-B and HLA-DR sharing; finally, the kidneys are allocated following a stepwise sorting based upon HLA-matching, HLA-immunization and waiting time.

The recipient, donor and transplant characteristics of the UW, HTK and EC groups were compared using the χ^2 test. Graft loss was defined as return to dialysis, graft nephrectomy or patient death, and survival probabilities were calculated by the Kaplan–Meier method [18]. To evaluate the influence of the preservation solutions when other prognostic factors were taken into account a two-step multivariate analysis using the Cox model was performed [19]: donor sex and age, cause of death of the donor, procurement procedure (multi-organ donor versus kidney-only donor), order of kidney transplant (first versus repeat), shipment – irrespective of the distance to be covered – of the donor kidney (yes versus no), cold ischaemia time, recipient sex and age, HLA-B,DR mismatch (broad HLA-antigens) and peak degree of immunization. By modelling an interaction factor between preservation solution and cold ischaemia time, the similar effect of each of the three preservation solutions over three time periods (0–24 h, 25–36 h, > 36 h) was assessed (yes versus no). In all Cox analyses, two-tailed p-values were used, with $p \leqslant 0.05$ considered as significant. For data handling SAS 6.08 was used while statistical analysis was performed with SPSS 6.0.

6.2. Results

6.2.1. *Descriptive analysis*
In this analysis, 4258 transplanted kidneys (28%) had been perfused using EC, 2963 (20%) with HTK and 7790 (52%) with UW (Table 3). Patients transplanted with a HTK-preserved kidney were, on average, significantly older (45 years) than patients receiving a EC- or UW-preserved kidney (44 and 43 years, respectively; $p = 0.01$). The HTK group included fewer patients with a peak immunization level of $\geq 6\%$ panel reactive antibodies (PRA) than the EC and UW group. The mean age of UW donors (34 years) was significantly lower than that of EC and HTK donors (41 and 43 years, respectively; $p = 0.000$). More multi-organ donors were found in the UW group (83%), whereas the EC and HTK group mainly consisted of kidney-only donors (78% and 62%; $p = 0.000$). The

main cause of death for the three groups differed significantly: most of the HTK and EC donors suffered cerebrovascular accidents (CVA; 48% and 44% respectively), in contrast to the UW donors of whom the majority died as a result of a head trauma (44%). The transplant characteristics showed no significant difference between the three groups.

6.2.2. *Graft survival in a univariate analysis*
The overall graft survival for UW-perfused kidneys was significantly better than for EC- and HTK-perfused kidneys during the 3-year post-transplant follow-up period (Fig. 1). Stratifying these curves according to cold ischaemia periods (Table 4), the EC-group showed the worst graft outcome in each of the three cold ischaemia periods (≤ 24 h, 25–36 h and > 36 h). No difference was seen between UW and HTK when the cold ischaemia time was $\leqslant 24$ h, but with more extended cold ischaemia periods, HTK was unable to keep up with the UW performance and the outcome approached that of EC grafts.

6.2.3. *Graft survival in a multivariate analysis*
Factors of prognostic importance for graft survival appeared to be (Table 5): recipient gender (male versus female) ($p < 0.0000$), recipient age ($p = 0.001$), peak %PRA ($p < 0.0000$), donor gender (male versus female) ($p = 0.02$), donor age ($p = 0.0001$), procurement procedure (multi-organ versus kidney only; $p = 0.0001$), order of transplantation (first versus repeat; $p = 0.01$), HLA-B,DR mismatch gradient (0 versus 1,2,3,4; $p < 0.0000$), shipment of the kidney (no versus yes; $p = 0.001$).

The preservation solution exerted an independent effect on the kidney graft survival: UW-preserved kidneys had less chance of graft failure (UW versus HTK, EC; $p = 0.03$). In addition, as the interaction term between preservation solution and cold ischaemia period was also significant ($p = 0.01$), the influence on graft survival of each preservation solution depended on the duration of the cold ischaemia time. The survival of UW-perfused kidneys was influenced less by cold ischaemia time than that of EC- and HTK-perfused kidneys.

6.3. Discussion and conclusion

When using cold storage as preservation, the best possible renal graft survival is currently obtained using UW solution rather than EC and HTK solutions. The current analysis of the Eurotransplant database clearly confirms this superiority of UW in a univariate as well as in a multivariate analysis.

Table 3. Recipient, donor and transplant characteristics of the EC, HTK and UW groups.

	EC ($n = 4258$)	HTK ($n = 2963$)	UW ($n = 7790$)	p
Recipient				
Gender				
Male	2622 (62%)	1824 (62%)	4748 (61%)	0.7
Female	1636 (38%)	1139 (38%)	3042 (39%)	
Mean age (years) (SE)	44 (0.1)	45 (0.1)	43 (0.1)	0.01
Peak pretransplant immunization				
0–5%	2429 (57%)	1834 (62%)	4674 (60%)	0.000
6–84%	1502 (36%)	962 (33%)	2556 (33%)	
≥ 85%	308 (7%)	150 (5%)	520 (7%)	
Not known	19	17	40	
Transplant order				
First	3703 (87%)	2568 (87%)	6712 (86%)	0.4
Repeat	555 (13%)	395 (13%)	1078 (14%)	
Donor				
Gender				
Male	2696 (63%)	1817 (61%)	4795 (62%)	0.1
Female	1562 (37%)	1146 (39%)	2995 (38%)	
Mean age (years) (SE)	41 (0.2)	43 (0.2)	34 (0.2)	0.000
Cause of death				
Head trauma	1701 (40%)	1026 (35%)	3396 (44%)	0.000
CVA	1885 (44%)	1435 (48%)	3288 (42%)	
Other	672 (16%)	502 (17%)	1106 (14%)	
Procurement procedure				
Multi-organ	951 (22%)	1133 (38%)	6426 (83%)	0.000
Kidney only	3307 (78%)	1830 (62%)	1346 (17%)	
Not known	–	–	18	
Transplant				
HLA-B,DR mismatch				
0	1092 (26%)	768 (26%)	2057 (27%)	0.2
1	1565 (37%)	1106 (37%)	2860 (37%)	
2	1391 (32%)	939 (32%)	2548 (32%)	
3	180 (4%)	130 (4%)	280 (3%)	
4	26 (1%)	19 (1%)	28 (1%)	
Not known	4	1	17	
Shipment of kidney				
Yes	1777 (42%)	1302 (44%)	3231 (42%)	0.06
No	2481 (58%)	1661 (56%)	4559 (58%)	
Mean cold ischaemia time (h) (SE)	24 (0.1)	23 (0.1)	23 (0.1)	0.1

SE = standard error of mean.

Particularly in multi-organ donors, UW is nowadays *the* solution to flush out all intra-abdominal organs, since it also correlates with the best graft survival in liver and pancreas transplantation (compared to EC; only a few data on HTK). One could argue that the beneficial effect of UW is due to its use in multi-organ donors, which are often the ideal donors (young male, better donor management). This is not true, since EC and HTK also show a better survival of kidneys procured from multi-organ donors [20].

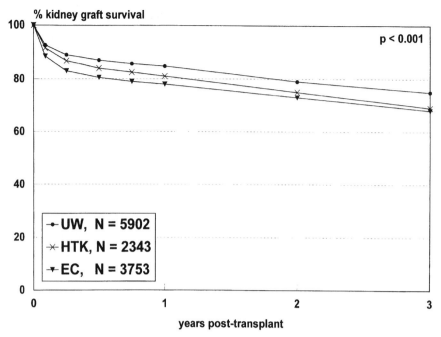

Figure 1. Kidney graft survival, stratified according to preservation solution (top line: UW; middle line: HTK; bottom line: EC).

Preservation solution		Cold ischaemia time (h)			
		0–24	25–36	> 36	Not known
EC solution					
n	3753	2190	1379	184	505
1 year	78	80 (0.9)	76 (1.2)	75 (3.2)	
2 years	73	75 (1)	71 (1.3)	71 (3.4)	
3 years	68	71 (1)	66 (1.4)	67 (3.7)	
HTK solution					
n	2343	1431	826	86	620
1 year	82	84 (1)	79 (1.5)	70 (5)	
2 years	75	78 (1)	72 (1.9)	64 (5.6)	
3 years	69	72 (1)	67 (2.3)		
UW solution					
n	5902	3672	1992	238	1888
1 year	85	85 (0.6)	85 (0.8)	84 (2.4)	
2 years	79	80 (0.8)	79 (1)	78 (2.9)	
3 years	75	75 (1)	75 (1.3)	75 (3.4)	

Table 4. Percentage kidney graft survival at 1, 2 and 3 years: preservation solution versus cold ischaemia time.

Standard error of mean in parentheses.

In kidney allocation systems, exchange of donor kidneys contributes to the goal of achieving the best overall graft survival. The penalty of exchange is often a longer cold ischaemia time: the median cold ischaemia times for transplants with locally procured and exchanged donor kidneys were 20 and 24 h, respectively (G.G. Persijn, personal communication). Though this difference is statistically significant, there is doubt about its clinical relevance. Cold storage of donor kidneys regularly extends beyond 24 h, placing

Table 5. Kidney graft survival: multivariate analysis.

Factors used in the multivariate analysis	p
Recipient gender (male versus female)	0.0000
Recipient age	0.001
Peak % PRA	0.0000
Transplantation (first versus repeat)	0.01
Donor gender (male versus female)	0.02
Donor age	0.0001
Donor cause of death (head trauma versus CVA, other)	0.8
Procurement procedure (MOD versus KOD)	0.0001
HLA-B,DR mismatch (0 versus 1, 2, 3, 4)	0.0000
Shipment of the kidney (no versus yes)	0.001
Cold ischaemia period (0–24 versus 25–36, > 36 h)	0.7
Preservation solution (UW versus HTK, EC)	0.03
Interaction term between preservation solution and cold ischaemia period	0.01

extra demands on the preservation solutions. The significant interaction factor between preservation solution and cold ischaemia time demonstrates that the effect of a solution depends on the cold ischaemia time. Beyond 24 h, the outcome of EC- and HTK-perfused donor kidneys is severely jeopardized compared with UW-perfused donor kidneys. The ability reliably to preserve donor kidneys, independent of the cold ischaemia period, underscores the value of UW solution. This is in agreement with the results of analysis of the CTS database [21]. Nevertheless, it should be noted that, when the cold ischaemia period is less than 24 h HTK seems to be an excellent alternative to the more expensive UW. Since hard data are still lacking on the transplant performance of HTK-perfused and stored livers and pancreata, HTK is only used instead of UW in kidney-only donors and donors from whom kidneys and thoracic organs will be procured.

Unfortunately, with the current donor procedure arrangements, one cannot anticipate the duration of cold ischaemia for the kidneys at the time one has to choose the preservation solution. Only upon the availability of a reliable donor HLA-typing prior to the organ procurement, will suitable recipients be identified much earlier, without off-setting the benefits of HLA-matching. Subsequently, by tuning logistics at the donor hospital as well as the recipient hospital, cold ischaemia time can be shortened [22]; only then can a more economical choice be made among equally successful preservation solutions.

7. Epilogue

Reliable organ preservation is a major factor in successful organ transplantation. With regard to renal transplantation, UW solution is to be preferred as flush-out and cold storage solution, demonstrating the best graft survival when compared with EC and HTK solutions.

References

1. Ploeg RJ. Principles in organ preservation. In: Ploeg RJ (ed.), Preservation of Kidney and Pancreas with the UW Solution. Thesis Leiden, 1991: 39–52.
2. Collins GM. Bravo-Shugarman MB. Terasaki PI. Kidney preservation for transplantation: initial perfusion and 30 hour ice storage. Lancet 1969; 2: 1219–22.
3. Belzer FO, Ashby BS, Dumphy JE. 24-hour and 72-hour preservation of canine kidneys. Lancet 1967; 2: 536–8.
4. Hoffmann RM, Belzer FO. Organ preservation: kidney, liver, pancreas. In: Philips MG (ed.), UNOS: Manual of Organ Procurement, Preservation and Distribution in Transplantation. Richmond, 1991: 105–19.
5. Rijksen JFWB. Die Probleme verschiedener Konservierungsflüssigkeiten in den Eurotransplant-Spenderzentren. Wisssenschaftliche Informationen Fresenius-Stiftung. Acta Nephrol 1977; 3: 93–6.
6. Sollinger HW. Vernon WB, D'Alessandro AM et al. Combined liver and pancreas procurement with Belzer – UW solution. Surgery 1989; 106: 685–91.
7. Groenewoud AF, Buchholz B, Gubernatis G et al. First results of the multicenter study on the HTK protection for kidney transplants. Transplant Proc 1990; 22: 2212.
8. Bretschneider HJ. Myocardial protection. Thorac Cardiovasc Surg 1980; 28: 285–302.
9. Ploeg RJ, Bockel van JH, Langendijk PTH et al. Effect of preservation solution on results of cadaveric kidney transplantation. Lancet 1992; 340: 129–37.
10. Ploeg RJ, Bockel van JH, Langendijk PTH et al. Clinical use of UW solution in liver and pancreas transplantation: a preliminary report. In: Ploeg RJ (ed.), Preservation of Kidney and Pancreas with the UW Solution. Thesis Leiden, 1991: 185–202.
11. Groenewoud AF, Thorogood J. Current status of the Eurotransplant multi-center study comparing kidney graft preservation with HTK, UW and EC solutions. Transplant Proc 1993; 25: 1582–5.
12. Porteous C, Stewart RM, Findlay J et al. Improved immediate renal allograft function following aggressive donor management and perfusion with UW solution. Transplant Proc 1991; 23: 2338–40.
13. Benoit G, Jaber N, Moukarzel M et al. Incidence of vascular complications in kidney transplantation: is there any interference with the nature of the perfusion solution? Clin Transplant 1994; 8: 485–7.
14. D'Alessandro AM, Kalayoglu M, Sollinger HW et al. Current status of organ preservation with University of Wisconsin solution. Arch Pathol Lab Med 1991; 115: 306–10.
15. Hölscher M, Groenewoud AF. Current status of the HTK solution of Bretschneider in organ preservation. Transplant Proc 1991; 5: 2334–7.
16. Sakagami K, Takasu S, Kawamura T et al. A comparison of University of Wisconsin and Euro-Collins' solutions for simple cold storage in non-heartbeating cadaveric kidney transplantation. Transplantation 1989; 49: 824–6.
17. Booster MH, van der Vusse GJ, Wijnen RMH et al. University of Wisconsin solution is superior to Histidine Tryptophan Ketoglutarate for preservation of ischemically damaged kidneys. Transplantation 1994; 58: 1–7.

18. Cox DR, Oakes D. Analysis of Survival Data. Chapman and Hall, London 1988.
19. Krzanowski WJ. Principles of multivariate analysis. Clarendon Press, Oxford 1988.
20. Smits JMA, De Meester J, Persijn GG. The outcome of kidney grafts from multiorgan donors and kidney-only donors. Transplantation 1996; 62: 767–71.

21. Opelz G. Collaborative Transplant Study Newsl 1993; 2: 2–3.
22. Gnant MFX, Rosenmayr A, Wamser P et al. Prenephrectomy tissue typing using donor lymph node cells: a reliable and safe way of shortening cadaver kidney ischemia time. Transplant Proc 1991; 23: 2685–6.

33 Primary dysfunction after orthotopic liver transplantation

RUTGER J. PLOEG

1. Introduction

In the last decade liver transplantation has emerged from clinical experimentation to become an accepted means of treatment for end stage liver disease [1–4]. The development of new immunosuppressants and enhanced modalities to treat postoperative rejection and infection have significantly increased patient and graft survival. The improved results mean that many adults and children with end stage liver disease are able to resume a nearly normal life after successful transplantation. In the last 10 years the number of liver transplants performed per year has increased from approximately 600 to more than 3000 in the USA and from 200 to 1500 in Europe. One of the factors which contributed significantly to this expansion was the introduction of the University of Wisconsin (UW) solution by Belzer and colleagues in 1986 [5–7]. With this new preservation solution the donor liver, pancreas, kidneys and small bowel could be flushed and cold-stored for a period sufficiently long to allow long distance procurement, organ sharing on an international scale, improved recipient preparation and implantation of organs without major detrimental effects on the immediate function after transplantation [8–10]. Also, with an increasing demand for donor livers suitable for pediatric recipients, livers could now be evaluated and reduced or even split during lengthy back-table procedures [11–13].

Despite these achievements, primary dysfunction of the liver persists to be a major complication immedi-

ately after orthotopic liver transplantation and may cause significant morbidity and mortality [14–16]. Well known and often described is the devastating complication of primary non-function (PNF), which leads to death of the patient unless an urgent retransplantation is performed. A persistent problem in this respect remains the lack of a clear definition of primary non-function. Due to differences in clinical assessment and access to donor organs for retransplantation between transplant centres, the reported incidence of primary non-function can vary substantially.

The occurrence of primary dysfunction immediately after transplantation should not be a surprise, since every transplanted liver carries the burden of a magnitude of potential injuries related to donor diagnosis, brain death, preservation, and reperfusion in the hostile environment of the recipient at time of transplantation. Many details of this complex process of injury, as well as the immediately required repair of the procured, preserved and transplanted organ, are still unclear. In the following paragraphs primary dysfunction in the clinical setting will be discussed, followed by a modest side step towards current views on how to ameliorate immediate function after liver transplantation.

2. Definitions of non-function: PNF, IPF and PDF?

In the past we have been confronted with a lack of agreement on the definition of primary non-function

G.M. Collins, J.M. Dubernard, W. Land and G.G. Persijn (eds). Procurement, Preservation and Allocation of Vascularized Organs 271–280
© 1997 Kluwer Academic Publishers.

(PNF) after liver transplantation. Although most experts in the field agree that PNF results in either retransplantation or death, no consensus was apparent regarding the time interval between actual transplantation and the definitive diagnosis of PNF, which could vary from 48 h to 14 days. To a certain extent, the definition of PNF in an individual centre seemed to be related to the availability of a new liver and the ability to retransplant the rapidly deteriorating patient. This resulted in markedly different reporting rates for the same event, adding to the confusion. It also became apparent that classifying recipients as either PNF or immediate function (IF) was too simple: a substantial number of recipients had a graft with just enough function to support life, but which displayed a substantial amount of hepatic injury. Many such patients finally recovered, some after extended morbidity and hospitalization, while others died weeks after transplantation.

For the purpose of clarification and better understanding, we suggested the use of the term initial poor function (IPF) in addition to primary non- (and never) function (PNF), and the term primary dysfunction (PDF) to describe both forms of inadequate function in the early period after liver transplantation [17]. We defined IPF as AST > 2000 IU/l, prothrombin time (PT) more than 16 s, and ammonia > 50 μmol/l on postoperative days 2–7. All three parameters had to be fulfilled, which probably underestimates the actual number of IPF livers. Patients with IPF either recovered, died or were retransplanted more than 7 days' post-transplant. PNF was defined as non-life-sustaining function of the liver requiring retransplantation or leading to death within 7 days after liver transplantation.

Poor function has been defined by several authors in a similar way [18–21]. In a well written review on this topic, Strasberg and his group stated that in most studies AST or ALT levels of > 2000–3500 IU/l were used to identify PDF in the first week after transplantation, revealing similar percentages [22]. They felt that using transaminases alone was undesirable and agreed with our discrimination of IPF using AST and PT; however, they doubted the extra benefit of including ammonia levels as a second indicator of biosynthetic function. After re-analysing our data their doubts appeared to be correct; we thus agree that AST and PT are sufficient to identify IPF. Strasberg also suggested modification of the definition of PNF to death or retransplantation within 14 days rather of 7 days after liver transplantation in recipients with IPF [22]. This remains questionable: primary non-function is by definition a description for the most extreme form of IPF and should be reserved for those grafts that show no life-supporting function at all after transplantation and, in retrospect, never have developed any life-supporting function. Recipients with PNF livers have to be re-listed as soon as possible for retransplantation and it is unlikely that these patients will survive more than one week post-transplant without a liver despite major intensive care. This is in contrast to initial poor functioning livers, which require additional support but are likely to recover eventually. Day-to-day review of the clinical condition and laboratory parameters within the first week post-transplant should reveal the trend towards either non- (and never) function or poor function with the potential of recovery that justifies a wait-and-see policy.

3. Towards clinical risk factor analyses

Primary non-function (PNF), the most serious form of primary dysfunction, occurs in 2–23% of patients and results in death unless an urgent retransplantation is performed, as mentioned above [9,23,24]. Less well recognized and defined as a separate clinical entity is initial poor function (IPF) of the liver, which represents borderline function immediately after liver transplantation. Livers with IPF will either recover after a prolonged period of dysfunction or lead to death or retransplantation at a later date. Primary dysfunction (PDF), including both PNF and IPF, is probably multifactorial [25]. Potential risk factors for PDF may include agonal events in the donor, procurement and preservation techniques, as well as recipient-related factors. As increasing numbers of liver transplants are performed in the USA and Europe due to significant expansion of recipient selection and less discrimination of donors, since donor resources remain limited, it is likely that the primary dysfunction rate will increase further [1,26,27]. To reduce the incidence of PDF and to improve patient and graft survival after liver transplantation it becomes important, therefore, to identify those risk factors associated with the occurrence of PNF and IPF. For this reason we developed a retrospective multivariate analysis model at the University of Wisconsin to evaluate a number of donor, preservation and recipient factors and their correlation with PNF and IPF.

3.1. Risk factors for primary dysfunction

In a series of 323 consecutive OLT performed at the University of Wisconsin, the effect of a large number of donor, preservation and recipient factors on PNF and IPF was analysed [17]. The relative contribution of each of these factors to the incidence of PDF was determined using a stepwise logistic regression model. Three month survival rate was calculated since effects of primary dysfunction and impact on survival should reveal themselves within the short term after liver transplantation.

3.1.1. *PDF: PNF, IPF and survival*

An important finding in the Wisconsin study was that the incidence of PDF was 22%, implying that 1 in 5 liver recipients will not have immediate life-sustaining liver function. In 6% of the livers with PDF, PNF occurred after liver transplantation. Despite the fact that the use of the UW solution has been shown to reduce the incidence of PNF [9,28], this number is considered high. Initial poor function was observed in 16% of the livers when strict criteria were applied containing the combination of significantly elevated hepatocellular enzymes and prolonged prothrombin time, reflecting inadequate synthetic function, and increased ammonia levels. The results showed that IPF is indeed a major complication after liver transplantation. Although not as devastating as PNF, IPF is associated with a significantly higher mortality (21%), graft failure rate (34%) and retransplantation rate (15%) within the first 3 months than that in patients with immediate liver function (7%, 12% and 9%, respectively; $p < 0.001$). These results were confirmed by Mor *et al.*, who analysed 365 OLT procedures and calculated a 13% incidence of IPF and a graft failure rate of 29% within the first 3 months [18]. When the UW solution was introduced in Europe, we performed a prospective multicentre study in a large number of European liver transplant centres to evaluate the effect of the new solu-

tion. The use of the UW solution in liver transplantation was found to be safe, effective and allowed significantly longer preservation times with increased organ sharing [29]. In a recent updated analysis, Porte *et al.* evaluated 303 consecutive liver transplants in 280 patients included in this multicentre study and found that PNF occurred in 7% and IPF in 14% [30]. Graft survival at 3 months was significantly adversely affected by four risk variables: retransplantation, blood group incompatibility, recipient diagnosis of acute hepatic failure and recipient age less than 16 years (Table 1).

3.1.2. *Donor factors*

When donor factors possibly contributing to PNF or IPF were evaluated in our Wisconsin study by univariate analysis, longer stay of the donor in the hospital (> 3 days), older donor age (> 49 years), and fatty changes in the donor liver biopsy resulted in a significantly higher PDF rate. Length of hospital stay was found to have a significant correlation with PDF in the univariate ($p < 0.05$) but not in the multivariate analysis. There has been a lot of speculation concerning the concept of starvation of potential donors since the nutritional status of the donor liver could have an important effect on outcome after transplantation and Intensive Care Unit patients are prone to malnutrition. Strasberg's group demonstrated that the degree of preservation injury strongly correlated with the nutritional status of the donor liver in the rat model [31], and similar results were obtained by Belzer's

Table 1. European Multicentre Study on UW solution in liver transplantation: multivariate analysis of risk variables for 3-month graft survival after first transplantation (*n* = 266, excluding technical failures).

Co-variate	Full model		Final model after backward elimination	
	RR	p-value	RR	p-value
Blood group match (incompatible vs identical)	3.55	0.03	3.81	0.01
Diagnosis (acute failure vs others)	1.16	0.78	NS	NS
Cold ischaemia time (> 18 h vs ≤ 18 h)	2.36	0.04	2.43	0.03
Recipient age (paediatric vs adult)	3.08	0.01	3.14	0.01
Donor age	1.03	0.02	1.03	0.01
Sex match				
Female to female	2.70	0.03	2.43	0.03
Male to female	2.33	0.04	2.17	0.03
Female to male (vs male to male)	1.32	0.60	1.00	

RR = relative risk; NS = not statistically significant.

group in rabbits [32]. In the clinical setting, the length of hospitalization of the donor has been shown to affect the incidence of PNF [33]. Obviously, length of stay is only one variable which represents a number of factors related to brain death, donor condition and donor management which have yet to be clarified.

In a number of series, the effect of donor age effect on outcome has been evaluated. Most studies have performed univariate analyses and have not been able to rule out confounding factors, e.g. recipient factors such as poor Child–Pugh status. In the Wisconsin study, donor age was evaluated as a continuous variable as well as a discrete variable (cohort analysis). In both analyses, older donor age significantly increased the incidence of PDF ($p < 0.009$). This corroborates earlier reports by UNOS showing significantly lower 1-year patient survival when livers were used from 45–55-year-old donors versus donors aged 15–45 [34]. However, a report by the Baylor group in Texas suggested that use of a liver from an aged donor (> 50) is as safe as the use of a young liver [18].

Portman has pointed out the hazard of transplanting a fatty liver [35]. D'Alessandro reported an increased risk of PNF when accepting livers with severe fatty infiltration [36]. Our multivariate analysis confirmed his earlier findings and showed an additional significant effect of moderate (30–60%) and severe (> 60%) fatty changes on the incidence of IPF. Later, these data were supported by Adam in Paris: following D'Alessandro's definition of fatty infiltration, the combined groups of moderate and massive fatty infiltration had a significantly higher PNF rate (13%) than the group of livers without signs of steatosis (2.5%) [37]. Mortality rose from 5.6% in recipients of normal grafts to 21% in the steatotic group. As a result of these data, many centres have stopped transplanting livers with more than moderate fatty changes. Since fatty changes are not always macroscopically visible, many teams have started to perform routine donor liver biopsies during procurement, before flush-out and cold storage of the organ.

Another variable is the donor diagnosis: the presence of intracranial haemorrhage in the donor was associated with a high rate of IPF showing a trend towards statistical significance, although it was difficult to speculate cause–effect relationship between this factor and IPF. Donor livers may also be injured as a result of the disease or injury leading to brain death through metabolic, endocrine or cardiovascular alterations [38,39]. It is also possible that interaction at this level of our univariate analysis has occurred with another variable, such as donor age, which could explain the significance of the effect. Further details are summarized in Table 2.

3.1.3. Cold ischaemia and preservation

When cold ischaemia-related factors were analysed a significant effect on IPF and PNF was seen with extended preservation, especially when cold storage times were longer than 18 h. As previously reported by the Pittsburgh group, successful transplantation is feasible following up to 34 h preservation with UW solution [24], and in Madison and other centres many livers have been transplanted after preservation times > 20 h without detrimental effects [8,28]. Nevertheless, the results caution against extended preservation of the liver, especially when this is not necessary, since prolonged cold storage is accompanied by a higher incidence of both IPF and PNF. From a clinical study it is almost impossible to conclude how much different components such as pre-preservation injury, cold preservation injury, rewarming injury and reperfusion injury contribute to the preservation time effect [25]. Cold ischaemia is a relative risk factor (Table 2). In the study by Adam et al. cold ischaemia time was evaluated in a cohort analysis and determined to be a risk factor when it extended beyond the arbitrary cut-off point of 12 h. No significance was reached, however, when cold ischaemia was calculated as a continuous variable ($p = 0.07$) [37]. In the European Multicentre study on UW solution in liver transplantation, we found that increased cold ischaemia times were associated with a trend ($p = 0.07$) towards lower graft survival (Fig. 1). In the cohort analysis, preservation over 18 h had an adverse effect on graft survival in first transplants. In retransplants cold ischaemia time was kept short, with a range of 2–14 h. Obviously, and despite its efficacy, use of UW solution will delay but not entirely prevent preservation-related PDF. We should, therefore, consider cold ischaemia time as a relative risk factor, although the duration of preservation at which this risk becomes significant remains unclear.

In the Wisconsin analysis no effect was seen on PDF when the duration of the anastomosis time during the transplant procedure was evaluated; however, the majority of livers was vascularized and reperfused within 60 min, which remains within the acceptable limits of warm ischaemia time tolerated by the liver [40].

Other factors such as local team procurement versus shipped-in organs and liver-only versus combined liver–pancreas retrieval had no effect on PDF in this series.

3.1.4. Recipient factors

When recipient factors are analysed, significant factors for occurrence of IPF or PNF were use of reduced-size livers, recipient age and renal insufficiency. Reduced-

Table 2. Effect of donor risk factors on primary dysfunction after 323 orthotopic liver transplantations at the University of Wisconsin, Madison.

	Post-transplant incidence (%)[a]			p[b]
	IF $(n = 250)$	IPF $(n = 53)$	PNF $(n = 20)$	
Diagnosis				
Trauma	86	9	5	
Miscellaneous	79	15	6	0.07
IC haemorrhage	67	23	10	
Hospital stay (d)				
< 3	80	16	4	
3–4	74	17	9	0.05
> 4	73	16	11	
Donor age (y)				
<16	83	13	4	
16–49	77	17	6	0.03
> 49	45	36	19	
Preservation time (h)				
1–6	83	14	3	
6–12	83	13	4	
12–17	74	18	8	0.004
> 17	62	27	11	
Liver biopsy:				
fatty changes				
None	81	14	5	
Mild (< 30%)	79	16	5	
Moderate				
(30–60%)	70	30	0	0.0001
Severe (> 60%)	0	20	80	

[a] IF: immediate function; IPF: initial poor function; PNF: primary nonfunction.
[b] Univariate analyses: p value shows significance for increased IPF and PNF per risk factor: χ^2 and Mantel–Haenzel χ^2.

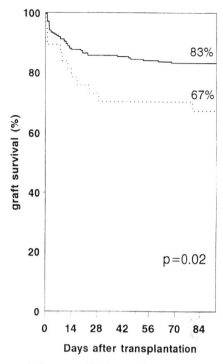

Figure 1. European Multicenter Study on UW solution in liver transplantation: Effect of cold ischemia time (CIT) on graft survival after first liver transplantations. Numbers of grafts at risk, with CIT $\leqslant$ 12 h: 148; CIT > 12 h: 118. Numbers of grafts at risk, with CIT $\leqslant$ 15 h: 197; CIT > 15 h: 64. Number of grafts at risk, with CIT $\leqslant$ 18 h: 234, CIT > 18h: 27 [30].

size liver transplants have been performed successfully at selected centres [41–44]. Initially, centres were reluctant and concerned about the potential for ischaemic damage and subsequent complications [42,45]. Since UW solution was introduced, the number of reduced-size liver transplants in paediatric recipients has significantly increased [46]. The increased incidence of PDF in this group demonstrated in the Wisconsin study is not a general finding (Otte, personal communication). A high IPF rate could be explained by reduction in liver mass with subsequent elevation of hepatocellular enzymes and slowly recovering synthetic function. Additional preparation and handling of reduced-size livers might also have caused ischaemic damage and

subsequent complications. Occurrence of PNF in a number of reduced-size liver series could, in retrospect, be explained partially by the use of older donor livers and use of fatty livers in the early part of these series and a donor–recipient weight ratio of more than 4–6:1.

Recipient age has a significant effect on primary dysfunction, although in an unexpected way. Advanced age has always been considered a relative contraindication to solid organ transplantation because of increased risk of cardiac or infectious complications and a higher mortality [47–49]. In contrast, however, univariate analysis showed that younger recipients suffered from more PDF than older patients. This confirmed the results reported by Pirsch *et al.*, who demonstrated that successful liver transplantation can be performed in recipients over 60 years of age with similar morbidity and patient or graft survival to that in younger patients [50]. The surprising finding that younger age is associated with a high PDF rate could be explained by interaction with the significant factor of reduced-size livers, which have been transplanted in young recipient group. This phenomenon shows the fallibility of univari-

Table 3. Effect of recipient risk factors on primary dysfunction after 323 orthotopic liver transplantations in the University of Wisconsin, Madison.

	Post-transplant incidence (%)[a]			p[b]
	IF ($n = 250$)	IPF ($n = 53$)	PNF ($n = 20$)	
Reduced liver				
No	81	14	5	0.0001
Yes	50	34	16	
Recipient age (years)				
< 16	71	23	6	
16–44	75	16	9	0.03
> 44	84	13	3	
Renal insufficiency				
No	79	15	6	0.02
Yes	52	37	11	

[a] IF: immediate function; IPF: initial poor function; PNF: primary nonfunction.
[b] Univariate analyses: χ^2 and Mantel–Haenzel χ^2.

ate analysis and reinforces the need for a multivariate analysis before any conclusions can be drawn. Finally, renal insufficiency prior to liver transplantation is associated with increased PDF after liver transplantation, illustrating other authors' findings that hepatorenal syndrome or renal insufficiency are predictors of a poor outcome after orthotopic liver transplantation (Table 3) [51–54].

3.1.5. *Perioperative factors*
It remains questionable whether perioperative factors are true primary and causal factors or just derivatives and sequelae related to donor, reperfusion and recipient factors. Of the perioperative factors in the univariate analysis, increased use of packed red blood cells and fresh frozen plasma correlate with a higher PDF rate. In contrast to other authors, our group concluded that it is not correct to define blood product use as a primary separate risk factor in a multivariate analysis. Like other perioperative factors such as anaesthesia, surgery and bypass time, the volume of blood products used is related to a large number of other causes and thus multifactorial. As a complex mixed factor, it should be regarded as an end-point or result of other chronologically earlier events. Blood product use will significantly depend on donor factors, surgical technique, recipient condition, etc. Inclusion would intro-

Table 4. The Wisconsin risk factor model: donor and recipient risk factors associated with increased incidence of primary nonfunction (PNF) and initial poor function (IPF) after orthotopic liver transplantation evaluated with a multivariate analysis using a (stepwise) logistic regression model.

	p
Reduced size livers	0.0001
Fatty donor liver biopsy[a]	0.001
Older donor age	0.009
Retransplantation	0.01
Renal insufficiency	0.02
Longer cold storage	0.02

[a] Subset $n = 158$ orthotopic liver transplantations with donor liver biopsies since 1987.

duce a possible bias in the multivariate analysis of risk factors for PDF after liver transplantation.

3.1.6. *Multivariate analysis*
When all donor and recipient factors possibly contributing to IPF and PNF were evaluated by multivariate analysis, the stepwise logistic regression model demonstrated that reduced-size livers, older donor age, moderate to severe fatty changes in the donor liver biopsy, retransplantation, renal insufficiency prior to liver transplantation and prolonged preservation times determined the incidence of IPF and PNF [17]. No interaction or interdependence was found between these factors (Table 4). Also, and surprisingly, no significant correlation was observed between the aetiology of liver disease, nutritional status, UNOS status, Child's–Pugh classification, and PDF. In studies by Alexander and Vaughn, UNOS status had a significant impact on 1-year survival [34] and, in contrast to our study, Mimeault also detected a relation between recipient medical status and IPF [55]. The lack of statistically significant correlation between some of these factors in our study and IPF or PNF does not necessarily prove lack of relationship between these variables and PDF.

4. Towards improvement of PDF

In the past decade, the understanding of the cellular basis for ischaemia and reperfusion-related injury has increased dramatically. Moreover, some findings in animal experiments have been in part confirmed by clinical studies after liver transplantation. Donor treatment to increase the tolerance to ischaemia and reperfusion injury of the liver may include nutritional support of the liver with glycogen [56,57], pretreatment with drugs such as chlorpromazine and dexamethasone [58,59], or protection with N-acetylcysteine [60]. On the other hand, pretreatment is a double edged sword: multiple organs are procured from > 50% of donors and drug manipulation might interfere with function of some of the other organs and have adverse effects. It might also be possible to suppress reperfusion injury in the recipient. The majority of rodent experiments have revealed some beneficial effects with the use of vasodilators [61], calcium channel blockers [62,63], inhibitors of eicosanoid metabolism [64,65] and with a number of scavengers of reactive oxygen species [66,67]. In the larger dog and pig model, or in the clinical situation, however, no improvement has been documented. Since causes of primary dysfunction after transplantation are multifactorial it is unlikely that treatment of the recipient only will result in ultimate success.

As a result of increased preservation times and prolonged cold ischaemic storage, structural changes occur in the various hepatic cell types. Most authors, however, believe that despite significant swelling of the hepatocytes, loss of viability leading to primary non-function is closely related to activation of Kupffer cells and injury of endothelial cells. Sinusoids become occluded as a consequence of the swelling of hepatocytes: this has been shown to be less dramatic in livers stored in UW solution than in EuroCollins' solution. After reperfusion hepatocyte swelling quickly reverses and only limited loss of hepatocyte viability is seen [68]. Lemasters' group has shown that oxygen consumption and carbohydrate metabolism remain within normal limits after extended times of preservation followed by reperfusion [69,70]. These findings have led to the speculation that dysfunction after transplantation is possibly not caused by damaged hepatocytes.

More dramatic is the ischaemia and reperfusion injury seen in sinusoidal endothelial cells. After short periods of cold storage the typical rounding of endothelial cells and retraction of the cytoplasm reverses; however, with longer preservation times denudation of the sinusoidal lining is found after reperfusion and livers lose their viability [71,72]. After 24 h of cold ischaemia in EuroCollins', reperfusion is followed by a 40% loss of viability of non-parenchymal cells as indicated by exclusion dye staining. The so-called reperfusion-induced endothelial cell killing is initiated after approximately 6–8 h of preservation in EuroCollins' reaching its maximum after 24 h. Preservation in UW solution has significantly increased the time of storage and made livers less vulnerable to reperfusion induced killing of endothelial cells [25,68].

Kupffer cells, the macrophages of the liver, appear to be relatively unharmed by cold ischaemia itself. On reperfusion, however, marked activation of Kupffer cells has been noted [69,73,74] and prominent structural changes are seen, with cell surface retraction, vacuole formation followed by degranulation. After 24 h of storage in EuroCollins' 100% of the Kupffer cells are activated on reperfusion. As a result of this activation, Kupffer cells release inflammatory mediators such as reactive oxygen species, including superoxide radicals and nitric oxide, and cytokines such as tumour necrosis factor, IL-1 and IL-6. Proteases and prostaglandins are also released [75–77].

An interesting approach by Thurman's group in North Carolina resulted in the development of the Carolina rinse solution [78]. This mildly acidic solution (pH 6.5) contains the electrolytes of Ringer's solution, antioxidants (allopurinol, desferroxamine, glutathione), substrates for ATP regeneration (fructose, glucose, insulin, adenosine), a calcium channel blocker (nicardipine) and hydroxyethyl starch. A significant reduction of activation of Kupffer cells and leukocyte accumulation, almost total abolition of endothelial cell killing and improved bile flow and microvascular blood flow were seen in the rat (transplant) model [79,80]. The concept of the Carolina rinse solution is in line with the ideas of Belzer and Southard that are best reflected in their choice of components for the UW solution [4]. To date, no additional beneficial effect of the Carolina rinse solution, when used together with UW solution, has been found in the larger animal model or clinically. Sanchez et al. tested the Carolina rinse solution and compared it with Plasmalyte prior to reperfusion in clinical liver transplantation [81]. No PNF occurred in either group with rather short cold ischaemia times of less than 9 h. Post-transplant AST, bilirubin, alkaline phosphatase and GGT levels in the group receiving livers treated with Carolina rinse solution were significantly lower than those in the control goup. Final conclusions, however, have to await completion of a larger clinical trial.

An entirely separate issue is the question concerning the effect of brain death itself on organ function in the donor. Only very limited research has been performed on this topic until now, and this has concentrated mainly on hormonal function. We have recently started to evaluate the hypothesis of potential predisposition towards organ injury during the period of prolonged and unphysiological brain death in the donor. Up-regulation of proto-oncogenes, cytokines and other precursors may very well in part be responsible for the initial 'formes frust' of ischaemic injury in transplantable organs. Subsequent preservation and reperfusion-related injury could then aggravate the damage and lead to primary dysfunction after liver transplantation.

5. Static cold storage or machine perfusion?

Currently, the predominant technique of preservation for the liver is static cold storage. Due to organ shortage, acceptance criteria for donor livers are less stringent. The use of marginal donors and livers with longer cold ischaemia times will increase the effect of ischaemia and reperfusion injury. It is questionable whether an improvement of the UW solution or another new preservation fluid will ameliorate this type of injury. After a certain preservation time, solutions used in static cold storage will not be able to reverse dominant catabolic processes and prevent time-dependent degradation of the liver: the limits of safe static cold storage have been reached. Therefore, maybe more emphasis should be directed towards Belzer's old concept of experimenting with hypothermic continuous machine perfusion for the liver. In clinical kidney transplantation, despite the significant reduction in delayed graft function (DGF) to 23% with UW solution [82], machine preservation is still associated with a lower DGF than the cold storage method. In the dog model, initially 5-day and later 7-day preservation and successful transplantation was possible using machine preservation [83,84]. Previously reported experiments by Pienaar et al. have shown successful liver transplantation after 72 h machine preservation in the dog model [85]. Hypothermic machine perfusion maintains the concentrations of ATP, glutathione, energy stores, cellular Na^+/H^+ ion pump activity, and calcium- and ATP-dependent cytoskeleton structure. Waste products are flushed away and diluted in the ocean effect of the volume of the preservation solution in the well of the machine perfusion system.

Preventing metabolic depression is the best way to increase the quality of the liver and prolong preservation time. Thus, upon reperfusion, the liver may be more capable of rapidly returning to normal function. Machine perfusion may also be able to salvage marginal livers procured because of an increasing demand for transplantable livers. In this respect, machine preservation could also be used to develop a viability assay based on analysing perfusate samples during preservation to distinguish viable from non-viable livers.

6. Summary

The results discussed above highlight the importance of immediate function of the liver after transplantation.

They also demonstrate the significant impact of PNF and IPF as two distinguished forms of primary dysfunction: PNF as a well known form of dysfunction and IPF of the liver as a separate form which we have tried to describe and define as a difficult intermediate group of malfunctioning livers.

In conclusion, initial poor function of livers (IPF) should be recognized as a separate clinical entity with its own significant effects. It is not the purpose of this discussion to advocate that all livers that involve a risk factor for IPF or PNF which is shown to be significant should be discarded and not transplanted. This would be rather unrealistic in the face of a persistent donor shortage which, unfortunately, requires compromise. The data provided should be used as background information to facilitate the clinical judgment of the responsible transplant team for the individual liver transplant recipient. On the other hand, one ought to realize that a combination of significant donor and recipient risk factors will certainly lead to a poor outcome after liver transplantation. If no risk factors are present, extended preservation with all its advantages, such as elective surgery, is justified. In the individual situation when a number of risk factors has to be accepted, preservation time is the only variable which can be controlled and should be kept as short as possible. In the near future we will hopefully, with the help of advanced techniques, be able to anticipate or even reverse ischaemia and reperfusion injury. This, however, will only be successful if we attempt to unravel as many risk factors as possible and include in our research the full sequence of potential liver injury related to the brain-dead donor, cold ischaemia time and, finally, the reperfusion in a hostile recipient environment.

Acknowledgements

I am indebted to my late mentor Dr. Folkert O. Belzer and the members of the Transplant Team at the Department of Surgery, University of Wisconsin, Madison, USA. I am also grateful to my colleagues and all participants in the European Multicentre Study on Organ Preservation with UW Solution who have contributed so much to our current clinical knowledge on organ procurement, preservation/reperfusion and outcome after transplantation.

References

1. Bismuth H, Ericzon BG, Rolles K et al. Hepatic transplantation in Europe. Lancet 1987; 2: 674–9.
2. First MR. Transplantation in the nineties. Transplantation 1992; 53: 1–5.
3. Starzl TE, Demetris AJ, van Thiel D. Liver transplantation. N Engl J Med 1989; 321: 1014–19.

4. Belzer FO, Southard JH. Principles of solid-organ preservation by cold storage. Transplantation 1988; 45: 673–9.

5. Wahlberg JA, Love RB, Landegaard L, Southard JH. Belzer FO. 72-hours' preservation of the canine pancreas. Transplantation 1987; 43: 5–8.

6. Ploeg RJ, Goossens D, McAnulty JF, Southard JH, Belzer FO. Successful 72-h storage of the dog kidney with UW solution. Transplantation 1988; 46:191–6.

7. Jamieson NV, Sundberg R, Lindell S, Southard JH, Belzer FO. Preservation of the canine liver for 24–48 hours using simple cold storage with UW solution. Transplantation 1988; 46: 517–25.

8. Kalayoglu M, Sollinger HW, Stratta RJ et al. Extended preservation of the liver for clinical transplantation. Lancet 1988; 1: 617–18.

9. Todo S, Nevy J, Yanaga K, Podesta L, Gordon RD, Starzl TE. Extended preservation of human liver grafts with UW solution. JAMA 1989; 261: 711–15.

10. Sollinger HW, Vernon WB, D'Alessandro AM, Kalayoglu M, Stratta RJ, Belzer FO. Combined liver and pancreas procurement with Belzer–UW solution. Surgery 1989; 106: 685.

11. Broelsch CE, Emond JC, Thistlethwaite JR, Rouch DA, Whitington PF, Lichtor JL. Liver transplantation with reduced-size donor organs. Transplantation 1988; 45: 519–24.

12. Pichlmayr R, Ringe B, Gubernatis G, Hauss J, Bunzendahl H. Transplantation einer Spenderleber auf zwei Empfänger (Splitting-Transplantation) – Eine neue Methode in der Weiterentwicklung der Lebersegmenttransplantation. Langenbecks Arch Chir 1988; 373: 127–30.

13. Emond JC, Whitington PF, Thistlethwaite JR, Cherqui D, Alonso EA, Woodle IS et al. Transplantation of two patients with one liver. Analysis of a preliminary experience with 'split-liver' grafting. Ann Surg 1990; 212: 14–22.

14. Gordon RD, Iwatsuki S, Esquivel CO et al. Liver transplantation. In Cerilli GJ (ed.), Organ Transplantation and Replacement. Lippincott, Philadelphia 1987, 511–16.

15. Shaw BW Jr, Gordon RD, Iwatsuki S, Starzl TE. Retransplantation of the liver. Semin Liver Dis 1985; 5: 394.

16. Demetris AJ, Sheahan DG. The role of the pathology department in a liver transplant program. Gastroenterol Clin North Am 1988; 17: 93–5.

17. Ploeg RJ, D'Alessandro AM, Knechtle SJ, Stegall MD, Pirsh JD, Hoffman RM, Saski T et al. Risk factors for primary dysfunction after liver transplantation: a multivariate analysis. Transplantation 1993; 55: 807–13.

18. Mor E, Klintmalm GB, Gonwa TA, Solomon H, Holman MJ, Gibbs JF, Watemberg I et al. The use of marginal donors for liver transplantation. Transplant Proc 1992; 53: 383–6.

19. Makowka L, Gordon RD, Todo S, Ohkohchi N, Marsh JW, Tzakis AG, Yokoi H et al. Analysis of donor criteria for the prediction of outcome in clinical liver transplantation. Transplant Proc 1987; 19: 2378–82.

20. Howard TK, Goran B, Klintmalm G, Cofer J, Husberg BS, Goldstein RM, Gonwa TA. The influence of preservation injury on rejection in the hepatic transplant recipient. Transplantation 1990; 49: 103–7.

21. Greig PD, Forster J, Superina RA, Strasberg SM, Mohamed M, Blendis LM, Taylor BR et al. Donor-specific factors predict graft function following liver transplantation. Transplant Proc 1990; 22: 2072–3.

22. Strasberg SM, Howard TK, Molmenti EP, Hertl M. Selecting the donor liver: risk factors for poor function after orthotopic liver transplantation. Hepatology 1994; 4: 829–38.

23. Greig PD, Woolf GM, Sinclair SB et al. Treatment of primary liver graft non-function with prostaglandin E1. Transplantation 1989; 48: 447–50.

24. Furukawa H, Todo S, Imventarza O et al. Effect of cold ischemia time on the early outcome of human hepatic allografts preserved with UW solution. Transplantation 1991; 51: 1000.

25. Clavien PA, Harvey PRC, Strasberg SM. Preservation and reperfusion injuries in liver allografts: an overview and synthesis of current studies. Transplantation 1992; 53: 957–62.

26. Belle SH, Detre KM, Beringer KC, Murphy JB, Vaughn WK. Liver transplantation in the United States: 1988–1989. In: Terasaki PI (ed.) Clinical Transplants 1990. UCLA Tissue Typing Laboratory, Los Angeles 1991; 11–14.

27. Otte JB. Recent developments in liver transplantation: lessons from 5-year experience. J Hepatol 1991; 12: 386–9.

28. D'Alessandro AM, Kalayoglu M, Sollinger HW et al. Experience with Belzer UW cold storage solution in human liver transplantation. Transplant Proc 1990; 22: 474–6.

29. Ploeg RJ, for the European Multicenter Trial. Preliminary results of the European Multicenter Study on UW solution in liver transplantation. Transplant Proc 1990; 22; 2185–8.

30. Porte RJ, Terpstra OT, Hansen BE, van Bockel JH, Thorogood J, Persijn GG, Hermans J, Ploeg RJ for the European Multicentre Study Group. Effect of UW solution on graft survival and function after liver transplantation. Transplantation 1996 (submitted).

31. Morgan GR, Sanabria JR, Clavien PA et al. Correlation of donor nutritional status with sinusoidal lining cell viability and liver function in the rat. Transplantation 1991; 51: 1176–88.

32. Boudjema KS, Lindell SL, Southard JH, Belzer FO. The effects of fasting on the quality of liver preservation by simple cold storage. Transplantation 1990; 50: 943–6.

33. Pruim J, van Woerden WF, Knol E et al. Donor data in liver grafts with primary non-function – a preliminary analysis by the European Liver Registry. Transplant Proc 1989; 21: 2383.

34. Alexander JW, Vaughn WK. The use of marginal donors for organ transplantation: influence of donor age on outcome. Transplantation 1991; 51: 135–9.

35. Portmann B, Wight DGD. Pathology of liver transplantation (excluding rejection). In: Calne R (ed.), Liver Transplantation. Grune and Stratton, Orlando 1987; p. 437–41.

36. D'Alessandro AM, Kalayoglu M, Sollinger HW et al. The predictive value of donor liver biopsies for the development of primary nonfunction after orthotopic liver transplantation. Transplantation 1991; 51: 157–61.

37. Adam R, Bismuth H, Diamond T, Ducot B, Morino M, Astarcioglu I, Johann M et al. Effect of extended cold ischemia with UW solution on graft function after liver transplantation. Lancet 1992; 340: 1373–6.

38. Wartofsky L, Burman KD. Alterations in thyroid function in patients with systemic illness: the 'euthyroid sick syndrome.' Gen Endocrinol Rev 1982; 3: 164.

39. Sazontseva IE, Kozlov IA, Moisuc YG, Ermolenko AE, Afonin VV, Ilnitskiy VV. Hormonal response to brain death. Transplant Proc 1991; 23: 2464–5.

40. Delva E, Camus Y, Nordlinger B et al. Vascular occlusions for liver resections. Operative management and tolerance to hepatic ischemia. Ann Surg 1989; 209: 211–15.

41. Bismuth H, Houssin D. Reduced-size orthotopic liver graft in hepatic transplantation in children. Surgery 1984; 95: 367–71.

42. Broelsch CE, Emond JC, Thistlethwaite JR et al. Liver transplantation with reduced-size donor organs. Transplantation 1988; 45: 519–23.

43. de Hemptinne B, de Ville de Goyet J, Kestens PH, Otte J. Volume reduction of the liver graft before orthotopic transplantation: report of a clinical experience in 11 cases. Transplant Proc 1987; 19: 3317–19.

44. Burdelski J, Schmidt K, Hoyer PF et al. Liver transplantation in children: the Hannover experience. Transplant Proc 1987; 19: 3277–8.

45. Broelsch CE, Emond JC, Thistlethwaite JR et al. Liver transplantation, including the concept of reduced-size liver transplants in children. Ann Surg 1988; 208: 410–15.

46. Kalayoglu M, D'Alessandro AM, Sollinger HW, Hoffman RM, Pirsch JD, Belzer FO. Experience with reduced-size liver transplantation. Surg Gynecol Obstet 1990; 171: 139–41.

47. Ost L, Groth CG, Lindholm B, Lundgren G, Magnusson G, Tillegard A. Cadaveric renal transplantation in patients of 60 years and above. Transplantation 1980; 30: 339–44.

48. Kock B, Kuhlback B, Ahonen J, Lindfors O, Lindstrom BL. Kidney transplantation in patients over 60 years of age. Scand J Urol Nephrol (Suppl) 1980; 54: 103–7.

49. Wedel N, Brynger H, Blohme I. Kidney transplantation in patients 60 years and older. Scand J Urol Nephrol (Suppl) 1980; 54: 106–10.

50. Pirsch JD, Kalayoglu M, D'Alessandro AM et al. Orthotopic liver transplantation in patients 60 years of age and older. Transplantation 1991; 51: 431–5.

51. McCauley J, Van Thiel DH, Starzl TE, Puschett JB. Acute and chronic renal failure in liver transplantation. Nephron 1990; 55: 121–6.

52. Gonwa TA, Morris CA, Goldstein RM, Husberg BS, Klintmalm GB. Long term survival and renal function following liver transplantation in patients with and without hepatorenal syndrome-experience in 300 patients. Transplantation 1991; 51: 428–32.

53. Cuervas-Mons V, Millan I, Gavaler JS, Starzl TE, Van Thiel DH. Prognostic value of preoperatively obtained clinical and laboratory data in predicting survival following orthotopic liver transplantation. Hepatology 1986; 6: 922–7.

54. Danovitch GM, Wilkinson AH, Colonna JO, Busuttil RW. Determinants of renal failure in patients receiving orthotopic liver transplants. Kidney Int 1987; 31: 195–9.

55. Mimeault R, Grant D, Ghent C, Duff J, Wall W. Analysis of donor and recipient variables and early graft function after orthotopic liver transplantation. Transplant Proc 1989; 21:3355.

56. Pattou F, Boudjema K, Kerr-Conte J, Wolf P, Jaeck D, Cinqualbre J. Rapid restoration of hepatic glycogen in donors before harvesting improves outcome of the pig liver graft. Transplant Proc 1994; 26: 23–4.

57. Cywes R, Greig PD, Morgan GR, Sanabria JR, Clavien P, Harvey PRC, Strasberg SM. Rapid donor liver nutritional enhancement in a large animal model. Hepatology 1992; 16: 1271–9.

58. Claesson K, Lindell S, Southard JH, Belzer FO. Chlorpromazine, quinicrine, and verapamil as donor pretreatment in liver preservation, tested in the isolated perfused rat liver. Cryobiology 1991; 28: 422–7.

59. Tokunaga Y, Wicomb WN, Conception W, Nakazato P, Collins GM, Esquivel CO. Successful 20-hour rat liver preservation with chlorpromazine in sodium lactobionate sucrose solution. Surgery 1991; 110: 80–6.

60. Nakano H, Boudjema K, Alexandre E, Imbs P, Chenard MP, Wolf P, Cinqualbre J, Jaeck D. Protective effects of N-acetylcysteine on hypothermic ischemia-reperfusion injury of rat liver. Hepatology 1995; 22: 539–45.

61. Anaise D, Ishimaru M, Madariaga J, Irisawa A, Lane B, Zeidan B, Sonoda K, Shabtai M, Waltzer WC, Rapaport FT. Protective effects of trifluoperazine on the microcirculation of cold-stored livers. Transplantation 1990; 50: 933–9.

62. Ar'Rajab W, Ahren B, Bengmark S. Improved liver preservation for transplantation due to calcium channel blockade. Transplantation 1991; 51: 965–6.

63. Hisanaga M, Nakajima Y, Wada T, Kanehiro H, Fukuoka T, Horikawa M, Yoshimura A, Kido K, Taki J, Aomatsu Y, Ueno M, Ko S, Nakano H. Protective effect of the calcium channel blocker diltiazem on hepatic function following warm ischemia. J Surg Res 1993; 55: 404–10.

64. Post S, Palma G, Gonzalez G, Rentsch M, Otto G, Menger MD. Role of eicosanoids in reperfusion injury in rat liver transplantation. Transplant Proc 1993; 25: 2547–51.

65. Urade M, Izumi R, Lyobe T, Iwasa K, Masutani H, Tani T, Yabushita K, Hashimoto T, Kiriyama M, Shimizu K, Yagi M, Miyazaki I. Changes of thromboxane B2 level in experimental orthotopic liver transplantation in swines: the effect of warm ischemia and thromboxane A2 synthetase inhibition. Transplant Proc 1993; 24: 1623–4.

66. Cosenza CA, Cramer DV, Cunneen SA, Tuso PJ, Wang HK, Makowka L. Protective efect of the lazaroid U74006F in cold ischemia-reperfusion injury of the liver. Hepatology 1994; 19: 418–25.

67. Goode HF, Webster NR, Howdle PD, Leek JP, Lodge JPA, Sadek SA, Walker BE. Reperfusion injury, antioxidants and hemodynamics during orthotopic liver transplantation. Hepatology 1994; 19: 354–9.

68. Caldwell-Kenkel JC, Thurman RG, Lemasters JJ. Selective loss of nonparenchymal cell viability after cold, ischemic storage of rat livers. Transplantation 1988; 45: 834–7.

69. Caldwell-Kenkel JC, Currin RT, Tanaka Y, Thurman RG, Lemasters JJ. Reperfusion injury to endothelial cells following cold ischemic storage of rat livers. Hepatology 1989; 10: 92–9.

70. Marzi I, Zhong Z, Lemasters JJ, Thurman RG. Evidence that graft survival is not related to parenchymal cell viability in rat liver transplantation: the importance of nonparenchymal cells. Transplantation 1989; 48: 463–8.

71. Myagkaya GL, Veen HA van, James J. Ultrastructural changes in the rat liver during Euro-Collins storage, compared with hypothermic in vitro ischemia. Virchows Arch B 1987; 53: 176–82.

72. MeKeown CMB, Edward V, Philips MJ, Harvey PR, Petrunka CN, Strasberg SM. Sinusoidal lining cell damage: the critical injury in cold preservation of liver allografts in the rat. Transplantation 1988; 46: 178–91.

73. Lemasters JJ, Caldwell-Kenkel JC, Currin RT, Tanaka Y, Marzi I, Thurman RG. Endothelial cell killing and activation of Kupffer cells following reperfusion of rat livers stored in Euro-Collins solution. In: Wisse E, Knook DL, Decker (eds.). Cells of the Hepatic Sinusoid. Vol 2. Kupffer Cell Foundation, Rijswijk 1989; pp. 277–80.

74. Caldwell-Kenkel JC, Currin RT, Tanaka Y, Thurman RG, Lemasters JJ. Kupffer cell activation and endothelial cell damage after storage of rat livers: effects of reperfusion. Hepatology 1991; 13: 83–95.

75. Lindert KA, Caldwell-Kenkel JC, Nukina S, Lemasters JJ, Thurman RG. Activation of Kupffer cells on reperfusion following hypoxia: particle phagocytosis in a low-flow, reflow model. Am J Physiol 1992; 262: G345–50.

76. Rymsa B, Wang JF, Groot H de. O_2-release by activated Kupffer cells upon reoxygenation. Am J Physiol 1991; 261: G602–7.

77. Colletti LM, Remick DG, Burtch GD, Kunkel SL, Strieter RM, Campbell DA. The role of tumor necrosis factor alpha in the pathophysiologic alterations following hepatic ischemia/reperfusion injury. J Clin Invest 1990; 85: 1936–43.

78. Currin RT, Toole JG, Thurman RG, Lemasters JJ. Evidence that Carolina rinse solution protects sinusoidal endothelial cells against reperfusion injury after cold ischemic storage of rat liver. Transplantation 1990; 50: 1076–8.

79. Gao W, Hijioka T, Lindert KA, Caldwell-Kenkel JC, Lemasters JJ, Thurman RG. Evidence that adenosine is a key component in Carolina rinse responsible for reducing graft failure after orthotopic liver transplantation in the rat. Transplantation 1991; 52: 992–8.

80. Post S, Rentsch M, Gonzalez AP, Palma P, Otto G, Menger MD. Effects of Carolina rinse and adenosine rinse on microvascular perfusion and intrahepatic leukocyte-endothelium interaction after liver transplantation in the rat. Transplantation 1993; 55: 972–7.

81. Sanchez-Urdazpal L, Gores GJ, Lemasters JJ, Thurman RG, Steers JL, Wahlstrom HE, Hay EI, Porayko MK, Wiesner RH, Krom RAF. Carolina rinse solution decreases liver injury during clinical liver transplantation. Transplant Proc 1993; 25: 1574–5.

82. Ploeg RJ, Bockel JH van, Langendijk PTH, Groenewegen M, Woude FJ van der, Persijn GG, Thorogood J, Hermans J (for the European Multicentre Study Group). Effect of preservation solution on results of cadaveric kidney transplantation. Lancet 1992; 340: 129–37.

83. McAnulty JF, Ploeg RJ, Southard JH, Belzer FO. Successful five-day perfusion preservation of the canine kidney. Transplantation 1989; 47; 37–41.

84. Schilling M, Saunder A, Southard JH, Belzer FO. Five-to-seven day kidney preservation with aspirin and furegrelate. Transplantation 1993; 55: 955–8.

85. Pienaar BH, Lindell SL, Gulik TM van, Southard JH, Belzer FO. Seventy-two-hour preservation of the canine liver by machine perfusion. Transplantation 1990; 49: 258–60.

34 | Results of intestinal transplantation

R. Margreiter

1. Introduction

Because of the large amount of lymphoid tissue in the small bowel, its immunogenicity is much greater than that of solid organs. In addition, graft-versus-host (GVH) disease has been identified as a major problem in animal experiments [1]. Alexis Carrel demonstrated the technical feasibility of intestinal transplantation 90 years ago and correctly predicted rejection to be the main obstacle [2]. Almost 70 years later the first series of successful small bowel transplants in animals was reported by Lillehei [3]. The same author published a clinical case of intestinal transplantation in 1967 [4], although the two first cases of intestinal transplantation had already been performed by Deterling and colleagues at the Boston Floating Hospital in 1964 [5]. Neither of these cases, however, has been reported in detail. Since the results of intestinal transplantations performed so far have been highly dependent on the type of immunosuppression used, it seems reasonable to break down the entire series of intestinal transplants according to immunosuppression.

2. Conventional immunosuppression

Between 1964 and 1970 a total of seven isolated intestinal transplants were performed using steroids and azathioprine as the primary immunosuppression. Technical failures and rejection were major problems and led to graft loss in all instances. Some basic data of these seven transplants are summarized in Table 1 [1].

3. Cyclosporin A

The availability of Cyclosporin renewed interest in bowel transplantation. Between 1983 and 1991 13 isolated small bowel transplants, five combined bowel

Table 1. Isolated intestinal transplants with conventional immunosuppression.

No.	Year	Centre	Graft	Source of the Graft	Outcome (Graft Survival)
1	1964	Boston	Segment ileum	Mother	Necrosis (12 h)
2	1964	Boston	ESB	Cadaver	Necrosis (2 days)
3	1967	Minnesota	ESB + colon	Cadaver	Necrosis (12 h)
4	1968	São Paulo	ESB	Cadaver	Necrosis (10 days)
5	1969	Paris	ESB + right colon	Cadaver	Rejection (26 days)
6	1969	Jackson, Mississippi	ESB	Mother	Necrosis (7 days)
7	1970	São Paulo	ESB	Cadaver	Necrosis (5 days)
8	1970	New York	Ileum	Sister	Died sepsis (76 days)

Abbreviation: ESB = entire small bowel.

G.M. Collins, J.M. Dubernard, W. Land and G.G. Persijn (eds). Procurement, Preservation and Allocation of Vascularized Organs 281–284
© 1997 Kluwer Academic Publishers.

Table 2. Isolated intestinal transplants with cyclosporin-based immunosuppression.

No.	Year	Centre	Immunosuppression	Source of the Graft	Outcome (Graft Survival)
1	1985	Toronto	CyA-Ster	Cadaver	Haemolysis (0 → A) Rejection, died (11 days)
2	1987	Chicago	CyA-Ster	Cadaver	Rejection (10 days)
3	1987	Paris	CyA-Ster	Cadaver	Thrombosis (3 h)
4	1987	Paris	CyA-Ster	Cadaver	Chronic rejection (6 months)
5	1987	Kiel	CyA-Ster-ATG	Mother	Rejection (12 days)
6	1988	London (Ontario)	CyA-Ster-Aza-ALG	Cadaver	Rejection (15 days)
7	1988	Kiel	CyA-Ster-ATG	Half-sister	Chronic rejection, renal failure, died 1993
8	1988	Paris	CyA-Ster-ALG	Cadaver	Chronic rejection (17 months)
9	1989	Paris	CyA-Ster-Aza-ALG	Cadaver	Rejection (2 months)
10	1989	Paris	CyA-Ster-Aza-ALG	Cadaver	Chronic rejection (36 months)
11	1989	Uppsala	CyA-Ster-Aza-ALG	Cadaver	Rejection, sepsis (56 days)
12	1990	Paris	CyA-Ster-Aza-ALG	Cadaver	Haemolysis, rejection (21 days)
13	1990	Paris	CyA-Ster-Aza-ALG	Cadaver	Perioperative death

CyA, cyclosporin A; Ster, steroids; ATG, antithymocyte globulin; ALG, antilymphocyte globulin.

and liver transplants and nine intestinal transplants as part of a multivisceral graft were carried out worldwide. The isolated intestinal transplants are summarized in Table 2. As can be seen, rejection was still the major cause of graft loss in this small series. There were, however, three survivors. The first patient to survive with a functioning intestinal transplant was transplanted in Kiel in 1988 [6]. This patient had to be treated for several acute rejection episodes and eventually died from renal failure and chronic rejection 5.5 years after transplantation (E. Schweizer, personal communication). Remarkable success was also reported from Paris, where one paediatric recipient lived free of total parenteral nutrition (TPN) for almost 3 years and another paediatric recipient survived for 17 months [7].

Eight combined liver–small bowel transplants have been performed under cyclosporin-based immunosuppression. The first such transplant was carried out in 1988 in London, Ontario, in a 41-year-old female suffering from short-gut syndrome and antithrombin III deficiency [8]. This patient lived for 5.5 years with excellent function of both grafts. Another patient from the same centre has now survived for more than 4 years. Two other patients died from infectious complications and one from a cerebrovascular accident (R.F.M. Wood, personal communication).

A total of nine multivisceral transplants were carried out in the cyclosporin era. Details are shown in Table 4. Six of these, including the first four cases, were children while the remaining three were adult recipients

Table 3. Combined liver/intestinal transplants with cyclosporin-based immunosuppression.

No.	Year	Centre	Immunosuppression	Outcome
1	1988	London (Ontario)	OKT3-CyA-Ster-Aza	Died (5 years)
2	1989	London (Ontario)	OKT3-CyA-Ster-Aza	Died, stroke (90 days)
3	1989	London (Ontario)	OKT3-CyA-Ster-Aza	Well (4, 5 years)
4	1991	Madison	OKT3-CyA-Ster-Aza	Died, multivisceral failure (52 days)
5	1992	Omaha	OKT3-CyA-Ster	Died, fungal sepsis (7 days)
6	1993	Omaha	OKT3-CyA-Ster	Died, rejection (410 days)
7	1993	Omaha	OKT3-CyA-Ster	Well > 1176 days
8	1993	Omaha	OKT3-CyA-Ster converted to FK 506	Died, rejection (530 days)

Cya, cyclosporin A; Ster, steroids; Aza, azathioprine.

Table 4. Multivisceral transplants with cyclosporin-based immunosuppression.

No.	Year	Centre	Age	Sex	Patient Survival	Cause of Death
1	1983	Pittsburgh	6.8	f	30 hours	Exsanguination
2	1986	Chicago	1.4	m	4 days	Exsanguination
3	1987	Pittsburgh	3.5	f	192 days	Lymphoma
4	1988	Chicago	0.7	m	109 days	Lymphoma
5	1989	Innsbruck	49	m	9 months	Tumour recurrence
6	1990	London (Ontario)	27	f	6.5 months	Lymphoma
7	1991	London (Ontario)	32	m	10.5 months	Lymphoma
8	1991	Strasbourg	1.5	m	7 months	Sepsis
9	1991	Strasbourg	0.7	m	5 months	Peritonitis

[9,10]. The first two children died perioperatively from exsanguination and the next two patients from lymphoma 192 and 109 days post-transplant. The first long-term survivor succumbed to tumour recurrence nine months after transplantation [11]. Two children transplanted in Strasbourg died of septic complications (K. Bondjema, personal communication). The high rate of lymphomas and infectious complications must be seen as a sign of overimmunosuppression. Most of these patients received monoclonal or polyclonal antibodies against lymphocytes in addition to the triple-drug regimen.

4. FK 506

A total of 30 isolated small bowel transplants, 48 combined liver–bowel transplants and 11 multivisceral transplants were performed with FK 506 as primary immunosuppression, the majority in Pittsburgh and Omaha. Exact figures are given in Table 5. By far the largest series has been produced by the Pittsburgh

Table 5. All types of intestinal transplants with FK 506-based immunosuppression.

	Isolated intestine	Liver + intestine	Multivisceral
Pittsburgh	22	29	11
Omaha	3	12	–
London (Ontario)	3	2	–
Paris	–	2	–
Cambridge	1	–	–
Innsbruck	1	–	–
	30	45	11

group, where between May 1990 and the end of 1993 a total of 62 intestinal transplants were performed in 34 paediatric recipients (mean age 3.8 ± 3.6 years) and 28 adult recipients (mean age 33.4 ± 9.5 years) [12, and S. Todo, personal communication]. Considering all types of intestinal transplant together, patient and graft survivals of 72% and 66% at 1 year and 53% and 34% at 4 years, respectively, were calculated. Actuarial 1-year graft and patient survival were 80% and 56% for the isolated intestinal group, 62% and 55% for the combined procedure and 82% and 82% for the multivisceral recipients. Whereas patient and graft survival in the latter group were identical, a few patients survived after the removal of a failing intestinal graft or underwent retransplantation of either the liver plus bowel or the multivisceral graft in one case each. In an attempt to improve graft function, the right colon was included in the intestinal graft in most patients from November 1992. Major causes of death were septic complications but not rejection. Only one patient was reported to have died from bowel leak and graft-versus-host (GVH) disease. Cytomegalovirus enteritis was a frequent complication in their series, as was lymphoproliferative disease. Nine of 32 paediatric cases developed lymphoma, which was highly associated with the use of OKT3 and was fatal in five children. At the time of the last report, 32 patients were at home, 30 of whom were TPN-free; 10 were still hospitalized, four of whom were TPN-free (R.F.M. Wood, personal communication).

The Omaha series includes four combined/small bowel transplants performed under cyclosporin A-based immunosuppression. 11 (nine paediatric) combined liver–small bowel and three isolated intestinal paediatric transplants receiving FK as prophylactic immunosuppressant. In the cyclosporin A group only one patient has become a long-term survivor, while six of the combined graft recipients taking FK 506 are alive with a functioning graft and one is alive with the small bowel graft removed. All three isolated bowel recipients are alive and well between 225 and 380 days post-transplant. From their entire patient population an actuarial 1-year survival of 70% for patients and 65% for the grafts was calculated. When the four cyclosporin patients are excluded, results are even better. Rejection was the major problem, and eventually the cause of death, during treatment with cyclosporin, whereas in the FK group anastomotic leak or perforation of the native stomach or duodenum or the transplanted bowel occurred in some patients. In their series no GVH disease was reported [13].

After FK 506 became available, a total of five intestinal transplants (two combined, three isolated, in two children and three adults) were performed in London (Ontario). Most remarkably, all of them survived and are reported to be well 1–12 months after grafting (R.F.M. Wood, personal communication).

Two combined liver–intestine transplants were performed in Paris. Unfortunately, no further information is available on these cases (C. Ricour, personal communication).

One successful isolated bowel transplant has been reported from Cambridge, and one was performed at our centre 5 months ago. Both patients are doing well [14].

5. Summary

Altogether, 124 intestinal transplants (51 isolated, 53 combined liver/intestinal transplants, 20 multivisceral) have been performed since 1964. Under conventional immunosuppression all attempts failed. When using cyclosporin A, steroids and azathioprine together with monoclonal or polyclonal antibodies against lymphocytes for induction therapy a few recipients became longterm survivors with functioning grafts. Rejection, however, was still the major cause of graft loss. In contrast, FK 506 led to a significant improvement in patient and graft survival. Experienced centres have achieved graft survival rates of 70% at one year.

Under FK 506 rejection appears to no longer be the major problem, but septic complications and lymphoproliferative disease develop. Interestingly, GVH disease does not seem to play a significant role in clinical intestinal transplantation. The preliminary results from the most recent series suggest that isolated intestinal and also combined liver–bowel transplants have become an option for selected patients with intestinal failure when long-term TPN is not possible. Even multivisceral transplants can now be considered for certain indications.

References

1. McAlister VC, DR Grant. Clinical small bowel transplantation. In: Grant DR, Wood RFM (eds), Small Bowel Transplantation. Edward Arnold, London 1994; 121–32.
2. Carrel A. The transplantation of organs. A preliminary communication. JAMA 1905; 45: 1645–6.
3. Lillehei RC, Goott B, Miller FA. The physiological response of the small bowel of the dog to ischemia including prolonged in vitro preservation of the bowel with successful replacement and survival. Ann Surg 1959; 150: 543–60.
4. Lillehei RC, Idezuki Y, Feemster JA et al. Transplantation of stomach intestine and pancreas: experimental and clinical observations. Surgery 1967; 62: 721–41.
5. Deterling R. Discussion of paper by Alican F, Hardy JD, Cayirili M et al. Intestinal transplantation: laboratory experience and a report of a clinical case. Am J Surg 1971; 121: 150.
6. Deltz E, Schroeder P, Gundlach M et al. Successful clinical small bowel transplantation. Transplan Proc 1990; 22: 2501.
7. Goulet O, Revillon Y, Brousse N et al. Successful small bowel transplantation in an infant. Transplantation 1992; 53: 940–3.
8. Grant D, Wall W, Mimeault R et al. Successful small bowel/liver transplantation. Lancet 1990; 335: 181–4.
9. Starzl TE, Rowe MI, Todo S et al. Transplantation of multiple abdominal viscera. JAMA 1989; 261: 1449–57.
10. Williams JW, Sankary HN, Foster PF et al. Splanchnic transplantation – an approach to the infant dependent on parenteral nutrition who develops irreversible liver disease. JAMA 1989; 261: 1458–62.
11. Margreiter R, Königsrainer A, Schmid T et al. Successful multivisceral transplantation. Transplant Proc 1992; 24: 1226–7.
12. Todo S, Tzakis A, Reyes K et al. Intestinal transplantation: 4-year experience. Transplant Proc 1995; 27: 1355–6.
13. Langnas AN, Antonson DL, Kaufman SS et al. Preliminary experience with intestinal transplantation in infants and children. Pediatrics 1996; 97: 443–8.
14. Calne RY, Pollard SG, Jamieson NV et al. Lancet 1993; 342: 58.

35 | Cardiac transplant survival in relation to preservation

M.M. Koerner, G. Tenderich, H. Posival, S. Wlost, H. Gromzik and R. Koerfer

Introduction

Almost three decades after the first successful orthotopic heart transplantation (HTx) in humans, cardiac transplantation has become an established therapeutical approach for endstage of heart failure, refractory to conventional therapy [1]. With the onset of brain death in the potential heart donor, significant deterioration of right and left ventricular function begins [2–6]. Because of the acceptance of extended donor criteria as well as the expected graft ischemic time, donor heart preservation plays a major role in early and late graft function [7,8] by protecting the electromechanically inactive heart. Various solutions have been used to produce a diastolic arrest in a hypothermic (4°C) environment. The overall ischemic time, as a sum of initial warm ischemia, cold ischemia during organ perfusion with preservation fluids, preservation time and warm ischemic time (time needed for revascularization), results in a depletion of adenosine triphosphate stores leading to a major shift in cell metabolism by initiating a cascade resulting in tissue damage during reperfusion [9]. In this context, attempts have been made to add different buffer systems, oxygen free radical inhibitors, oxygen etc. to the preservation solution. In order to minimize cellular edema, some solutions are kept hyperosmolar. As there are signs that ischemia may increase gene expression of cytokines, upregulation of adhesion molecules and major histocompatibility complex expression, facilitating an augmentation of specific alloimmune response after transplantation, attempts have been made to influence the immunological response [9–15]. In cardiac transplantation, a maximum ischemic time of 13 h for adults [16] and 10 h for children [17] has led to the development of different devices for permanent perfusion with the aim of further increasing the maximum ischemic time [18]. Forty-two years after the first successful application of cardioplegic solution [19], there is still controversial discussion about the composition of an optimal cardioplegic solution including blood cardioplegia and warm reperfusion [20], as well as its administration: high volume versus low volume versus a combination of both methods [21].

Results

The different types of preservation solutions can be divided into two groups: extracellular solutions (high $Na^+ > 100$ mmol/l, high sodium > 100 mmol/l) and intracellular solutions (high potassium > 100 mmol/l). Table 1 shows the composition of currently used preservation solutions. In general, intracellular solutions are thought to provide better protection over longer storage periods and have become more attractive for heart preservation, in spite of the potassium-induced (Ca^{2+} influx) vasoconstriction [23]. Numerous studies have been performed comparing the different kinds of cardioplegic solutions. Optimal organ (heart) preservation may decrease the postoperative inotropic support, need for defibrillation and myocardial pacing, decrease morbidity and help to alleviate the developing donor shortage by permitting the use of marginal donor hearts. Furthermore, it extends the period of preservation time, currently accepted as 5–6 h in the adult [24] and up to 10 h in children [17]. A comparison of intracellular solutions for myocardial preservation showed that HTK-Bretschneider solution (HTK) produced the best recovery of human atrial myocardium after a 24-h preservation period, compared with Euro-Collins (EC)

G.M. Collins, J.M. Dubernard, W. Land and G.G. Persijn (eds). Procurement, Preservation and Allocation of Vascularized Organs 285–291
© 1997 Kluwer Academic Publishers.

Table 1. Composition of preservation solutions (Wicomb *et al.* [8], modified by Koerner and Tenderich)

Components (mmol/L)	SU2	STH2 (1)	HTK4	Euro-Collins	UW	ROE's solution[39]	Cardiol II
Potassium	17	16	10	115	125	20	125
Sodium	14.5	140 (120)	15	10	35	27	40
Magnesium	—	16	4	30	5	6	4
Calcium	—	1.2	—	—	—	—	—
Chloride	17.4	139 (160)	50	15	—	—	—
Bicarbonate	14.5	10	—	10	—	+	—
Phosphate	—	—	—	57.5	25	—	25
Lactobionate	—	—	—	—	100	—	100
Raffinose	—	—	—	—	30	—	30
Glutathione	—	—	—	—	3	—	—
PEG	—	—	—	—	—	—	50 g/l
HES	—	—	—	—	50 g/l	—	—
Adenosine	—	—	—	—	5	—	—
Insulin	—	—	—	—	100 U/l	—	—
Decadron	—	—	—	—	8 mg/l	—	—
Penicillin	—	—	—	—	133 mg/l	—	—
Allopurinol	—	—	—	—	1	—	—
Desferal	—	—	—	—	—	—	7.1 μmol/l
Nitroglycerine	—	—	—	—	—	—	2.5 mg/l
Histidine	—	—	180	—	—	—	—
Histidine HCl	—	—	18	—	—	—	—
Mannitol	72	—	30	—	—	—	—
Tryptophan	—	—	2	—	—	—	—
Ketoglutarate	—	—	1	—	—	—	—
Glucose (mg)	250	—	—	182	—	—	—
pH (at 4°C)	7.8	7.8	7.1	7.0	7.4	7.4	7.8
Methylprednisolone (mg)	—	—	—	—	—	250	—
Dextrose (mg)	—	—	—	—	—	50	—

SU = Stanford University solution, STH = St. Thomas Hospital solution, HTK = Bretschneider solution, UW = University of Wisconsin solution, PEG = polyethylene glycol, HES = hydroxyethyl starch

and University of Wisconsin solution (UW) [25]. In a clinical multicenter study in 600 heart transplant patients, satisfactory results could be shown with HTK provided the ischemic time did not exceed 4 h [26]. Comparing the intracellular Euro-Collins solution (EC) with St. Thomas solution (ST) in a randomized trial in 62 transplantations, a tendency towards early postoperative improvement could be demonstrated by EC preservation. Hemodynamic follow-up one year posttransplant did not show any significant difference between the two preservation solutions [27]. Comparing UW with crystalloid cardioplegia and cooling storage (CCS) in a randomized blinded prospective clinical trial in 16 patients, no clinical differences in the early postoperative course could be demonstrated [28]. Only enzymatic analysis showed better myocardial protection as well as earlier recovery of electrical activity in the UW group [29]. Recently published data about 14 heart transplant patients with

an organ preservation time between 10 and 13 h preserved with St. Thomas crystalloid cardioplegia showed a 75% survival rate 1 year and 71% 5 years after transplantation [16]. In a retrospective analysis of 200 patients after cardiac transplantation, comparing preservation with UW (intracellular) and Stanford (extracellular) solution, UW storage was associated with an increased incidence of graft vasculopathy versus Stanford extracellular preservation solution.

As demonstrated, there is controversy about the clinical application of the different preservation solutions. Currently available protocols show partly excellent results even for long-term preservation [16]. Attempts to improve preservation solutions by adding viral vectors to mediate gene transfer, altering the immune response [30–32], are under investigation. Further modification includes the administration of leukocyte-depleted reperfusion [33], adenosine [34], thromboxane A$_2$ receptor antagonists [35], dipyri-

287

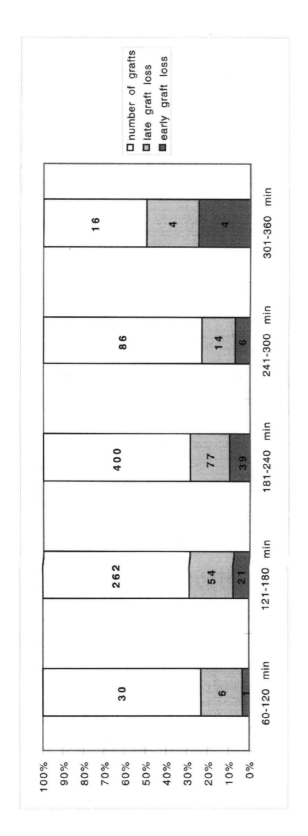

Figure 1. Ischemic time in relation to early (*n* = 70; 8.8%) and late graft loss (*n* = 153; 9.3%) in 794 cardiac transplant procedures with HTK preservation

288

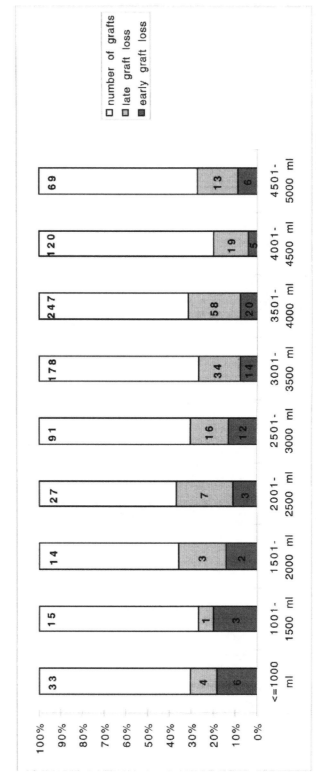

Figure 2. Volume of cardioplegia in relation to early and late graft loss ($n = 223$) in 794 cardiac transplant procedures with HTK preservation

damole and platelet-activating factor receptor antagonists [36]. Hibernating induction triggers like D-Ala2-Leu5-encephalin can increase ischemic tolerance by influencing cell metabolism via opioid receptors [37]. Furthermore, different reperfusion protocols try to limit perfusion-induced damage to the myocardial microvessels by lowering the perfusion pressure, administration of oxygen free radical scavengers, retrograde second warm shot of cardioplegia [20,38] and substrate enhancement [8].

Single center experience with HTK preservation

Material and methods

Between March 1989 and December 1996, 801 grafts ranging from 3 days up to 65 years (mean 52 y) were transplanted in 794 recipients (666 men, 128 women; ages 3 days to 77 y, mean 49.6 y) and retrospectively analysed considering early and late graft loss in relation to ischemic time and cardioplegia volume as well as cumulative survival. All allografts preserved with HTK-Bretschneider solution, a low-potassium histidine-buffered tryptophane-ketoglutarate cardioplegia (Custodiol provided by Dr Franz Koehler, Alsbach Chemie GmbH, Bergstr., Germany), high volume pressure-controlled were included (we excluded 7 grafts: 6 preserved with UW, 1 with St. Thomas, because explantation was not performed by our team). Up to the end of the first year of life in infants, 10–12 ml/g heart weight of HKT solution were applied over 3–4 minutes. We performed gravity perfusion, beginning with 20–30 mmHg, and reduced to 15–20 mmHg after cardiac arrest. In adults, perfusion pressure should be 80 mmHg. However, of utmost importance is the total amount of cardioplegia.

Results

Ischemic time ranged from 88–332 min (mean 193.7 ± 43.5 min); the duration of the perfusion time ranged from 44–595 min (mean 104 ± 49.9 min). Some very long perfusion times could be explained by bridging a failing graft to retransplantation (retransplantation rate $n = 11$; 1.34%).

Volumes of the HTK solution ranged from 350–5000 ml (mean 3521.9 ± 905.9 ml). Comparing different ischemic times in relation to early and late graft loss, we found comparable results with an ischemic time ranging from 60–300 min. Extended ischemic times over 5 h up to 6 h resulted in an increased early and late graft failure (Figure 1).

Comparing different amounts of cardiac preservation solution ranging from 350–5000 ml, we found comparable results in the different groups regarding to the different amounts of HTK (Figure 2).

Our cumulative survival curve with an early graft loss of 9% and a late graft loss of 20% justifies our current cardiac preservation protocol (Figure 3).

Remarks

This single center study, with all its limitations of a retrospective analysis, demonstrates that donor heart preservation with HTK solution provides the

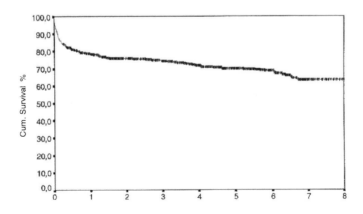

Figure 3. Cardiac transplantation between March 1989 and December 1996 — graft survival up to April 1997; ($n = 794$ with HTK-Bretschneider preservation (801 minus 7 grafts (6 with UW and 1 with St. Thomas))

possibility of extending ischemic time over 5 hours with an early and late graft loss comparable to or even lower than published international results in pediatric and adult recipients [1,17]. HTK is effective for distance heart procurement to minimize the donor heart shortage. It is obviously feasible to preserve marginal hearts. Prospective randomized multicenter studies could elucidate the open questions concerning the different preservation protocols.

Acknowledgements

The authors wish to thank Professor U. Raute-Kreinsen and Professor W. Lang (Dept. of Pathology) for their diagnostic support; Ms S. Traut for her technical help in producing the manuscript; the German Association of Organ Recipients (reg. Ass.) for major grant support; the Eurotransplant International Foundation at Leiden (the Netherlands) and all collaborating European Transplant Centers for their fruitful cooperation; and, last but not least, the donors and their relatives for their gift of life.

References

1. Hosenpud JD, Novick RJ, Breen TJ, Keck B, Daily P. The registry of the International Society for Heart and Lung Transplantation: twelfth official report – 1995. J Heart Lung Transplant. 1995; 14: 805–15.
2. Bittner HB, Kendall SWH, Chen EP, Van Trigt P. The combined effects of brain death and cardiac graft preservation on cardiopulmonary hemodynamics and function before and after subsequent heart transplantation. J Heart Lung Transplant. 1996; 15: 764–77.
3. Novitzky D. Selection and management of cardiac allograft donors. Curr Opin Cardiol. 1996; 11: 174–82.
4. Novitzky D, Cooper D, Morrel D, Isaacs S. Change from aerobic to anaerobic metabolism after brain death and reversal following triiodothyronine therapy. Transplantation. 1988; 45: 32–6.
5. Baldwin JC, Anderson JL, Boucek MM, et al. Task Force 2: Donor guidelines. Bethesda Conference Nov. 1992. JACC. 1993; 22: 15–20.
6. Novitzky D, Cooper D, Reichart B. Hemodynamic and metabolic responses to hormonal therapy in brain-dead potential organ donors. Transplantation. 1987; 43: 852–4.
7. Phillips MG, ed. Organ Procurement, Preservation and Distribution in Transplantation. Richmond: UNOS; 1991: 86–7.
8. Wicomb WN, Portnoy VF, Collins GM. Advances in heart storage. In Cooper DKC et al., editors. The Transplantation and Replacement of Thoracic Organs. Dordrecht: Kluwer; 1997: 675–87.
9. Land W, Messmer K. The impact of ischemia/reperfusion injury on specific and non-specific, early and late chronic events after organ transplantation. Transplant Rev. 1996; 10(2): 108–27.
10. Kamikubo Y. Cardiac dysfunction and endogenous cytokines in global ischemia and reperfusion injury. Hokkaido Igaku Zasshi. 1993; 68: 813.
11. Halloran PF, Batiuk TD, Goes NB, et al. Strategies to improve the immunologic management of organ transplants. Clin Transplant. 1995; 9: 227.
12. Winn RK, Mihelcic D, Vedder NB, et al. Monoclonal antibodies to leukocyte and endothelial adhesion molecules attenuate ischemia–reperfusion injury. Behring Inst Mitt. 1993; 92: 229.
13. Arfors KE, Lundberg C, Lindbom L, et al. A monoclonal antibody to the membrane glycoprotein complex CD18 inhibits polymorphonuclear leukocyte accumulation and plasma leakage in vivo. Blood. 1987; 69: 338.
14. Simpson PJ, Todd RF III, Fontane JC, et al. Reduction of experimental canine myocardial reperfusion injury by a monoclonal antibody (Anti-Mo-1, Anti-CD11b) that inhibits leukocyte adhesion. J Clin Invest. 1988; 81: 624.
15. Ma XL, Tsao PS, Lefer AM. Antibody to CD18 exerts endothelial and cardiac protective effects in myocardial ischemia in the rat. Circulation. 1992; 86: 279.
16. Obadia JF, Girard C, Ferrara R, Chuyel M, Chassignolle JF, Dureau G. Long conservation organs in heart transplantation: Postoperative results and long-term follow-up in fourteen patients. J Heart Lung Transplant. 1997; 16: 256–9.
17. Alonso de Begona J, Gundry SR, Razzouk AJ, Boucek MM, Bailey LL. Prolonged ischemic times in pediatric heart transplantation: Early and late results. Transplant Proc. 1993; 25(1): 1645–8.
18. Wicomb WN, Cooper DKC, Barnard CN. Twenty-four-hour preservation of the pig heart by a portable hypothermic perfusion system. Transplantation. 1982; 34(5): 246–50.
19. Melrose DG, Dreyer B, Bentall HH, Baker JB. Elective cardiac arrest: preliminary communication. Lancet. 1955; 269: 21–2.
20. Bracamonte L, Pavie A, Fraysee JB, et al. Blood cardioplegia and warm reperfusion in heart transplantation: Improvement of myocardial function and clinical recovery (abstract). J Heart Transpl. 1990; 9: 69.
21. Preusse CJ, Winter J, Gebhard MM, Nordbeck H, Schulte HD, Bircks W. Myocardial equilibration procedures with high-volume cardioplegia. Presented at the 7th Asian Congress of Thoracic and Cardiovascular Surgery, Nov 17–21, 1985, Bangkok. Thai J Surg. 1986.
22. Wicomb WN, Holl JD, Avery J, Collins GM. Optimal cardioplegia and 24-hour heart storage with simplified UW solution containing polyethylene glycol. Transplantation. 1990; 49: 261.
23. Jeevanandam V, Auteri JS, Sanchez JA, et al. Cardiac transplantation after prolonged graft preservation with the University of Wisconsin solution. J Thorac Cardiovasc Surg. 1992; 104–224.
24. Starling RC, Hammer DF, Binkley PF, et al. Adenine nucleotide content in cold preserved human donor hearts and subsequent cardiac performance after orthotopic heart transplantation. J Heart Lung Transplant. 1991; 10: 508–17.
25. Hendry PJ, Labow RS, Keon WJ. A comparison of intracellular solutions for donor heart preservation. J Thorac Cardiovasc Surg. 1993; 105: 667–73.
26. Stein DG, Drinkwater DC, Laks H, et al. Cardiac preservation in patients undergoing transplantation. J Thorac Cardiovasc Surg. 1991; 102: 657–65.
27. Reichenspurner H, Russ C, Überfuhr P, et al. Myocardial preservation using HTK solution for heart transplantation. Eur J Cardio-thorac Surg. 1993; 7: 414–19.
28. Weyand M, Hermann G, Konertz W, Bernhard A, Scheld HH. Long-term function of Euro-Collins-preserved human cardiac allografts. Transplant Proc. 1992; 24(5): 2011–12.
29. Jeevanandam V, Barr ML, Auteri JS, et al. University of Wisconsin solution versus crystalloid cardioplegia for human donor heart preservation. J Thorac Cardiovasc Surg. 1992; 103: 194–9.
30. Gojo S, Niwaya K, Taniguchi S, Kitamura S. Gene transfer into the donor heart during cold preservation for heart transplantation. Ann Thorac Surg. [In press].

31. Csete MW, Drazan KE. van Bree M, *et al.* Adenovirus-mediated gene transfer in the transplant setting. I. Conditions for expression of transferred genes in cold-preserved hepatocytes. Transplantation. 1994; 57: 1502–7.

32. Shaked A, Csete ME, Drazan KE, *et al.* Adenovirus-mediated gene transfer in the transplant setting. II Successful expression of transferred cDNA in a syngeneic liver grafts. Transplantation. 1994; 57: 1508–11.

33. Pillai R, Bando K, Schueler S, *et al.* Leucocyte depletion results in excellent heart–lung function after 12 hours of storage. Ann Thorac Surg. 1990; 50: 211.

34. Forman MB, Velasco CE. Role of adenosine in the treatment of myocardial stunning. Cardiovasc Drug Ther. 1991; 5: 901.

35. Bryne JG, Appleyard RF, Sun S, Couper GS, Cohn LH. Thromboxane A2 mediates reperfusion injury after heart preservation. J Heart Lung Transplant. 1993; 12: 256.

36. Sawa Y, Schaper J. Roth M, *et al.* Platelet-activating factor plays an important role in reperfusion injury in the myocardium. J Thorac Cardiovasc Surg. 1984; 10850: 211.

37. Bolling SF, Su TP. Childs KF. *et al.* The use of hibernation induction triggers for cardiac transplant preservation. Transplantation. 1997; 63: 326–9.

38. Carrier M, Leung TK. Solymoss BC. Cartier R, Leclerc Y, Pelletier LC. Clinical trial of retrograde warm blood reperfusion versus standard cold topical irrigation of transplant hearts. Ann Thorac Surg. 1996; 61: 1310–5.

39. Kawauchi M, Gundry SR. de Begona A. *et al.* Prolonged preservation of human pediatric hearts for transplantation: Correlation of ischemic time and subsequent function. J Heart Lung Transplant. 1993; 12: 55–8.

Section IV
Ethics and Legislation in Organ Donation

36 | Voluntarism and coercion in living organ donation

ROBERT A. SELLS

1. Introduction

Renal transplantation has become the definitive treatment for end stage renal failure in those patients fit enough to benefit from it. It gives patients a better quality of life, free from dialysis, spares patients and the health service the costs of providing dialysis systems, and it lightens the load and economic pressure on renal units which face increasing demands while remaining under-resourced [1].

The dominant influence on transplant practice has always been the societal attitudes to the rights of individuals to donate, as well as to receive, an organ transplant. The ethical approach to organ donation is conditioned principally by those rules which seek to confer benefit while preserving autonomy; what is and is not 'ethical' will be determined by the balance between clinical utilitarian demand (saving lives in a cost-effective way) and respect for the individual's right to donate or not to donate in life or after death.

In practice the great majority of renal transplants are obtained from cadaveric donors. This source of organs is supplemented by a small number (15% in Western countries) of kidneys taken from altruistically motivated, living, healthy relatives. However, the relentless increase in the number of potential organ transplant recipients has produced a continuing and increasing deficit in cadaveric organ donors. In many Western countries we have reached the limit of the number of cadaveric organs that may be retrieved for transplant purposes. Several organ distribution agencies in Europe have reported a plateau in the number of cadaver organs of all types retrieved during the 3 years up to 1993. For instance in the USA between 1988 and 1991, the number of transplant candidates on waiting lists increased by 55%, when the number of donors increased only by 16%; by the end of March 1993 > 30 000 potential recipients awaited transplantation [2,3]. A report from Sweden reports a fall in the chances of receiving a renal transplant from 46% to 39% over the years 1965–1987 [4].

The scarcity of cadaveric organs has led to an increase in the number of kidneys transplanted from living donors. In many poor countries, where chronic dialysis cannot be provided outside the private sector and where cadaver donors are infrequently available due to cultural or legal restrictions, the only chance of preventing death from end stage renal failure may be a living related, or a paid unrelated kidney donor transplant. In a few centres in Germany and Japan, a shortage of cadaveric livers has led to segmental liver transplants being donated from parents to their children [5,6]. Segmental pancreas transplants have also been performed from living related donors to diabetic siblings or offspring [7]. Given the increasing success of living donor transplants as judged by graft and patient survival, and given the scarcity of cadaveric organs, live donor transplants must be regarded as a regrettable necessity. There is a widely held view in the transplant profession that the only justification for the use of living donors in renal transplantation is the continuing shortage of cadaveric donors [8].

In some countries, however, the poor and socially disadvantaged have come to be regarded as an expandable resource from whom organs may be bought. In addition, relatives of dialysis patients may well feel pressurized by feelings of guilt into offering a kidney to their unfortunate family member. This situation has produced a lively debate within the medical and legal profession on the coercive influences brought to bear

G.M. Collins, J.M. Dubernard, W. Land and G.G. Persijn (eds). Procurement, Preservation and Allocation of Vascularized Organs 295–300
© 1997 Kluwer Academic Publishers.

on healthy living people by the plight of chronically sick patients who could be cured by a transplant. Must living organ donation always be a voluntary act? Or is financial gain, or other coercion, ever justifiable as a means of bridging the gap between the supply and the demand for kidneys?

2. Coercion of related altruistic donors

A foundation stone of clinical transplantation has been altruistic donation of kidneys from living relatives: we have insisted on unconstrained, voluntary transplant donation. Societies which support the development of transplantation have generally refused to assign a monetary value to a transplantable organ or tissue: the gift of a transplant is therefore priceless, and legal control now exists in the West to prevent payments for living related organs. There is no legal or other enforceable obligation to donate an organ during life to a relative. Nonetheless, while a relative may experience a strong sense of duty to donate for compassionate reasons there may also be financial or other social implications of chronic ill health in the recipient which affects the whole family.

The terms 'obligation' and 'duty' are frequently used in the debate about this subject [9]. An obligation is an externally applied constriction of an individual's right to choose not to donate. I would include in this category blackmail (within families as well as between unrelated people), the use of organs from criminals in custody whose voluntariness is compromised by the need to shorten their sentence by agreeing to donate, and in all cases when a person sells one of his organs during life (see below). Duty, however, I would define as an internal motivation arising from love, friendship with, or respect for, another individual. A sense of duty can be sufficiently strong in a person as to make it difficult to distinguish between duty and obligation. So long as the individual still has the freedom to choose not to give, then the motivation could be defined as a sense of duty, rather than the result of an externally applied obligation. However, a no less well motivated relative may have decided not to donate when the hazards were pointed out to him and, in these cases, refusal to donate may only be decided after much agonizing thought and self examination. In both the donor and the non-donor within such a family, the exercise of choice has taken place: the organ can be withheld (at the cost of harming the recipient) or can be given (at the cost of hurting the donor). It is, of course, the recipient's

plight which has forced the dilemma on the relatives; and in practice the degree of motivation experienced by the eventual donor is usually proportional to the strength of his or her relationship with the recipient.

When considering a possible living related kidney donation, the transplant surgeon has to handle the situation with great care. Any attempt at coercion, such as forceful presentation of the medical advantages of transplantation, should be avoided. An enquiry of the recipient or his family as to whether or not a member of the family has offered to donate a kidney need not be coercive, and is frequently followed by an offer which leads to a living related organ donation. It is the doctor's duty under these circumstances to preserve voluntarism, to let the members of the family decide for themselves, and to relieve all the family members of any external sense of compulsion to donate.

The altruistic living donor must, of course, give informed consent, which can only be obtained if he has a proper understanding of the risks involved. The risk of unilateral nephrectomy causing early postoperative death in a healthy donor has been assessed at about 1 in 4000 (J. Utting, personal communication). This theoretical figure has been derived from an estimate of the risk of pulmonary embolus in a healthy person, combined with the possibility of an unforeseeable, idiosyncratic, fatal response to anaesthetic agents. Levy et al. have reported an incidence of death of 1 in 1600 donors [10]. To date, no donor deaths have been reported following segmental related pancreas transplantation, although 13% of donors have developed pancreatic leakage, abscess or intra-abdominal fluid collection [7]. The long-term effects of hemi-pancreatectomy on a healthy donor may however be significant: pancreatic endocrine function in healthy human pancreas donors has been studied [11] and in 75 first-degree relatives who submitted to this operation, beta cell reserve appears to be significantly decreased, although donors generally maintained normoglycaemia. Segmental resection of liver for transplantation from parents to children is a technically demanding procedure. The potential for hepatic complications such as secondary haemorrhage and thrombosis, as well as postoperative abnormal liver function, is obviously present after this procedure, although no donor deaths have yet been reported. Busuttil has predicted a mortality rate of 1–2% [12].

Because of the risk, and the inevitable discomfort and inconvenience of a major operation, the donation of organs by mentally incompetent adults and children has raised serious ethical issues concerning possible exploitation arising from consent provided by surrogates or guardians. The ethical consensus is that these patients should not be used as living related donors of non-regenerative organs. Nine Canadian provinces have enacted legislation which prohibits minors and mentally incompetent adults from making live donations [13].

Altruistic organ donation by a family member or an 'emotionally related person' (wife or friend) may be, and usually is, psychologically beneficial to the donor: Roberta Simmons [14] tested the state of mind of such donors, 5–9 years after altruistic voluntary donation, using standard psychological testing, and compared them with a group of non-donor controls. Few (8%) regretted their act, and donors scored higher in self-esteem and low depressive affect after donation than before, irrespective of whether the transplant failed or not. We have no data with which to judge the consequences of donation under compulsion, but can speculate that such cases will be less likely to result in such beneficial outcomes.

It is the surgeon's responsibility to ensure that the donor is medically, as well as psychologically, suited to the procedure, that the risks of donation are acceptably small, that the donated organ is healthy, and that the expectation of success in the recipient is reasonable. These strict criteria must obviously include a thorough medical examination, and an assessment of cardiorespiratory function. It is generally thought advisable, and in some countries mandatory, to obtain a psychiatric evaluation of the donor's motivation and his ability to understand the risks of the operation, which have to be discussed frankly and repeatedly with the transplant surgeon.

3. The payment of living non-related donors for their organs

Financial rewards for organ donation represent the most difficult and contentious aspect of transplant ethics to date. The first publicized cases of commerce in organs were examples of rampant commercialism practised in developing countries: surgeons, some of them from the West, were reported to have transplanted organs from supposed related donors into private, fee-paying recipients. It subsequently became clear that the recipients had paid the donors who were actually unrelated, and extensive networks were revealed of organ procurement agencies involving middlemen who searched the local Indian population for fit potential donors. These people were tissue typed and matched to recipients who were able to pay large

fees for their organs. The hallmarks of this trafficking were that middlemen were involved and took a large proportion of the fee. Surgeons were alleged to have been making a lot of money out of the trade, and in those centres where such procedures were performed 'underground' there was no proper medical screening of the donors. Informed consent rules were being ignored, no independent review of the procedures was conducted, the postoperative care of the donor was substandard and often resulted in serious morbidity. The Transplantation Society condemned these practices, threatening with expulsion any member who willingly took part in the sale of organs [15]. Legislation against organ trade was rapidly promulgated in most countries [16]. Despite these measures the practice has persisted, and Salahudeen in 1991 [17] published the results of living related organ transplants from Indian donors in Bombay to fee-paying Arab immigrants. The survival figures for the transplants were relatively poor, and a significant number of patients suffered HIV infection vectored by unscreened donor tissue. These practices are conducted by doctors who appear to have abandoned professional and ethical standards of care, and operations performed under these circumstances are now universally condemned.

A safer and less ethically offensive system of paid organ donation has been suggested by Reddy et al. [18]. Faced with a seemingly unending stream of fatally ill renal patients for whom no care could be provided, in a country where a mere 3.7% of the total national budget is allocated to health and family welfare (a negligible proportion of which is given for the treatment of renal failure), this group of doctors in Madras decided purposely to accept healthy donors wishing to sell their kidneys and who were demonstrably fit and free of transmissible disease. Dr Reddy and colleagues plead that the inevitable death of a recipient can be prevented by a safe operation on a volunteer donor, who would receive a solatium. In the universal sense everyone would benefit: in addition to the restoration of life to the recipients, the donor would be paid a sum of £1000 and given 3 years' medical insurance free. In introducing this practice of the 'rewarded gift', no offence was deemed to have been committed, as the operation was done in good faith, proper informed consent had been obtained from the donor, the operation was performed in order to save the life of the patient, and the payment of a solatium was within Indian law. However, the majority of these patients were private, fee-paying individuals, and therefore the 'rewarded gift' was not available to the vast majority of non-paying recipients.

The response to this form of coercion world-wide has varied according to the local availability of cadaver organ donation, and of dialysis. In America, where healthcare is provided on a fee-paying or insurance basis, some authors, mainly economists and lawyers, have stated that perhaps, under some conditions, financial incentives for donation might be acceptable for living unrelated organ donation. Blumstein [19] has taken a strong view that altruistic donation is not a pre-requisite of organ transplantation between living people and he laments the insistence on the exclusion of commercial incentives which could augment the supply of organs available. This is in direct confrontation to the view expressed by the World Health Organization [16], which in 1991 issued guiding principles on human organ transplantation and recommended that in the light of the principles of distributive justice and equity, donated organs should be made available to patients on the basis of medical needs, and not on the basis of financial or other considerations. WHO also ruled against physicians being involved in transplantation if they had reason to believe that the organs concerned had been the subject of commercial transactions, since the body and its parts cannot be the subject of commercial transactions, and all giving or receiving of payments should be prohibited. However, the reimbursement of reasonable expenses incurred in the donation by the donor should not be prohibited.

What are doctors to make of this evident conflict between those representing the economic interests of the healthcare providers in developed countries on the one hand, and the traditional medical view on the other that commodification of the human living body is objectionable and that altruism should remain the traditional basic foundation stone of organ donation?

Progress in this debate has been helped by reflections on some recently defined basic ethical principles. A moral philosophical view states that the principles of autonomy, beneficence and non-maleficence are satisfied in part by the act of organ donation [20]: selling an organ is a self-determined act and is beneficial in a universal sense, in that the transaction leads to improvement in the health of the recipient, and financial benefit to the donor and his family. Self-harm *per se* is not enough to forbid donation (living related donors are, after all, used in the West) and risk-taking *per se* is not irrational, neither is it forbidden (there is no law against rock climbing or deep sea diving). The philosophical view continues, the mere existence of risk cannot permit a general prohibition which curtails the freedom of all to sell their organs [21].

The consensus medical response to this line of thinking could be summarized as follows:

1. A full understanding of the risks is essential for properly informed consent to any form of surgery; since paid organ donors will always be relatively poor, and may be underprivileged and under-educated, the donor's full understanding of these risks cannot be guaranteed. Laws are therefore required to protect these individuals from exploitation. Such legislation, of course, places a definite limitation on the freedom of everyone, in order to prevent the possibility of exploitation of some.

2. We believe that operations should be performed for therapeutic indications, and not for the acquisition of money.

3. A rewarded donor from an impoverished background cannot be presumed to give proper voluntary consent since the coercive influence of a substantial payment is likely to distort the balance of risk versus benefit in a person's mind, and in conditions of severe impoverishment could amount to a compulsion to donate, on behalf of improvement in life-style of the donor's family.

4. In a free market for organs, profit is the first objective and medical standards will fall, no matter how well-regulated the market is.

5. 'Legal' paid donation would undermine altruistic donation.

6. Traffick in organs divides society, in that the donor will always be relatively poor and the recipient relatively rich.

7. Commodification of the body is objectionable.

The problem about basing our ethical attitudes on deontological or ethical theory is that the application of rules derived therefrom may be impossible in those countries where ethical niceties are likely to be subjugated by the impelling desire of the potential recipient to stay alive, and the disinclination of very poor people to refuse the chance to improve their lot and that of their families by selling a kidney. In India, where this market is flourishing, the relatively well-off recipient will always be able to find a willing paid donor. The Indian government has passed a law based on a report [22] which recommends the outlawing of paid organ donation.

Much of the comment on the situation in India concerning financial coercion has emanated from the West. Some doctors and philosophers have recognized the important contextual differences which, they believe, should form the basis of judicious ethical guidance. Such guidance should reflect not only basic ethical principles but the very significant differences in opportunity for and access to life-saving treatment in different cultures. Dossetor and Manickaval [23] have stated that organ sales could be justifiable in two carefully defined circumstances:

(1) Indirect altruism: it would be morally acceptable for a donor to sell his kidney provided the money was spent improving the health of a third party individual.

(2) Mandated altruism: the wealthy recipient should pay an additional sum (above the payment for the donor) to provide treatment for another renal failure patient who would otherwise die.

I have also suggested elsewhere [24] that these two principles of indirect altruism and mandated altruism could be combined with a system of third party review of hospitals where paid donation is practised, which would separate the financial issues, and consequent ethical tensions, from the hospital and the medical practitioner where these paid organ donor transplants are performed. It is suggested that a local 'Donors' Trust' could be established, the trustees being chosen by local officials and experts in the law and social work. The Trust would be paid by the recipient of a 'paid for' organ, and by the hospital where the operation was performed; in addition, the Trust could raise charitable funds and government grants to develop local dialysis centres and to promote cadaver transplantation. The donor and the recipient would be independently examined by social workers employed by the Trust and the fee and the solatium would be calculated by the Trust, for each individual. If a member of the donor's family was in dire need of expensive medical treatment which could not otherwise be afforded, then that extra sum would be included in the solatium. The recipient would also have to pay the costs and salaries to the hospital.

I personally believe that the development of the principles of mandated altruism and indirect altruism must be permissible in a country where any form of organ transplantation free of coercion is at present unattainable. Western doctors are comfortable with the rejection of all forms of payment for organs in the West; such an attitude is affordable in countries where dialysis is more or less freely available, and the infrastructural, social, and religious environment is conducive to cadaver donation. Perhaps, though, a more libertarian view should be taken when advising doctors working in poor countries about the ethical standards to which they should conform.

Perhaps the most difficult aspect of this debate is the knowledge that the ethical principles may be easily agreed, but their consistent application through legislation and social and cultural acceptance, will be a difficult goal to reach. It is not so much the differences in ethical approach which divides the East and the West in this issue, as the flagrant abuse of ethical principles in transplant surgery which appears to be so difficult to prohibit in those countries where the market in organs has flourished.

References

1. McGeown MG. Prevalence of advanced renal failure in Northern Ireland. Br Med J 1990; 301: 900–3.
2. Grenvik A. Brain death and organ transplantation: a forty year review. *Opuscula Med* 37: 33–39.
3. Evans RW, Orians CE, Asher NL. Potential supply of organ donors: an assessment of the efficiency of organ procurement efforts in the United States. *JAMA* 1992; 267: 339–46.
4. Hylander B, Lundblad H, Kjellstrand CM. Changing patient characteristics and chronic haemodialysis. Scand J Urol Nephrol 1991; 25: 59–63.
5. Emond JC, Heffron TG, Kortz EO, Gonzales-Vallinir Contis JC, Black DD, Whittington PF. Improved results of living related liver transplantation with routine application in a paediatric programme. Transplantation 1993; 55: 835–40.
6. Tanaka K, Uemoto S, Tokunaga Y, Fujita S, Sano K, Nishizawa T, Sawad H, Schriahase I, Kim HJ, Yamaoka Y. Surgical techniques and innovations in living related liver transplantation. Ann Surg 1993; 217: 82–91.
7. Sutherland D. Single pancreas transplantation. In: Groth CG (ed.). Pancreatic Transplantation. WB Saunders and Co, Philadelphia 1988; p. 177.
8. British Transplantation Society recommendations on the use of living kidney donors in the United Kingdom. Br Med J 1986; 293: 257–8.
9. Sells RA. Voluntarism of consent in both related and unrelated living organ donors. In: Land W, Dossetor JB (eds), Organ Replacement Therapy: Ethics, Justice and Commerce. Springer-Verlag, Munich 1991; pp. 18–24.
10. Levy *et al.* Ann Intern Med 1986; 106: 719.
11. Seaquist ER, Robertson RP. Effects of hemi-pancreatectomy on pancreatic alpha and beta cell function in healthy donors. Clin Invest 1992; 89: 1761–6.
12. Busuttil RW. Living related liver donation. Transplant Proc 1991; 23: 43–5.
13. Jones M. Medical Negligence. Sweet and Maxwell, London 1991; p. 264.
14. Simmons R. Long-term reactions of renal recipients and donors. In: Levy NB (ed.), Psychonephrology. Plenum, New York 1983; pp. 275–87.
15. The Council of the Transplantation Society. Lancet 1985; 2: 715.
16. World Health Organization. 1991. Human Organ Transplantation: a report on the development under the auspices of WHO.
17. Salahudeen AK, Woods HF, Pingle A, Neur-El-Hudea Sulayman M, Shakuntela K, Mandakumar M, Yahya TM, Daar AS. High mortality among recipients of bought living unrelated donor kidneys. Lancet 1990; 336: 725–8.
18. Reddy KC, Thiagarajan CM, Shunmugasundarm D, Jayachandran R, Nayar P, Thomas S, Ramachandran V. Unconventional renal transplantation in India. Transplant Proc 1990; 22: 910–11.
19. Blumstein JF. Governments' role in organ transplantation policy. In: Blumstein J, Sloan F (eds), Organ Transplantation, Policy, Issues and Prospects. Duke University Press, Durham and London 1989.
20. Beecham T, Childress J. Principles of Bio-medical Ethics, 2nd ed. Oxford University Press, New York, 1983.

21. Radcliffe-Richards J. In: Kjellstrand CM, Dossetor JB (eds), Ethical Problems in Dialysis and Transplantation. Kluwer, Dordrecht 1992; p. 53.

22. Singhvi LM, Jain SC, Nundy S, Vas CJ. Report of the Group Constituted to Examine the Proposal for Enactment of Legislation for the Use of Human Organs and Their Donation for Therapeutic Purposes. All India Institute of Medical Sciences, New Delhi 1991.

23. Manickaval V. In: Kjellstrand CM, Dossetor JB (eds), Ethical Problems in Dialysis and Transplantation. Kluwer, Dordrecht 1992; p. 61.

24. Sells RA. Some ethical issues in organ retrieval 1982–1992. Transplant Proc 1992; 24: 2401–3.

37 | Reimbursement, 'rewarded gifting', financial incentives and commercialism in living organ donation

A.S. Daar, Th. Gutmann and W. Land

1. Introduction

Organ transplantation is among the most impressive achievements of modern biomedicine. The field has gained clinical maturity in only four decades, but this very rapid rate of development has resulted in disparities between technology on the one hand and the handling of its implications on the other. The very success of transplantation has raised important societal concerns. In the future some other area may become the main issue, but today the main issue is organ shortage. The shortage may be relative, but the problem is world-wide and is increasing. Its ramifications are still evolving. Honest individuals and teams throughout the world are working hard to find solutions to the shortage problem while unscrupulous individuals and teams are exploiting the shortage to enrich themselves. This chapter is an attempt to distinguish the work of the former from that of the latter.

The subjects of this chapter are exceedingly complex and are not near a solution. Knee-jerk responses and bland condemnations have not been effec-

tive in stopping unethical practice in the past. What is needed is more of a debate and a dialogue to enable understanding of the issues. If we are to approach the subject with intellectual honesty then today all we can hope for is a clarification of the issues involved, avoidance of terminological confusion and an understanding of the context in which the debate takes place. To do this we must have a brief history of events and how they have shaped the debate. We can then dissect the components of the debate. If at the end there are some new questions to be answered then this chapter will have served its purpose.

2. Development of the debate: a historical perspective

Clinical organ transplantation began in the mid 1950s, initially with kidney transplants between living identical twins, since at that time chemical immunosuppression was not available. Azathioprine

G.M. Collins, J.M. Dubernard, W. Land and G.G. Persijn (eds), Procurement, Preservation and Allocation of Vascularized Organs 301–316
© 1997 Kluwer Academic Publishers.

and steroids began to be used in the early 1960s, leading to allotransplantation whereby non-identical siblings, other family members and cadaver donors became possible sources for organs. The resultant expansion in transplant activity is well recorded in the reports of the Transplant Registry and it is interesting when we look back today that a sizeable proportion of those kidneys came from living non-related donors [e.g. 1–3. See also reviews 4–6].

There is little to indicate the existence of unethical behaviour in those early days, but it must be remembered that the ethical milieu has changed drastically since then, not only in medicine but generally. It is difficult to comprehend today, for example, that anyone could have allowed some of the microbiological or radiation studies carried out by the USA Government at that time. It is difficult to understand how some physicians could have allowed poor Americans with syphilis to go untreated in order to observe the long term effects of spirochaetal infections: this is, however, exactly what was done in the USA in the post war years. In the field of transplantation, it would now be unacceptable to ask prisoners to become donors, but this was practised in the USA and was obviously acceptable. There is, however, little to indicate that in the 1960s, when transplantation was practically confined to the USA and Europe, that there was any trafficking or commerce in organs. In 1970, however, the Transplantation Society felt this was an important enough danger to declare that the sale of organs by donors living or dead is indefensible under any circumstances [7].

The question of commerce began to surface in the early 1980s. This became almost inevitable for several reasons – first, graft and patient survival was improved as a result of deliberate blood transfusions and the advent of cyclosporin A, second, a large number of renal transplant units were opened in many countries, including in many developing countries, third there was an increase in demand for organs and fourth, living non-related donors began to be used after a period when this had stopped because of the successful introduction of cadaver donation based on brain-death criteria.

Trading in organs began to be reported. It is important to remember that even in those early days of commerce in organs, this was already an international issue. Not only was there evidence, mainly in the lay press, that trafficking and commerce were taking place in developing countries such as those in Latin America and India, but attempts to cash in on the demand for organs were also being made by entrepreneurs in Europe and the USA. For example, in Germany, Count

Rainer Rene Adelmann zu Adelmannsfelden styling himself a 'specialist in legal loopholes', set up an Organ Bureau offering US$30–40 000 for a kidney to unfortunate people who had debt problems and who were identified through bankruptcy notices in newspapers. An American physician in Virginia also tried to establish a similar enterprise in the USA.

It is not difficult to guess the profession's reaction to these developments. This was totally justifiable and understandable: there were sensational stories and reports in the media, and politicians were also beginning to look into the question. Furthermore, members of the profession were on the one hand genuinely concerned at the effects of commerce on the whole enterprise of cadaver donation, perceived to be motivated by altruism, and on the other by a genuine revulsion at the thought of the commodification of the human body. Laws were enacted banning commerce, and professional guidelines from practically all transplantation societies adopted the same attitude. It is again important to understand that the outcry and its response were mainly in those countries that had dialysis facilities and could afford to dialyse patients who had no donors. In developing countries such as India, the international outcry had the effect of driving commercial donation/transplantation underground – a situation similar to that which occurred in response to bans on alcohol and on abortion in Western countries. Transplantation in those countries did not stop, despite an absence of cadaver donation. In one Latin American study which asked 'In your country, is paid organ donation acceptable?' the answer from 13 countries was a unanimous 'No'. The answer to the question 'In your country, is paid organ donation suspected to occur?' was more revealing: five of the 13 countries said 'Yes' [8]. The fact that in many cases paid living organ donation occurred in family donations began to illustrate some of the complexities of the whole series of questions about buying/selling/incentives/compensation etc.

In 1985 the Transplantation Society published its guidelines forbidding payment for organs and members of the society abide by the guidelines on pain of expulsion.

2.1. The origins of 'rewarded gifting'

A meeting was held in Pittsburgh in 1987 to honour Dr Tom Starzl, one of the pioneers of organ transplantation. One of the speakers there was a Dr C.T. Patel who eloquently argued that the circumstances prevalent in India warranted a second look at, and perhaps a redefinition of, the question of payments [9].

Essentially his argument was that India was poor, had no public dialysis facilities to make an impact, and cadaver donation was non-existent. Patients paid others to donate kidneys to them in order to save their lives. As far as we are aware, this was the first time that someone came from a country actually practising commerce, and defended the practice at a public scientific meeting. However, what Dr Patel was proposing was not justification of commerce in human organs. He was making a more profound statement when he went on to generalize: 'Kidney donation is a good act. It is the gift of life. The financial incentive to promote such an act is moral and justified.' At some point he used the terms 'gifting, with reward' and the term 'rewarded gifting' entered the lexicon of transplantation. I found it fascinating that at the same conference Dr Francis Moore, obviously against the practice of commerce, seemed also to introduce a shade of grey when he said 'selling of kidneys from living donors, evidently a common practice in India, finds a *negative response in our society unless the recipients are chosen without respect to ability to pay, i.e. some form of government subsidy*' (our italics) [10].

2.2. The era of open debate: definitions

For many of us the mid 1980s was an era of confusion, but also an era when we began to find the correct questions to ask. Fear of the consequences conditioned many views. For example at the first major debate of this issue by the Transplantation Society at its XIIth International Congress in Sydney in 1988 it was noted that we have our prejudices, and these are to some extent coloured and informed by the prevailing conditions in the countries where we practise. While I believe there is a distinct difference between 'rewarded gifting' and 'rampant commercialization', I am worried about opening floodgates, for the consequences could be bad. And I ask myself: even if societal acceptance is the ultimate arbiter of ethics where do we, as a profession, draw the line? [11]. Two other significant developments occurred at that conference. Peter Little, who at that time was a nephrologist in charge of a kidney transplant programme in Baghdad, pointed out that the Transplantation Society should not see itself as the only arbiter of ethics, since its council was made up exclusively of people from the developed rich Western world and could not understand or represent the views of those from the poorer developing world, who made up the bulk of mankind [12]. Dr Little was not the only person critical of the Society. Dr Raj Yadav, from India, also decried the tendency of the Society to criticize without making an effort to understand, or even to

agree to visit India to help Indians in their efforts to establish cadaver kidney donation.

The other significant event was the reference by Robert Sells to the work of a group in Madras that was performing paid kidney transplantation allegedly without many of the features of rampant commercialism [13]. Dr Reddy and his colleagues in Madras were apparently not using brokers. They claimed to have adequate checks and balances, including psychiatric evaluation of the potential donors and, more significantly, they provided health insurance for the donor for 3 years after the donation. These and other features of this programme, e.g. fixed payments to donors themselves (£1000 sterling at that time) allowed the group, while not claiming to be introducing 'rewarded gifting', to claim that their version was much more acceptable than the Bombay version of uncontrolled, unchecked commercialism, where the bulk of the money paid for the organ went to the broker or middleman.

It seemed at this stage that the confusion was only being compounded. There seemed a clear need for more detailed discussion, clarification and hopefully understanding. The opportunity arose at a conference organized by Dr John Dossetor and Dr Calvin Stiller in Ottawa in 1989. Entitled *Ethics, Justice and Commerce in Transplantation: A Global View*, this was a pivotal conference which brought together perspectives from around the world, and involved philosophers, ethicists, lawyers and neurologists in addition to divisions involved in transplantation. At the conference Daar *et al.* [14] presented a simple classification of the ethical and practical issues of living donor kidney transplantation. The aim was to facilitate discussion by clarifying what was being discussed. Category VI (criminally coerced donation) became important a little later when it became obvious that rumours, while not yet substantiated, were increasing to suggest that criminal activity (surreptitious organ removal, murder, kidnappings) were taking place. Indeed the United Nations soon after appointed Professor Vitit Muntarbhorn of Thailand to investigate these allegations.

The organizers in Ottawa also invited Dr Reddy, who attended with his colleague Dr Thiagarajan. In two separate presentations [15,16] they defended vigorously their practice in Madras, the overall message being that they were primarily acting to benefit their patients, who had no choice other than death. Their results, they claimed, were excellent under the circumstances. The then President of the Transplantation Society, Professor Richard Batchelor, was invited by the Indian participants to send a team to India to study the situation at first hand. He chose Sells and Daar, who were both members of the Ethics Committee of the Transplantation Society, to represent the Society. They went to India, had extensive discussions, saw at first hand what was happening, interviewed donors and recipients and participated in a conference of the Indian Society of Urology in Bangalore, at which the issue of rampant commercialism and 'rewarded gifting' was discussed under the chairmanship of Dr Eli Friedman. They subsequently presented their findings and recommendations to the Council of the Society during the next (XIIIth) International Congress of the Transplantation Society in San Francisco in 1990 [17]. In essence, they recommended that the Society, rather than condemning the Indians, should try actively to help them develop cadaver donation and transplantation. These recommendations were agreed to in principle by the Society at a general assembly during the conference in San Francisco. Several members, notably Dr Sells, have actually implemented the recommendations and, for example, have arranged scholarships and grants to train young Indian surgeons in cadaver kidney transplantation.

India, however, is not the only country involved, although historically it has been at the forefront of this debate. Other countries have also been involved, including the Philippines, Iraq, Latin American countries, Egypt (see [18]); and, more recently, South Korea. A very well publicized case in London, UK, is thought by many to have been only the tip of the iceberg. It involved the sale of their kidneys by poor Turkish peasants who were actually flown to London from Turkey and at the private Humana Hospital had their kidneys removed for transplantation into rich British recipients at the same hospital. The media uproar resulted in a law in Britain which allows non-related living donation only under the most extreme of circumstances. Indeed, the law established a new regulatory authority known as the Unrelated Living Transplant Regulatory Authority (ULTRA). The political response was criticized by many as being unnecessarily hasty. Philosophers responded in various ways. At least one philosopher, Dr Janet Radcliffe-Richards, argued strongly that there was nothing wrong with buying and selling of organs under the circumstances pertaining to the poor Turks in London. This and the professional/ethical and other legal responses are discussed later.

In 1990 Walter Land and John Dossetor organized another very important and influential conference in Munich. Entitled *Organ Replacement Therapy: Ethics, Justice and Commerce* it was viewed as Ottawa II. The book resulting from that conference [19] is a landmark publication that goes a long way towards explaining some of the complexities of this issue. During that conference, an additional dimension was added by Dr L.R. Cohen's strong advocacy of the ethical virtues of a futures market in cadaveric organs [20].

3. A discussion of the issues

3.1. Some common concepts

What do we agree about? Concepts probably supportable by the majority, are:

(1) A fundamental assumption underlying all discussion of this subject must be the sanctity of human life. The issues raised from this axiom are discussed below.

(2) The dialogue itself must continue until a breakthrough makes it irrelevant. This would happen if there more resources were available world-wide and rates of cadaver donation improved dramatically (with public support); or when xenotransplantation was really successful. Currently, some of the most important thinkers and practitioners continue to participate in the debate. Even accepting the premise that our fundamental duty is to ban commerce and trading in human organs and tissues, that position can only translate into successful, long term practice if it is based on informed, public discussion and if it seriously considers where in fact the line is to be drawn; if it looks at alternatives without emotion; and if it is very clear what are the overall goals, aims and objectives of public policy.

(3) It is probably easier to control and regulate cadaver donation than living donation.

(4) The discussion should be approached in a way which will isolate individual issues, to be dealt with in depth. This will avoid confusion and emotion.

3.2. The issues raised

The very nature of life, of the body and its parts, and of the relationships between different individuals and between individuals and their governing structures need to be considered. At the same time, the meaning of freedom, of self-determination, and the conditions upon which these can be infringed will inform the debate upon the nature of consent (to organ donation; to surgery; to the donation of organs by related cadavers; [is presumed consent really ethical? See [21]] and will influence the details of legislation. An examination needs to be made of the psychological and emotional basis for the act of donation on the part of the living donor and the relatives of the cadaver 'donor'. An understanding has to be gained regarding the nature of incentives and what criteria constitute a deterioration of incentives to the realm of coercion. In the end, where will the decisions come from: the profession?; the bioethics establishment?; the religious authorities?; the law? It has been claimed that societal acceptance is the final arbiter of ethics, but what are we as professionals to do if we do not agree, and where do we draw the line?

Even if we leave religion aside, there will always be disagreement as to whether the primary philosophical approach to this debate should be deontological or consequentialist (see [22].) What if the two approaches produce different conclusions? The very nature of ethics will be raised: is it universal, regional or situational? It might be necessary to come to a real understanding of the relationship between principles on the one hand and their application in individual circumstances on the other. The very fact that we now have professional ethicists employed in hospitals suggests that 'principlism' alone is inadequate: we have to struggle with the details.

3.3. The context

Little takes place in a total vacuum. The context in which today's debate unfolds has rarely been emphasized. It is not even clear to many transplant surgeons today that the Hippocratic approach to the issues of donation, and especially of allocation, has been superseded by the discipline of bioethics. Indeed the birth of the bioethics establishment itself (especially in the USA) was nurtured by a shortage of haemodialysis facilities in the 1950s and 1960s. The implications of bioethics, involving as it does not only professional ethicists but philosophers, lawyers, religious scholars, economists, health policy experts/consultants, anthropologists, academics etc., is that the role of the professional transplant clinician has been diminished. This is exactly why knee jerk, intuitive or emotional responses will now not be adequate. The situation is compounded by the fact that, as medical professionals, we are not yet prepared intellectually or by training to discuss many of the issues with the people who influence public policy. Unfortunately this also happens to coincide with a period when the traditional awe and respect of the profession by the public has been eroding substantially.

With respect to bioethics itself, one of the most important characteristics of its teenage development has been its secularization [23]. The very basis of 'moral'

behaviour has always been and will continue to be discussed, but with secularization the rules of the game will continue to change. With radical pluralism we are all moral strangers, and how can moral strangers enter into civilized discourse? Commonality is to be found in only mutual respect and limited democracy [24]. Societal ethics, as opposed to professional ethics, are here to stay, especially in the field of transplantation [25]. We must learn the rules quickly.

The shortage of organs, itself contributed to by the success of transplantation, must also be seen against the background of escalating health care costs and economic constraints. Even the wealthiest countries in the world will have to prioritize those services to be funded from public sources, if they have not done so already. This will only mean one thing in the future: the erosion of the luxury of 'ethical behaviour' and the ascendency of economists and accountants in formulating health care policy.

Members of the medical and related professions themselves, by their behaviour, may be inadvertently contributing to the context of this debate. The obligation from them must, at a minimum, be that their behaviour is consistent with the principles they espouse. In the analysis of the basis of donation the theme of 'altruism' recurs. This term is always used in referring to living donors, or to the relatives of a potential deceased donor. If an enterprise is to be predicated on such an illusory (in today's society) value, should it be restricted only to the act of donation? Why is the profession itself not to be held up to such a high and sublime moral value? This phenomenon was aptly summarized by Dickens, who pointed out that it may be incongruous and hypocritical that when hospitals make money from transplantation, physicians and associated health professionals advance careers and incomes, drug companies profiteer and the medical industrial complex is enriched, only the original donor of tissues is expected to be altruistic [26]. Indeed, even the pilots and airline staff who carry donated organs are paid for their troubles [27]. It can be argued that if we do not volunteer our services on an altruistic basis then we should at least restrain ourselves from emphasizing altruism as the basis for motivation to donate. In any case, motivation is very complex in any human enterprise, and altruism has been over-rated [28]. It may be time that the material benefits derived by transplant surgeons from transplantation should become an ethical issue in its own right. It is also important to realize that the adoption of the predominant paradigm against any form of payment for organs, and the resulting legislation, occurred before there had been significant public debate.

3.4. Arguments against payment for organs

These have taken various forms. Those from among
the profession have generally condemned any payment
on the basis that buying and selling of organs is repug-
nant, repulsive, unethical and immoral. Others have
felt that the most important argument is that the donor
as an individual is likely to be poor and will be exploitable; this argument, of course, extends to the
donors being poor as a class, exploitable by the rich as
a class. Poverty itself is a form of coercion – and so the
donation is coerced. Trafficking in organs will divide
society. It has been pointed out, by us among many
others [29], that the results of rampant commercialism
are likely to be poor, mainly because the institutions
involved do not act according to the best interests of
the donor and recipient but are simply using them to
enrich themselves. The profit motive precludes good
medical care and application of strict medical criteria
of selection. Furthermore, availability of such transplants would tend to inhibit development of cadaver
programmes and even of those programmes trying to
encourage intrafamily donation. This is a purely consequentialist argument but one that at present is
applicable.

Others have relied on Kantian arguments that selling
organs commodifies the human body (which must be
assumed to have some sanctity) and thereby degrades
the donor to a 'thing'. The monotheistic religions will
probably argue along similar lines. It can also be
argued, of course, that paying/selling/buying will
inevitably undermine the whole edifice of modern-day
organ donation based on altruism. Similarly, if donating an organ is based upon the principle of gifting [30]
then it is a contradiction in terms [31] to make any
payment for the organ.

There are also some specific arguments applicable to
surgeons and also related to the question of consent
[32]. These include:

(1) Surgeons should operate on patients based only on
    therapeutic (physical or psychological) benefit, not
    to materially enrich the subject.
(2) A donor who is paid is being given an incentive,
    which if he is poor enough will amount to coer-
    cion. He can therefore not give proper voluntary
    consent. Poor people may also be pressurized by
    their needy families or by third parties into selling
    their organs. Such lack of voluntarism in consent
    would be hard to detect.
(3) A scenario which has apparently been described in
    South America may come to pass: a poor person
    may wish to buy his family out of poverty by
    selling all his organs, including vital ones.

Many of the consequentialist reasoning, of course,
depends upon the 'slippery slope' argument – that once
any payment, no matter how small, is allowed, then
this will inevitably lead to all the other personal, professional and societal evils alluded to above. This, of
course, leads to the question of whether such transactions can be regulated. Some feel that the strongest
argument against the sale of organs is the inability to
regulate such transactions [33].

3.5. Arguments in favour of some form of payment for organs

These have been expressed by various commentators
at different times in different contexts. They are juxta-
posed here to the preceding section to demonstrate the
complexity of the issues, arguments and counter-
arguments.

In the first instance is the issue of self-determination.
This is a particularly strong argument in Western
secular societies which, at least since the Enlighten-
ment, have tended to emphasize the rights of the individual over the society he finds himself/herself in.
Surely a person who has the right to climb the north
face of the Eiger or to become rich by taking part in
Formula 1 racing has the right to give up an organ and
to receive payment for it? Whether others will judge
him a vendor or a donor will not bother this individual,
who will wish to determine what right society has to
deter him, even if his action entails harm to himself. In
the Western liberal tradition of ethical and political
thought, respect for a person's autonomy means
respect for his unfettered voluntary choice as the sole
rightful determinant of his actions except where the
interests of others need protection [34]. Since utilitar-
ianism is as valid as, if not more valid than, other
philosophical approaches, such an individual would
feel entitled to claim that he is increasing the overall
good, welfare and thriving of society by increasing the
numbers of organs available for transplantation. The
onus to show the opposite (i.e. that numbers of organs
would be reduced) falls then to those who hold the
opposite viewpoint; the latter would have to demonstrate, in addition, that alternate methods of organ
procurement are more effective in the long run.

This individual will also be entitled to claim that
since he is a free agent, and is not donating under circumstances of potential family pressure, that he
demonstrates true voluntarism – and voluntarism is
surely a major component of legal consent [35,36]. It
therefore seems wrong to assert that in a market system
for the procurement of organs free and informed
consent by the donor is no longer possible. If it is said

that the prospect of financial reward pressures an individual into making a choice which is not truly free, one should also take into account that most individuals make important decisions throughout their lives, especially those decisions concerning their work, which reflect a need for money. Yet such decisions are generally regarded as being freely made.

Many philosophers have pointed out that there are no compelling arguments against the sale of organs *per se* [24,37], but that it is the potential abuse of the practice, especially if only the rich then receive organs from the poor (exploitation), which makes this practice unacceptable. The immediate response then is that you do not 'throw away the baby with the bath water' – you try and regulate the practice, introducing mechanisms whereby the ability to pay for an organ should not deter any needy recipient from obtaining an organ [10]. It should be the abuse, not the practice, that should be banned; the practice should be regulated. Perhaps the best arguments along these lines have been put forward by the philosopher Janet Radcliffe-Richards in relation to the uproar that greeted reports of the purchasing of kidneys in London from poor peasants from Turkey. Amongst other things, she has commented that the question of poverty being a coercive force is untenable, and even if entertained, forbidding something altogether because of the danger of coercion is extremely difficult to justify because it involves placing a certain limitation on the freedom of everyone in order to prevent the possibility of limitation of the freedom of some. She argues that although direct altruism is a good ideal, and that it may be best if a kidney is offered out of love for a relative, that this does not in the least suggest that what is less than best is necessarily wrong.

In addition, many persons who voluntarily try to sell their organs may even be exclusively altruistically motivated, e.g. towards their family, a phenomenon which is discussed below [39]. If we admit that, we will also recognize that the question of self-degradation depends on whether the person who sells an organ evaluates his/her action as self-degradation or not, and this may depend on several circumstances. Is it really self-evident that the young Turkish father who had arranged to sell a kidney in order to pay for urgent hospital treatment for his little daughter would have violated his dignity and self-respect to a greater degree by selling an organ than by letting his daughter die?

Donation within families is also not without potential pitfalls. As has been pointed out by us previously [35], there are potentials for what are considered unacceptable practices in the family donor situation also, where both coercion (psychological 'moral bullying and other assorted pressures') and payment can and do take place. If the willing and the subtly coerced can be distinguished in the family context, they can also be distinguished in other contexts. If we believe we cannot, we would have to give up living related donation completely, as did the Munich group in the late 1980s [35].

Those who favour the regulation of commerce, whether in the living donor or cadaver situation, have pointed out that the slippery slope argument is philosophically a weak basis on which to build public policy. Risks of all types are controlled by legislation, guidelines and regulations: examples include alcohol and driving (an example of where society does not over-react to every potential abuse) and nuclear power. In market economies, unequal bargaining situations are quite customary, and the commodification of the body and its power of labour, regulated by open markets, is a normal, even a basic phenomenon (generally in cases without a comparable gain of medical values as in the field of organ transplantation). Our societies' reaction is usually not to ban such markets, but to build in checks and balances, as e.g. minimum wage laws, protection of labour laws and Social Security systems.

Although there have been sporadic attempts to establish commercial organizations to deal in live donor organs in the West, these have often been by individuals outside the profession, outside of academia and motivated by a personal desire for enrichment, such as Count Rainer Adelmann in Germany. In the cadaver situation, on the other hand, especially in the USA respectable members of academia and of the health policy establishment have openly written in favour of commercial arrangements, e.g. a futures market. These advocates have included Brams [40], Perry [41], Peters [42], Schwindt & Vining [43], Hansmann [44] and more recently, Cohen [20] and Blumstein [45].

3.6. Documentation of a crisis unfolding: the ostrich syndrome

An important reason for continuing the debate and looking for the boundaries of ethical practice is that unethical and sometimes criminal transplant and related activity is not only continuing but is increasing. This has become an international issue, which in the end has the potential to harm transplantation in every country. Indeed, the whole concept of transplantation *per se* is already being questioned.

In November and December 1992 a British-Canadian documentary film aired on television in Europe and North America alleged that Moscow has now become a major centre for obtaining organs and tissues for commercial transplants both in Moscow and for export abroad for transplantation, for research and for other commercial activities. The makers of the programme claimed that one Russian company sold 700 kidneys, hearts and lungs, 1400 livers, 18000 thymus glands, 2000 eyes and 3000 pairs of testicles (which are used for rejuvenating cream). Documents showed that a Russian company had agreed to supply foreign customers with 600 kidneys at $20 000 each. Bruce Harris of Covenant House, the London-based international child-care agency, who was an investigator for the programme, claimed to have copies of commercial contracts for organs between a Russian company and clients in Germany, Italy and Israel. Businessmen in Britain, Italy and Turkey had proposed joint ventures to undertake low cost transplants for foreigners in Moscow, where a kidney transplant can be obtained for as little as $80 000 [46].

Accusations were also made in the film that illegal/criminal acquisition of organs occurred in Honduras and Argentina. Judy Jackson, the Canadian director of the film, is quoted as saying 'Hospitals in the US are vying with each other for organs and one major transplant hospital went to Brazil to offer equipment for livers'. The film accuses a Moscow surgeon of using a false manifest in the name Eurotransplant to export organs. In a broadcast of the film in Germany in December 1993 the Eurotransplant Foundation is accused of accepting organs from donors from Moscow, from donors who did not fulfil brain-death criteria. Eurotransplant was said to have offered those organs for transplantation without mentioning their origins. These accusations forced Eurotransplant to initiate a lawsuit against Spiegel-TV GmbH in Germany to stop it from further transmission of the programme. The court in Dusseldorf allowed the claim on 21st December 1993. Eurotransplant issued a press communique to the Deutsche Presse Agentur for publication on 15th January 1994 [47].

A Reuter article in April 1994 quoted Italian magistrate/prosecutor Carlo Maria Capristo in the southern Italian port city of Bari who claimed that the Mafia was probably involved in the trafficking of corneas from Eastern Europe to Italy. A total of 43 people were being investigated for trafficking in corneas and other organs and it was claimed that doctors, hospital officials and businessmen were involved in the investigation, which began in November 1993 when two nurses at a Rome hospital told magistrates that the eye of a deceased patient had been removed and replaced with glass. The report claimed that a cornea transplant in Italy costs $7000 [48].

In April 1994 there was a major scare against foreigners in Guatemala, who were suspected of being involved in the kidnapping of children for illegal adoption and to obtain organs for transplantation. An American woman, June Weinstock, was severely beaten up and was unconscious on a ventilator in hospital [49].

A French television film with the title 'Voleurs d'Organs' produced some evidence that patients in the psychiatric asylum of Montes de Oca, near Buenos Aires, Argentina, had killed for the purpose of selling their organs, especially corneas. The makers of the film claim (and present a surviving witness) that some people were abducted and killed for their organs in Bogota and that some children from the slums were criminally deprived of their corneas after having been brought to the hospital for treatment of diarrhoea etc. The film alleges that there obviously is an organ market, especially for corneas, in Bogota and in the Mexican town of Tijuana. In Tijuana the film-makers were offered a kidney for US$15 000. There are also accusations in the film that black market corneas from Colombia are transplanted in France.

In France, the enthusiasm with which transplant surgeons have approached donation seems to have had a negative impact. Control over transplant regulation in France has now passed from the hands of France Transplant, the professional body, to the government directly. What effect this will have in the future and whether the 'presumed consent/opting out' law will continue is unclear. In the short term, cadaver kidney donation rates have dramatically fallen in France and in several other European countries [50].

In South Korea, a gang organized to traffick in human organs for transplantation was recently arrested. Kidneys can be bought openly in Bombay; there are reports that it is also possible to buy organs in Egypt and Iraq [18,51].

3.7. Living non-related donation as an issue

In 1984, three Nobel prizewinners (Peter Medewar, Jean Dausset and George Snell) wrote to President Reagan to suggest that no transplant should ever be performed between unrelated individuals. These three individuals were all eminent scientists in the field of transplantation, and they certainly had a right to express their opinion. However, whose views were they representing? What was the basis for their advice? What qualifies a person trained in the sciences to advise on matters that clearly have much larger, societal implications? What debates took place prior to their advice to Reagan? We believe that this was another example of a knee-jerk response that is subsequently difficult to support.

We have recently reviewed the subject of living genetically non-related donors from several viewpoints

[6,52]; our conclusion, based upon documented facts and the writings of ethicists, philosophers and professionals and also based on precedence within the profession, was that provided certain guidelines are followed there is nothing intrinsically wrong with donation by well-motivated individuals who are not related to the recipient. The following is a summary of the analysis by us and by others.

3.7.1. Consent

There is no reason to assume that consent will be invalid. There is reason to believe that voluntarism is more likely [35,36] than in family situations. The ethical principle that underlies the requirement of informed consent is the principle of respect for autonomy. In bioethical discussions today, there is a widespread consensus that it is important to start with a general presumption in favour of this principle [53]. This implies the conclusion that the donor (...) has a right to take a reasonable risk in order to achieve substantial benefit for the recipient. This is true even if the donor and recipient are not related [54]. Moreover, we have to admit that the risk–benefit ratio of any proposed living donor transplant is determined ultimately by personal value judgments and that these judgments should generally be made by the one most affected by the outcome – the prospective donor [55]. There is, however, a possibility for conflict between autonomy for donors and autonomy for medical professionals. In such cases, the autonomy of a transplant professional or group to decide the appropriateness of a given donor–recipient transplant, based on analysis of the potential risks and benefits, has equivalent or greater primacy than that of the donor [54].

3.7.2. Vulnerability/exploitation

A wife or husband or close friend is not more likely to be exploited than is a genetically related donor. This fear profoundly fails as a convincing argument [56].

3.7.3. Commerce

The fear that commerce will inevitably ensue (the slippery slope) is also unsupportable [56]. In theory every possible evil is possible: it is not donation by a nonrelative which should be condemned, but the abuse that might ensue from trafficking. Abuse can be regulated against by rational agents: the right model here may be the Warnock Committee's report. This did not ban all surrogate mothering arrangements, but only commercial surrogacy arrangements [38].

3.7.4. Increasing organ donation

We have argued that such donations do indeed have the potential of increasing organ donation [57]. This utilitarian argument in favour of living non-related kidney donation has also been made by others [56,4]. In fact, in the early days of renal transplantation such donors were used almost routinely and they made a significant contribution [1,5]. In the 1972 report of the Registry of Human Transplantation, 10% of the 1488 transplants were from such donors. (See [6].)

3.7.5. Moral rights of potential recipients

While it is virtually impossible to provide all potential recipients with a cadaveric organ within a limited period of time, it seems hard, if not impossible, to justify withholding an organ that could be donated to a severely ill person by a close friend who is histocompatible, altruistically motivated and voluntarily consenting, just because the donor is not related to the recipient. The potential recipient has a moral right not to be excluded from therapeutic measures without compelling reasons. As long as we do not violate other basic moral principles, we have the duty to maximize the recipient's chances of receiving curative, palliative or even life saving treatment.

3.7.6. Altruism

If we argue that altruism is the basis for donation, then why exclude all but the very few? It seems odd to emphasize altruism and then circumscribe its opportunity for expression [56]. Although a few people would not support donation by a spouse, the majority do, in fact, accept that this form of donation is completely supportable. Donation by a spouse acknowledges altruism to be mediated by significant and powerful emotions, which are not plausibly confined to genetic or even legal relations. In fact we could argue that a complete definition of altruism would emphasize the lack of a relationship (and therefore the possibility of a direct benefit): strangers would in fact make the best altruists. This is reflected in category III of the classification of living donors. After all, in the cadaver donor situation, it is (almost) always a stranger whose organs are used; it is strangers who consent to the donation; card carriers agree to donate to strangers when they die. What, then, is the logic of denying living persons the right to exercise this prerogative?

3.7.7. Consistency and regeneration

We allow living individuals to donate blood and bone marrow to unrelated, often unknown, recipients. Why not, say, a kidney? The argument that marrow and blood are regenerating tissues while kidneys are not is counterbalanced by the fact that kidneys are paired and that there are no unacceptable short- or long-term risks of donating a kidney. If this argument is extended, to be consistent, we would have to disallow living genetically related donation, and few would accept this. Furthermore it seems an artificial construct to base ethical acceptability on the basis of regeneration. The underlying principle is to avoid harm. *Primum non nocere* as a principle is acceptable to the living donor, whether related or not, but it is not the only rule or value to be considered. The most relevant moral principles in medical ethics today are (1) respect for persons, including their autonomous choices and actions; (2) beneficence, including both the obligation to benefit others (positive beneficence) and to maximize good consequences – i.e. to do the greatest good for the greatest number (utility); (3) justice, the principle of fair and equitable distribution of benefits and burdens; and finally (4) nonmaleficence (*non nocere*), the obligation not to inflict harm [54,58]. With regard to the living donor, *primun non nocere* as a principle is, to a measured extent, breached since the nephrectomy does carry a small risk for the donor. Since this is, however, at the donor's request and for the physical benefit of another individual, this infringement of the principle of nonmaleficence is generally outweighed by the principles of beneficence and respect for the donor's autonomy and by the fact that, with regard to both donor and recipient, the overall risk–benefit relationship is increased. In any case, this shows once more the impotence of Hippocratic fundamentalism in the transplant setting.

3.7.8. *Results*

This is a key consideration: it would be difficult completely to justify living non-related donation if the results were not good. They are, however, excellent [6] whether donor-specific transfusions are used or not, ... and they are in fact better than the results of cadaver donor renal transplantation. What is more important, there is no evidence from centres reporting their results, and where the practice was adopted not for the benefit of the doctors but for the benefit of the patients, that there has been any deterioration to a situation of paid organ donation. There is also no evidence to indicate that such donation *per se* has impaired the development of either cadaveric or living related donation. There is evidence, on the contrary, that successful cadaver programmes can be established after the availability of living non-related donation: this has happened in Iran (I. Fazel, personal communication).

3.7.9. *Beneficial outcome*

The goal of transplantation, as indeed of any ethical medical enterprise, is to bring about a beneficial outcome. It is easy to understand the benefit to the recipient. It is also easy to understand the benefit to the institution (doctors, laboratories, hospital board etc.) whether it be a for-profit or non-profit organization. The fact that pharmaceutical companies derive a beneficial outcome is also undoubted. Health care providers, usually the government, also benefit financially by not having to pay for dialysis. Studies have repeatedly shown that living donors derive significant benefit from the act of donation. For many, it is perhaps the single most important (humanitarian) act in their lives. The vast majority would be willing to donate again, even if the transplant had failed. Is it illogical, therefore, to argue for the extension of beneficial outcome to the living donor, be that individual genetically related or not to the recipient? Elsewhere this has been the argument for the financial benefit of the donor – here it is an argument for the psychological, spiritual and moral uplifting of the donor.

3.7.10. *Public opinion*

A small number of studies have looked at this question (see [6] for review). It seems clear that the majority of the public are in favour. It seems doubtful whether the public will ever be against any enterprise such as this, which benefits everyone.

3.7.11. *Professional opinion*

Again, a survey of American transplant institutions has shown that, in principle, the majority are in favour of such donation, although at the time of the study (1989) many were still reluctant to accept such donors [59].

For all these arguments, we confirm the conclusion that where there is a demonstrable and enduring relationship, living non-related donation is ethically acceptable. Indeed, at both the Ottawa [60] and the Munich (Resolution no.5 [19]) conferences, there was consensus supporting donation by voluntary living donors. When not genetically related they can also be called emotionally related. The extension to altruistic strangers seems obvious.

4. The response to the question of commerce

4.1. Professional/ethical response

No respectable body of professionals has accepted rampant commerce as the basis for donation and transplantation. The following examples document the overwhelming negative response. The 1971 Committee on Morals and Ethics of The Transplantation Society stated: 'The sale of organs by donors living or dead is indefensible under any circumstances' [7]. The 1985 Transplantation Society Guidelines declared 'It must be established by the patient and the transplant team alike that the motives of the donor are altruistic and in the best interest of the recipient and self serving or for profit. Active solicitation of living unrelated donors for profit is unacceptable. It should be clearly understood that no payment to the donor by the recipient, the recipient's relatives or any other supporting organization, can be allowed. However, reimbursement for loss of work earnings and any other expenses related to donation is acceptable.' Special resolution: 'No transplant surgeon/team shall be involved directly or indirectly in the buying or selling of organs/tissues or in any transplant activity aimed at commercial gain to himself/herself or an associated hospital or institute. Violation of these guidelines by any member of The Transplantation Society may be cause for expulsion from the Society' [61].

The World Health Organization considers, 'Such trade is inconsistent with the most basic human values and contravenes the Universal Declaration of Human Rights and the spirit of the WHO Constitution' [62]. According to European Health Ministers 1987: 'A human organ must not be offered for profit by any organ exchange organization, organ banking centre or by any other organization or individual whatsoever' [62]. A statement from the Conference on Ethics, Justice and Commerce; A Global View. Ottawa Aug. 20–24 1989 was: 'The buying and selling of human organs and tissues for transplantation is unacceptable' [60]. Similar feelings were expressed at the Conference on Organ Replacement Therapy: Ethics, Justice and Commerce. Munich, December 11–14, 1990: 'The Congress supports maintaining a prohibition of commerce to obtain organs or tissues for allotransplantation' [19] Resolution #2.

Similar sentiments have also been expressed by regional transplantation societies around the world.

4.2. Legal response

A large number of countries, including some with little or no transplant activity, have now included on their statute books laws banning commerce in organs for transplantation. WHO has recently published a book [63] which includes the legislative response to various issues of transplantation, including the question of protection of minors and other disadvantaged and vulnerable individuals, and the different types of consent. This subject is discussed in more detail in Chapter 38.

Although transplantation has spread rapidly, many countries do not yet have specific laws on transplantation. However, transplantation rarely operates in a legal vacuum. Laws from the past often exist to regulate, for example, the legal status of dead bodies, and criteria of death have been developed regarding religious and public health concerns, for instance, that affect the transfer of body parts into living recipients [64]. Some developing countries, e.g. Argentina and South Africa, have had laws enabling transplantation for a long time, and more recently several developing countries have enacted specific organ transplant legislation. A major survey of organ transplant legislation in 16 Latin American countries was recently published by the Pan American Health Organization [65]. This review looked at the universally important transplant issues such as those above, and reviewed the 'required request' system, recipient selection, determination of death, conflict of interest, funding, donor compensation and international sharing of organs. In March 1987 the Council of Arab Ministers of Health adopted a Unified Arab Draft Law which, it is hoped, will be a model for both living donor and cadaver donor transplantation [62,66].

Regarding the question of commercialism, WHO has recently published a report on developments in the field of transplantation under its auspices between 1987 and 1991 [62]. A large number of developing countries in the Americas, Europe, Eastern Mediterranean, Africa (e.g. Malawi, Zimbabwe), Western Pacific (Singapore) and South East Asia (Indonesia, Sri Lanka) already have some legislation; others have non-statutory measures (Hong Kong, Israel, Malta and Saudi Arabia), while in some jurisdictions (notably India, but also Israel and the Philippines) new legislation is either pending or in preparation [67]. Egypt has adopted a resolution by the General Assembly of the Egyptian Society of Nephrology (effective as of June 30, 1992) authorizing living donor transplantation only between consanguineous relatives. Hong Kong issued on 27th March 1992 a Human Organ Transplant Bill prohibiting commerce and establishing a Human Organ Transplant Board (perhaps modelled on the British system) to approve genetically unrelated living transplants, which would otherwise be illegal. In 1991 Israel proposed an insertion of new provisions in its Public Health Ordinance that would ban commerce. Finally, WHO itself adopted in May 1992 its Guiding Principles on Human Organ Transplants [62,67], with important definitions and clarifications, and any country wishing to develop transplant legislation would be advised to look to this for guidance. Furthermore, the Office of Health Legislation, World

Health Organization, 1211 Geneva 27, Switzerland has details on computer of most of the laws already enacted and its Chief, S.S. Fluss, would be happy to assist any country or organization in this matter.

5. An acceptable approach to the issues raised

It seems obvious that the issues raised are exceedingly complex, and each could form the basis of serious and prolonged discussion by experts from several disciplines. In our introduction, we said that the purpose of this chapter was to try and distinguish the work of those honestly trying to help their patients from the work of those trying to enrich themselves at the expense of their patients. How does one approach this subject? We pointed out during the brief historical review that initially the response to the question of payments for organs was an explicit and emphatic No. This was the overall view, the dominant set of values, the paradigm. The introduction of the concept of some form of payment being ethically acceptable, that in the right circumstances this would not diminish the value of the 'gift' of the donated organ [9], opened a new chapter. Intellectual honesty demanded serious and unimpeded discussion of the issues. There was, however, a lot of confusion and honest discussion seemed unlikely, especially since the subject engendered a lot of emotion. We believe the confusion/ difficulties arose as result of:

(1) the novelty of the idea;
(2) the emotionally charged atmosphere in the late 1980s when the buying and selling of organs was being documented, mainly in the lay press;
(3) the decision-makers coming among the profession and brought up on complete prohibition of payment. They genuinely feared the slippery slope;
(4) there was a significant change to bioethics: societal versus professional values were just coming to the attention of many people in the profession [25], and they were unprepared for this and also feared its implications on their traditional territory;
(5) the term 'rewarded gifting' seemed to many to be a contradiction in terms [18], was essentially the same as commerce [68], was a terminological subterfuge [69]. We have since pointed out that the concept of a 'gift' is not as simplistic as would appear on superficial analysis. Gifts play an important role in society and are consciously or

subconsciously governed by certain requirements/ rules, but essentially they do involve the need for reciprocation in order to be meaningful (See [70]);
(6) the opportunity for serious discussion was absent. 'Ethics', if it appeared at all in the programme of professional congresses, was genuinely paid only lip service, and the discussion was unlikely to be an interdisciplinary one;
(7) the nature of the subject was such that open and honest debate was unusual. Many believed that any 'weakening' on the part of the professional could have resulted in that individual being considered beyond the pale of the profession;
(8) many people in the West assumed this had nothing really to do with them. It seemed a problem for Indians or others in developing countries and was unlikely to come calling at their doorstep.

In 1989, Daar and colleagues introduced at the Ottawa conference a classification that was meant to deal with some of the difficulties mentioned above [11]. It took into account the realities of living kidney donation, the debate going on, and was simple enough to be able to isolate issues to be discussed without confusing them with other categories. It pointed out the grossly acceptable from the grossly unacceptable and in its latest form [71] it clearly delineates the 'grey area' into which any new proposal could be entered for discussion. The criteria that seem obvious for inclusion in the grey area include:

(1) a clearly thought out idea;
(2) the proposals are predominantly for the benefit of the patients, not the doctors or their institutions (we believe this difference in context is the fundamental essence of the discussion);
(3) it should use a framework of ethical/moral/ philosophical principles;
(4) take into account the realities on the ground. It should be clear that whereas fundamental principles are not compromisable or situational, their application to individual situations needs careful thought and weighing of prevailing circumstances.

In 1991 this basic classification was accepted by members of the Ethics Committee of the Transplantation Society as the basis for discussion of this complex subject.

5.1. Ideas currently in the grey area

Despite the fact that 'rewarded gifting' may be supportable, we have now abandoned the term because of all its emotional associations. Nevertheless, we have previously attempted to distinguish between compensated donation and donation with incentive [57]. It should be made quite clear that compensation for genuine expenses incurred in the process of donation by the donor, including lost income and hospital expenses incurred or to be incurred, is acceptable. There is difficulty in working out this compensation in practice (e.g. how much income is lost by a millionaire businessman on a particular day?; does a temporarily unemployed clerk deserve any payment?; who should be making these payments and what mechanisms can be set up to organize this?) and it is unclear what should be compensated for (see below under 'pain money').

The advantage of dividing this category into compensated donation and donation with incentive was the resultant focus on the issue of incentives the appropriateness of which can then be discussed seriously without confusion with other issues.

Taking into account the differences pertaining to the economic and social reality between the developed (rich, advanced, dialysis freely available, well-developed cadaver donation) and the developing (poor, less advanced, no dialysis and no cadaver donation: a good example would be India) worlds, Dossetor and Manickavel [72] and Dossetor [39] have concluded that, although there may be some truth in the argument that extreme poverty may be coercive and that completely unregulated commerce could result in exploitation of the poor by the rich, the burden to benefit ratio in the East is such that payment for organs should be allowed if this could be supervised by honest professionals and members of the public, provided that:

(1) the donor has a genuine altruistic motive for wanting the money e.g. to pay for treatment of a daughter who has leukaemia (indirect altruism); and
(2) the recipient pays not only for the donation/organ but also for improving the conditions where the donor came from (water supply; education or preventive measures; establishing and running of cadaver programmes etc.) This has been called 'mandated philanthropy'.

Sells has written about a variation he calls 'the donor trust' [73,74]. This echoes some of the ideas above; it also makes it possible for poor recipients to be able to obtain organs for transplantation. It would ensure fair payment to the donor and adequate remuneration to the doctors and their institution. It would apply mainly to economically less fortunate countries which have no dialysis or cadaver donation.

The Interdisciplinary Lebendspende (living donor) group in Munich, based at the Ludwig-Maximilians-University, is made up of one transplant professional, together with theologists, psychologists, a lawyer and a legal philosopher. It has looked at the appropriateness of the concept of 'Schmerzensgeld'. Inspired by the legal term of Schmerzensgeld (pain money or smart money, i.e. compensation for personal suffering), which originates from the context of actions for illegal damages, a financial reward could be paid not for the organ, but for the pain and trouble an organ donor has to endure. Such a reward would still fall under the category of 'compensated donation'. It would be closer to removing disincentives than to providing financial incentives and it would preserve the socio-cultural meaning of the act of donation. This *quid pro quo*, paid to related and non-related or emotionally related donors as well, could comprise indirect payments (insurances etc.) as well as a certain amount of cash. In this model, incentives would still be directed not to the sale of the organ itself, but to the act of altruistic or, at least, not financially motivated giving. There seems to be nothing wrong with such payments to donors who, in the eyes of the transplant professional or group, act voluntarily and, at least partially, with altruistic or related motives. This model seems acceptable, desirable and probably sufficient at least for developed countries which have the cultural and legal resources to provide sufficient controls, checks and balances for such a system.

Prof. Gilbert Thiel of the University of Basel has already begun exploring the possibility of offering medical insurance to living donors.

In addition to the above, the following observations and experience are relevant to this discussion. We make no judgement as to their ethical correctness, since serious debate has not taken place and information is limited.

In Iran, a very large number of transplants have been described as occurring under the umbrella of 'rewarded gifting' [75]. It is claimed that doctors and their institutions do not participate in any way in negotiations between donors and recipients. The majority of donations are said to involve altruistic motives, and donors have included voluntary soldiers. The consent obtained from donors and recipients specified that no commerce was involved. The doctors do not profit from carrying out the transplant. The results have been acceptable; there has been no reported overt commercialism and, more significantly, this practice has not stopped the development of cadaver donation, which only awaited the acceptance by religious authorities to get off the ground.

The work of the Madras group led by Dr Reddy [13,15,16] was first brought to the attention of the profession by Sells at the 11th International Congress of the Transplantation Society in Sydney in August 1988 [13]. Reddy and his colleagues have claimed that their programme, which involves payment of about US$ 2000 to living unrelated donors for kidneys, is meant to benefit the recipient; medical criteria are paramount in the selection; psychological enquiry and counselling are available to the donors; poor recipients are (occasionally) transplanted free of charge; medical insurance and follow up are available to the donor for at least 3 years and, quite importantly, no middlemen or brokers are involved. In at least three publications in the scientific literature members of this group have eloquently defended this practice of 'unconventional' transplantation. They have evolved terminology such as 'consideration' and 'solatium' for the payment to donors and have talked about the situation and the culture in India (including the concept of *Dharma*) as justifying their practice. One of their papers was subtitled *To buy or let die*. The same authors, however, have indicated their reservations that such a programme is not likely to function generally in India: there was a danger in maintaining the crucial contextual difference before the enterprise was used for the benefit and profit of doctors, brokers and middlemen [6]. These authors have also avoided the now shunned terminology 'rewarded gifting', although they were first used as an example of such a system.

In a careful study performed in Canada the attitudes of the public, of medical students at McGill University and of medical personnel was evaluated in relation to the question of buying an organ by one of two theoretical recipients. The first theoretical recipient (David) lived near Montreal in Canada, where dialysis is available. The second (Varum) was in Madras, India, where there were no alternatives to transplantation. This was an interesting study which bears close scrutiny; it is also a study whose results are amenable to several interpretations. Essentially there was a majority in favour of purchase from amongst the public for both David (69% yes rate) and Varum (74% yes rate). Medical students had a 'yes' rate of 51% and 57%; medical personnel, especially the transplanters, were less liberal (23% and 27%). What was interesting for this discussion, however, was the observation that the majority from all groups were particularly concerned about the question of the regulation of any such practice. It is also important to note that the responses for David and Varum were not too dissimilar [33]. This focuses the discussion then on the question of regulation, rather than on other issues.

In the USA, particularly in relation to cadaver donation, there have been ideas proposed by eminent academics in favour of open commercialization [45] and even of 'futures' markets [20]. Blumstein [45] has, in addition, pointed out the discrepancy that exists in the way that the whole of the transplant enterprise is organized in the USA (restrictive) compared with the way health care in general has (up to now) been organized (profit and incentive driven). Note, however, that there are financial incentives in the organ procurement system in the USA, but the incentives are meant for the procurers (i.e. medical and technical personnel etc.), and not for the donors. Incentives in the USA have also been supported by the National Kidney Foundation [76] and the United Network on Organ Sharing (UNOS) working group on donation [77]. Some form of incentives for living donors has also been backed by, among others, a former President of the (International) Transplantation Society [78].

6. Conclusion

The subject(s) under discussion are more complex and admit of more subtleties than would appear on superficial analysis. The issues have implications beyond the territory normally handled by physicians alone, and their discussion necessarily now involves all participants in the new discipline of bioethics. We have presented a historical unfolding of the debate and attempted to put it in context, showing thereby that the debate does need to attain a degree of refinement, the participants having to some extent 'lost innocence' [74].

If there is one underlying difference between what is acceptable and what is not, we believe that this difference does reside in the contextual shift between these: on the one hand an enterprise predicated upon profits for doctors, agents and institutions, using the patient as the tool for that enterprise; and on the other, an honest attempt to do what professionals have always been trained to do, which is to serve the interests of our patients as well as possible, not enriching ourselves unduly at the expense of our patients. Others have pointed out that there are differences between well endowed countries and less well endowed countries: what is unacceptable in the former may be acceptable, with safeguards, in the latter.

On the part of the donor, an operational question to consider might be whether the individual is still a 'donor' or has become a 'vendor' [28] – remembering, of course, that there is a strong school of thought among secular philosophers that sees no moral wrong in the selling of organs. As with many ethical debates, it is the premise with which one embarks on the debate that influences its outcome and so long as the premises differ, the outcome will differ. The professional today is caught between the bioethics establishment on one side and the society at large on the other. Both may come to a conclusion that he/she finds difficult to live with and ultimately he/she may have to fall back on a strictly professional code of conduct: a surgeon does not have to operate under conditions that he/she finds ethically unacceptable. The question therefore reverts to where do we, as professionals, draw the line? It may boil down to a question of virtue, of not confusing our interests with those of our patients.

References

1. Payne R, Perkins HA, Kountz SL et al. Unrelated kidney transplantation and matching for HL-A antigens. Transplant Proc 1971; 3: 1036–41.
2. Kountz SL, Perkins HA, Payne R et al. Transplant Proc 1970; 2: 427.
3. Starzl TE, Schroter GPJ, Hartmann NJ et al. Long term (25 year) survival after renal hemotransplantation – the world experience. Transplant Proc 1990; 22: 2361–5.
4. Levey AS, Hou S, Bush HL Jr. Kidney transplantation from unrelated living donors. N Engl J Med 1986; 314: 914–16.
5. Tilney NL, Hollenberg NK. Use of living donors in renal transplantation. Transplant Rev 1987; 1: 225–38.
6. Daar AS, Sells RA. Living non-related donor renal transplantation – a reappraisal. Transplant Rev 1990; 4: 238–40.
7. Committee on Morals and Ethics, Transplantation Society. Ann Intern Med 1971; 75: 631–3.
8. Santiago-Delpin EA. Organ donation and transplantation in Latin America. Transplant Proc 1991; 23: 2516–18.
9. Patel CT. Live renal donation: a viewpoint. Transplant Proc 1988; 20: 1068–70.
10. Moore FD. The ethical revolution: ancient assumptions remodelled under pressure of transplantation: Transplant Proc 1988; 20: 1061–7.
11. Daar AS, Salahudeen AK, Pingle A. Woods HF. Ethics and commerce in live donor renal transplantation: classification of the issues. Transplant Proc 1990; 22: 922–4.
12. Little PJ. McMullin JP, MacDonald A. Live donor renal transplantation in Iraq. Transplant Proc 1989; 21: 1400–1.
13. Sells RA. Ethics and priorities of organ procurement and allocation. Transplant Proc 1989; 21: 1391–4.
14. Daar AS. Ethics issues – a Middle East perspective. Transplant Proc 1989; 21: 1402–4.
15. Reddy KC. Organ donation for consideration: an Indian viewpoint. In: Land W, Dossetor JB (ed). Organ Replacement Therapy: Ethics, Justice, Commerce. Springer-Verlag, Berlin 1991; pp. 173–80.
16. Thiangarajan CM. Reddy KC. Shunmugasundaran D. Jayachandran R, Nayar P. Thomas S, Ramachandran V. The practice of unconventional renal transplantation (UCRT) at a single centre in India. Transplant Proc 1990; 22: 912–14.
17. Daar AS, Sells RA. The problems of paid organ donation in India. Report on behalf of the Ethics Committee of the Transplantation Society to the President and Council of the Transplant. Society XIII Int Congress of the Transplant. Soc San Francisco, August 1990.
18. Abouna GM, Sabawi MM, Kumar MSA and Samhan M. The negative impact of paid organ donation. In: Land W and
Dossetor JB (eds). Organ Replacement Therapy: Ethics, Justice, Commerce. Springer-Verlag Berlin, 1991; pp. 164–72.
19. Land W, Dossetor JB (eds). Organ Replacement Therapy, Ethics, Justice, Commerce. Springer-Verlag, Berlin, 1991.
20. Cohen LR. The ethical virtues of a futures market in cadaveric organs. In: Land W and Dossetor JB (eds). Organ Replacement Therapy: Ethics, Justice, Commerce, Springer-Verlag Berlin, 1991; pp. 302–10.
21. Caplan AL. Requests, gifts and obligations: the ethics of organ procurement. Transplant Proc 1986; 18: 49–56.
22. Gutmann Th. Living kidney transplantation: aspects of legal philosophy. Transplantationsmedizin 1993; 5: 75–87.
23. Hanford JT. Religion, medical ethics and transplants. J Med Humanities 1993; 14: 33–8.
24. Engelhardt HT Jr. Is there a universal system of ethics or are ethics culture-specific? In: Land W and Dossetor JB (eds). Organ Replacement Therapy: Ethics, Justice, Commerce, Springer-Verlag Berlin, 1991; pp. 147–53.
25. Veatch RM. Theories of medical ethics: the professional model compared with the societal model. In: Land W, Dossetor JB (eds), Organ Replacement Therapy: Ethics, Justice, Commerce, Springer-Verlag Berlin, 1991; pp. 3–8.
26. Dickens BM. Human rights and commerce in health care. Transplant Proc 1990; 22: 904–5.
27. Peters TG. The regulation of human tissue and organs. Washington DC Transplant News, 1990; 192: 5.
28. Childress JF. The body as property: some philosophical reflections. Transplant Proc 1992; 24: 2143–8.
29. Slahudeen AK, Woods HF. Pingle A, Nur-el-Huda Suleyman M, Shakuntala K. Nadakumar M, Yahya TM, Daar AS. High mortality among recipients of bought living-unrelated donor kidneys. Lancet 1990; 336: 725–8.
30. Morris & Sells 1985.
31. Abouna GM, Kumar MSA, Samhan M, Dadah SK, John P, Sabawi NM. Commercialization in human organs: a Middle East perspective. Transplant Proc 1990; 22: 918–21.
32. Sells RA. Voluntarism of consent in both related and unrelated living organ donors. In: Land W, Dossetor JB (eds). Organ Replacement Therapy: Ethics, Justice, Commerce, Springer-Verlag Berlin, 1991; pp. 18–24.
33. Guttman A, Guttman RD. Attitudes of health care professionals and the public towards the sale of kidneys transplantation. J Med Ethics 1993, 19: 148–53.
34. Feinberg J. Harm to Self. The Moral Limits of the Criminal Law, Vol. III. Oxford University Press: Oxford, 1986.
35. Land W. The problem of living organ donation: facts, thoughts and reflections. Transplant Int 1989; 2: 168–79.
36. Land W. Das belohnte Geschenk? Überlegungen zur Organspende von gesunden Menschen. Klett-Cotta Stuttgart, Merkur, 1991; 45: Heft 2, 120–9.
37. Radcliff-Richards J. From him that hath not. In: Land W, Dossetor JB (eds). Organ Replacement Therapy: Ethics, Justice, Commerce. Springer-Verlag Berlin, 1991; pp. 190–6.
38. Warnock M (ed.) A Question of Life. The Warnock Report on Human Fertilisation and Embryology. Basil Blackwell, Oxford 1985; p. 65.
39. Dossetor JB. Rewarded gifting: is it ever ethically acceptable? Transplant Proc 1992; 24: 2092–4.
40. Brams M. Transplantable human organs: should their sale be authorized by State statutes? Am J Law Med 1977; 3: 183–96.
41. Perry C. Human organs and the open market. Ethics 1980; 91: 63–71.
42. Peters DA. Marketing organs for transplantation. Dialysis Transplant 1984; 13: 40–2.
43. Schwindt R. Vining AR. Proposal for a future delivery market for transplant organs. J Health Politics Policy Law 1986; 11: 483–500.
44. Hansmann H. The economics and ethics of markets for human organs. In: Blumstein JF. Sloan FA (eds). Organ Transplantation Policy: Issues and Prospects. Duke University Press, Durham 1989; pp. 57–85.

45. Blumstein JF. The case for commerce in organ transplantation. Transplant Proc 1992; 24: 2190–7.
46. Boadle 1993.
47. Persijn G, Cohen B. Press communiqué; reproduced in Eurotransplant News 1994; 3.
48. Reuters 1994.
49. Time (International Edition). Guatemala. Dangerous rumours, suspicious rise over the origin of anti foreigner hostility that provoked assault on American Women. Reported by Trish O'Kane, written by Laura Lopez. 35, 18 April 1994.
50. Eurotransplant. Introduction by B. Cohen. Eurotransplant News 1994; 116: 1.
51. Friedlander MM, Gofrit O, Eid A. Unrelated-living-donor kidney transplantation. Lancet 1992, 342: 1061–2.
52. Daar AS. The case for using living non-related donors to alleviate the worldwide shortage of cadaver kidneys for transplantation. Ann Acad Med Singapore 1991; 20: 443–52.
53. Childress JF. The place of autonomy in bioethics. Hastings Cent Rep 1990; 20: 12–17.
54. United Network for Organ Sharing 1991 Ethics Committee. Ethics of organ transplantation from living donors. Transplant Proc 1992; 24: 2236–7.
55. Spital AL. The ethics of unconventional living organ donation. Clin Transplant 1991; 5: 322–6.
56. Evans M. Organ donations should not be restricted to relatives. J Med Ethics 1989; 15: 17–20.
57. Daar AS. Rewarded gifting and rampant commercialism in perspective: is there a difference? In: Land W, Dossetor J (eds), Organ Replacement Therapy: Ethics, Justice, Commerce, Springer-Verlag Berlin, 1991; pp. 181–9.
58. Beauchamp TL, Childress JF. Principles of Biomedical Ethics, 3rd edn. Oxford University Press, Oxford, 1989.
59. Spital A. Unconventional living kidney donors – attitudes and use among transplant centers. Transplantation 1989; 48: 243–8.
60. Conference on Ethics, Justice and Commerce: a global view, report by the Progress Committee, Epilogue. Transplant Proc 1990; 22: 1054.
61. Council of the Transplantation Society. Commercialisation in transplantation: the problem and some guidelines for practice. Lancet 1985; ii: 715–16.
62. WHO Guiding Principles. In: Human Organ Transplantation: A report on developments under the auspices of WHO (1987–1991). WHO, Geneva, 1991.
63. WHO. Legislative Responses to Organ Transplantation. Kluwer Academic Publishers, Dordrecht 1993.
64. Dickens BM. Legal aspects of transplantation: judicial issues. Transplant Proc 1992; 24: 2118–19.
65. Fuenzalida-Fuelma HL. Organ transplantation: the Latin American legislative response. Bull Pan Am Health Org 1990; 24: 425–45.
66. Daar AS. Current practice and the legal, ethical and religious status of postmortem organ donation in the Islamic world. In: Land W, Dossetor J (eds), Organ Replacement Therapy: Ethics, Justice, Commerce. Springer-Verlag, Berlin, 1991; pp. 291–9.
67. Fluss SS. Legal aspects of transplantation: emerging trends in international and national legislation. Transplant Proc 1992; 24: 2121–2.
68. May W. In discussion of session on commerce in human organs. Transplant Proc 1990; 22: 937.
69. Colabawalla BN. Letter to the Editor. Lancet 1990; 2:
70. Daar AS. Cross-cultural perspectives in transplantation – a view from the borderline. In: Levine RJ, Andreopoulos J. Days DS (eds), Organ Transplantation and Human Rights: Cross-Cultural Perspectives. 1995; in press.
71. Daar AS. 1992.
72. Dossetor JB, Manichavel V. Ethics in organ donation: contracts in two cultures. Transplant Proc 1991; 23: 2508–11.
73. Sells RA. Towards an affordable ethic. Transplant Proc 1992; 24: 2095–6.
74. Sells RA. Resolving the conflict in traditional ethics which arises from our demand for organs (Vancouver SOS Conference 1993). Transplant Proc 1993, 25: 2983–4.
75. Simforoosh N, Amir Ansari B, Bassiri A, Gol S. Social aspects of kidney donations in 300 living related and unrelated renal transplantations. In: Land W, Dossetor J (eds), Organ Replacement Therapy: Ethics, Justice, Commerce. Springer-Verlag Berlin, 1991; pp. 77–82.
76. NFK. Consensus conference on financial incentives, New Orleans, Chair: N. Feduska, 1991;
77. Kittur DS, Hogan MM, Thukral VK, McGaw LJ, Alexander JW. Incentives for organ donation? Lancet 1991; 338: 1441–3.
78. Monaco AP. Comment: a transplant surgeon's view on social factors in organ transplantation. Transplant Proc 1989; 21: 3403–6.

38 | International legislation in living organ donation

Thomas Gutmann and Bernhard Gerok

1. Introduction

All over the world, living organ donation makes an important contribution to expansive organ procurement. Almost everywhere transplantation surgery is guided by national and international ethical codices. During the last two decades, many states have passed acts and decrees to establish legal regulations in the field of organ transplantation; the majority of these provisions also address organ donation by living adults or even minors. The creation of clear rules, the elimination of legal confusion, and the official endorsement of personal autonomy are some of the advantages of express legal permission for living organ donation [1]. Moreover, according to most theories of democracy, substantial regulations, especially those directly concerning basic moral or human rights, should be defined by the legitimized legislator and not be delegated to social subgroups such as, for example, medical organizations.

Despite fundamental differences in the cultural, philosophical and legal traditions within the international community of states, an analysis not only of the European [2,3], but of the world-wide legislative patterns demonstrates common underlying principles and, in general, a common approach to the ethical and social issues involved. Of course, there can be differences between the legal provisions required by formal laws and executive decrees dealing with organ transplantation on the one hand and codes of medical ethics and medical practice on the other hand. However, it may be of interest to examine the full range of legal provisions by which different countries try to find solutions for at least some of the basic problems of living organ donation which have been defined by the growing international discussion about medical ethics.

2. Informed consent

The main concern of international legislation in living organ donation is to ensure that informed consent to the removal is voluntarily given by the potential donor. Although this seems to be self-evident, the statutes of Belgium [4], Spain [6] and Tunisia [7] prescribe that the donor must give his/her consent expressly, freely and consciously. In Greece [8], Finland [9], the Russian Federation [10], Libya [11] and Viet Nam [10] the transplantation laws provide that the consent shall be given on a voluntary basis, while in Yugoslavia the consent is supposed to be given 'without compulsion' [11]. Mexico seems to make even higher demands because it prescribes that there must not be any 'physical or moral coercion' of the living donor [12]. Pursuant to the transplantation act of the Russian Federation, any person who coerces a living donor to consent to removal of organs and/or tissues shall be liable to criminal proceedings [10]. Of course, most countries provide criminal prosecution and consequences within the civil law in the case of intimidation and duress.

According to the transplantation laws in Cyprus [13], Denmark [7], France [45], Greece [8], Hungary [14], Italy [2], Norway [2], Romania [15], the Russian Federation [10], Sweden [2], Turkey [6], Costa Rica [16], Panama [8] and Venezuela [17] the potential donor

G.M. Collins, J.M. Dubernard, W. Land and G.G. Persijn (eds). Procurement, Preservation and Allocation of Vascularized Organs 317–324
© 1997 Kluwer Academic Publishers.

must have been duly informed by a physician of the nature of the intervention, its consequences and the risks before giving his/her consent. A more comprehensive provision is to be found in Spain [6] (and similarly in Belgium [4], Germany [48], Luxemburg [2] and Tunisia [7]): The law specifies that the information provided shall concern the foreseeable physical, mental and psychological consequences, the possible effects of the donation on the donor's personal, family and professional life, and the benefits which it is hoped the recipient will derive from the transplantation. Finland prescribes that the information is to be given by a physician who shall not be the physician caring for the recipient [9].

To ensure respect for the donor's autonomy, it seems appropriate to prescribe that his/her decision to give away an organ may be withdrawn right up to the moment of the operation. With regard (only) to explicit regulations in transplantation statutes, the donor may at any time revoke the consent which s/he has given in Belgium [4], Finland [9], France [45], Germany [42], Greece [8], Romania [15], Yugoslavia [11], Algeria [9], Kuwait [48], Argentina [5], Bolivia [18], Panama [8], Sri Lanka [49] and Australia [1]. Beyond that Hungary [14], Spain [19] and Tunisia [7] guarantee expressly that this may take place without any formality. Of course, such withdrawal of consent by the donor shall not make him subject to any claims whatsoever. At least Hungary [14], Spain [19], Argentina [5], Mexico [12] and Venezuela [17] prescribe that the primary donor may revoke consent at any time without incurring any liability.

3. Formal requirements for the donor's consent

The 1996 Council of Europe Convention on Human Rights and Biomedicine prescribes that the donor's consent has to be given expressly and specifically either in written form or before an official body [46]. In Cyprus [13], Denmark [7], Finland [9], Luxembourg [2], Romania [15], the Russian Federation [10], Sweden [2], Yugoslavia [11], Argentina, Chile, Colombia, Guatemala [20], Panama [8], Peru [20], Viet Nam [10] and Australia [1] the donor's consent already has to be given in writing. South Africa orders written consent to be given only for the removal of non-replaceable tissues [22].

In Belgium, consent shall be given in writing before a witness that has attained the age of majority [4]; in Romania [15], Algeria [9], Kuwait [48] and Costa Rica [16] in writing before two witnesses. Hungary [14] and Bolivia [20] provide a declaration in the presence of a notary; in Mexico [12] express consent is to be given

in writing in presence of a notary public or two appropriate witnesses. Italy [2], Spain [6] and Sri Lanka [49] prescribe that consent must be given in writing and in the presence of a specified public authority. In France, the donor even has to give his consent before the president of a superior court or a judge assigned by him [45]. In Greece, the donor's declaration of willingness must be made in notarial form, or on a form on which the police authority has confirmed the authenticity of the signature of the potential donor or orally, recorded and in the presence of two witnesses [8]. Finally Australia intended that the consent must be given in the absence of family and friends to avoid duress [1].

Some countries provide procedural safeguards to secure informed consent. In Germany [42] the medical information has to be given in the presence of a further physician who is neither involved in the removal or the transplantation of the donor's organ nor subject to directives of a physician involved in these measures. The content of the information given and the statement of consent must be written down and signed by the donor, the physician and the further physician. In Manitoba (Canada) an agreement to the removal of tissue from a person's own body while living 'is not valid unless a physician who does not have and has never had an association with any person benefiting or likely to benefit from the consent certifies in writing that the person giving the consent has been advised of and understands the nature and effect of the procedure authorized by the consent' [22]. While in Venezuela the donor needs a favourable psychiatric assessment by the relevant department of the establishment or hospital centre [17], there is a still more complicated procedure in Spain: the donor's physical and mental state of health shall be confirmed by a physician other than the one who is to carry out the removal procedure. The donor's consent to the removal of the organ shall be valid only if, all other requirements aside, it is given in writing in presence of a magistrate, the first named physician, the physician who is to carry out the removal procedure, and a person within the health centre specially licensed for authorizing the procedure. Any of these persons may validly oppose the donation and, consequently, the removal of the organ, despite the fact that all of the requirements have been formally satisfied, if s/he harbours any doubt that the donor's consent has been given expressly, freely, consciously and without any bias [19].

4. Minors and incompetents

Not all countries ban outright the removal of organs from a minor and/or mentally disabled person. Some of them allow it on certain conditions and attempt to provide procedural safeguards for the individuals at risk. Today, not many countries with transplantation laws fail to deal with the issue at all.

In general, there are two opposing attitudes towards this problem. On the one hand, laws of total pro- hibition have the advantage of certainty and maximize the overall legal protection of these groups of persons. On the other hand, however, the removal of a body part from a minor can be ethically justified in exceptional cases, while total prohibition can be unjust because its inflexibility fails to take account of the dif- ference beween mature and immature minors. In very exceptional cases even tragic injustice could be done by a blanket ban [1]. However, as the Final Report of the US Task Force on Organ Transplantation suggests, there should at least be a 'heavy presumption against using children (especially preadolescent children) and mentally retarded persons' as sources of non- regenerative organs, especially kidneys, because they are usually unable to give valid consent. The Task Force suggests that there should be an independent judicial review of any proposal to remove such an organ from an incompetent person [23]. Moreover it seems appropriate that such an authority should only, if at all, approve the removal of an organ from an incompetent person after having received an extensive report by an independent expert in (child) psychology.

In Cyprus [13] and Italy [2] a potential donor has to be legally competent. In Austria [2], France [45], Germany [42], the Russian Federation [10], Argentina [5], Chile, Colombia and Guatemala [20] s/he must be legally competent and over 18 years of age, i.e have reached the age of majority (as provided in Greece [8], Spain [6], Tunisia [7], Argentina [20], Mexico [12] and Panama [8]). In Costa Rica a living donor must have reached the age of majority [16], while in Honduras and Sri Lanka [49] he has to be over 21 years [20]. Pursuant to the enactments in Romania [15], Algeria [9] and, similarly, Manitoba (Canada) [22] and Bolivia [18], the adult donor has to be capable of exercising proper judgement.

As the Australian Code [1], the 1978 model code of the Council of Europe contained a general prohibition of taking non-regenerative tissue from the legally incapacitated, but a mechanism was provided which allowed removal in special cases: 'The removal of sub- stances which cannot regenerate, from legally incapac- itated persons is forbidden. However, a state may permit such a removal in a special case justified for therapeutic or diagnostic reasons if the donor, having the capacity of understanding, has given his consent, if his legal representative and an appropriate authority

have authorized removal and if the donor and the recipient are closely genetically related. [...] A removal of substances which presents foreseeable sub- stantial risk to the life or the health of the donor who is a legally incapacitated person is forbidden' [21].

In Denmark, the intervention may be performed on a person under 18 years of age with his/her consent, if there are special reasons for doing so and provided that such consent has received the approval of the person exercising parental authority [7]. In Norway, the European country with the highest proportion of living renal donors with regard to the total number of kidney transplantations per year in Europe (1990: 49% [24]), persons under 18 years of age may give their consent with the endorsement of their guardian and the person who has parental custody under special circumstances and if the operation is also approved by the Directorate of the Health Services [2].

In Luxembourg, a removal is possible in the case of minors for the benefit of the donor's brother or sister if s/he has given consent in writing and his/her legal representative as well as a committee of three experts, appointed by the Minister of Health, give the author- ization for the removal [2].

Similarly in Sweden no distinction is made between organs that regenerate and those that do not. Under ex- traordinary circumstances, the National Board of Health and Welfare may give its permission for removal of an organ from a minor or a person unable to give his/her consent, if the operation is not being performed against the donor's own wishes [2].

In Turkey, however, the removal of an organ or tissue from a person who is under 18 years of age or who is legally incompetent is permissible in cases where the person has drawn up and signed a document in the presence of at least two witnesses and in the absence of pressure of any kind, or where the person has given an oral undertaking in the presence of at least two witnesses and has then signed a declaration which is countersigned by a physician [6]. Although in the same law physicians are required to refuse to remove any organ or tissue from persons unable to take their decision for mental or psychological reasons, the Turkish regulation does not seem sufficient for an adequate protection of these groups of potential donors.

Some enactments are more restrictive and provide exceptions only in the case of regenerative tissues, as is suggested by the World Health Organisation's *Guiding Principles on Human Organ Transplantation* [25]. In this sense, the 1996 Council of Europe Convention on Human Rights and Biomedicine pre- scribes that the removal of regenerative tissue from a person who does not have the capacity to consent may be authorised by national law provided that (a) there is no compatible donor available who has the capacity to consent, (b) the recipient is a brother or a sister of the donor, (c) the donation has the potential to be life-saving for the recipient, (d) authorisation is given specifically and in writing by his or her representative or an authority or person or body provided for by the law and (e) the potential donor concerned does not object [46]. In Finland, persons under 18 years of age may only donate renewable tissues provided that the consent in writing of the person's guardian and trustee and the approval of the National Board of Health are obtained. The National Board requires the submission of not only a surgical and psychiatric report but also a report by an expert in child psychology or paediatrics [9]. Similarly, in Manitoba (Canada) regenerative tissues may be transplanted from a person who is under the age of 16 years, with this person's consent only where the proposed recipient of the tissue would die without the transplant; the risk to the life and health of the person giving the consent is relatively unsubstantial; the person giving the consent is a member of the immediate family of the proposed recipient of the tissue; a parent or a legal guardian consents to the transplant of the tissue and the transplant is recommended by an independent physician and approved by a certain Court upon an application therefore [22].

The law in France attempts to prevent minor donors from being misused by a similar procedure. A minor may donate bone marrow if s/he is the brother or the sister of the recipient. The substance may be removed only with the consent of the person's legal representatives given before the president of a superior court or a judge assigned by him, and after authorization has been given by a committee made up of at least three experts, including two physicians, one of whom shall be a paediatrician. The experts are appointed at national level. Where it is possible to obtain the views of the minor, refusal by the latter to agree to removal of the organ has to be respected [45]. Also in Greece only bone marrow may exceptionally be removed from minors, provided that the donor and the recipient are fully histocompatible siblings and consent has been obtained from the person legally responsible for them [8]. In Yugoslavia, a bone marrow donor may be a minor. In this case only the parents may give consent to the donation on his/her behalf [11]. South Africa forbids the removal of any tissue from a person who is mentally ill and the removal of non-regenerative tissues from minors, but allows the removal of replaceable substances when consent has been granted by the parents or guardians of the minor [22]. Belgium prescribes that if the removal from living persons of organs

and tissues does not normally have serious effects on the donor, or if the organs or tissues are regenerable and intended for transplantation to a brother or a sister, donation may be made by a person who has not attained 18 years of age. This shall require the prior consent of the donor if s/he has attained 15 years of age, and the prior consent of the person(s) whose consent to the marriage of a minor is requested. In all cases where the donor is over 18 years of age but has not attained 21 years, the consent of the person(s) whose consent to the marriage of a minor is required in accordance with the civil code has to be obtained for the removal of both renewable and not renewable tissues and organs [4].

5. Donors in coercive situations

A general provision is to be found in the transplantation act of the Russian Federation, pursuant to which no organ may be removed for transplantation purposes from persons who are dependent upon the recipient, either because of their functions or in any other manner [10]. As a prisoner is in a coercive situation by definition, prisoners should not be considered a group from which it is legally or ethically appropriate to obtain living unrelated donation [26]. Nevertheless, only few laws cover this issue: The Bolivian statute deals with the question of potential donors under special disciplinary conditions and prescribes that prisoners and other persons detained in closed institutions may not donate organs or tissues, except of their own free will to blood relatives or relatives by marriage, and subject to the approval of the competent authority [18]. Panama [8], Colombia, Guatemala, and Paraguay [20] exclude prisoners, and, in general, any person who is subject to a restriction on his/her legal rights, from organ donation.

6. Further consents required

If the donor is married, the removal of organs from living persons requires the consent of the spouse residing with the donor in both Belgium [4] and Turkey [6]. However, considering the basic ethical principle of respect for the autonomy of the patient, here: the donor, such a legal veto power for the donor's spouse does not seem justified.

7. Recipient's informed consent

In medical ethics, it is unanimously agreed upon that the recipient's right to refuse an organ, which is founded on the basic ethical principle of respect for his/her autonomy, takes precedence by all means [27]. Nevertheless some countries laid down expressly the need to obtain the recipient's informed consent. Hungary [14], Romania [15], Spain [6] and Bolivia [18] require the express (the Russian Federation [10], Yugoslavia [11] and Venezuela [17]: the written) permission by (in Greece [8]: no objection on the part of) the recipient or, in the case of a mentally or legally incompetent person, that of the relatives in charge of him. Algeria [9] provides the recipient's expression of consent in the presence of the physician who is head of the medical service, and of two witnesses. In Romania [15] and the Russian Federation [10] there are explicit exceptions from this rule for those special cases, where a delay in carrying out the appropriate intervention would threaten the recipient's life and it is impossible to obtain consent. In most other countries the legal systems also permit proxy decision making in such cases.

8. Safety of donors

Nearly all countries forbid the removal if there is an increased risk for the donor. The degree of risk allowed and evaluation of the risks vary between the countries. The model code of the Council of Europe suggests 'Where removal of substances presents a foreseeable substantial risk to the life or the health of the donor, a removal may only be permitted exceptionally when it is justified by the motivations of the donor, the family relationship with the recipient and the medical requirements of the case. However, a state can prohibit such removal' [21]. This is done by the transplantation acts of Austria [2], Germany [42], Cyprus [13], Denmark [7], Finland [9], Greece [8], Norway [2], the Russian Federation [10], Spain [19], Sweden [2] and Yugoslavia [11], which forbid removals that entail any serious and manifest risks to the donor's life or health. In Libya [11] it has to be determined that 'no harm' will be caused to the living donor. Similarly, the statutes in Argentina [5], Ecuador [10,13], Panama [8] and Venezuela [17] proscribe that only one of two paired organs, or anatomical materials the removal of which does not entail any reasonably foreseeable risk that the donor will die or be completely and permanently disabled, may be removed. Pursuant to the laws in Romania [15], Turkey [6], Algeria [9] and Tunisia [7] the operation at least must not endanger the life of the donor. Finally, there is a special paternalistic rule in Bolivia [18,20], Colombia, Guatemala, Honduras, and Paraguay [20], since pregnant women may not donate organs or tissues under any circumstances in these countries.

In general, the removal of organs and tissues, especially when they are non-regenerative, is only allowed for diagnostic or therapeutic purposes. Beyond that, some statutes focus on the recipient's need of the transplant. Belgian law proscribes that if the removal of organs and tissues from living persons may affect the donor, or if such organs and tissues are non-regenerable, removal may only be performed if the recipient's life is in danger and if the transplantation of organs or tissues from a deceased person could not produce an equally satisfactory result [4]. For example in Romania [15], the Russian Federation [10], Algeria [9] and Ecuador [13] organs may be removed from living donors only if the recipient suffers from a disease for which the transplant is the only means of prolonging or improving his life. As suggested by the World Health Organisation's *Guiding Principles on Human Organ Transplantation* [25], some countries, such as Mexico, prescribe expressly that except in the case of blood and its components, the procurement of organs and tissues from human beings for therapeutic purposes shall preferably be from the bodies of deceased persons [11].

In some states, special procedures are required in order to maximize the donor's security. In Finland every willing living donor needs the approval of the National Board of Health. The application for approval shall be accompanied by a report by experts in transplantation surgery and psychiatry which may only be dispensed with in applications concerning the removal of renewable tissues [9]. According to the Canadian Draft Uniform Act, no transplant may be carried out before an independent assessment conducted by not fewer than three persons, of whom one shall be a physician and none had an association with either the donor or the recipient [47]. In Ecuador, prior to the transplant the donor shall present a favourable medical opinion by a physician concerning his/her state of health, a favourable medical opinion by a psychiatrist concerning his/her state of mental health and a favourable medical opinion by a psychologist concerning the probable consequences of the transplant for his/her personality [13]. In Italy, a report containing a favourable technical-medical opinion is to be forwarded to the provincial medical officer and the magistrate for authorization to carry out the transplantation [2]. Pursuant to the statutes in Romania [15], the Russian Federation [10] and Algeria [9] a medical commission specially established within the hospital facility shall decide whether the removal or transplantation is necessary and shall authorize the intervention. The Syrian Arab Republic requires a commission comprising three medical specialists to decide whether removal of an organ constitutes a danger to the donor's life and to decide the need of the recipient for the transplant [4]. In Hungary a similar decision has to be made in each individual case by a joint appraisal of a specially designated group of three physicians not involved in the removal and transplantation procedures [14]. In South Africa the removal of a tissue from a living donor shall not be effected without the written authority of a medical practitioner in charge of the hospital concerned, who does not perform the transplantation or take part therein [22]. Similarly, in Spain, the physical and mental conditions of the donor must be certified by a doctor other than the one carrying out the operation [2].

9. Living non-related organ donation

Many countries seek a genetically related donor for reasons of tissue compatibility and to avoid possible abuse by donors whose motives are of a financial nature rather than altruistic, but only a few countries make it a legal requirement. Normally, on the level of the formal transplantation statutes, at least spouses and adopted children are accepted as recipients in exceptional cases.

The model code of the Council of Europe suggested that the '[r]emoval of substances which cannot regenerate must be confined to transplantation between genetically related persons except in exceptional cases where there are good chances of success' [21]. In the UK the recipient must be genetically related to the living donor (in a defined degree), and proof of this relationship must be genetically established before transplantation. In cases where this is not possible, an application must be made to a committee of 12 persons appointed by the Secretary of State for Health (*Unrelated Live Transplant Regulation Authority*), to seek their approval for transplantation. Reports by the physicians in charge of the donor and the recipient shall be submitted to the Authority as well as a report from an independent assessor confirming that the donation is not made under any pressure and that the donation is a bona fide gift with no financial or material gains [13,28]. In France, the donor has to be the recipient's parent, child or sibling for the removal of other substances than bone marrow. In urgent cases, also spouses are accepted [45]. In the Russian Federation, the removal of organs from a living donor is authorized only if there exists a genetic relationship with the recipient (other than in cases of bone marrow grafts) [10]. The decree in Honduras permits only siblings of the living donor to be recipients [20]. In Argentina living donors are accepted up to fourth degree of relationship only [29], and also in Costa Rica

a potential living donor may act as such only for the benefit of a relative up to the fourth degree of consanguinity or up to the third degree of affinity, or of his/her spouse [16]. In Venezuela, the recipient's parents as well as any adult children and siblings shall be accepted as living donors for therapeutic purposes; the National Executive, however, may define other acceptable groups of persons who are of age [17]. The World Health Organisation's *Guiding Principles on Human Organ Transplantation* suggest that donors of non-regenerative organs should be genetically related to the recipients [25].

Some of the principal objections to non-related donation, however, seem to be misdirected. The basic theoretical ethical problem with living organ donation is the balancing of the donor's autonomy with the societal need to maximize non-maleficence to him/her [26]. With regard to the respect for the donor's autonomy, we first have to admit that 's/he has a right to take a reasonable risk in order to achieve substantial benefits for the recipient. This is true even if the donor and the recipient are not related' [26]. If it is the general legislative goal to ensure that the donor's consent is voluntarily given, it should be taken into account that family members are probably more vulnerable to undue pressure than friends. Moreover, there is no reason to believe that 'emotionally related' persons, as spouses, living partners or close friends who are willing to donate an organ are generally motivated by financial gain. Finally, as long as it is virtually impossible to provide all potential recipients with a cadaveric organ within a limited period of time, it seems hard to justify to withhold an organ that could be donated to a severely ill person by a close friend who is histocompatible, altruistically motivated and voluntarily consenting. Therefore a growing number of transplant surgeons and medical ethicists conclude that non-related, and especially 'emotionally related' donation should be welcomed where clinically appropriate and truly voluntary (see e.g. [30–36, 44]). The Final Report of the US Task Force on Organ Transplantation came to a similar conclusion. 'There is no reason to exclude all living unrelated donors, such as spouses and friends, but special care should be taken to ensure that the decision to donate is informed, voluntary, and altruistic and special emphasis should be placed on histocompatibility' [23].

Summing up, the available evidence suggests that decisions about the acceptability of living related and unrelated donors should be made on a case-by-case basis [32,37]. Therefore a comprehensive legal prohibition of living unrelated or even emotionally related donation does not seem justified. For this reason, e.g.

the German draft transplantation law seeks 'safety by procedure' [43]. The removal of non-regenerative organs will be permissible only for the purpose of transplanting them to relatives of the first and second degree, to spouses, fiancés and to other persons in an obvious close personal relationship with the donor. The removal of an organ of a living person must not be performed before an expert commission (including a physician, a person who has attained the qualifications necessary to become a judge, and a person who is experienced in psychological questions) has given an expert report on whether there are any actual grounds for supposing that the donor's consent was not given freely or the organ is subject of forbidden trafficking in organs [42]. A minor problem connected with this issue is anonymity. The model code of the Council of Europe suggests that the anonymity of the donor and of the recipient must be respected except where there is a close personal or family relationship between the two [21]. Equivalent provisions are to be found in France [45], where anonymity can be set aside for therapeutical reasons, and in Turkey [6]. Spain, however, seems to prescribe without an exception that 'the recipient's anonymity must be guaranteed' [6,19]. The statutes of Cyprus [13] and Greece [2] try to prevent the divulgation of the identity of the living donor to the recipient and vice versa. This requirement does not seem to be very significant, because living donors in most cases are in close personal or consanguineous relationship with the recipient.

10. Commercialization

In 1991, the World Health Organisation published an exhaustive review of international and national legislation, codes and other measures to combat commercialism in the use of human organs and tissues for therapeutic purposes [38–40], which cannot be reported here. (For recent developments see [10,11,40, 42,45,46].) This analysis reveals a broad international consensus on this issue and shows that most of the countries which have passed legislation in the field of organ transplantation provide that the human body and its parts must not be subject of commercial transactions. Many enactments provide that persons violating these laws are liable to punishment. In a number of states, advertising the need for or availability of organs, with a view to offering or seeking payment, is prohibited. Many statutes (including the model code of the Council of Europe [21]) expressly allow that loss of earnings and any expenses caused by the removal or preceding examination may be refunded, but not all states do so.

International ethical discussion has now begun to recognize that there are decisive differences between rampant commercialism on the one hand and different concepts of 'rewarded gifting' on the other [41]. Compensation may comprise more than just refunding the loss of earnings, and, in certain circumstances, there may even be ethically justified ways to increase financial incentives to donate an organ without crossing into sales. These possibilities merit further exploration.

In many national legal regulations, however, there is a lack of distinction between the concepts of compensation and commercialization, and many provisions, as for example the World Health Organisation's *Guiding Principles* that suggest that 'giving or receiving payment (including any other compensation or reward) should be prohibited' [25] may seem to be a case of throwing out the baby with the bathwater.

Acknowledgements

The authors wish to thank the Kester-Haeusler-Stiftung, Fuerstenfeldbruck, for its financial support of the research work leading to this article. We would also like to thank the Bibliothek des Deutschen Bundestags.

References

1. Scott R. The Body as Property. Viking, New York 1981: pp. 235–64.
2. Council of Europe. Conference of European Health Ministers; 1987 Nov 16–17; Paris. Organ Transplantation. Current Legislation in Council of Europe Member States and Finland and Results of European Co-operation. Council of Europe, Strasbourg 1987.
3. Wolfslast G. Legal aspects of organ transplantation. An overview of European law. J Heart Lung Transplant 1991; 11: 160–3.
4. Int Dig Hlth Leg 38 (1987).
5. Int Dig Hlth Leg 28 (1977).
6. Int Dig Hlth Leg 31 (1980).
7. Int Dig Hlth Leg 42 (1991).
8. Int Dig Hlth Leg 35 (1984).
9. Int Dig Hlth Leg 36 (1985).
10. Int Dig Hlth Leg 44 (1993).
11. Int Dig Hlth Leg 43 (1992).
12. Int Dig Hlth Leg 37 (1986).
13. Int Dig Hlth Leg 40 (1989).
14. Int Dig Hlth Leg 24 (1973).
15. Int Dig Hlth Leg 30 (1979).
16. Int Dig Hlth Leg 27 (1976).
17. Int Dig Hlth Leg 23 (1972).
18. Int Dig Hlth Leg 34 (1983).
19. Int Dig Hlth Leg 32 (1981).
20. Fuenzalida-Puelma HL. Organ transplantation. The Latin American legislative response. In: World Health Organisation. Informal Consultation on Organ Transplantation; 1990 May 2–4; Geneva. WHO. Geneva 1990. Appendix.

21. Council of Europe. Resolution 78 (29) on harmonisation of legislations of member states relating to removal, grafting and transplantation of human substances, Strasbourg 1978.
22. Int Dig Hlth Leg 41 (1990).
23. Task Force on Organ Transplantation. Organ Transplantation. Issues and Recommendations. US Department of Health and Human Services, Washington 1986.
24. Land W, Cohen B. Postmortem and living organ donation in Europe. Transplant laws and activities. Transplant Proc 1992; 24: 2165–7.
25. World Health Organisation. Guiding principles on human organ transplantations. Lancet 1991; 337: 1470–1.
26. United Network for Organ Sharing 1991 Ethics Committee. Ethics of organ transplantation from living donors. Transplant Proc 1992; 24: 2236–7.
27. United Network for Organ Sharing 1991 Ethics Committee. General principles for allocating human organs and tissues. Transplant Proc 1992; 24: 2227–35.
28. Thomas G, Ryall M, Taber SM. Ethical dilemmas in transplantation. Transplant Proc 1992; 24: 2099.
29. Cantarovich F. Legal aspects of transplantation in Argentina. Transplant Proc 1992; 24: 2123–4.
30. Daar AS, Sells RA. Living not-related donor renal transplantation – a reappraisal. Transplant Rev 1990; 4: 128–40.
31. Evans M. Organ donations should not be restricted to relatives. J Med Ethics 1989; 15: 17–20.
32. Land W. The problem of living organ donation. Facts, thoughts and reflections. Transplant Int 1989; 2: 168–79.
33. Spital AL. The ethics of unconventional living organ donation. Clin Transplant 1991; 5: 322–6.
34. Spital AL. Unrelated living donors. Should they be used? Transplant Proc 1992; 24: 2215–17.
35. Lamb D. Organ Transplants and Ethics. Routledge, London 1990.
36. Blake PG, Cardella CJ. Kidney donation by living unrelated donors [Editorial]. Can Med Assoc J 1989; 141: 773–5.
37. Childress JF. The gift of life. Ethical problems and policies in obtaining and distributing organs for transplantation. Primary care. Clin Office Practices 1986; 13: 379–94.
38. World Health Organisation. Human Organ Transplantation. A Report on Developments under the auspices of World Health Organisation (1987-1991). WHO, Geneva 1991.
39. Fluss SS. Preventing commercial transactions in human organs and tissues. An international overview of regulatory and ad-ministrative measures. In: Land W, Dossetor JE (eds), Organ Replacement Therapy. Ethics, Justice, Commerce. Springer, Berlin 1991; pp. 154–63.
40. Fluss SS. Legal aspects of transplantation. Emerging trends in international action and national legislation. Transplant Proc 1992; 24: 2121–2.
41. Daar AS, Gutmann Th, Land W. Chapter 37 in this volume.
42. German Draft Transplantation Law (Entwurf eines Gesetzes über die Spende, Entnahme und Übertragung von Organen), BT-Drs. 13/4355, 16/4/1996, not yet passed.
43. Gutmann Th, Elsaesser A, Gruendel J, Land W, Schneewind KA, Schroth U. Living Kidney Donation: Safety by Procedure. Clin Transplant 1994: 356–7.
44. Spital A. Do U.S. transplant centers encourage emotionally related kidney donation? Transplantation 1996; 61: 374–7.
45. France, Loi 94-654 relative au don et à l'utilisation des éléments et produits du corps, à l'assistance médicale à la procréation et au diagnostic prénatal (29/7/1994), J.O 30/7/1994.
46. Council of Europe, Convention for the Protection of Human Rights and Dignity of the Human Being with Regard to the Application of Biology and Medicine (Convention on Human Rights and Biomedicine), CDBI (96) 26, 6/6/1996, passed in November 1996.
47. Canada. The Uniform Human Tissue Donation Act (Draft 1990).
48. Kuwait. Decree-Law No. 55 of 20 December 1987 on organ transplantation (publ. 27/12/1987, No. 1751:3-4).
49. Sri Lanka. The Transplantation of Human Tissues Act, No. 48 of 1987.

After this article had been received by the editors, the World Health Organization has published an uncommented global collection of laws and regulations dealing with organ transplantation. The book contains materials that mostly had originally been published in the WHO's *International Digest of Health Legislation*: World Heath Organization. Legislative Responses to Organ Transplantation. Dordrecht: Martinus Nijhoff Publisher, 1994.

39 Psychological aspects in living organ donation

KLAUS A. SCHNEEWIND

1. Introduction: the challenge of living kidney transplantation

The number of kidneys transplanted from living donors varies considerably in different countries. According to a survey published by the European Dialysis and Transplant Association [1], 1018 kidney transplantations performed in West Germany in 1983 involved cadaver donors, and only 35 persons received their replacement organ from a living donor. In contrast, in the USA during the same period, 1796 out of a total of 6129 kidney transplantations (29.3%) were carried out using grafts from living donors [2]. The number of living kidney transplantations was, therefore, about nine times higher in the USA than in West Germany.

Based on statistics dating from 1990, the proportion of kidney tranplantations from living donors in Europe is highest in Norway (49%), Greece (40%), Denmark (24.7%) and Sweden (23.5%), whereas Germany (1.7%), Spain (1.3%) and Portugal (0%) belong to the countries with the lowest living kidney transplantation rate [3]. As a consequence, empirical evidence concerning living kidney transplantation rests mainly on studies from the USA and Scandinavian countries.

At a time when there is an increasing shortage of postmortem organs that can be transplanted, living kidney transplantation has become a major treatment option for chronic renal disease. On the other hand, the danger of a more or less aggressive commercialization of organ replacement and singular reports on criminal acts of forced kidney explantation have led to many objections to living organ donation, from both the public and experts. Some recent publications on the issue of living organ donation show that this matter is more complicated than it seems at first sight [4,5]. More importantly, close scrutiny of legal and ethical considerations has shown that, in principle, there are no objections against practising living kidney transplantation [5].

The present contribution does not intend to discuss the pros and cons of living kidney donation. Rather, I am convinced that, within the premises of legally and ethically acceptable action, it is vitally important to take stock and expand our knowledge concerning the antecedents, concomitants and consequences of living kidney transplantation. I further believe that, based on this kind of empirical evidence, it will be easier to decide whether and under which circumstances the treatment option of living kidney transplantation can responsibly be recommended. With this in mind, the present contribution will particularly focus on the psychological aspects of the processes and outcomes of living kidney transplantation. More specifically, some of the published research concerning the psychological impact of transplantation on the recipient and the donor, as well as on their relationship, will be reviewed. In a final section I shall briefly outline some desiderata for future research that might lead to a better understanding of the psychological processes of those who are involved, as recipients or donors, in living kidney transplantation.

G.M. Collins, J.M. Dubernard, W. Land and G.G. Persijn (eds). Procurement, Preservation and Allocation of Vascularized Organs 325–330
© 1997 Kluwer Academic Publishers.

2. Psychological effects of living kidney transplantation

On a world-wide scale there is an amazing paucity of published research studies addressing the effects of living kidney transplantation. Apart from clinical case studies, research evidence stemming from controlled studies that are based on sound methodological standards (i.e. quasi-experimental or prospective longitudinal designs) are even more scarce. In the following a selective review of the available findings focusing on three aspects, the recipient's perspective, the donor's perspective and the recipient–donor relationship, will be presented.

2.1. The recipient's perspective

It has generally been found that transplanted patients, as opposed to patients receiving dialysis, experience a considerable improvement in their physical and psychological well-being. Nevertheless transplanted patients still believe that they are chronically ill and live under many restraints [6]. Katschnig and Konieczna [7] found that 80% of transplanted patients but only 33% of dialysed patients felt that their physical condition was 'excellent' or 'good'. With respect to mental and emotional well-being about two-thirds of transplanted patients and one-third of those on dialysis had a positive outlook. Moreover, dialysed patients were more irritable, despondent and more pessimistic about their future than transplanted patients.

These findings do not allow differentiation between patients who underwent postmortem versus living kidney transplantation. It is thus impossible to disentangle differential long term effects concerning the psychological adaptation of these two groups of transplanted patients. One of the rare prospective long-term studies was published by Simmons [8], who followed a sample of 148 renal recipients and their donors over a period of up to 9 years. When comparing indices of physical, emotional and social well-being longitudinally the author found marked improvements in the years after the transplantation. Four-fifths of the transplanted men had entered the labour force or were engaged in some kind of job training. In addition, 5–9 years after transplantation these men reported decidedly fewer problems with sexual impotence than before transplantation. It should be noted, however, that only one-third of the transplanted patients were rated as being in good health.

Although there is some evidence that graft rejection is less prevalent in living kidney than in postmortem transplantation [9] the psychological aspects on organ rejection are far from being well-understood. A few cases have been documented attesting to the recipient's increased feelings of guilt and self-denigration as a consequence of organ rejection. However, these effects might be due to individual differences in certain personality dispositions that existed prior to the transplantation or even prior to the onset of renal disease. Some data that seem to corroborate this hypothesis point in this direction. In one study, Pommer et al. [10] compared a group of 23 successfully versus a group of 10 unsuccessfully transplanted patients using personality data that were assessed prior to the transplantation. The authors found that patients of the latter group had less optimistic expectations concerning the transplantation, were less likely to undergo a second transplantation in case of a failure of the first one, and proved to be more submissive, rigid and depressive in various personality tests. Although the methodological rigour of this study can certainly be improved, this kind of prospective longitudinal research will contribute to unravelling the psychological determinants which, in addition to medical aspects, have an impact on the probability of graft rejection.

2.2. The donor's perspective

Turning to research that has focused on the psychological aspects of the donor, it should first be noted that almost all of the published studies refer to genetically related living donors. In one of the most comprehensive studies to date Smith et al. [11] interviewed 536 living kidney donors from nine transplantation centres in the USA. In this multicentre study most of the donors (59.8%) were siblings, and about one-third of the donors were parents who agreed to donate a kidney for the benefit of one of their children. However, transplantation from a child to a parent was found in only 5.5% of the sample, and more remote familial relationships between donor and recipient (e.g. uncle–nephew) were observed in just 1.3% of all cases.

So far, a series of independent studies has unequivocally concluded that there are usually no detrimental effects for the donors following explantation of a kidney. In the multicentre study by Smith et al. [11] only two of 536 donors reported more or less serious medical complications. More than 92% of the subjects in this study contended that the explantation had no impact on their physical health at all. Bennet and Harrison [12] found similar results in their long-term study on 300 donors: 295 of their subjects reported that the explantation had left their physical and mental health unchanged.

These findings were further corroborated in a careful long-term study by Simmons and her collaborators [8,13]. In this study, 135 donors, all of whom were genetically related to the recipients, were followed over a period of up to 9 years using multiple assessments at different times. It is particularly noteworthy that this study also had a control group consisting of 65 so-called non-donors, i.e. family members who had been eligible for donation but for several reasons, including personal unwillingness, were excluded from becoming actual donors. A major finding was that the donors received higher scores on a self-esteem scale than did the non-donors. More importantly, this effect remained stable even 5–9 years after the transplantation.

Of special interest is the question of whether the family member's decision to donate a kidney was made of their own free will. In Simmons' longitudinal study the majority of donors (and also non-donors), i.e. 57% of all potential donors, reported that they made their decision on a voluntary basis [14]. In the Smith et al. [11] multicentre study 86% of the donors said that they were not influenced by family members or friends, and 94% denied that they had experienced any pressure from the medical personnel to make a pro-donation decision. In fact, if there was any attempt to influence the potential donor's decision it was in the opposite direction, i.e. convincing him or her to refrain from donation. This was especially the case with adolescents and mothers caring for dependent children.

Another interesting question is how the donors arrive at their decision. Simmons et al. [13] were able to isolate three types of decision making, which they called the moral, the rational, and the delay (or stepwise rational) decision models. These authors found that about two-thirds of their sample of living kidney donors made their decision according to the moral model, i.e. they spontaneously agreed to donate when they were asked whether they are ready to do so. Another 25% went through a rational decision-making process comprising a sequence of activities like collecting relevant information, evaluating different options and finally selecting one of the options. Only a very small subgroup of the sample, i.e. 5%, behaved according to the third model, first postponing the decision for a while and then proceeding along the line of the rational model. These findings can be interpreted in terms of a strong internalized norm of mutual solidarity within the family system. It should be mentioned, however, that there is also a substantial number of non-donors in the family unit [13]. Moreover, voluntariness might, at least in part, refer to what Fellner and Marshall [15] have called the 'myth of informed consent'. In any case, it seems to be appropriate to scrutinize the decision to voluntarily donate a kidney in some detail before the actual transplantation is being initiated.

As has already been mentioned, there are almost no published studies on the psychological aspects of living kidney donation that refer to non-related donors. Nevertheless, some authors are rather explicit about the advantages of non-related living organ donation [16,17] while others present a more balanced treatment of this issue, including the case of 'rewarded gifting' [3,18].

The only study that the present author was able to locate dates back more than 20 years [19]. In this study 18 non-related living kidney donors underwent an extensive assessment procedure, including an in-depth analysis of personality processes and social relations. Upon careful inspection of the data the authors arrived at an extremely positive view of these donors' personality structure [20]. This particular group of donors had a highly positive outlook on life, and they were mainly motivated by the idea of making a substantial contribution to preserving the life of a physically endangered person. It is also worth mentioning that the underlying motivation was less altruistic than egocentric in nature – although in a positive sense: these donors derived a high sense of self-efficacy and self-esteem from their decision to donate. These findings correspond nicely with the results that Simmons [8] reported in the comparison of her sample of genetically related donors and non-donors.

Since the database on non-related living kidney donation is extremely small we definitely need more research evidence on the multiple factors underlying the motivation of non-related living organ donors, including personality, social relations and also financial aspects that might influence a person's decision to donate. Despite a threatening commercialization of organ transplantation it should be noted that, in principle, there are no legal or ethical reasons in support of an unqualified prohibition of non-related organ donation [21–23].

2.3. The relationship between recipient and donor

A series of studies has looked at the quality of the relationship between recipient and donor. In the Smith et al. [11] multicentre study the majority of the donors (56%) reported a very close pretransplantation relationship with the recipient. After the transplantation 42% of the donors indicated that their relationship with the recipient had improved either 'slightly' or 'considerably' and only 1.5% reported that the quality of their relationship had deteriorated.

While the findings of the multicentre study are based on retrospective data the design of Simmons' [8] longitudinal study allowed for a long-term prospective data collection. Thus, prior to the transplantation 59% of the donors and 55% of the recipients reported that their relationship was 'very close'. Shortly after the transplantation the corresponding scores increased considerably to 77% for the donors and 86% for the recipients. One year later these values stabilized at 71% for the donors and 77% for the recipients. It should be noted, however, that the quality of the relationship of the donor–recipient dyad was clearly moderated by the success or failure of the transplantation. When the transplantation was unsuccessful the recipients reported four times as many difficulties with the donors than in the case of a successful transplantation. Conversely, successfully as opposed to unsuccessfully transplanted recipients referred to the relationship with their donors as 'particularly close' almost twice as often [24]. In some cases, however, the donor–recipient relationship might become considerably strained. There was some evidence that this might even include suicide on the part of the donor if the graft had been rejected or the recipient had died [25]. Even though outcomes such as these might be attributed to specific personality characteristics and life circumstances that existed prior to the transplantation it points to the importance of a careful psychodiagnostic assessment of both the donor and the recipient as well as their relationship that also takes into account the possibility of a transplantation failure.

Since most living kidney transplantations involve donors from the family the selection of an appropriate donor might be associated with a heightened level of conflict within the family system. Simmons et al. [14] found that in 21 out of 79 cases the search for a kidney donor within the family led to considerable intrafamilial tensions. Competition and rivalry seem to be dominant themes. The authors also found that the task of looking for and selecting an appropriate donor within the nuclear or extended family is often taken over by a particular family member who is respected as the family's 'opinion leader'. In some cases the family's 'black sheep' was selected as donor to give him or her the opportunity to pay for the debts of former 'deviance' from the family rules and to become reintegrated into the family system. The issue of living kidney donation also often served as a welcome means to cool down existing conflicts and tensions within the family system. However, some observations, based on clinical case studies, indicate that pre-existing relationship problems might exacerbate the patient's adaptation to his or her post-transplantation life. In an early study Eisendrath [26] reported that eight of 11 patients who died as a consequence of transplantation suffered from strong feelings of being neglected by their families, whereas no such pattern was found among successfully transplanted patients. In a similar vein, Basch [27] observed in a small sample of nine patients that relationship problems which existed prior to transplantation became even more pronounced after the transplantation had been performed.

It is especially noteworthy that pre- and post-transplantation effects are not confined to the donor–recipient relationship but can also be observed with respect to other persons (e.g. non-donating family members, spouses, friends) who are only indirectly involved in the transplantation process. These persons more or less strongly influence the process of donor selection and the change of relationships that occur in the post-transplantation phase. Of particular interest is the role of non-donors within the family system. For example, Simmons et al. [13] found that the spouses of potential donors often objected to the explantation of their partner's kidney, thus undermining the willingness of a family member who, on principle, was ready to donate. Moreover, intimate personal relationships might be affected after the patient has received a new kidney. Smith et al. [11] found that one-third of those patients who divorced after transplantation reported that the fact that they underwent a transplantation was a factor in the divorce. In any case, these data attest to the importance of conceiving the transplantation process as a systemic event that has multiple effects within the network of close personal relationships.

A special group of potential donors are the spouses of patients with chronic renal disease. For several reasons, however, this group of emotionally related persons has not yet been considered as donors [3] although, as mentioned above, there are no compelling legal or ethical reasons to exclude this particular group of potential donors from donation [21–23]. It should be considered, however, that transplantation decisions involving spouses or committed long-term partners have to take into account special aspects of relationship quality and corresponding expectations. Moreover, the couple's relationship history has been found to be particularly important when the transition from an often extended period of dialysis to transplantation takes place [28,29]. There are some indications that within a couple system where one partner, due to his or her chronic renal disease, is highly dependent on the other partner both spouses co-construct a particular kind of their relationship. For example, Balck et al.

[28] found that although marital satisfaction was higher in a group of couples with one dialysed partner than in a control group without chronic disease, the former group showed less mutual openness and communication. The authors believe that this finding might reflect a particular coping strategy to prevent the couple from becoming involved in too much disagreement and conflict which, in turn, might jeopardize the equilibrium that the spouses have established in their mutually dependent relationship. Evidence from other fields of chronic disease, such as coronary heart disease and heart transplantation, suggests that the patient's regained freedom of movement can considerably disturb the balance of the marital system established in the pre transplantation period [30,31].

In summary, the available research evidence suggests that the relationship between donor and recipient, within a familial or otherwise emotionally close relationship context, plays an important role in the search for and selection of potential donors as well as in the post-transplantation adaptation process. Although in most cases the quality of the donor–recipient relationship proved to be mutually satisfying or changed for the better in the post-transplantation phase there are also particular relationship constellations that need special attention in order to prevent negative outcomes. Quite paradoxically, under certain circumstances the less positive effects on the relationship level might be triggered by the overall beneficial effects that successfully transplanted patients usually experience. Therefore, the prospective impact of transplantation on the future relationship development of those who are involved in the transplantation process and its consequences should be carefully scrutinized during the pre-transplantation phase.

3. Some desiderata for future research

Given the conceptual and methodological progress that has been made in recent years in the field of health psychology and behavioural medicine [32,33] the following considerations are believed to contribute to a better understanding of the psychological processes that are involved in the adaptation to living kidney transplantation.

3.1. Dynamic contextual models

Modern stress theory views the occurrence of chronic diseases (e.g. chronic renal dysfunction) as an enduring physical stressor that affects the patient as well as

relevant persons within the patient's relationship context. Within this framework, living kidney transplantation can be conceived as a critical life event that activates specific coping behaviours on the part of the recipient and the donor which, in turn, are partly determined by the coping styles that both persons acquired prior to transplantation. Thus, coping is an individual and joint process of finding a new personal and interpersonal balance in view of changed opportunities and restraints that are associated with the transition to transplantation and the time that follows. Depending on the quality and appropriateness of the coping behaviours and the consequences they generate, the outcome will be a more or less successful adaptation to the transplantation procedure itself and to new challenges that follow the transplantation event. It is suggested that future psychological research in the area of living kidney transplantation should be based on dynamic contextual models of this kind [34].

3.2. Prospective longitudinal designs

One of the implications of dynamic contextual models is that they are inherently longitudinal in nature. It is recommended that longitudinal research designs should cover a sufficiently long period of time from pre- to post-transplantation to trace the developmental (and adaptational) paths for recipients, donors and their relationship. In addition, it would be particularly revealing to compare the processes and outcomes of the adaptation to transplantation across different recipient–donor constellations implying, for instance, biologically related, emotionally related and non-related donors.

3.3. Transplantation counselling

It is further suggested that the selection of potential donors should be based on a rational counselling model. The purpose of this approach is to ensure the optimum discussion of information and clarification concerning medical, legal, economical and psychological implications of the transplantation process and its consequences [34]. The final goal of such an unbiased counselling process would be to create a situation where both the recipient and the potential donor are in a position to decide for themselves whether the transplantation should be performed or not.

It is hoped that empirical studies that are organized along these lines will advance our understanding of the psychological processes of decision making and adaptation in living organ transplantation.

References

1. Davison AM (ed.). Proceedings of the European Dialysis and Transplant Association European Renal Association. Volume 21. London. 1985.

2. End-Stage Renal Desease Network Coordinating Council. Program Report 1984. National Forum of End-Stage Renal Disease Networks, Tampa 1985.

3. Land W. Lebendspende von Organen – derzeitiger Stand der internationalen Debatte. Z Tx Med 1993; 5: 59–63.

4. Land W, Dossetor JB (eds). Organ Replacement Therapy: Ethics, Justice, Commerce. Springer, New York, 1991.

5. Special issue. Z Tx Med 1993; 5: 50–96.

6. Beard BH. The quality of life before and after renal transplantation. Dis Nerv Sys 1971; 32: 24–31.

7. Katschnig H, Konieczna T. Die psychosoziale Situation chronisch hämodialysierter und nierentransplantierter Patienten und ihrer Angehörigen. Unpublished research report, Ludwig Boltzmann-Institut, Wien, 1982.

8. Simmons RG. Long-term reactions of renal recipients and donors. In Levy NB (ed.), Psychonephrology II. Plenum Press, New York 1983; pp. 275–87.

9. Land W. Medizinische Aspekte der Lebendspende: Nutzen/Risiko-Abwägung. Z Tx Med 1993; 5: 52–6.

10. Pommer W, Diedrichs P, Hummel M, Kratzer P, Offerman G, Molzahn M. Patients' expectations from renal grafting and transplantation outcome. Psychother Psychosom 1985; 44: 95–102.

11. Smith MD, Kapell DF, Province HA, Robson AM, Dutton S, Guzmann T, Hoff J, Shelton L, Cameron E, Emerson W, Glass NR, Hopkins J, Peterson C. Living-related kidney donors: a multicenter study of donor education, socioeconomic adjustment and rehabilitation. Am J Kidney Dis 1986; 8: 23–33.

12. Bennet AH, Harrison JH. Experience with living familial renal donors. Sug Gyenecol Obstet 1974; 39: 894–98.

13. Simmons RG, Klein SD, Simmons RL. Gift of Life: The Social and Psychological Impact of Organ Transplantation. Wiley, New York 1977.

14. Simmons RG, Hickey K, Kjellstrand CH, Simmons RL. Donors and non-donors: the role in kidney transplantation. Semin Psychiatry 1971; 3: 102–15.

15. Fellner CH, Marshall JR. Kidney donors: the myth of informed consent. Am J Psychiatry 1979; 126: 1245–51.

16. Fellner CH. Organ donation: for whose sake? Ann Intern Med 1973; 79: 589–92.

17. Levey AS, Hou S, Bush HL. Kidney transplantation from unrelated living donors. Time to reclaim a discarded opportunity. N Engl J Med 1986; 314: 914–16.

18. Daar AS. Rewarded gifting and rampant commercialism in perspective: is there a difference? In: Land W, Dossetor JB (eds), Organ Replacement Therapy: Ethics, Justice, Commerce. Springer, New York 1991; pp. 181–9.

19. Sadler HH, Davison L, Caroll C. The living genetically unrelated kidney donor. Semin Psychiatry 1971; 3: 86–101.

20. Sadler HH. The motivation of living donors. Transplant Proc 1973; 5: 1121–3.

21. Gutmann Th. Rechtsphilosophische Aspekte der Lebendspende von Nieren. Z Tx Med 1993; 5: 75–87.

22. Elsässer A. Ethische Probleme bei Lebendspende von Organen I. Z Tx Med 1993; 5: 65–9.

23. Gründel J. Ethische Probleme bei Lebendspende von Organen II. Z Tx Med 1993; 5: 70–4.

24. Simmons RG. Psychological reactions to giving a kidney. In: Levy NB (ed.), Psychonephrology I. Plenum Press, New York 1981; pp. 227–45.

25. Weizer N, Weizman A, Shapira Z, Yussim A, Munitz H. Suicide by related kidney donors following the recipient's death. Psychother Psychosom 1989; 51: 216–19.

26. Eisendrath RM. The role of grief and fear in the death of kidney transplant patients. Am J Psychiatry 1969; 126: 81–7.

27. Basch SH. The intrapsychic integration of a new organ. Psychoanal Quart 1973; 42: 364–84.

28. Balck F, Koch U, Speidel H. Psychonephrologie. Springer, Berlin 1985.

29. Koch U, Wenz C. Lebendnierentransplantation aus psychologischer Sicht. In Albert FW (ed.), Praxis der Nierentransplantation II. Schattauer, Stuttgart 1989; pp. 75–87.

30. Bunzel B. Herztransplantation: Pschosoziale Grundlagen und Forschungsergebnisse zur Lebensqualität. Thieme, Stuttgart 1993.

31. Waltz M, Badura B, Pfaff H, Schott T. Marriage and the psychological consequences of heart attack: a longitudinal study of adaptation to chronic illness after 3 years. Soc Sci Med 1988; 27: 149–58.

32. Green J, Shellenberger R. The Dynamics of Health and Wellness. Holt, Reinhart and Winston, Fort Worth 1991.

33. Schwarzer R. Psychologie des Gesundheitsverhaltens. Hogrefe, Göttingen 1992.

34. Schneewind KA. Psychologische Aspekte der Lebendnierenspende. Z Tx Med 1993; 5: 89–96.

40 | Brain death

H. ANGSTWURM

Knowledge of brain death and the understanding of its significance as a definitive sign of death are two of the basic principles of transplantation medicine. However, the possibility of transplanting organs of dead persons has not given rise to a new concept or to a new definition of death, nor does it have any influence on the determination of death. There is only one human death, and the definition of death pertains only to the person involved (only those affected can define and confirm it).

1. Signs of death

Death can be biologically and hence medically determined only as a permanent loss of vital signs. These signs can be grouped into the various life units affected – cells, tissues, organs, organisms, populations and biozones. Similarly, the signs of death can be differentiated. Following the hierarchy to which life units are subject, a higher unit presupposes a lower unit. However, the reverse is not always true: a lower unit does not always presuppose a higher one. Consequently, without living cells there can be no other life; living cells alone do not represent a living organ and living organs alone do not represent a living organism. While there is no question that a living thing whose last cell has died is dead, it is just as certain that death had occurred before then. A living thing as an organism, as a functional unit of a whole, is more than only the sum total of its cells, tissues and organs. The human being as a living being, as an organism, can be dead even when some of the parts of the body such as organs or tissues are still alive or being artificially kept alive. The difference between the organism, the living

'human being' as a functional unit of the whole, and its individual parts is clearly seen in the permanent loss of brain function.

2. Brain death

'Brain death' means that the entire brain – the cerebrum, cerebellum and brain stem – has died, but that the natural effects of this event on the other organs have been prevented by intensive care treatment, including controlled ventilation. Brain death means:

pathogenetically: an increase in intracranial pressure leading to cessation of brain circulation;
morphologically: an ischaemic infarct of the entire brain;
functionally: the complete and irreversible loss of all brain function.

The definition of brain death pertains only to the person involved, it has nothing to do with any purpose and certainly not any interests of others. It represents a natural phenomenon, since it is the finalization of the individual's illness and, being natural, it is not variable according to need. The definition of brain death excludes all malformations and injuries, however severe they might be, which cause only partial loss of brain activity, as well as states of temporary loss of brain function, and hence the corresponding stages of embryonic development.

The diagnosis of brain death is made according to its definition. The clinician uses the functional definition of brain death. He knows that the brain becomes inactive before brain circulation ceases. The chance of brain function returning can be ruled out by

G.M. Collins, J.M. Dubernard, W. Land and G.G. Persijn (eds). Procurement, Preservation and Allocation of Vascularized Organs 331–332
© 1997 Kluwer Academic Publishers.

excluding any remediable conditions, and by either observation or technical findings that confirm the presence of brain damage so severe that general, not only personal, experience would deem recovery impossible. The diagnosis confirms an already existent stage. For this reason the diagnosis is not a matter of judgement, or of making a decision, or of assessing the further course of the condition; nor is it a purely legally binding but perhaps reversible declaration of death.

3. Brain death as a sign of death

The complete and irreversible loss of brainfunction biologically means the loss of:

independence as a functional unit, as a whole (autonomy as organism);
the ability of function automatically as a functional unit, as a whole (spontaneity as organism);
the ability to select individual functions from the whole as functional unit;
the correlation between the whole as functional unit and its surroundings (adaptation and disassociation as a whole);
unity of the individual functions and their interrelations with the whole as functional unit (integration).

In human beings this loss at the same time means the loss of the essential physical basis of one's bodily and spiritual existence in this world.

On the one hand, brain death destroys the autonomous, self-determining and, out of reasons deep within oneself, the automatically functioning life unit and order. It destroys the organism as a functional unit of the whole. What remains is a collection of organs which no longer belong to a unit of a higher order and are no longer combined as a whole, and which from now on can only function by means of constant support from outside. On the other hand, brain death destroys the individual's physical basis for every spiritual feeling. He is no longer able to make, process, and respond to a perception or observation; he can no longer create, pursue, and express a thought, or reflect on something and communicate what he thinks; he no longer can sense and show emotion, never again will he be able to make a decision. Thus, through the irreparable cessation of his brain function, the individual has lost two properties of his life as an organism endowed with a mind.

4. Difficulties in understanding brain death as a sign of death

Nevertheless, it can prove difficult to understand the complete and permanent loss of brain function as a definitive sign of death. Unlike rigor mortis, livor mortis, and signs of decay and putrefaction, brain death can only be determined and distinguished from the death-like state of an intensively treated individual by means of specific tests. Moreover, complete and irreversible loss of brain function usually affects individuals who up until that point had been healthy, very often within the first days after an accident or a dramatic illness. For that reason, those who find it difficult to recognize permanent and complete loss of brain function as a sign of death deserve as much empathy, tolerance and understanding as we can show them. With objectivity and openness much can be done to improve the knowledge of brain death and the understanding of its significance as a sign of death.

An experience such as the death of another human being, a puzzle like the meaning of death, a fight like that against death as life's enemy, and the fear that each of us has of death all push the capacity of medicine and the power of physicians past their limits. In facing the phenomenon of death, we all need help from philosophers, theologists and pastor. Last but not least, we all need human compassion.

41 | A survey of religious attitudes towards organ donation and transplantation

A.S. DAAR

1. Religious considerations

Questions regarding religious teachings on organ donation, particularly with respect to cadaver donation, are often raised. More often than not, however, religious constraints are more imagined than real. In the past few years, a number of authors and religious authorities from the major world religions have commented on many aspects of these questions. I have tried below to capture and encapsulate the essence of those discussions relating specifically to transplantation. The major monotheistic religions of the West (Judaism, Christianity and Islam), because of their shared origins, have similar conceptions of creation, of man's relation to God, of the material and the spiritual, of the soul, of the essential sanctity of life and of death and eschatology. Although religious discourse, sources (canonical literature), justifications, examples used, emphases and lines of authority vary, all three religions in general support living organ donation, cadaver organ donation and the establishment of death using brain-death criteria. All three generally accept that the diagnosis of physical death is best left to the physician. Hinduism and Buddhism both encourage living and post mortem organ donation. However, the tradition of Shinto, even though linked to Buddhist rituals, has not been able to encourage the development of cadaver organ donation in Japan; this may be a problem also in other traditions.

Islam is discussed in some detail because of my closer familiarity with the religion.

2. Judaism [1–3]

Jewish law (halachah) is at once permanent (in the sense that the scriptures and Talmudic texts may not be altered) and unremittingly adaptable to needs posed by given circumstances. The important issues for debate among Rabbinic authorities have included desecration of the body after death, prohibition against deriving any benefit from a corpse and responsibility to accord the deceased full burial. Judaism ascribes supreme value to every moment of life, regardless of its quality or likely duration. It is therefore not surprising that one of the most important of the 613 commandments is the crucial commandment to save life. This over-rules every other commandment except for three prohibitions: abandoning the worship of God, forbidden sexual acts and killing another person (i.e. one may not take a life at the expense of another). Transplantation of a kidney has been accepted as a life-

G.M. Collins, J.M. Dubernard, W. Land and G.G. Persijn (eds). Procurement, Preservation and Allocation of Vascularized Organs 333–338
© 1997 Kluwer Academic Publishers.

saving procedure (as, interestingly, is corneal transplantation because of the traditional teaching that the blind are considered extremely impaired and in danger of losing life) [3]. Hence, the consensus is that the saving of life, limb or function is of such paramount importance that it effectively over-rides these constraints, provided that the post mortem donor is treated with respect, is not mutilated and all remaining parts are buried with the deceased.

Because of the absolute requirement that a life may not be saved at the expense of another, it is important that death of the donor should not be hastened to benefit the recipient. In the late 1980s, there was a swing in halachic opinion toward the acceptance of brain death as the decisive marking of life's termination. The Chief Rabbinate in Israel has accepted the declaration of brain death as a criterion for the establishment of death under certain conditions. In Israel, three (not two) physicians must constitute the committee, and at least one objective test must be performed. These changes now mean that Jews are not only allowed to donate but are obliged to do so, i.e. it is now a *mizveh*, a commandment to do that (compare this concept with the idea of Fardh Kifaya in the section on Islam below). Even ultraorthodox Jews now sometimes tolerate organ transplantation. Furthermore, Israeli law in the early 1990s did not require consent from the family, who only needed to be informed of the intention to remove organs, although the family does have the right to object. Living-donor transplantation is permitted, part of the justification being the superior results, but there is no obligation on the donor to place himself or herself at significant risk, and living donors should not be coerced.

3. Christianity [4–9]

Man was created in the image of God (*imago Dei*), who blew his own breath (*ruach Jahwe*) into the body of his creature, thus transfiguring him and making man different from the rest of creation (Genesis 2:7). The body and soul together are the 'person'. Every human being is an individual person, independent of his social standing, achievements or health. His dignity is inalienable. The body, though, is important: it is at the core of traditional Christian belief in the Incarnation ('in flesh becoming'), the Passion, Death and Resurrection of Christ. The body will also be resurrected in the future. Therefore, even though the cadaver is no longer the person, its handling requires respect, care and ritual reverence. The voluntary readiness to donate one's organs as a means of saving the life of a sick

person is not only legitimate but is also a magnanimous act of charity, generosity and love. The donor acts here with ethical responsibility.

The brain is neither the seat of the soul nor the 'origin' of the intellect. The Christian doctrine of the departure of the soul from the body at the moment of death would seem to support the concept of brain death. In 1957, Pope Pius XII declared that in case of prolonged coma (instances that we would now perhaps understand to constitute brain death), the soul might already have left the body and no 'extraordinary means' of support would be required, and he emphasized that the determination of death should be left to the physicians [5].

On August 31, 1990, the German Bishops Conference and the Council of the Evangelical Church in Germany published a common declaration welcoming transplantation and encouraging and justifying organ donation [7]. On June 10, 1991, Pope John Paul II delivered an address at the Vatican to the participants of the First International Congress of the Society for Organ Sharing. In this extremely important address [9] he made it clear that the Roman Catholic Church supports organ transplantation, and he concluded by quoting Jesus: 'Give, and it will be given to you, good measure, pressed down, shaken together, running over, will be put in your lap' (Luke 6:38).

Certain German commentators, including the Protestant ethicist Ch. Kupatt, have recently reopened the debate on the widely-held acceptance of brain death criteria as being diagnostic of death [10].

4. Islam

4.1. Introduction

Over a billion people in the world are Muslims; most live in developing countries, where rates of renal failure are high and transplantation is increasing. To most Muslims, religion plays a major role in their lives. It is not surprising, therefore, if questions related to religion often arise when discussing transplantation with Muslims. Below are the kind of issues that are often raised. Many Muslims are themselves often not familiar with religious rulings and opinions on transplantation.

4.2. The questions

What is Islam's conception of disease?
Does Islam accept modern therapies such as transplantation? Does it encourage transplantation?

What are Islam's teachings that would encourage donation?

Is a Muslim a fatalist who need not seek therapy for major illness?

What is the conception of the relationship of man to man, and of man to Allah?

What is the meaning of life, and what is death? Who diagnoses death?

If there is a day of judgment, of resurrection, what happens if a part of the body is missing?

Is it permissible to cut up a dead body to remove an organ?

Have there been any official rulings about donation and transplantation? If so, what is the legal process?

Should the donor sell his/her organs for transplantation?

What is practised in Muslim countries?

Looking ahead to xenotransplantation: what if the donor is a pig? (since the pig is considered ritually unclean in Islam, it is forbidden as food in the same way that it is forbidden to eat pork in Judaism).

4.3. The answers

4.3.1. *Nature of disease: obligation to seek treatment*
Islam does not subscribe to the 'punishment' theory of disease causation. Diseases have causes other than retributive divine intervention. Life is sacred, and must be preserved whenever possible. To seek self-preservation through modern scientific treatment is therefore an obligation. Organ failure, just like any other disease, must be treated if possible; if the best method of treatment is transplantation, then that is not only acceptable, but must be encouraged and the authorities must provide for the therapy, provided this is not harmful to others. Primarily, however, disease must be prevented if possible and health is to be promoted.

4.3.2. *Qualities conducive to transplantation*
Islam encourages the following qualities which are supportive and conducive to organ donation. These are:

1. Altruism. For example, the faithful are described in the Quran as: 'They give priority over themselves even though they are needy.'
2. Generosity. For example, 'In the society of the faithful, donations should be in generous supply and should be the fruit of faith and love of God and his subject' [16].
3. Duty. For example, 'The donation of body fluids or organs, such as blood transfusion to the bleeding or a kidney transplant to the patient with bilateral ir-

reparable renal damage, ... is *Fardh Kifaya*, a duty that donors fulfil on behalf of society' [16].
4. Charity. For example, the Quran says, 'And whosoever saves a human life it is as though he has saved all mankind' and if the living are able to donate, then the dead are even more so; and no harm will afflict the cadaver if the heart, kidneys, eyes or arteries are taken to be put to good use in a living person. This is indeed a charity' [16].
5. Responsibility. For example, Umar ibnul Khattab, the second Islamic Khalifa decreed, 'If a man ... dies of hunger ... the community should pay his *fidiah* [money ransom] as if they had killed him'. 'The individual patient is the collective responsibility of society, which has to ensure his health needs by any means [while] inflicting no harm to others' [16].
6. Cooperation. For example, 'The faithful in their mutual love and compassion are like the body ... if one member complains of an ailment, all others will rally in response' (Tradition of the Prophet). 'The faithful, to one another, are like the blocks in a whole building ... they fortify one another' (Tradition of the Prophet).
7. Public health education.

Islam discourages exploitation and compulsion.

4.3.3. *Allah, man and the gift of life*
Man is encouraged to live in peace with fellow man: Muslims in a community constitute an *Umma*, which requires mutual cooperation and support to thrive. While altruism is encouraged and minimal risk is acceptable, significant harm to oneself while alive is not encouraged in order to help another. The person is made up of the physical body and the soul. Not much knowledge has been given to man regarding the soul, except that Allah breathes His spirit into the foetus to make it a complete human being and death occurs when the soul has departed from the body; the exact moment of this occurrence is beyond man's perception. Life is a gift from God and it must not be forgotten that everything in life, including the body, belongs to God. Abuse of the body and suicide are therefore sinful.

4.3.4. *Islamic law*
Islamic law is the Shariah, which is at once permanent and yet capable of responding to every challenge, including issues in transplantation. The basis of Shariah is the Quran and the Sunna, i.e. the sayings, actions and rulings of the Prophet Mohammed [Peace be upon him]. The fundamental principles of jurisprudence when an issue arises that requires a decision are:

Need and necessity are equivalent;
Necessity allows 'prohibited' matters;
Injurious 'harm' should be removed;
Prevention of evil has priority over obtaining benefit;
The greater benefit prevails over the lesser benefit [17].

4.3.5. Rulings on transplantation by religious authorities

Based upon these principles and the foregoing attributes expected of a Muslim, the majority of Islamic legal scholars have concluded that transplantation of organs as treatment for otherwise lethal end stage organ failure is a good thing. Donation by living donors and by cadaveric donors is not only permitted but is encouraged. The senior Ulamaa (Scholars) Commission of Saudi Arabia in Fatwa (legal ruling) no. 99, dated 9.11.1402 (25 August 1982) resolved by majority the following: 'The permissibility to remove an organ or part thereof from a dead person for the benefit of a Muslim, should the need arise, should the removal cause no dissatisfaction, and should transplantation seem likely to be successful.'

In Egypt, the Grand Mufti, Gad al Haq, decreed in Fatwa no. 1323 of 5 December 1979 that it is permissible to donate organs from the living, provided no harm was done, the donation was done freely, in good faith and for the love of God and the human fraternity. He also allowed cadaver donation provided there was a will of testament or the consent of relatives of the deceased. In cases of unidentified corpses, an order from the Magistrate should be obtained prior to removal of the organs.

The Third International Conference of Islamic Jurists, at their meeting in Amman, Jordan, on 16 October 1986, in Resolution no. 5, declared in favour of using brain death criteria to establish death, as follows: 'A person [is] considered legally dead, and all the Sharia's principles can be applied, when one of the following signs is established: 1. Complete stoppage of the heart and breathing, and the doctors decide that it is irretrievable. 2. Complete stoppage of all the vital functions of the brain, and the doctors decide it is irreversible, and the brain has started to degenerate.'

It must be remembered that Islam is not monolithic and allows for differences of opinion in details. At various stages there have been minority opinions, requiring cessation of the circulation and respiration, for death to be diagnosed. Nevertheless, the Fourth International Conference of Islamic Jurists, meeting in Jeddah in 1988, endorsed all previous Fatwas, including the landmark Fatwa no. 5 (above) of 1986 which allowed the use of brain death criteria to diagnose death. In addition, the 1988 conference clearly rejected

any trafficking or trading in human organs, and re-stressed the principle of altruism [13].

4.3.6. Xenotransplantation

If ever the day came when xenotransplantation was possible, this would easily be justified in Islamic law, even if the donor was a pig. I have discussed this extensively elsewhere [18] but one fact is enough to put this question to rest. Over 900 years ago tooth and bone transplantation was practised in Muslim countries (Al Bar 1991). Porcine bones at that time gave better results than bones from other species for grafting, and despite the injunction against the eating of pig flesh, jurists accepted the use of these porcine bones.

4.3.7. Draft law on human organ transplants

Muslim Arab countries have actually taken the lead in trying to formulate international legal norms: the 12th session of the Council of Arab Ministers of Health meeting in Khartoum, Sudan, 14–16 March 1987, responding to a WHO call, promulgated the Unified Arab Draft Law on Human Organ Transplants (A.40/INF.DOC/6-30 April 1987). Article 1 states: Specialist physicians may perform surgical operations to transplant organs from a living or dead person to another person for the purpose of maintaining life, according to the conditions and procedures laid down in this law. Article 5 states: 'organ transplants may be performed from a dead body, provided that consent is obtained from the next of kin, under the following conditions: 1. Death has been definitely established by a committee of three specialist physicians, including a neurologist. The physician who is to perform the operation must not be a member of the committee. 2. The deceased, while alive, did not object to the removal of any organ from his body.'

4.4. Summary

In summary, disease must be prevented if possible, but when it develops, every available scientific method must be sought for its healing. Transplantation is considered a valid method of treatment, particularly to save lives. Both cadaver and live donor transplants are permitted, provided that there is no compulsion or exploitation and there is adequate informed consent. Organs should not be the object of trading or trafficking. Brain death criteria to establish death have been accepted by the majority of Muslim jurists. Individual scholars may hold different opinions; what I have described above is the majority opinion, as reflected in actual practice in Muslim countries, particularly in the Middle East, where transplantation is now practised in almost all countries. Saudi Arabia performed the first cadaveric kidney transplantation in 1984 [19] and has a very active cadaver programme based upon brain death criteria. Oman has a similar law (Ministerial decree), which has allowed us to use cadaver organs based on brain death criteria; Turkey has similar laws. Not only kidneys, but now liver and heart transplants are being performed in Muslim countries. The question regarding waking up with some organs missing on the day of judgment/resurrection can be dealt with by the following logical argument: surely if Allah is powerful enough to be able to create a whole person in the first place, then Allah is more than capable of reconstituting him again if the need arose, for Allah is the creator of all the Universe, and he cherishes and cares for his creatures, especially man, whom he has designated his vice-regent on earth.

5. Hinduism [20]

The main philosophy of the religion is based on The Law of Karma and reincarnation. This has direct relevance to transplantation. The soul is immortal, occupying a new body with each incarnation, but without erasure of the experiences of previous births. The physical body, because it is made up of the basic universal elements of earth, water and air should be returned to these basic elements through cremation. However, the dead are respected and gracefully mourned, and the body must be respected, cleaned and escorted for cremation.

Hindu methodology contains traditions whereby human body parts were used to benefit other humans and society. There is nothing in the religion to indicate that organs from either the living or the post mortem donor could not be used to alleviate suffering, especially because one of the basic themes of the Hindu religion is to help those who are suffering. The Lord Krishna has said that whatever we do today will decide what we will become tomorrow. Thus religion *per se* is unlikely to contraindicate either living or cadaveric donation in India.

6. Buddhism [21]

At the absolute level, the body is but a conglomeration of matter and mind, and any sense of permanence is but an illusion, as is our notion of life itself. Death is the 'temporary end of a temporary phenomenon', to be followed by rebirth when there is a new mind–body partnership. Thus, there is nothing intrinsically sacro-

sanct or holy about the human body, alive or dead, and its disposal after death does not make much difference. However, the ideal of the social good (*attha samhita*) encourages the decent treatment of the dead for reasons of love, respect, gratitude or example. Donation for transplantation while alive or after death is seen as an act of generosity (*alobha*), which is (itself) described as a moral mental property contributing to the achievement of Nirvana (Parinibbana), the *summum bonum* in Buddhism, and as an example of compassion (*karuna*), one of the four guidelines to social living. Thus, transplantation from the living or the dead is allowed, as is xenotransplantation. Psychological aspects need to be given particular attention because the mental quality of the donor could influence the recipient's course.

7. Shinto

Shinto is as old as Japanese culture, and as a religion gives both ethical and ethnic identity to the Japanese. In Japan, Buddhism itself has been influenced by the native Shinto tradition and by other Japanese folk beliefs, which are different from those of China or Korea. In Shinto, the central value is purity: all gods are pleased with purity and angered by impurity and pollution. Death is the ultimate polluted matter. The dead body is so impure, polluted and dangerous that it must be expelled quickly; contaminated persons and things must be decontaminated by specific purification rites. The dead body is so impure, in fact, that Shinto has not even developed theories or rites to handle it, but Buddhism has developed rituals and ceremonies for the dead, and it is these that are used.

The dead, however, go on to become deified in the system of ancestor worship (Shinto is theanthropic). Dead spirits are worshipped for either 33 or 49 years, after which they lose their personal identity, become extremely pure and end up as the community's guardian gods, who are then worshipped as such. Amaterasu, the god of the sun and also the paramount god of Shinto, is believed to be the primary ancestor of the Japanese Royal Family.

The word *itai* (the remains), as opposed to *shitai* (the dead body), embraces a sense of identification of a continuing relationship between the bereaved and the recently dead person. *Itai* (or *go-itai* to indicate politeness and respect) has its own hopes and requests, and in order to avoid misfortune, the bereaved must not only guess and grant these requests but also avoid any injury to *itai*. It thus becomes clear why it is difficult in Japan to obtain consent from bereaved families for organ donation, dissection or diagnostic post mortem examinations; these are all regarded as injury to *itai*. In fact, even if a person has indicated a willingness to donate his body to a medical school, the family members often refuse consent for dissection. They do this because they want to avoid injury to the *itai* by their own will, as this injury to the *itai* makes the dead person's soul more miserable than ignoring the person's living will.

The difficulties inherent to transplantation and especially regarding the question of brain death have been discussed in some detail by Ohnuki-Tierney ([22], see also comment on this article by Daar[24]).

8. References

1. Weiss DM. 1990; Organ transplantation, medical ethics and Jewish Law. Transplant Proc 1988; 20: 1071–5.
2. Bulka RP. Jewish perspective on organ transplantation. Transplant Proc 1990; 22: 945–6.
3. Aiallam. General discussion on the dilemma of postmortem organ donation. In: Land W, Dossetor JB (eds), Organ Replacement Therapy: Ethics, Justice and Commerce. Springer-Verlag, Berlin 1991; pp. 319–20.
4. Scorsone S. Christianity and the significance of the human body. Transplant Proc 1990; 22: 943–4.
5. Sass HM. Philosophical arguments in accepting brain death criteria. In: Land W, Dossetor JB (eds), Organ Replacement Therapy: Ethics, Justice and Commerce. Springer-Verlag, Berlin 1991; pp. 249–58.
6. Angstwurm, H. Brain death as death of a human being: a matter of image of man. In: Land W, Dossetor JB (eds), Organ Replacement Therapy: Ethics, Justice and Commerce. Springer-Verlag, Berlin 1991; pp. 241–4.
7. Grundel J. Theological aspects of brain death with regard to the death of a person. In: Land W, Dossetor JB (eds), Organ Replacement Therapy: Ethics, Justice and Commerce. Springer-Verlag, Berlin 1991; pp. 245–8.
8. Teo B. Organ transplantation: a Christian viewpoint. Transplant Proc 1992; 24: 2114–15.
9. Pope John Paul, II. Special message on organ donation. Address of the Holy Father to the participants of the Society for Organ Sharing, June 20, 1991. Transplant Proc 1991; 23: xvii–xviii.
10. Kupatt Ch. Anmerkungen zur Selbsstbestimmung uber den eigenen Korper aus protestantischer Sicht. Symposium zur Lebendspende von Organen Programm. Munchen, 26–28 Oktober, 1995.
11. Sachedina AA. Islamic views on organ transplantation. Transplant Proc 1988; 20: 1084–8.
12. Sahin AF. Islamic transplantation ethics. Transplant Proc 1990; 22: 939.
13. Al Bar MA. Islamic view on organ transplantation. In: Abouna GM, Kumar MSA, White AG (eds), Proceedings of the 2nd International Conference of Middle East Society of Organ Transplantation, Kuwait, 11–15 March, 1990. Kluwer Academic Publishers, Lancaster 1991; pp. 574–8.
14. Daar AS. Current practice and the legal, ethical and religious status of post-mortem organ donation in the Islamic world. In: Land W, Dossetor JB (eds), Organ Replacement Therapy: Ethics, Justice, Commerce. Springer-Verlag, Berlin 1991; pp. 295–9.
15. Sellami MM. Islamic position on organ donation and transplantation. Transplant Proc 1993; 25: 2307–9.
16. Islamic Code of Medical Ethics. The Kuwait Document (1981). International Organisation of Islamic Medicine, 1st Edition, Kuwait IOMS [Copies in Arabic and English can be obtained from the present author].
17. Al Qattan M. In: Abomelha MS (ed.), The Juristic Ijitihad Regarding Transplantation of Organs in Organ Transplantation: Proceedings of a Symposium held in Riyadh, December 1984. Medical Education Services, Oxford 1984; pp. 1–4.
18. Daar AS. Xenotransplantation and religion: the major monotheistic religions. Xeno 1994; 2: 61–4.
19. Al Otaibi K, Al Khader A, Abomelha MS. First Saudi Cadaver Donation. Saudi Med J 1985; 6: 217.
20. Trivedi HL. Hindu religious view in context of transplantation of organs from cadavers. Transplant Proc 1990; 22: 942.
21. Sugunasiri SHJ. The Buddhist view concerning the dead body. Transplant Proc 1990; 22: 947–9.
22. Ohnuki-Tierney, E. Brain death and organ transplantation: cultural bases of medical technology. Curr Anthropol 1994; 35: 233–42.
23. Namihira, E. Shinto concept concerning the dead human body. Transplant Proc 1990; 22: 940–1.
24. Daar AS. Brain death and organ transplantation. Curr Anthropol 1994; 35: 245–6.

Further reading

Daar AS. Transplantation in developing countries. In: Morris PJ (ed.), Kidney Transplantation, Principles and Practice. 4th edn. Saunders, Philadelphia 1994; 478–503.

Hathout H. Islamic basis for biomedical ethics. In: Pellegrino E, Mazzarella P, Corsi P (eds), Transcultural dimensions in medical ethics. University Publishing Company, Frederick 1992; pp. 58–72.

Rahman C, Snine A, El Kadi A. Islamic code of medical professional ethics. In: Veatch RM (ed.) Cross Cultural Perspectives in Medical Ethics: Readings. Jones and Bartlett Publishers, Boston 1989; pp. 120–6.

Yaseen MN. The rulings for the donation of human organs in the light of Sharia rules and medical facts. Arab Law Quarterly 1990 5(1): 49–89.

42 | Philosophical arguments for accepting the brain death criterion

DIETER BIRNBACHER

1. Introduction

The so-called brain death criterion according to which a man is dead when his total brain has completely and irreversibly ceased to function is now widely accepted and has been widely introduced into legislation and professional codes. It is not to be overlooked, however, that here is also a good deal of scepticism and, in some quarters, direct opposition to the criterion, reinforcing otherwise motivated reservations to the medical practice of organ transplantation, and often resulting in its downright rejection. Scepticism regarding the brain death criterion is sometimes disqualified by medical researchers and clinicians as a case of pure 'irrationality'. However, the matter is too important, practically and theoretically, to be dealt with in this manner. If, as Hans Jonas and a few other philosophers and theologians have suspected, there is a substantial probability that the practice of explanting organs from a brain-dead body under artificial respiration amounts to no less than vivisection or even murder, the consequence would certainly have to be that the practice is immediately stopped and put under heavy legal sanctions. Theoretically, the challenging of the brain death criterion by its opponents is a welcome occasion to reflect anew, and perhaps more systematically and more critically, on its anthropological and general philosophical foundations.

2. Definition of death versus criteria of death

A suitable starting point for a critical examination of the adequacy of the brain death criterion is the dis-tinction introduced by Culver and Gert [1] between definition, criteria and tests of death. This distinction is important because judgements on the adequacy, certainty and reliability of these different kinds of indicators follow very different criteria. A testing procedure designed to show that a certain criterion is met must be empirically well founded if it is to function properly. Similarly, a criterion (or operational definition) must correspond to the state of scientific knowledge, i.e. to the best-established scientific theory in the field, in order for it to function as a reliable indicator of the state of affairs for which it is a criterion. Defining conditions, on the other hand, are not amenable to justification in empirical or (narrowly defined) scientific terms but require for their validation reasons of a different sort: reasons of adequacy (in the case of well-established concepts) or (in the case of not fully established concepts) reasons of theoretical or practical usefulness. This implies that definitions cannot be ascertained in the same way as criteria and testing procedures. It also implies that they cannot be 'uncertain' [2, p. 233] in the way empirical or theoretical hypotheses can be uncertain. The only thing experience, including scientific experience, can show is that certain conditions obtain. It cannot show which concepts are suited to describe these conditions. The empirical generalizations and scientific theories underlying our tests and criteria can be true or false, well-confirmed or ill-confirmed, certain or uncertain. Our definitions, however, can only be suitable or unsuitable, adequate or inadequate, practical or impractical.

Two conclusions immediately follow: first, however great the importance of scientific results for the acceptability of criteria of death and the tests associated with

G.M. Collins, J.M. Dubernard, W. Land and G.G. Persijn (eds), Procurement, Preservation and Allocation of Vascularized Organs 339–342
© 1997 Kluwer Academic Publishers.

them, it would be illusory to expect science to provide an 'objective' definition of human death. Second, the acceptability of a given criterion of death can only be assessed in reference to an underlying definition of death. Anyone who rejects the underlying definition of death will generally also reject the corresponding criterion, not for the reason that the criterion is not sufficiently certain in scientific terms but for the reason that it is an indicator for something different from what it should be an indicator for. In fact, the most frequent criticisms of the brain death criterion are not generally aimed at the scientific validity of the criterion as such but at the definition of death presupposed by this criterion: whatever this criterion is a criterion for, it is not, according to this view, a criterion for the death of a person. The primary task of a philosophical justification of the brain death criterion is, therefore, to address the question of the definition of death, of what constitutes the death of a human being.

3. The death of a human individual

It was said above that conceptual questions can and must be answered by considerations either of adequacy or of practical usefulness. Obviously, great dangers would be imminent if we had to follow the second course and to give a merely pragmatic definition of a concept so central to our perception of (and dealings with) ourselves and other persons as the concept of death. Fortunately, there is no need to resort to this doubtful option. An explication of the concept of death can be securely based on well established and widely shared conceptual intuitions. Even if the borders of the concept, as with all non-scientific concepts, are not so neatly defined as to leave absolutely no question undecided, the core content of the concept can be expressed by the following four propositions.

First, the subject of death is the human individual as a complex entity composed of body and mind – man as an animal normally endowed with both consciousness and self-consciousness. This is the answer to the 'attributive question' distinguished by Linke *et al.* [3]. That this answer is not as trivial as it sounds becomes evident when it is contrasted with two possible alternatives: that the subject of human death is the human body, and that the subject of death is the person, where 'person' is understood in a narrower sense than that of the full human individual. Both alternative answers are deficient in that they take partial aspects as absolutes and are far from capturing the content of the concept of the human individual embedded in our culture. The

human individual is not only body, but a unity of both physical and mental aspects. To be dead or living is not a property of the human body but of the full human individual. It is the human individual as a complex whole that is born, grows old, and finally dies.

The same has to be said of the 'personal' aspect of the human individual which, again, is only one aspect and not the complex whole. The concept of the person, insofar it is not simply an equivalent of 'human individual', has a variety of senses most of which are constructs within certain philosophical, theological or legal systems, and which were never assimilated into everyday language. This is true, for example, of the metaphysical (or platonic) concept of a person as an immaterial spiritual substance which is able to survive the death of the physical individual with the prospect of being 're-embodied' at a later stage of its existence. The same holds for the mentalistic and the (even narrower) 'cognivistic' concept of a person according to which the person begins (and ceases) to exist with the beginning (and irreversible loss) of the capacity for consciousness, or with the beginning (and irreversible loss) of the capacity for self-consciousness and thinking (as in [4], ch. 4). In both of these senses, the death of the person can occur long before the death of the human individual as a complete entity. An even more extreme example is the Lockean (legalistic) concept of the person, according to which one and the same individual can embody, in its lifetime, a number of different 'persons', each responsible for the actions which it can consciously remember ([5], book 2, ch. 27). None of these highly constructive concepts of the person corresponds to the conceptual role of the subject of life and death in its primary and non-metaphorical sense. As even Robert M. Veatch, a well-known advocate of a higher brain definition of death, admits, there seems to be no absurdity or impossibility in the thought that someone could have irreversibly lost personhood, whatever that may mean, and still be alive ([6], p. 175). The subject of life and death is the empirical, bodily individual. It is not identical with a metaphysical entity more or less inaccessible to experience, nor with certain of its coming and going capacities (like its capacity for consciousness, self-consciousness or thought), however characteristic these capacities may be for the species of which it is a member.

Second, for the human individual as an animal composed of body and mind there is only one death. This is one reason to doubt whether the familiar expression 'brain death' is really fortunate. This expression may easily be taken to suggest that there is more than one death: brain death, heart death, clinical death etc. That, however, would be a misunderstanding. The complete and irreversible cessation of brain functioning is not a special kind of death but only one more criterion for the same state of affairs, 'death', which continues to be indicated, outside the critical care unit, by the traditional criteria of irreversible cessation of heart activity, circulation and respiration.

Third, that a human individual is dead means that he or she has irreversibly lost the capacity of conscious experience as well as of bodily functions as far as these are centrally controlled. By his nature man (like other mammals) is an entity with both mental and physical properties. Life and death are, accordingly, distinguished by the functioning and non-functioning of two systems: of consciousness and of the physical organism. The irreversible non-functioning of one of these systems is not by itself sufficient to call a man dead. A man in irreversible coma is not dead as long as he goes on living as a biological organism. Even the irreversible loss of the capacity (possessed by the brain) to integrate the various bodily functions into the unity of the organism would not be sufficient to call a man dead if the process of consciousness continued, for example if (contrary to fact) consciousness depended on the activity of the heart. Even in this hypothetical case only one of the two necessary conditions of death would be fulfilled.

Finally, that a man is dead does not mean that every single organ or component of his organism has ceased to function. The line between life and death is drawn, rather, by the fact that the individual organs and organ systems are no longer centrally controlled and no longer integrated into the whole of an organism. The physical aspect of death is the disintegration of the organism rather than the cessation of all life and growth processes in its parts and subsystems. It is essential, furthermore, that these activities of control and integration are exercised by the organism itself. If computers should be developed one day with the capacity of exercising these integrative functions even after complete loss of brain function (thus making a dead man act as a living one) this would in no way falsify the proposition that the man is dead.

If, as I think, these four conditions are inherent in the traditional concept of death, it becomes clear that neither the brain death nor the heart death criterion are by themselves able to tell us anything about what the death of a human individual is. Both are criteria, and not definitions, of death. That is why accepting the brain death criterion does not mean 'redefining' death but only recognizing one further criterion for the same fact that is traditionally indicated by the criteria of irreversible heart and respiration failure.

4. Brain death as a criterion of death

A definition in the full sense must be expected to characterize its object under all possible circumstances. For a criterion, on the other hand, it is sufficient to indicate its object under the circumstances actually obtaining. In a hypothetical world in which both consciousness and the integration and central control of bodily functions depended on the heart instead of the brain, failure of brain function would not by itself be a sufficient criterion of death, just as in the real world the loss of one's own heart is not by itself a sufficient criterion of death. In the real world, however, both consciousness and the integration of bodily functions are dependent on the function of the brain. It is, therefore, universally the case that when the brain has completely and irreversibly ceased to function the defining conditions of death (irreversible loss of consciousness and irreversible loss of integration of bodily functions into the whole of an organism) are fulfilled.

With this, we have a further reason to reject Hans Jonas' thesis that the brain death criterion is a conceptual innovation based on a purely pragmatic stipulation. Once the above explication of the concept of death is accepted, it is seen to be based on a scientifically well established theory of the necessary conditions of the integration of bodily functions and of consciousness. Integration of bodily functions into the whole of the human organism is only achieved by the functioning human brain. It is true that the artificially respired human body is capable of reflexes and certain movements (due to continuing spinal activity) even after irreversible loss of brain function, but these are no longer integrated into the whole of an organism. The same is true for consciousness. The empirical evidence clearly shows that a functioning brain is a necessary, and presumably also sufficient, condition of all conscious states and activities.

5. The standard arguments against the brain death criterion

One of the most frequent criticisms of the brain death criterion is that it is hardly more than a pragmatic convention, ultimately guided by interests, especially the interest in procuring organs from brain-dead critical care patients for transplantation. Against this it must be said that the practical usefulness of a criterion is no reason to doubt its adequacy. The fact that a criterion serves a purpose does not by itself derogate its validity, just as a technical application of a scientific theory does not derogate (but rather confirms) its truth. If what was said above is right, the justification of the brain death criterion is independent of any considerations of interests. Both the brain death criterion and the definition of death underlying it can stand alone and have their own plausibility. The historical fact that attention was drawn to the criterion, by the Harvard Committee of 1968, in the context of organ transplantation (as well as of decisions to withhold medical treatment), does not in any way detract from its material adequacy.

Another objection to the brain death criterion is that it seems to have the unacceptable consequence that we cannot say of an individual that it was, or lived, before birth, as a human embryo at a stage at which the embryo is not yet capable of consciousness or of central control and integration of bodily functions. It may be argued that it is not evident that the defining conditions and criteria for the end of life can be applied, without qualification, to the beginning of life. An answer to the question of when a life ends does not necessarily prejudge the answer to the more difficult question of when a life begins (cf. [7]).

The fiercest opposition to brain death comes from those who want the criteria of death to be, as it were, phenomenal instead of scientific, openly visible instead of hidden and merely inferred. They refer to the fact that the outer appearance of artificially respirated patients whose brain has completely and irreversibly lost its function (and who are, according to the brain death criterion, dead) is not significantly different from that of living critical care patients similarly treated. Against this it must be said that outer appearance, impressions and spontaneous reactions are not the proper basis for factual judgements, especially not for judgements with the practical import of judgements of life and death.

6. Ethical consequences

The criteria and the definition of death can be, and must be, justified without resorting to practical, including ethical, considerations. Nor can they by themselves serve as a normative basis for ethical postulates of whatever kind. The ethical norms which regulate how to deal with patients at the borders of life have to be justified independently. The brain death criterion implies no more (and no less) than that a human individual is to be dealt with as dead after his brain has completely and irreversibly ceased to function, and that an individual to which none of the criteria of death applies has to be dealt with as living. That this statement is of some practical importance can be seen in the case of the anencephalous neonate. Contrary to the opinion of some authors that anencephalous neonates without cortex constitute a 'special case' because they are unable to develop an 'inner mental life', the absence of conscious experience is clearly not sufficient to declare these children 'dead'. In so far as the residual brain is able to control at least the vegetative functions, they are living human individuals and have to be treated as such.

References

1. Culver CM, Gert B. Philosophy in Medicine. Conceptual and Ethical Issues in Medicine and Psychiatry. Oxford University Press, Oxford 1982: pp. 179–94.
2. Jonas H. Gehirntod und menschliche Organbank: Zur pragmatischen Umdefinierung des Todes. In: Jonas H, Technik, Medizin und Ethik. Zur Praxis des Prinzips Verantwortung. Insel, Frankfurt 1985; pp. 219–41.
3. Linke DB, Kurthen M et al. Der Hirntod: Testung, Kriterienfindung, Definition, Attribution und Personkonzept. In: Toellner R (ed.), Organtransplantation. Gustav Fischer, Stuttgart, 1991; pp. 73–9.
4. Singer P. Practical Ethics. Cambridge University Press, Cambridge 1979.
5. Locke J. An essay concerning human understanding (1690).
6. Veatch RM. Whole-brain, neocortical, and higher brain related concepts. In: Zaner RM (ed.). Death: Beyond Whole-Brain Criteria. Kluwer, Dordrecht 1988: pp. 171–86.
7. Lockwood M. When does a life begin? In: Lockwood M (ed.), Moral Dilemmas in Modern Medicine. Oxford University Press, Oxford 1985; pp. 9–31.

43 | Legal and judicial aspects of post mortem organ donation

BERNARD M. DICKENS

1. Introduction

Countries, and often separate jurisdictions within countries, have their own distinctive legal approaches to post mortem recovery (or 'procurement') of organs for transplantation. This study offers a general overview of principles that the laws of various jurisdictions address, illustrated selectively by instances with which the author is familiar. These are drawn primarily from the Anglo-American legal system, meaning the Common law system, less from the European-derived Civil law system and not, for instance, from a legal system immediately based on religious texts such as Islamic law. Although laws will respond to issues according to their own principles, a common set of issues has emerged from the medical ability to transplant tissues from bodies of the dead, and to preserve such tissues pending their implantation or other disposal. Accordingly, the study presents questions rather than answers that will appear in similar form before the legislatures and judicial courts of the world.

The important questions of human dignity and social justice raised by the medical and related means to recover and preserve transplantable cadaveric materials lead into the no less important question of their allocation among potential recipients whose lives they may prolong, but this study concerns only recovery and preservation. Further, although legislation in many countries draws distinctions between 'organs' and 'tissues', this study will address them together and distinguish laws regarding their uses only when neces-

sary. Organs are commonly understood as tissue structures that living bodies cannot replace if they are removed, while tissues are materials such as blood and bone marrow that the body naturally regenerates. The distinction is of vital concern to living donors, but of less concern regarding dead bodies. Issues regarding recovery of sperm, ova and both viable and non-viable embryos and foetuses from recently deceased persons are profound, but not relevant to organ transplantation. Similarly, the 1990 judgment of the Supreme Court of California in the *Moore* case [1] has raised considerable legal interest in the use of tissues from both living and deceased donors for biotechnological research and commercial development, but these interests lie beyond the immediate concern in transplantation.

2. Legal approaches to death

The universal experience of human death generates responses in every medium of individual, social and cultural expression. Laws based on religious or moral principles reflect this conditioning in their approaches to death. The Common law reflects its Judaeo-Christian heritage and moral sentiment regarding a person's criminal infliction of death on another, but the Common law is a legal system based primarily on property and inheritance. Less attention is paid to the inherent qualities or rights of people than to their property; people are a means by which property is owned, possessed, protected and transferred. Death is

G.M. Collins, J.M. Dubernard, W. Land and G.G. Persijn (eds). Procurement, Preservation and Allocation of Vascularized Organs 343–357
© 1997 Kluwer Academic Publishers.

considered a legal status. The time of a person's death marks the point at which other legal events occur, such as the inheritance of an estate by survivors or the process of distribution of the estate, a body may (and in a relatively short time must) be buried, cremated or otherwise disposed of in accordance with law, payment becomes due on a life insurance policy, the deceased's rights to take or to continue legal action cease and dependents' claims for wrongful death begin. It also marks the point under modern legislation at which organs may be recovered for posthumous transplantation.

The legal status of death arises when the legal criteria of death are satisfied. The criteria are based on observations that medically qualified persons have the capacity to make, although in many circumstances lay persons could apply the criteria too. Classically, the criteria of death were the cessation of respiration and blood circulation. Satisfaction of the criteria was evidenced by a body's lack of breathing and heartbeat. Medical means now exist to determine the absence of respiration and pulse with a high degree of scientific precision, but death was clearly determinable in earlier times by unscientific tests. Imprecision contributed to horror stories of living persons being treated as dead and apparently dead people reviving, and to people's superstitious fears of being buried alive, but imprecision was no obstacle to the criteria being applied with legal effect.

Death determined by cardiovascular criteria was considered an event rather than a process, and classical law defined an act as homicidal if the act caused death that occurred within a year and a day of the act. The modern expression of this rule for instance in the Criminal Code of Canada, section 227, is that: 'No person commits culpable homicide ... unless the death occurs within one year and one day from the time of the occurrence of the last event by means of which the person caused or contributed to the cause of death'. Outside criminal liability, the law's interest was less in scientific precision than in resolving whether death occurred before or after another event, such as the death of another person.

The relativity of death is illustrated in the common circumstance when a childless husband and wife make mutual wills. The husband leaves his estate to his wife, but if she dies before he dies, he leaves his estate (which may include what he inherits at her earlier death) to his family. The wife similarly leaves her estate to her husband, but if he dies before she does, her estate including his goes to her family. If the couple die in a common disaster, such as a motor vehicle or aircraft accident, each family will seek evidence that the other's member died first. In the absence of evidence, the law applies the presumption as to *commorientes*, deeming the older to have died before the younger. If the state levies death duties or an estate tax, its revenue authorities might also want evidence of which of the two died first if that affects amounts payable.

Criteria of death based on absence of respiration and blood circulation have proven difficult to apply now that these functions can be sustained by mechanical means. Artificial ventilators and heart–lung machines are applied to patients expected to recover or who are conscious; their inability to maintain respiration and heartbeat spontaneously clearly does not render them dead in law. When such mechanical means were applied to unconscious, brain-damaged patients, however, the issue arose of whether they may legally be classified as dead. Advantage came to be taken of the evolution of a neurological criterion of death in addition to classical cardiovascular criteria, and its recognition in law. The new brain death criterion has been particularly advantageous for recovery of transplantable organs, but it did not originate for this purpose.

An incentive to develop additional tests of death was the imprecision of respiration and pulsation criteria notwithstanding scientific and biotechnological developments, and a continuing popular dread of being buried alive. Machines might fail to detect shallow breathing and very faint heartbeat, associated perhaps with deep coma and drug-induced states. An early legal acceptance of the brain death criterion occurred in 1967, in a case arising in California [2]. A husband whose wife was suffering from terminal cancer fired five revolver shots into her head before using the weapon on himself. Medical evidence showed that she continued to bleed profusely, whereas he appeared not to have bled at all from his fatal injury. By classical cardiovascular tests, her bleeding would show she was alive because her heart was beating, while he was dead. The court resolving an insurance policy claim accepted, however, that the wife's severe brain damage was not only incompatible with survival, but that it had caused an immediate and irreversible end to her vital functions, and that she had died before her husband.

The first express judicial embracing of brain death linked to transplantable organ recovery in the Common law world is often ascribed to a judicial direction given to a jury in Virginia in 1972 [3]. A victim of serious cranial injuries suffered in a fall was placed on a ventilator, but when the electroencephalogram showed total absence of neocortical activity, the attending physicians considered him dead, stopped ventilation and immediately removed his heart for transplantation. The victim's brother sued the physicians, claiming that the patient was still breathing and therefore alive while his heart was being removed. The judge directed the jury that they could apply either classical cardiovascular tests of death or the new neurological criteria, and the jury found the physicians not liable for causing death.

Before judicial acceptance of brain death criteria, several American state legislatures had introduced versions of the celebrated 1968 recommendations of the Ad Hoc Committee of the Harvard Medical School [4]. Legislatures in many countries have subsequently defined death through legislation, for instance by adding brain death criteria to pre-existing cardiovascular criteria, or replacing the latter by the former. Regarding transplantation, some legislatures have not proposed new legal criteria but have deferred to medical practice. For instance in Canada, the Human Tissue Gift Act of Ontario provides in section 7(1) that: 'For the purposes of a post mortem transplant, the fact of death shall be determined by at least two physicians in accordance with accepted medical practice'. This elastic legal criterion of 'accepted medical practice' is applied through expert medical witnesses testifying in court about what medical practice is accepted, and a court of authority recognizing a practice as accepted within the medical community. A practice need not be uniform to be accepted. An old practice may remain accepted by a respected minority of practitioners even though general practice may apply a newer criterion of death, and an innovative criterion may be adequately accepted even though most practitioners do not use it and it remains contentious in medical professional assessment. For instance, this legal formula could accommodate the recent proposal emerging from the University of Pittsburgh Medical Center to forgo exclusive reliance on brain death tests and seek to recover organs as soon as possible from 'non-heart-beating donors', even though the proposal is controversial on medical, ethical, and in some jurisdictions legal grounds [5].

3. The legal management of cadavers

While the royal courts were in the historical process of developing the classical Common law, they did not enjoy the dominance and exclusive jurisdiction that they have now achieved. Considerable concurrent power was exercised by religious or ecclesiastical courts. After the English Reformation of the sixteenth century ended the influence of Roman Catholic institutions, Anglican ecclesiastic courts had jurisdiction in matters affecting churches, consecrated burial grounds and management of dead bodies. The response of the Common law was simply to confirm that, since dead bodies were not property, they were not part of deceased persons' estates, and that bodies were controlled by executors of estates responsible for burial costs and not inherited by those who gained ownership of the estates. The 'no property' rule concerning dead bodies may not have been absolute in earlier times [8], but it has come to be widely accepted as the relevant modern law. Some courts have said that family members possess a 'quasi-property' interest in a dead body, however, for the purpose of burial or cremation.

Although mismanagement of a dead body is not a crime against the deceased or those who inherited his or her property, it became recognized as a crime, meaning a wrong against society, deliberately to cause indignity to a dead body. Preparation of a body for burial, including embalming, is not an offence when undertaken with respect, but employing a body for medical education or scientific research is more problematic. Modern laws address the need for these uses of cadavers through legislation that permits their supply to approved centres, but their use there for unapproved purposes or in disrespectful ways can result in criminal proceedings. Cutting dead bodies for removal of organs for transplantation is similarly protected by legislation, which provides the legal scheme under which bodies become controlled by hospital or similar facilities where transplantable materials may be removed. Legislation is also the basis on which individuals may give legal effect to their preferences regarding posthumous recovery and use of their organs for transplantation, medical education and scientific research.

The legislation adopted in some jurisdictions deals only with availability of cadavers for recovery of transplantable organs, and has no provisions on donations from living persons. For instance in the USA, all states have adopted close variants of the Uniform Anatomical Gift Act, which defines an anatomical gift as 'a donation of all or part of a human body to take effect upon or after death'. The legislation therefore applies only to a 'decedent', defined as 'a deceased individual and includes a stillborn infant or fetus'. In the absence of evidence of a decedent's contrary wish, family members may donate organs from a cadaver, but it is not clear whether anyone except the mother may consent to recovery of organs from a stillborn or aborted foetus. Where legislation also covers living as well as post mortem donation, a gift of organs from an aborted foetus may be considered a live donation of her tissues by the mother.

Although the Common law does not treat cadavers as property in most cases, there are some exceptional instances in which bodies are preserved and have a distinctive characteristic that may warrant legal protection by a property interest. For instance, the embalmed body of the great English philosopher, political scientist and social reformer Jeremy Bentham (1748–1832) preserved by University College in the University of London, may be considered the property of the college. In 1905, the Supreme Court of Oklahoma indicated that a cadaver lawfully acquired for the benefit of science may be property [7]. Whether organs removed from a cadaver may be considered as property will be discussed below; it may seem curious to conclude that an organ from a dead body is legal property when the body itself is not [8].

4. Post mortem organ donation legislation

Some countries' laws reflect cultural or religious objections to the removal of organs from bodies of the dead, associated perhaps with convictions about resurrection and spiritual destiny after death. Where legislation exists that allows post mortem recovery of transplantable organs, it tends to fall into one of two general legislative patterns, namely 'opting-in' or express consent laws, and 'opting-out' or implied consent laws. The former are more traditional, and remain common in Anglo-Saxon jurisdictions. The latter are becoming more prevalent in especially Western European countries [9], and are frequently favoured by transplant physicians not only because they seem to facilitate recovery of transplantable organs but also because they present the enterprise of organ recovery and transplantation as a benefit society may legitimately promote.

The two patterns reflect contrasting philosophies. Opting-in laws permit individuals before death, or family members after death, expressly to donate cadaveric organs as an expression of altruism and autonomy. They suggest, however, that donation is an exceptional act and that the norm is that bodies are buried intact. Opting-out laws treat cadaveric organs as a public asset, but permit individuals who object to their own or deceased family members' organs being removed, perhaps because of their religious, spiritual or cultural beliefs, to prohibit organ recovery. This permission preserves personal autonomy, but it may require individuals who object to organ recovery to identify themselves to health or other public or quasi-public authorities, and to place their personal religious or other convictions on record. Opting-out laws require individuals to explain why they decline participation in an act of public altruism.

Opting-in laws may be reinforced by legal provisions that require health personnel or facilities to ask eligible individuals whether they are willing to do so. These 'required request' provisions will be outlined below.

4.1. Opting-in laws

Early models of legislation that permit individuals to donate their organs for transplantation after death are laws limited to recovery of corneas, the first human body part to become transplanted on a significant scale. The legislation now empowers not only individuals to approve post mortem acquisition of any of their organs, but also specified family members of a deceased person to consent to acquisition, provided that the deceased when living had not expressed disapproval of recovery of his or her body tissues following death. Further, when patients apparently close to death have not expressed consent to their organs being recovered post mortem for transplantation but have not shown any resistance to this prospect, and physicians or other health-care attendants cannot request their consent, for instance because they are unconscious or not able to form or express a choice, physicians or others may discuss organ recovery with their relatives before death. Any consent that appropriate family members give prior to death to posthumous acquisition of organs can be acted on as promptly as possible when death occurs, to maximize utility of recovered organs.

Although the concept to which legislation of this nature gives effect is relatively uncomplicated in principle, experience of legislation in operation discloses a number of areas of legal uncertainty. An initial concern is how clearly a person must express consent to opt-in to posthumous donation, and how that consent should be recorded. A common practice has been to attach a general and brief donation card to another significant document, particularly a vehicle driver's licence. Where this is the established form, it tends to exclude those ineligible to hold a driver's licence. If ineligibility is due to immature age this may be acceptable, since young people tend to be further from anticipated death than others and may not have developed mature awareness of adult responsibilities. If sudden death occurs, parents are often available to decide on donations. In many countries and cultures, however, this form of declaration may also exclude women where it is not usual or socially acceptable for women to be vehicle owners or drivers. In recent years, organizations have been formed to promote post mortem organ donation, and they produce separate donation forms or cards that are easily available to and portable by anyone without regard to an extraneous condition such as possession of a driver's licence.

A functional disadvantage of attaching a donor declaration to a driver's licence is that, in the event of sudden death, whether or not in a vehicle accident, police may establish the victim's identity by reference to the licence, and retain it among other possessions in police custody without communicating its contents to ambulance or hospital personnel. Accordingly, when death is medically confirmed and relatives are being traced and contacted, hospital staff able to recover and preserve organs, and perhaps prepare a prospective recipient for transplantation, remain unaware of the deceased person's earlier consent to organ retrieval. Further, when ambulance personnel have a choice to transport a victim either to a hospital that can recover organs or to one that cannot, their choice of the latter will frustrate the victim's intention to donate. Realization of the significance of the victim's declaration to donate has resulted in police being trained to look for a declaration when they seek to discover a victim's identity or take custody of his or her possessions, but experience continues to show that opportunities of organ recovery are lost due to inadequate searches for declarations and communication of positive findings.

Mechanical recording of data relevant to individuals' health care, and computer-assisted linkage and retrieval of such data, offer the promise of reducing the chances of a declaration of posthumous donation being unavailable at a donor's death. Donors are also increasingly urged on completion of a donation form to give copies to their family or personal physician and other regular health-service providers, to any hospital or clinic they attend for health care, to lawyers or spiritual counsellors and particularly to closer family members who are likely to be contacted in the event of their sudden illness or death. A disincentive is that a family member may be distressed to learn of prospective donation, particularly if this is contrary to a family's religious traditions.

Some family members, and prospective donors, may fear that hospital staff admitting and treating a patient identified as a potential source of transplantable organs may be ambivalent about the patient's survival, and not undertake procedures that might prolong his or her life if they would render organs unavailable for transplantation on death. Confidence in medical ethics and the integrity of health facility administration may not be sufficient to overcome this fear, particularly when, as is common in the USA, hospitals are run with the goal of making commercial profits for investors. A response may be for individuals to inform family members that they have no objection to their organs being recovered for transplantation following their deaths, but not to complete or carry a donor declaration.

A legal concern comparable to that of recording consent to posthumous organ donation is recording refusal of consent. Legislation usually empowers surviving family members to approve physicians' or hospitals' acquisition of organs for transplantation from deceased relatives who did not, while living, make declarations of donation. The legal condition of such approval is that the deceased left no evidence that they did not wish their bodies to be used in this way. Evidence would exist in a prohibitive sustained religious faith, in burial instructions incompatible with organ removal, or, for instance, in clearly communicated disapproval of donation. A communication to a family member or a health or other service provider who proves not to be available when unexpected death occurs, and a request for posthumous donation is made to a person eligible to donate who is available, may fail to achieve its purpose. Accordingly, while the opting-in pattern of legislation appears to require donors to take the initiative to declare donation in some suitable way, it may also require people who do not want their organs to be removed after death to demonstrate their refusal in a way that reasonably anticipates the unforeseeable circumstances of their deaths.

Legislation almost invariably provides that a defined family member commits no offence if he or she consents in good faith to posthumous organ recovery from a deceased person who had in life expressed an objection of which the consenting family member is unaware. Similarly, a hospital or other facility involved in removing or transplanting an organ on such a family member's consent incurs no legal liability, provided that its relevant officers and staff had no independent evidence of the deceased person's objection. A procedure should be in place in a facility that recovers organs after death to ensure that any patients' objections to organ recovery expressed to officers or staff members are truly recorded. Facilities should be no less vigilant to record refusals to opt in than they are to record consents to donate. A person's explicit refusal expressed and recorded in one facility risks frustration if the person is admitted, perhaps involuntarily, to another institution. Mechanical access to medical or health information shared among health facilities within an area will contribute to the effectiveness of patients' declarations both to consent and to decline to consent to posthumous organ donation.

Legislation usually provides that a person's competent declaration of post mortem donation, made in accordance with the legislated provisions, is legally effective and in itself adequate to empower appropriate authorities to recover organs for transplantation. Not only is additional consent of family members not required, but they have no legal power to veto such a donation. Despite this legal reassurance, however, there is considerable evidence that many health care personnel and facilities will not take organs on deceased persons' declarations when family members or any one emotionally close to such persons object [10].

Accommodation of family members' objections to implementation of a deceased person's donation is perhaps an unavoidable dysfunction of a legal rule which is sound in itself. Legislation usually provides that medical determination of a potential donor's death and surgical removal of organs shall be performed by physicians who have no commitment to or involvement with a prospective recipient. The provision is ethically designed to preclude any conflict of interest in diagnosis of death and management of the patient in the process and aftermath of death. It maintains confidence in medical attendants' allegiance only to the interests and dignity of the dying patient. Such medical and related personnel should have no divided loyalties between prospective organ donors and prospective recipients. The fact that they work in facilities that have active transplantation programmes and with colleagues who promote posthumous organ recovery may itself create pressures and inducements to maximize organ retrieval. However, personnel involved with potential donors as patients tend to remain engaged with their family members following donors' deaths, and committed to family members' successful management of bereavement and grief. When organ recovery legally permitted by the deceased would cause distress to family members and obstruct their recovery from mourning, physicians and other personnel may consider it preferable not to act on the deceased patient's donation. Wastage of recoverable organs may be considered necessary for surviving family members' well-being.

Potential recipients of legally donated organs appear to have little if any legal status to enforce deceased donors' organ gifts over donors' family members' objections. They may have no status as individuals to compel facility personnel to retrieve donated organs, even when they are patients in the same facilities as

deceased donors' bodies and enjoy priority in the allocation of organs offered without any specific designation to them. Legislation that renders a patient's declaration full legal authority to recover organs after death remains only permissive; it does not oblige facilities or personnel eligible to acquire suitable organs to do so. It is not negligent for facility personnel to favour deceased donors' family members over potential recipients of organs, since personnel have no legal duty of care to them that compels disregard for the interests of bereaved relatives of donors. Hospital and other institutions appear to have more legal responsibilities to patients than to relatives of deceased patients, but declining donations in order to serve the well-being in bereavement of deceased donors' family members may constitute legitimate preventive community health care. Facility personnel who decline offered organs have no duties of care in negligence law and no fiduciary duties towards potential recipients, because of the legislated and ethical disconnection between personnel who manage a potential donor's terminal care and determination of death, and patients eligible to receive donated organs.

Courts might be more sympathetic to a patient acting against a hospital or similar facility in a representative capacity on behalf of a class of patients who are potential organ recipients. The patient might seek a declaration or order against the facility's refusal or failure to have a system to record terminal patients' consent to posthumous donation, and to apply a protocol for recovery of such donated organs. A jurisdiction's rules on initiation of litigation might permit potential recipients and perhaps their dependents to act as a class, or activist organizations to proceed in their own right, to require a particular facility or facilities in general to have arrangements to give effect to patients' posthumous donations. Rules on court procedure and standing to sue differ among jurisdictions, and within a single jurisdiction may be influenced by attitudes towards consumer protection, deference to medical and hospital autonomy, the status of health facilities as governmental, public or private institutions and, for instance, activists' interests and alternative means to advance their purposes.

The legislation that implements the opting-in system permits prospective donors, whether individuals in anticipation of their own deaths or their family members afterwards, to set conditions or limitations to donation. They may donate some identified organs but not others, donate for instance to a specific hospital or university-affiliated institution as opposed to others, or for treatment of patients affected by a particular disease or dysfunction. It can be difficult to determine, however, the extent to which a donor's specification can be accommodated by the general legal context of donation. Revelations of allocations of scarce organs to foreign patients who pay high medical fees may deter prospective donors from opting in, because, while they are altruistic towards those with whom they feel common bonds, they feel no commitment to assist strangers. An option that retains the altruistic gesture is to donate on the condition that the recipient be a patient from the donor's own country, region or community.

Such a donation may prove to assist no patient qualified according to the donor's specification, and result in waste of a potentially life-enhancing resource. A legal challenge concerns whether the donation violates or offends legal provisions on non-discrimination that are binding on private individuals or public health facilities. A donor who limits recipients on grounds of their race, religion, origin or other characteristic unrelated to sickness or need may compel a physician or, for instance, health facility administrator to confront and resolve a complex legal and ethical challenge, speedily and without warning, while a prospective recipient's survival depends on the response to a deceased donor's perhaps obscurely phrased or clearly xenophobic or bigoted specification.

A possible response is to decline donations that discriminate among recipients. This may be appealing, but may also result in unnecessary deaths of qualified patients while not protecting the interests or well-being of patients who are not qualified. The response may be defensible on the reasoning that potential donors who are not legally permitted to select recipients may prefer to donate without discrimination rather than not donate at all. There is experience, however, to the contrary. In the United States, African-American or black people are over-represented among patients who require transplantations and under-represented among donors [11]. Physiological features such as high blood pressure may explain the former, but the latter has been related in part to a perception among the black population that any organs they donated would benefit primarily non-black recipients, who in general enjoy better access to health services than black people, particularly those who are socioeconomically disadvantaged. Pioneering transplantation of hearts from black donors to white recipients in South Africa reinforced this perception. It has been suggested that if black donors could be assured of black recipients, the black population would be more disposed to make posthumous donations. White donors who limit recipients to white people may violate antidiscrimination laws, but it may be questioned whether allowing black donors to specify black

recipients may be lawful under affirmative action programmes or exceptions designed to advance the interests of under-privileged minority populations. The conclusion that such specification is unlawful may maintain the prevailing low level of black people's donations.

The legal requirement that, in order to be effective, a donation must be made without coercion or undue inducement may appear more relevant to living than post mortem donations. The inducement of financial payment is addressed below with legal provisions for the exclusion of commerce.

Family members of a deceased person may be subject to both coercion and over-inducement to consent to posthumous recovery of transplantable organs. Pressure may be exerted by health professionals, officers of transplantation facilities and, for instance, family members of likely recipients. Legislation on 'required request' (below) may suggest that health personnel and facilities are required to obtain a high proportion of consents. Inducements may come from the same sources in the form not simply of payment but of other advantages offered to donors, such as access for themselves or others for whom they care to health services otherwise inaccessible to them. A family member's donation based on appreciation of a facility's services or a health care provider's dedication, or on gratitude for the care rendered to the deceased, has not been deliberately induced, but the distinction between an adequately autonomous donation and a consent a donor was conditioned or manipulated to provide may be narrow. Since a physician or facility that has recovered organs on the basis of a consent that the physician or facility had improperly procured is liable to suffer in a number of legal and disciplinary proceedings, they have strong self-protective incentives to prevent both coercion and over-inducement of family members to make donations.

4.2. Opting-out laws

A number of countries, predominantly in Western Europe, have considered legislation appropriate that authorizes removal of organs from cadavers unless in life the deceased had expressed an objection, and thereby opted out of automatic liability to posthumous organ recovery for transplantation. In France, for instance, Law No. 76-1181 provides [12, p. 200] in section 2 that: 'Organs may be removed for therapeutic or scientific purposes from cadavers of persons who have not, during their lifetime, indicated their refusal to permit such a procedure. However, where the cadaver is that of a minor or of an incompetent person, organs may be removed for transplantation purposes only with the authorization of the person's legal representative'. Separate legislation of 1949 governs corneal grafting (see Act No. 49–890), and the national Public Health Code governs recovery for therapeutic purposes of blood and blood plasma.

To give effect to the 1976 enactment, Decree No. 78–501 [12] prescribes that persons who wish to prohibit organ removal from their bodies after death may formulate the prohibition in any manner. A person admitted to a hospital that is specially licensed to remove organs from bodies following death may record a prohibition at any time in a register to be kept for this purpose. If the person is or becomes incapable of expressing views, any indication found on his or her person, among his or her personal effects or elsewhere that suggests that he or she would prohibit the removal of organs following death must be entered in the register. Anyone who can testify that a hospitalized person is opposed to organ removal after death must enter in the register a substantiated statement to this effect, indicating the manner in which the prohibition was expressed, the circumstances under which it was given, and, where appropriate, its extent. Physicians responsible for recovery of cadaveric organs must, if not already aware of a particular deceased person's prohibition, ensure that there is no entry in the register indicating the person's opposition, and similarly ensure that the deceased was not a minor nor mentally incompetent. If the deceased was a minor or mentally incapable of expressing his or her wishes, organs may be removed only on written authorization of the deceased's legal representative, entered in the register. In this regard, there must be opting in by the representative before but also possibly following the deceased person's death. Physicians who remove cadaveric organs must present a detailed report on the operation, the condition of the body and of the organs removed, and avoid removal of organs if this would leave or create uncertainty as to the cause of death.

Details of the central concept expressed in the French legislation differ among countries. In Belgium, for instance, the Law of 13 June 1986 [12, pp. 133–7] provides in section 10(1) that: 'Organs and tissues for transplantation, and for the preparation of therapeutic substances ... may be removed from the body of any person recorded in the Register of the Population or any person recorded for more than six months in the Aliens Register, unless it is established that an objection to such a removal has been expressed.

'It shall be a requirement, in the case of persons other than those mentioned above, that they have explicitly expressed their consent to the removal'.

Capable persons aged 18 years and over may express objections, but a younger person who is capable to demonstrate objection or, during his or her lifetime, a close relative living with the youth may also record the youth's opposition to posthumous removal of organs and/or tissues. Legal representatives, guardians or closest relatives of persons whose mental condition prevents them from making their wishes known may express objection during such persons' lifetimes. Objections to posthumous organ and tissue removal made by capable persons or on their behalf must be signed and dated, and transmitted to the Data Processing and Information Centre of the Ministry of Public Health and Family Affairs [12, p. 137].

It may be questionable in ethics and in law regarding civil liberties and privacy whether persons who object to posthumous organ recovery should be required to record this fact in governmental or hospital registers. If their objection is based on religious or philosophical grounds, such as a belief in reincarnation that requires their bodies to be buried intact, this provision requires them to record their most profound convictions in government registries. Giving such information to hospital authorities is less objectionable, since knowledge of this nature permits hospitals to treat patients and their dead bodies according to patients' religious requirements, for instance concerning dietary practices and notifications and procedures on death. The objections remain, however, that when posthumous donation is deemed to be a public benefit, objectors become identifiable as people who propose to withhold that benefit, and that persons who have recorded objections may fear that hospitals will disfavour them as recipients of life-preserving transplanted organs.

Singapore's Law No. 15 of 1987 [12, p. 310] is unusually explicit in this regard. In the multiracial society of Singapore, composed of people of Malay, Chinese, Indian and European extraction, ethnic and religious affiliations are more apparent than in most countries. The law prohibits trading in any human organ and in blood, but its provisions otherwise apply only to kidneys. Other legislation may apply to other organ removals from deceased persons. Section 5(1) of the law permits a designated officer of a government or specially approved private hospital to authorize 'the removal of any organ [i.e. kidney] from the body of a person who had died in the hospital for the purpose of the transplantation of the organ'. Section 5(2) provides that no such authority shall be given, however, unless death was caused by accident or injuries caused by accident, or if the person now deceased had registered an objection with the state's Director of Medical Services, or was neither a citizen nor permanent resident of Singapore. If the person was aged under 21 years or was not of sound mind, authorization can be given only with consent of a parent or guardian. Consistently with a designated officer's inability to authorize kidney removal in the case of non-accidental death, such as death due to disease or natural death, no authorization is possible if the deceased person was above 60 years of age. Section 5(2) (g) also prohibits authorization of kidney removal from the body of a deceased person 'who is a Muslim'.

The special relevance of actual objection and presumed objection under section 5(2) (g) to posthumous kidney recovery concerns section 12 of the Law, which governs recipients of organs. This provides that: 'in the selection of a proposed recipient of any organ removed pursuant to section 5 – (a) a person who has not registered any objection with the Director [to posthumous donation] ... shall have priority over a person who has registered such objection (s. 12 (1))'. A person who withdrew a registered objection shall have the same priority as a person who has not so objected over a person whose objection is registered 'at the expiration of two years from the date of receipt of the withdrawal by the Director' (s. 12 (1) (b)). Further, 'a person referred to in section 5(2) (g) [that is, 'a Muslim'] shall have priority over a person who has registered such objection only if he has made a gift of his organ, to take effect upon his death, under section 3 of the Medical (Therapy, Education and Research) Act' at or within a specified time (s. 12 (2) (a)). Accordingly, Muslims who opt in to posthumous kidney donation have priority over other Muslims, and also over non-Muslims who have opted out, and the same priority as a non-objecting non-Muslim. When a Muslim opts in to posthumous donation after the time specified in section 12(2) (a), however, his or her equal priority with non-objecting, non-Muslims arises 'at the expiration of two years from the date of such gift ' (s. 12(2) (c)), presumably to prevent a sick Muslim from opting in for the purpose of gaining immediate eligibility and priority as a kidney recipient over other Muslims who have not opted in, and over objecting non-Muslims.

The justice of this distinctive accommodation of Muslims is ultimately to be evaluated in the context of the local culture and of the perceptions of the state's Muslim community. A person's objection to post mortem donation does not necessarily extend to *in vivo* receipt of a transplanted organ. In prioritizing the entitlement to receive kidney transplantation of passive non-Muslims over passive Muslims, and requiring the latter to declare and register their willingness to donate their kidneys in order to enjoy the same priority as non-objecting non-Muslims, the legislation is liable to scrutiny under international human rights conventions that prohibit discrimination on grounds of race, religion and ethnic origins. Against this, however, if the need to opt out of posthumous donation by registration with a governmental agency is considered oppressive, even when the register 'shall not be open to inspection by the public' (s. 10 (2)), Muslims may not necessarily be considered to suffer any disadvantage against others. For Muslims to be identified as such may not be oppressive in a multiracial society where an individual's ethnicity and presumptive religious affiliation are readily apparent, but if Muslims are subject to religious precepts against posthumous surrender of organs it may be objectionable for a Muslim to have to record dissent from doctrines of his or her religious faith, particularly if non-conformity renders a believer liable to religious sanctions or recrimination.

Accordingly, the legal problems and legal and ethical concerns that are raised by legislation and its interpretation implementing the opting-in system of cadaveric organ recovery are not obviated by adoption of the opting-out system. The problems are different in character, but not necessarily different in degree of complexity or the challenge they pose to the achievement of justice.

4.3. Required request laws

Some jurisdictions that have followed the opting-in pattern of laws have recognized the limitations of depending on individuals to take initiatives to offer their bodies after death for organ recovery. Particularly in the USA, they have imposed legal responsibilities on physicians or hospital administrators to ask eligible individuals if they would agree to posthumous donation, forcing them either to consent or to refuse. In this way, laws based on the opting-in approach are applied through the mediation of physicians, hospital administrators or others to require those who are eligible to consent to organ donation expressly to decline if they oppose donation, in the style of opting-out legislation.

In the USA, the National Conference of Commissioners on Uniform State Laws drafts model legislation that it recommends should be enacted in each of the different states. Uniform draft Acts tend to be widely adopted by states, often with variations that reflect the traditions and legislative dynamics of the various states. Drafts often include options for the language that states may consider. In 1987, the Commissioners proposed the Uniform Anatomical Gift Act [12, p. 388] designed to govern 'donation of all or part of a human body to take effect upon or after death' (s. 1 (1)). Section 5 of the uniform draft Act, addressing routine inquiry and required request, provides that: '(a) On or before [a patient's] admission to a hospital, or as soon as possible thereafter, a person designated by the hospital shall ask each patient who is at least [18] years of age "Are you an organ or tissue donor?" If the answer is affirmative the person shall request a copy of the document of gift. If the answer is negative or there is no answer and the attending physician consents, the person designated shall discuss with the patient the option to make or refuse to make an anatomical gift. The answer to the question, an available copy of the document of gift or refusal to make an anatomical gift, and any other relevant information, must be placed in the patient's medical record. (b) If, at or near the time of death of a patient, there is no medical record that the patient has made or refused to make an anatomical gift, the hospital [administrator] or a representative ... shall discuss [i.e. with family members] the option to make or refuse to make an anatomical gift and request the making of an anatomical gift ... The request must be made with reasonable discretion and sensitivity to the circumstances of the family. A request is not required if the gift is not suitable, based upon accepted medical standards, for a purpose specified [i.e. transplantation, therapy, medical or dental education, research, or advancement of medical or dental science]. An entry must be made in the medical record of the patient, stating the name and affiliation of the individual making the request, and of the name, response, and relationship to the patient of the person to whom the request was made'.

Beyond this requirement that an appropriate family member be requested to consider making a gift of the patient's organs following death, the uniform draft Act identifies a range of persons who shall make a reasonable search for a document or other information showing whether a gift has been made, including police, fire and emergency rescue personnel who find a person dead or close to death, and hospital personnel, and directs what shall be done with any document found.

It is interesting that the uniform draft Act disfavours failure to comply with its provision on routine inquiry and required request being subject to direct legal penalty. Section 5 (f) provides that: 'A person who fails to discharge the duties imposed by this section is not subject to criminal or civil liability but is subject to appropriate administrative sanctions'. This may reflect a deference to health professionals and hospital management personnel that finds it distasteful that they should be liable to judicial proceedings, and an attempt to discourage malpractice and related liability claims. Individual states are free to recognize such liabilities, but may rely on administrative sanctions such as reprimands, suspensions, demotions and similar professional disciplinary procedures and, for instance, loss or suspension of hospital accreditation by accrediting agencies.

The draft provision addresses only hospital personnel and admitted patients, but physicians are encouraged to include similar routine inquiries of patients they see in their private offices or surgeries, and hospitals are encouraged to extend such routine inquiries to outpatient, emergency, minor surgery and similar services that do not require admission to the hospital.

4.4. The law of necessity and rescue

Concepts of human dignity and self-determination, reinforced by the special reverence family members feel towards bodies of their recently deceased loved ones, support rejection of the attitude that human bodies after death can be treated as a source of spare parts for community use [9, p. 621]. Opting-in laws give effect to these concepts, but laws implementing the opting-out approach are also solicitous of objections to organ recovery both by persons anticipating their own deaths and in significant cases by relatives in the absence of objection by the persons now deceased. In Denmark, Italy, Sweden and Norway [9, p. 621, n. 138], for instance, removal is unlawful if relatives of deceased persons object to it for their own reasons. In contrast, Finnish law No. 355 of 26 April 1985 [12, p. 195] provides that if the deceased consented to removal, 'the procedure may be carried out despite the objection of the relatives' (s. 4).

Laws that are supported because they protect individuals' and families' expectations that deceased bodies for which they care are treated with respect for their wishes, and not plundered for transplantable and otherwise usable materials, are challenged, however, by legal claims of access to organs and tissues in order to preserve existing lives. Reverence and protection for the dead are derived from reverence for and protection of the living. It must be asked whether the regard properly paid to individuals' posthumous self-determination and families' natural protectiveness of deceased members' wishes and of their own sensitivities at a time of bereavement and grief can justify another's death that transplantation of an organ recovered from the deceased could have forestalled.

Neither persons anticipating their own deaths nor relatives of those who have died have legal duties to potential recipients of organs. Legal claims may be advanced, however, that physicians and those who assist them do not merit punishment for taking organs in defiance of the opposition expressed by persons now deceased and their relatives, in order to preserve others' lives.

Many countries in the Civil law tradition impose positive duties of reasonable rescue [9, p. 362], but rescue in defiance of legal objections to removing organs from dead bodies may not be considered reasonable or justified. An initiative to save a life by unauthorized recovery of an organ may, however, go unpunished in Civil and Common law jurisdictions, under legal doctrines on voluntary rescue and on necessity. A leading Common law decision on necessity is the English case of *R. v. Bourne* [13]. A physician who terminated a pregnancy to save not the life of a pregnant woman but her health, fearing that continuation of pregnancy would cause her to become 'a mental wreck', was held not to be convictable of criminal abortion if he acted in good faith for that purpose. The criminal law the physician was acquitted of violating carried a sentence of up to life imprisonment. Laws prohibiting non-consensual removal of organs from cadavers invariably impose lesser punishments. It may appear that if a physician can act against a heavily sanctioned law to preserve a person's health, a physician can act against a lesser sanctioned law to preserve a person's life.

The Common law doctrine on necessity provides that, although the risk of danger may be perceived subjectively, the proportionality of the response must be validated objectively [14]. That is, a physician will not be legally liable if, having honestly determined a patient to be at risk of death without organ transplantation, he or she acts in a manner that strikes an objectively favourable balance between the value that the violated law serves and the competing interest or value the defendant felt bound to protect. Betraying a deceased person's wish to be buried intact and/or defying a family's wish that a cadaver not be cut for organ removal may be considered tolerable for the purpose of saving a patient's life, or of making the attempt. In cultures where religious or other beliefs lay heavy emphasis on the importance of burial intact, however, the objective assessment of proportionality might be differently resolved.

Acceptance of the necessity defence is limited to exceptional cases where individuals react in the face of a sudden appearance of danger. The doctrine cannot apply to exonerate a physician or other person who determines systematically or in advance of a sudden emergency to disregard inconvenient or disrespected laws. Further, noting the distinction that justifiable conduct is legally permitted, in contrast to excusable conduct, which is legally wrong but, in the circumstances of the particular case does not warrant a criminal or a civil legal sanction, courts have held that the doctrine of necessity may only excuse wrongful conduct from punishment. Necessity does not render it lawful or just [14]. Although a physician or other person may accordingly escape criminal and civil liability for taking a cadaveric organ for transplantation in defiance of the deceased person's objections and/or those of the person's family members, the act is legally wrong, and may legitimately result in professional and other disciplinary sanctions of an administrative nature.

5. The prohibition of commerce in cadaveric organs

At the request of the World Health Assembly in 1987, the World Health Organisation prepared Guiding Principles on Human Organ Transplantation [12, p. 468] that the World Health Assembly endorsed in May 1991 and recommended member states to reflect in their national policies. The original incentive for the Guiding Principles was that the Assembly was 'concerned at the trade for profit in human organs among living human beings' [12, p. 468]. The WHO study recognized the potential for commerce in cadaveric organs as well, however, and proposed the following principles:

Guiding Principle 5: The human body and its parts cannot be the subject of commercial transactions. Accordingly, giving or receiving payment (including any other compensation or reward) for organs should be prohibited.

Guiding Principle 6: Advertising the need for or availability of organs, with a view to offering or seeking payment, should be prohibited.

Guiding Principle 7: It should be prohibited for physicians and other health professionals to engage in organ transplantation procedures if they have reason to believe that the organs concerned have been the subject of commercial transactions.

Guiding Principle 8: It should be prohibited for any person or facility involved in organ transplantation procedures to receive any payment that exceeds a justifiable fee for the services rendered.

Guiding Principle 9: In the light of the principles of distributive justice and equity, donated organs should be made available to patients on the basis of medical need and not on the basis of financial or other considerations.

Implementation of these principles would require many states to develop their prevailing practices and their legislation for this purpose, but many countries have laws already in place that prohibit commerce in human organs and tissues, although blood and blood constituents are usually exempted from this prohibition. Indeed, the WHO Guiding Principles do not deal with blood or blood constituents for transfusion purposes, nor with reproductive tissues including sperm and ova.

Prohibitory legislation is of differing levels of detail. French Law No. 76–1181 [12, p. 200] simply provides that 'removal of organs ... shall not give rise to any remuneration' (s. 3). In contrast, following sensationalized accounts of young residents of impoverished countries coming to London for commercial donation of their organs to wealthy recipients, the UK enacted the Human Organ Transplants Act 1989 'to prohibit commercial dealings in human organs intended for transplantation; [and] to restrict the transplanting of such organs between persons who are not genetically related' [12, p. 375]. This Act creates criminal offences when human organs are bought or sold, and offered or advertised for purchase or sale, 'organ' being defined as 'any part of a human body consisting of a structured arrangement of tissues which, if wholly removed, cannot be replicated by the body' (s. 7(2)). Conditioned by its origins, the Act is primarily oriented to the control of donations made by living donors, but the prohibition applies to persons receiving or seeking payment while alive in exchange for a promise to consent to posthumous donation, and to family members receiving or seeking payment to consent to donations from bodies of deceased relatives who had expressed no objection.

The objection to people sacrificing their physical integrity to donate organs for payment is not fully rational in light of the comparable risks individuals are legally entitled to take for employment or other reward [15], and inapplicable to people being paid for providing the chance that, after their death, the organs and other tissues of their bodies will be transplantable. The objection is similarly inapplicable when family members can consent to organ recovery from a deceased person, however much it may be preferred that they be inspired by altruism. Those capable of consenting to organ recovery are denied the power to profit under the Act, and are protected from commercial temptations, but different intermediaries may be paid. For instance, the French prohibition of

remuneration to donors is 'without prejudice to the reimbursement of any costs that such procedures may entail' [12, p. 200], and the UK prohibition of payment: 'does not include any payment for defraying or reimbursing (a) the cost of removing, transporting or preserving the organ to be supplied; or (b) any expenses or loss of earnings incurred by a person so far as reasonably and directly attributable to his supplying an organ from his body' (s. 1 (3)) [12, p. 375].

Accordingly, entrepreneurs are permitted and even encouraged to be involved in supplying organ donation services, but donors, whether of their own organs from their living bodies or from their bodies after death, or of their deceased relatives' bodies, are prohibited from seeking or accepting payment, and no one may offer another person payment as an inducement to consent to donation from his or her own body while alive or after death, or from the body of a deceased relative.

It has been seen that the basis of legal prohibition of commerce is to preserve human dignity lest the human body and its organs may become mere commodities of trade, to prevent individuals engaging in unsavoury transactions analogized to prostituting their bodies, and to protect them from being tempted by reward to violate their bodily integrity. The prohibition may also cost lives, however, since reliance on altruism of potential donors provides an inadequate supply of organs available for life-prolonging transplantation [16]. It has been observed that tolerance of commerce might not increase the number of organs available, and might deter altruistic cadaveric donations by tarnishing and devaluing the virtue of donation [17]. Nevertheless, particularly in the USA, where health care is often perceived as a service available like any other in the market place, a vigorous modern literature has emerged that advocates the merits of payment to increase supply of organs, and so prolong lives, invoking the market principle that payment induces supply [18,19].

Inducing cadaveric donation by the offer of reward does not result in people treating their living bodies disrespectfully, being tempted to imprudence, or suffering posthumous indignity or mutilation; the process of removal of cadaveric organs is the same for both altruistic and rewarded donation. Commodification may not arise when payments are modest, and standardization of payment eliminates competitive bidding. Family members' paid consents to organ recovery from bodies of deceased relatives may appear mercenary, but people may more acceptably be paid to promise availability of their organs on death. Payment may not be in money but, for instance, in relief from terminal care or burial expenses. Such payments that benefit survivors rather than donors themselves are consistent with principles of altruism, which in this case benefits both the unknown recipients of organs and the deceased person's family members. Accordingly, arguments may be expected to continue that some form of payment may be tolerable for cadaveric donation without risking the harms that gave rise to demands for legal prohibition of payments.

The requirement that all countries should outlaw rewards for donation has been condemned in some cases as ethical or cultural imperialism. It is claimed that the requirement reflects the perceptions of Western materialistic countries that payment signifies commerce, commodification and exploitation of poor and vulnerable people [20]. In other cultures, however, the practice of gift exchange reflects stable traditions of mutual regard and recognition of relative status; not to return a gift appropriately would constitute an insult, a denigration of the gift itself and violation of an important norm of social cohesion. Gift exchanges outside commerce may have ceased to be familiar in industrialized, non-traditional societies, but elsewhere donation of an organ, by a living donor or the family of a deceased person, would socially be expected to be reciprocated in a culturally regulated form [21]. Exploitation, oppression and injustice may be present in traditional societies no less than in others, but, it is claimed, legally to prohibit any form of payment on the ground that it axiomatically imports a loss of human dignity is culturally insensitive.

6. Confidentiality

Living persons will rarely donate organs such as kidneys to strangers, but will confine this sacrifice to the service of another for whom they specially care. Naturally replaceable body materials such as blood, sperm and perhaps bone marrow may be donated, however, to unknown recipients. In the case of cadaveric donations, whether by persons in anticipation of their own deaths or by donors of organs from deceased relatives, donations are almost invariably required by law to be mutually anonymous. Families of deceased donors are unable directly to assert any moral or other claims against recipients, and recipients cannot directly discharge any moral or other obligations they may feel they owe donors or their families. Posthumous donation contributes to the well-being and health of society itself rather than of identifiable individuals, and recipients may express gratitude through reciprocal social altruism rather than private return gestures.

Donation becomes impersonal, and serves society. It is in this spirit that many countries have institutionalized the disciplined pursuit of social benefit through the adoption of opting-out laws, which also include provisions to ensure confidentiality that prevent linkage of particular donors with particular recipients. With the growing practices of multiple organ recovery from single cadaveric donors, and organ segment transplantation, a single donor may be the source of organs transplanted into numerous recipients.

Legislation mandating preservation of confidentiality of particular donors and recipients of transplanted materials usually has suitably guarded exceptions through which information on donation or receipt of organs can be given to courts of law, coroners' courts, health professional licensing and disciplinary tribunals, other administrative tribunals, police offers and, for instance, medical researchers. Hospitals are usually expected to be able to link recipients to donated organs, for instance for therapeutic follow-up and warning if conditions are subsequently discovered in donors that may affect recipients. Some laws also permit disclosure simply with the consent of affected persons such as recipients, but prohibit linkage of such recipients with particular cadaveric donors. Where registers are kept such as of donation consents or conditions, access to them will be carefully guarded and protected through legal sanctions. Entry on such a register does not establish, of course, that donation actually occurred.

Mechanical data handling has progressed to facilitate reciprocal tracing between donors of cadaveric organs and recipients, which creates a need for legal protection of confidentiality against improper linkage. Absolute confidentiality such as through legally compelled destruction of data is undesirable, however, because post-transplantation knowledge acquired about the cadaveric source of an organ may be essential to share with a recipient or a recipient's physician. For instance, realization that the deceased person suffered from an infection transmissible through transplantation should lead to a recipient being warned, offered appropriate tests and treated as medically indicated. Expanding knowledge of genetic characteristics and predispositions may similarly show advantages of being able to link cadaveric sources of organs with recipients. At the same time, however, such knowledge also shows with what care confidentiality must be protected, since knowledge of a cadaver's genetic status may disclose knowledge of the deceased person's living family members such as children, brothers, sisters and parents [22].

7. Legal control of cadaveric organs outside the body

Organs within living and deceased persons are parts of them, and have no separate legal identity as property. The question arises, however, of their status and control in preservation or in transit between the cadaver and the intended recipient. In the much-discussed *Moore* case [1] the Supreme Court of California dismissed a living person's claim to pursue remedies for misuse of his property when, without disclosure and therefore without the plaintiff's informed consent, tissues were taken from him for research and development of a commercial product of biotechnology. The Court expressly reserved the right to find property interests in such tissues, however, in an appropriate case [1, p. 493].

An objection to recognition of organs outside bodies as property is the fear that this would lead to commerce and its perceived related evils, but property rights can exist in materials prohibited from trade, such as papers containing state secrets. Indeed, recognition of property rights may provide a legal means to protect materials from becoming objects of commerce [23]. Further, it is fallacious to believe that when commerce in property is denied, potentials for earning perhaps suspect rewards are foreclosed. In many countries where sperm donation is precluded from commerce, for instance, donors are paid. Payment is not for the product itself, however, but for the service of making it available [24]. Classifying donation as a service transaction rather than a commodity transaction takes it outside the prohibition against selling materials from human bodies, and makes the legal question of property ownership of less relevance.

A value of recognizing a property right in a cadaveric organ outside the body is that the right might belong to a hospital or organ recovery agency that could treat the organ appropriately, and disregard directions on its use from uninformed persons and those motivated by self-interest. As opposed to this, however, denying a hospital the right of control by recognizing another agency's or person's claim would compel the hospital to manage the organ appropriately, particularly to serve the purpose for which it was donated, and be legally accountable for its due preservation and use, affording protection against its damage through negligence or misjudgment [23].

If a donor gave his or her organs to a particular hospital, university or similar institution to be recovered posthumously, or family members made a gift of organs to a specific institution, such institution would seem to enjoy greatest if not exclusive legal power over their preservation and use. This is subject, of course, to any legislated provisions, for instance giving rights of control and allocation to other agencies [25]. Laws applying the opting-out system of organ recovery are more likely than others to operate through centralized agencies that control recovery and allocation of organs. When no institution is named as recipient under the opting-in system, however, and donation is made for no more specific purpose than for 'transplantation', 'scientific research' and/or 'medical education', a hospital or other agency possessing the organ may be considered not its legal owner, but only the holder of another's property, and be obliged to keep and use it for the purpose for which possession was given. The owner of the property, to whom the holder owes accountability, will be the legal executor of the deceased donor's estate. When the deceased neither made nor objected to a donation, the family member legally entitled to give consent to donation will be the owner. The legal essence of the ownership consists not in the ability to use or sell the organ, but in the ability to direct its proper use and prevent its misuse by others, and to compel accountability by the right to obtain legal remedies for misuse.

References

1. Moore v. Regents of the University of California, 793 P. 2d 479 (Cal. 1990).
2. United Trust Co. v. Pyke, 427 P. 2d 67 (Cal. 1967).
3. Tucker v. Lower, Richmond, VA No 2831, May 1972, discussed in Converse R. But when did he die?: *Tucker* v. *Lower* and the brain death concept. San Diego Law R. 1975; 12: 424–35.
4. Beecher H. A definition of irreversible coma. Special Communication: Report of the Ad Hoc Committee of the Harvard Medical School to Examine the Definition of Brain Death. JAMA 1968; 205: 337–40.
5. Lynn J. Are the patients who become organ donors under the Pittsburgh protocol for 'non-heart-beating donors' really dead? Kennedy Inst Ethics J. 1993; 3: 167–78, and see other articles in this edition of this journal.
6. Matthews P. Whose body?: people as property. Curr Legal Probl 1983: 193–225.
7. Long v. Chicago, R.I. and P. Railway Co. 86 P. 289 (Okl 1905), at p. 291.
8. Dickens BM. The control of living body materials. Univ Toronto Law J. 1977; 27: 142–98.
9. Giesen D. International Medical Malpractice Law. Martinus Nijhoff, Dordrecht 1988; pp. 619–23.
10. Mason JK, McCall Smith RA. Law and Medical Ethics, 4th edn. Butterworths, London 1994; p. 304.
11. Callender CO, Bayton JA, Yeager C *et al.* Attitudes among blacks toward donating kidneys for transplantation: a pilot project. J Natl Med Assoc 1982; 74: 807–9.
12. World Health Organization. Legislative Responses to Organ Transplantation. Martinus Nijhoff, Dordrecht 1994.
13. [1939] 1 K.B. 687 (Central Criminal Court, London).
14. Perka v. The Queen (1984) 14 C.C.C. (3d) 385 (Sup Ct Canada).

15. Radcliffe-Richards J. From him that hath not. In: Land W, Dossetor JB (eds), Organ Replacement Therapy: Ethics, Justice, Commerce. Springer-Verlag, Berlin 1991; pp. 190–6.

16. Spurr SJ. The shortage of transplantable organs: an analysis and a proposal. Law Policy 1993; 15: 355–95.

17. Abouna GM, Sabawi MM, Kumar MSA, Samhan M. The negative impact of paid organ donation. In: Land W, Dossetor JB (eds), Organ Replacement Therapy: Ethics, Justice, Commerce. Springer-Verlag, Berlin 1991; pp. 164–72.

18. Cohen LR. Increasing the supply of transplant organs; the virtues of a futures market. George Washington Law R 1989; 58: 1–51.

19. Blair RD, Kaserman DL. The economics and ethics of alternative cadaveric organ procurement policies. Yale J Regulation 1991; 8: 403–52.

20. Reddy KC. Organ donation for consideration: an Indian viewpoint. In: Land W, Dossetor JB (eds), Organ Replacement Therapy: Ethics, Justice, Commerce. Springer-Verlag, Berlin 1991; pp. 173–80.

21. Simmons KG, Klein SD, Simmons R. Gift of Life: The Social and Psychological Impact of Organ Transplantation. Wiley, New York 1977.

22. American Association for the Advancement of Science. The genome, ethics and the law: issues in genetic testing. Washington DC: AAAS Publication No. 92–115, 1992.

23. Dickens BM. Living tissue and organ donors and property law; More on *Moore*. J Contemp Health Law Policy 1992; 8: 73–93.

24. Dickens BM. The control of living body materials. Univ Toronto Law J 1977; 27: 142–98.

25. Dworkin G, Kennedy I. Human tissue: rights in the body and its parts. Med Law R 1993; 1: 291–319.

44 The dilemma of organ allocation: the combination of a therapeutic modality for an ill individual with the distribution of a scarce valuable public (health) good

WALTER LAND

1. Participation of the public in setting organ allocation policy – a 'must' in view of public transplant crises?

Transparent, equitable and fair allocation of organs removed from cadaver donors represents one of the most burning and still unsolved ethical issues in modern transplant medicine. All efforts to solve the problem on the basis of the professional model of medical ethics in a most agreeable way have failed so far. On the other hand, the problem is supposed to be solved successfully only on the basis of the societal model [1]. It is becoming increasingly evident that society has to share responsibility with the professionals in the field of equitable organ allocation. Accordingly, the call for participation of the society in the responsibility of organ allocation policies became recently louder and louder. This claim appears to be justified for one simple reason: post mortem organ donation depends entirely on the voluntary willingness of all members of a society: if the society agrees to donate organs after death and if society accepts all problems and facts surrounding post mortem organ do-

nation (e.g. recognition of brain death as death of a person, acceptance of simultaneous removal of 10 different donor organs from one deceased individual), then society should have the right and should be allowed to have a special interest in knowing how these organs are distributed and which patients will benefit from them.

There has traditionally been reluctance of members of national and international transplant societies to allow the public to participate actively in the global field of post mortem organ donation, including the setting of organ allocation policies. This attitude changed, however, particularly in view of the 'receipt' in terms of a real punishment; and the occurrence of international transplant crises which are characterized by vanishing confidence and trust of the public in the ethical probity of transplant surgeons and physicians. These public crises, occurring in, for instance, Germany and France at the time of writing this article, have been associated with a drastic fall in numbers of suitable donor organs by about 20%. Admittedly, other issues and phenomena, such as commerce in organ allocation in India, use of criminals as organ donors in China etc., have also contributed to the development of such public transplant crises. Nevertheless, the

G.M. Collins, J.M. Dubernard, W. Land and G.G. Persijn (eds). Procurement, Preservation and Allocation of Vascularized Organs 359–365
© 1997 Kluwer Academic Publishers.

definite lack of transparency in post mortem organ allocation policies should not be underestimated as a factor inducing mistrust within a community. In this situation, professionals working in the field of organ transplantation should try to react and undertake everything to restore public trust. Such reactions could include discussions of allocation problems operating on four levels: the ownership of donor organs; structure of the public participation; the transplant centre waiting lists versus regional (state) waiting lists; and organ allocation policies in the light of the three major modern theories of justice. These points will be discussed briefly below.

2. Ownership of cadaveric donor organs and allocation policy

The issue of ownership of transplantable organs is of utmost importance since the claim of making allocative decisions may be deduced from the issue of ownership. At the international conference on Ethics, Justice and Commerce in Organ Replacement Therapy in Munich, Dec. 1990, Congress resolution No. 8 claimed: 'Cadaveric organs procured within a community should be considered assets of the community, and the community rather than just the medical profession should determine their allocation through announced criteria' [2]. In the view of the participants, this wise resolution was in sharp contrast to the common conceptions about this issue during the past 20 years.

The history of development and establishment of post mortem organ procurement over the past two decades has been dominated by the profession-derived assumption that transplant surgeons and physicians (or institutions involved in organ procurement) are supposed to obtain (lawful) ownership of transplantable organs. This natural and, for professionals, convincing attitude of transplant surgeons and physicians culminated in the establishment and acceptance of the so-called 'local donor': transplantable organs which had been removed by explant surgeons of a (given) transplant centre from a cadaveric donor in their hospital or in a peripheral cooperating non-transplant hospital 'belonged' primarily and preferentially to the transplant team of that particular centre.

Many transplant centres all over the world claimed to have a right to set up own allocation policies in regard to these 'own' organs, particularly in the sense of treating their own patients on their own waiting lists. It has to be mentioned here that these self-made allocation policies of a centre in regard to organs from local donors did not usually violate the existing alloca-

tion rules of the official organ exchange institutions (organ procurement agencies) such as Eurotransplant in Europe. Those organ allocation rules represent superficial rules which determine the frame of allocation and are more or less guidelines which leave plenty of room for own allocative decisions of the centres on the basis of their own discretion. The practice of using a local donor is associated – quite naturally – with a violation of ethical values such as distributive justice, equity, equal access for all patients – values which appear to become more and more important in the field of organ allocation policies particularly from the public's point of view.

There is also a danger that such practice will lead to an increase of current public transplant crises since it carries the risk of a fight for cadaveric organs between competing transplant centres, as discussed by Guttmann [3]: '... in regions with multiple transplant centres that obtain donors from non-transplant hospitals, the ability to keep a kidney for one's own programme leads to competitive behaviour and "control of donors". Transfer or access to donors becomes the ticket to keeping at least one kidney, regardless of the allocation scheme. This is effected by professional connections, official and unofficial, rather than any logical principle of relationship.' The local donor practice – a policy in sharp contrast to congress resolution No. 8 (see above) – has been vehemently defended in the past by presenting the 'motivation and fairness' argument: local activities of transplant centres in the field of post mortem organ procurement (e.g. education of the public; contacts and cooperation with non-transplanting peripheral neighbour-hospitals) can only be maintained and/or maximized if transplantable organs from local donors are preferentially used for patients from the waiting list of that particular centre. The motivation of members of a transplant centre to do this unpleasant job is provided by the incentive of being able to treat their own patients (thus running a big 'prestige' transplant programme eventually in competition with other centres). Admittedly, this motivation argument may be regarded as acceptable on the basis of the paternalistic principle of the Hippocratic tradition. However, in view of the current multinational transplant crises it has to be criticized, because its practical meaning certainly contributes to the steadily-increasing mistrust of the public towards post mortem organ donation/allocation. The German and French populations are currently extremely sensitized against this whole matter so that the awareness of the existence of a transplant-centre controlled, decision-making mechanism of organ allocation, which potentially may bypass allocation systems based on medical, juridical and social factors, could totally kill their willingness to accept transplant medicine.

Thus, under the global and superior viewpoint to regain the trust and confidence of the public in the ethical probity of transplant surgeons and physicians, the practice of regarding cadaver organs as in the ownership of members of the transplant centre should be abandoned.

3. How can the public participate in setting allocation policy?

One of the recent well recognized and more widely accepted prerequisites for a fair and just organ allocation system is the discrimination between medical and justice-based factors. Medical allocation factors can be just factors, but are not necessarily so. Medical factors are established by professionals; justice factors, however, can only be worked out under close cooperation between professionals and the public. Indeed, it is becoming increasingly clear that the public has to be involved in the establishment of a fair setting of an equitable organ allocation system for a simple reason: organ transplantation represents on one hand a therapeutic modality (with responsibility only on the side of the professionals); on the other hand a distribution/allocation of a scarce valuable common good in which society is extremely interested.

Although there appears to be growing agreement amongst professionals that the public should be involved in the process of setting allocation policies in general, there is still a heavy debate on the issue of how intensive should this participation be. The current debate is here characterized by two completely different extreme opinions. At one extreme, there is the statement of complete and rigorous refusal of any competence of transplant professionals to make allocative decisions; at the other extreme, the statement of complete and rigorous refusal of any competence of non-professionals (= the public) to participate in allocative decision making.

The first opinion was put forward by Veatch [4], who saw no reason why the medical professional should be empowered at all to make allocative decisions. One argument is that the clinician (e.g. the liver transplant surgeon) is strongly committed to the welfare of his or her patient and therefore, because he does not see the clinical state of all the other patients waiting for a liver transplant at other transplant centres, he may come up with the wrong allocation decision. The second opinion was articulated by liver and heart transplant surgeons when addressing clinical urgency as a decisive alloca-

tion factor. Assuming that the clinical status of patient (A) and patient (B), both waiting for a liver transplant , is in favour of patient (A), he is supposed to receive the next available liver. The clinical status of patient (B) might, however, change within minutes (acute oesophageal bleeding), so that the next available liver must go to him. This kind of an acute allocative decision can only be made by the liver transplant surgeon him/herself and never by a non-professional: the surgeon who makes the urgent bed-side decision is fully responsible for the outcome of the operation.

All arguments in favour of the one or the other extreme position are well supported. Nevertheless, there seems to be a way by which both different opinions could be put together in a reasonable approach to the problem.

In terms of a close cooperation between professionals and the public. liver surgeons, for example, could establish a formula of organ allocation which weighs and balances clinical criteria such as urgency, expected medical benefit, need, equity, centre balance, and so forth and provide certain scores per each criterion. This formula, worked out in advance together with the public, enables a liver transplant surgeon to make his/her acute and proper allocative bed-side decision in the middle of the night at an urgent situation in full agreement with the 'public voice' but fully responsible on his/her own.

Accordingly, in kidney transplantation, the cooperation between professionals and a public body could lead to the design of a kidney allocation formula which includes. as well as medical factors, urgency factors and e.g. certain social factors. Those social factors, however, have been established on an individual patient basis prior to admission to the waiting list under appropriate assessment by the public board. When a surgeon accepts a kidney for a certain patient in the middle of the night. he is able to rely on the assessment which has been previously established by both the professional and the public board. The public compatibility of such an allocation policy worked out in close cooperation between professionals and the public could be further fortified if the public was allowed to supervise the system retrospectively in terms of a public surveillance of profession-oriented organ allocation systems.

One of the critical questions in the context of such a debate has always been: who is the public? Certainly, this is a still unanswered question. Nevertheless one could start to answer this issue by creating a committee consisting of e.g. a social worker, a nurse, a member of the community. representatives of the press and media, a representative of the dialysis group patients, a representative of a previously transplanted patients' group and so forth. Of course, as already pointed out above, such a group should not suddenly meet in the middle of the night to help the transplant surgeon in his/her allocative decision-making process at the bedside but rather should cooperate with the professionals in establishing guidelines for an appropriate allocative policy.

4. Is there a fair and just organ allocation in regard to the existence of transplant centre waiting lists?

The increasingly loud call for a guarantee of equal access for all patients within a region, state or nation to available donor organs, associated with growing efforts to include criteria of distributive justice in the daily practice of organ allocation, has focused the attention of health politicians and others on the problem of transplant centre waiting lists. The problem here is that instead and in view of a common allocation policy at the meso-allocation level, which is valid and in force for a certain number of transplant centres within a defined organ exchange area, the allocation of organs at the microallocation level differs from centre to centre within that particular area.

The reason for this paradoxical situation is illustrated by presenting the allocation policy of kidney transplants as applied in Germany*. The rules concern mandatory sharing and optional sharing: mandatory sharing has to be performed when (a) a recipient with a six HLA-antigen match is available at another transplant centre of this area and (b) there is no recipient with at least two HLA-DR (on DR/one B) compatibilities on the centre's own waiting list. If neither (a) or (b) is relevant, the kidneys can be kept at the centre where they were procured, with the expectation that they will be transplanted to recipients with optimal or good HLA matches. This latter situation is mostly encountered and accounts for the majority of uses of kidneys procured locally. Although allocation of these kidneys to patients on the centre's own list is expected and supposed to follow the dogma of best HLA matches, it leaves plenty of room for discretion for the medical colleagues responsible for local allocative decision-making. In addition to the use of medical factor, HLA matching, other allocative principles may be con-

sidered in this situation, such as the fidelity principle, the queuing principle, ability to pay principle (private patients), the squeaky wheel principle, and last but not least, the need of the 'programme' principle [5]. The policy of how many and what other principles of organ allocation from this list are used differs from centre to centre and depends entirely on the composition of the transplant team involved and charged with responsibility. Ultimately, the responsibility lies in the hands of the leader of the transplant programme.

Since different transplant centres, particularly in one common region, are in competition as far as recruitment of patients for a waiting list, application for funds, gaining of prestige and reputation etc. are concerned, their major goal must be to present successful transplant programmes. One important prerequisite for a successful programme, however, is a high number of transplanted patients. In addition, at least in Germany and other European countries, a high number of kidney transplantations/year has also to be performed in order to reach sufficient and efficient financial support by the insurance companies: fewer transplantations than expected and originally calculated jeopardize continuation of financial support of the programme.

A summary of the situation presented here clearly indicates that the centre-controlled kidney allocation policy of organs removed from local donors differs from centre to centre depending on the centre's policy to use, in addition to the medical allocation factors, other principles. Interestingly enough, variation in a centre's allocation policy is not possible if a kidney transplant is offered to the centre by Eurotransplant directly. This offer which is always directed to a particular given patient on the centre's waiting list, follows strictly and exclusively the principle of an optimal HLA match.

The practice of different centre-controlled allocation policies in regard to the use of organs from local donors leads automatically to distributive injustice and inequality of organ allocation in regard to all patients who are waiting for a kidney transplant on the separate centre's waiting list within that particular area/region. We are dealing here with an international problem which has also already been addressed by health politicians. For instance, Senator Edward Kennedy (USA) claimed: 'A patient waiting for an organ in one state should not have a substantially longer or shorter waiting time than a patient in similar condition in another state' [6]. Many arguments call for common state/regional waiting lists (e.g. regions of about 10–15

---

*Meanwhile, these allocation rules have been replaced by a strict, transparent scoring system (Eurotransplant) which guarantees an optical degree of fair, centre-independent, patient-oriented allocation.

million inhabitants). This alone would guarantee a successful approach to distributive justice and equality in the daily practice of allocating organs for all patients of that particular state/region. Another advantage of such common regional waiting lists appears to be evident: the adoption and introduction of 'scoring systems' for optimal organ allocation, including potential social factors, seem to be more realistic from the logistical point of view. Last but not least, such a system would contribute to an increase in the credibility of transplant professionals in view of the public.

5. Organ allocation and the role of the three major modern theories of justice: utilitarianism, egalitarianism and libertarianism

The search for an organ allocation system which provides a maximum of distributive justice poses another problem: which of the three major modern theories of justice should predominantly be followed in the field of organ allocation? In order to answer this question properly, a short look at their role and their potential meaning in the field of organ transplantation appears to be indicated. It seems of interest to sort out those aspects of each theory which would promise some merits when discussed in regard to a reasonable practice of organ allocation. The following considerations are closely based on the work of Churchill [7].

5.1. Utilitarianism

Utilitarian theories reference the rightness or wrongness of actions or policies to the good or bad consequences they generate. While egalitarian theories emphasize intrinsic worth, utilitarian approaches avoid judging policies by the intention of such policies and make judgements of rightness based on the empirical results. Right acts and policies are those which result in the most good achieved, or the greatest net happiness for the greatest number [7]. Current policies in kidney transplantation follow utilitarian theories extensively. A single principle – HLA-matching – rather than a complex work of rules and maxims, references to outcomes and events, namely long graft survival times (associated with a minimum of transplant rejections) in the largest number of kidney transplant recipients. In fact, many multicentre as well as single centre studies have clearly shown that both short-term and long-term kidney allograft survival is statistically

positively influenced by HLA matching. Controversial papers on this matter have been and are still being published, however. The main advantage of the utilitarian approach in kidney allocation, besides its simplicity, is that it fits very nicely into the conceptions of tissue typers and transplant clinicians who believe in the value of HLA-matching. Nevertheless, it has to be stressed that many absurdities are associated with this type of allocation policy [3].

The main disadvantage of the utilitarian approach in the sense of using the HLA match principle is its distributive injustice with regard to the varying waiting time of patients for a suitable renal transplant. For example, the principle of a good HLA match as a main medical allocation factor may allow that, within a period of 8 years, a particular patient has been transplanted thrice (always with a good HLA match), whereas during the same time period, another patient is still waiting for his/her first allograft (because e.g. of a rare HLA constellation). Another disadvantage becomes evident: a standard for justice which is referenced solely to outcomes must rely on the ability to predict outcomes on an individual basis correctly. All transplant clinicians, however, know very well that this dogma is not always guaranteed in transplanted patients. A kidney allocated and transplanted to a patient because of a six HLA antigen match (an ideal immunological situation with long graft survival expectancy) may be lost at the second postoperative day as a result of primary venous thrombosis.

The question which has to be raised at this point has been formulated by Churchill [7] – does the emphasis on the greatest happiness mean that great suffering for a few can be tolerated so long as the vast majority benefit? Would this encourage neglect of patients to achieve the greater social good?

Perhaps these questions indicate why the utilitarian theory of justice cannot satisfy the public completely (nor all patients), although it is well accepted by the majority of transplant professionals because it sounds so reasonable for medical doctors.

5.2. Egalitarianism

'Egalitarian theories emphasize similarities or equalities amongst persons. Such theories typically embrace sections of intrinsic worth, that is, those aspects of persons which are not instrumental to achieving some other good, but in terms of which persons are to be valued for their own sake. Egalitarian theories of health care distribution focus on the need for services as the basic criterion in allocation, rather than money, insurance, social class or other factors ... Egalitarian theories are supported by recognition not only of the equal intrinsic worth of persons, but by a com-mon human vulner-ability to disease, disability and death ...' [7].

Rawls [8] contends that inequalities in the distribution of the primary goods of a society can be tolerated only if these inequalities are to everyone's advantage. Inequalities in allocation of scarce transplantable organs in terms of a simpler definition can, indeed, be encountered frequently: there are certain categories/groups of patients who are preferentially transplanted in comparison to other patient categories/groups. As a result, there are groups of patients who either experience extremely long waiting times or are not transplanted at all. Such inequalities are either due to the pure application and nature of medical allocation factors only (worked out by the professionals), such as HLA matching/certain clinical urgency states, or due to centre-dependent modification of allocation rules which diverge from generally accepted rules within an organ exchange region. Classical examples of inequalities in this sense include the existence of a rare HLA pattern in a group of patients which prevents kidney transplantation due to a lack of HLA-compatibilities, and lack of a standardized, generally accepted evaluation of a clinical urgency state in heart/liver transplantation. The definition of clinical urgency (followed by preferred allocation of a heart/liver) is based on the individual assessment of the programme director of a heart/liver transplant programme, and thus may vary from centre to centre. There will also be more frequent use of kidneys from local donors with a loose application of good HLA matching in one centre (leading to more rapid transplantation of patients of that centre's waiting list) in comparison to another centre which sticks strictly to an optimal HLA-match as prerequisite for any transplantation. It is obvious from those examples, and there are many more, that allocation of organs at the present does not follow the principle of 'intrinsic worth' of patients. Egalitarian approaches are not favoured by professionals, but might be favoured by the public, who do not see organ transplantation as a therapeutic modality only but also as a distribution of a scarce common health care good. Nevertheless, egalitarian approaches should at least be discussed by transplant clinicians. Such appoaches would include the discussion of only one single transplantation trial per patient (hard to accept by medical doctors since retransplantation belongs to the therapeutic repertoire of every transplant clinician and acts as an allocation factor in terms of the fidelity principle). In addition, the establishment of a clearcut standardization of clinical urgency status in heart and liver transplantation (with supervision by an ethical committee) should also be considered.

Surveillance of a standardized allocation policy of each transplant centre within a region would also contribute to the acceptance of egalitarian ideas in the field of organ allocation. Altogether, the introduction of at least some conceptions of egalitarians into the current practice of organ allocation would certainly contribute to a decrease of public mistrust.

5.3. Libertarianism

'Libertarian approaches to justice stand in stark contrast to the two previously discussed. Whereas both egalitarian and utilitarian approaches present alternative conceptions of the common good, libertarian thinking denies the existence of a common good altogether ... Libertarianism, as the name suggests, values liberty, and the cardinal virtues -- courage, loyalty, respect for others, beneficence – are not also valued, but only liberty is a fundamental right' [7].

Sade [9], a convinced libertarian, claims that since a physician owns his professional skills, he is entitled to do with them as he pleases. The strengths of libertarian thinking are obvious, at least to many Americans. The US health care system is basically libertarian in orientation [7]. In Europe, in regard to our past and current allocation policies, libertarian features can definitely be found. The preferential use of organs from a local donor by certain explant teams, as mentioned above, is just one example. Perhaps, there is still room for a libertarian approach of organ allocation in situations of acute developing clinical urgencies (e.g. in heart and liver transplantation) when the responsible transplant surgeon has to make a definite final bed-side decision for his/her patient without considering other patients on the waiting lists. Such libertarian approaches should, however, really be restricted to such clinically urgent situations and should not become a feature of general allocation policies, at least not in Europe. In view of the current public transplant crises, libertarian theories would certainly increase the public's mistrust and weaken the transplanters' credibility. Perhaps, the time may return when the current problems are solved, to reconsider libertarian approaches in the field of organ allocation in an extremely balanced way, since they are very attractive for a majority of transplant clinicians.

References

1. Veatch RM. Theories of medical ethics: the professional model compared with the societal model. In: Lands W, Dossetor JB (eds), Organ Replacement Therapy: Ethics, Justice, Commerce. Springer-Verlag, Berlin 1991; pp. 3–12.

2. Congress Resolutions. In: Lands W, Dossetor JB (eds), Organ Replacement Therapy: Ethics, Justice, Commerce. Springer-Verlag, Berlin 1991; p. 556.

3. Guttmann RD. Facing organ allocation issues: an insider's view from the New World. In: Lands W, Dossetor JB (eds), Organ Replacement Therapy: Ethics, Justice, Commerce. Springer-Verlag, Berlin 1991; pp. 410–18.

4. Veatch RM. Who empowers medical doctors to make allocative decisions for dialysis and organ transplantation? In: Lands W, Dossetor JB (eds), Organ Replacement Therapy: Ethics, Justice, Commerce. Springer-Verlag, Berlin 1991; pp. 331–6.

5. Dossetor, JB. Principles used in organ allocation. In: Lands W, Dossetor JB (eds), Organ Replacement Therapy:

Ethics, Justice, Commerce. Springer-Verlag, Berlin 1991; pp. 393–8.

6. Warren J. Transplant Newsl 1993; 3: 82.

7. Churchill LR. Theories of justice. In: Kjellstrand CM, Dossetor JB (eds). Ethical Problems in Dialysis and Transplantation. Kluwer Academic Publishers. Dordrecht 1992; pp. 21–34.

8. Rawls J. A theory of medical ethics. Harvard University Press, Cambridge, MA 1971.

9. Sade R. Medical care as a right: a refutation. N Engl J Med 1971; 285: 1288.

45 | Living unrelated kidney transplantation

GIL THIEL

1. Introduction

The first experience with living unrelated kidney transplantation was reported in 1967 from the transplant centre in Denver, where 23 out of the first 75 living kidney donor transplants were from unrelated volunteers [1]. Although not stated in the paper, some of the volunteers were prisoners, who deliberately offered one kidney to unknown recipients in order to reduce their sentence. This form of living kidney donation would nowadays be called LURD (living unrelated renal donation), which includes all forms of living kidney donations, including purchased kidneys. Emotionally related living kidney donations (ERLKD), however, are a very distinct subgroup of LURD, to which this chapter is solely devoted.

ERLKD is the donation of a kidney by a non-blood-related donor to a recipient with whom the donor is emotionally closely linked. The motive for the donation must be credible on close examination and must be free from material reasons (monetary payment, debt reimbursement, gift, etc.). The donation must occur voluntarily, without any form of external pressure. A typical example of a donor is the recipient's spouse or partner. However, it can also be much more far-reaching: it could include the father-in-law, the aunt of the wife, childhood friend, etc. ERLKD is a form of LURD but, by definition, excludes all LURDs that are based on a purchased kidney or on an emotionally unrelated volunteer's kidney.

The history of ERLKD in Europe has not yet been well documented. In particular, it is not known when and where isolated cases of ERLKD took place. Of the three European centres which have officially included ERLKD in their regular practice, the first ERLKD occurred in Rome on 12 December 1983 (D. Alfani, personal communication), in Oslo on 3 October 1984 (A. Jacobsen, personal communication), and in Basel on 16 May 1991. LURDs, however, were sporadically performed in Brussels as early as 1966 [2] and most probably also in other European centres. It is interesting to note that ERLKD is prohibited by law in France today and was also meant to be prohibited in the first draft of the new German transplantation law in 1994 – this has meanwhile been altered.

Relatively few LURDs have been carried out in Europe in 1995, to our knowledge 45. In the annual report of Eurotransplant of 1995 twelve ERLKDs are mentioned (Freiburg i.Brg. 3, Innsbruck 2, München 2, Rotterdam 2, Bruxelles 1 and Halle 1) in contrast to 211 living related kidney transplantations (5.7%). During 1995 another 14 ERLKDs were performed in Oslo, 11 in Rome and 8 in Switzerland (7 in Basel and one in Bern). No ERLKD was performed in France or Spain in 1995. Thus, there are large differences from country to country and from centre to centre.

A dynamic development away from prohibition and towards general acceptance is taking place, a move which would have seemed unthinkable a few years ago. For example, since the 1970s in German-speaking areas, living donations have been viewed as unethical because they can cause harm to healthy donors (*primum nil nocere*). Since the International Congress on Ethics and Transplantation in Munich in 1990 [3] it has become clear, to the surprise of many nephrologists, that professional ethical philosophers have fewer difficulties with voluntary living donations than with the removal of an organ from a cadaver.

G.M. Collins, J.M. Dubernard, W. Land and G.G. Persijn (eds). Procurement, Preservation and Allocation of Vascularized Organs 367–373
© 1997 Kluwer Academic Publishers.

2. Arguments in favour of ERLKD

The main arguments for and against ERLKD are partly shared with those for living donations in general. There are seven main arguments in favour of ERLKD:

1. The increasing waiting list for cadaveric kidneys (with the exception of Spain) and the stagnating or decreasing number of cadaver organ donations.
2. The positive transplantation results of ERLKD, with > 90% success rates after one year, despite poor HLA matches [2,4–9]. Recently, however, excellent results of spouse transplantation have been reported by two international registries [10,11] (Figures 1 and 2). A good outcome of living kidney donation despite a zero HLA match has also been described [12].
3. The strong motivation of the ERLKD donor, comparable to that of parents donating to their children.

4. There is often a direct personal advantage for the donor. Spouses in particular profit directly from the success of the transplantation, in a manner that cannot be compared with the donation between siblings. When we informed the first non-blood-related Swiss donor in 1991 that we would accept her as a donor for her brother or sister but not for her husband, she answered spontaneously, 'You cannot imagine how much I would rather donate a kidney to my husband than to one of my brothers or sisters. I share the fate of his illness with him everyday.' For us, this broke down the barrier against non-blood-related living donations.
5. The possibility, with proper planning, of by-passing dialysis completely, i.e. opting for ERLKD or relative living donation instead of dialysis as soon as kidney replacement therapy is needed. Whenever a chronic progressive renal insufficiency is diagnosed, and the estimated time before dialysis is one or two years, we start the search for a related living donor or a possible

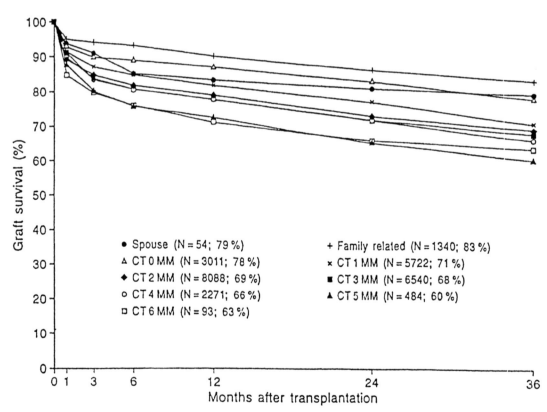

Figure 1. Results of kidney graft with spousal donors (Eurotransplant). Survival of spouse-donated renal grafts compared with first renal cadaveric transplantation. At 3 years spouse donors have the same graft survival as cadaveric first renal transplant (CT) with zero HLA mismatches (0MM).

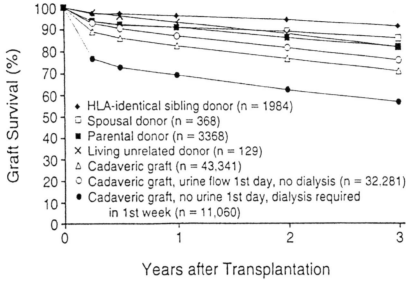

Figure 2. Results of first kidney grafts from spousal donors (UNOS). Up to 3 years from the United Network for Organ Sharing (UNOS) [11]. The living unrelated donors did not include spouses. Spousal donors did at least as well the non-HLA-identical sibling donors.

ERLKD. If dialysis can be avoided, the resulting advantages are substantial for the affected person (quality of life, no time loss due to dialysis treatment, maintained full employment etc.), for the health insurance companies (elimination of dialysis costs), and for the state (elimination of disability allowances). Patients suffering from progressive renal failure and their family and friends should be encouraged to consider ERLKD.

6. The experience that a donation between non-blood-related but emotionally linked people causes much fewer psychological problems than transplantation between siblings. Siblings may not have lived together for many years, may share inherited problems, or may have spouses that do not get along with each other.

7. Surprisingly, ERLKD also raises far fewer ethical objections and psychological resistance from the medical and nursing staff within a hospital than does a cadaver kidney transplantation programme with its associated problems about the diagnosis and care of the brain-dead and their use as organ donors.

3. Arguments against ERLKD

There are also seven main arguments against ERLKD and living donation in general:

1. *Primum nil nocere* is the oldest and strongest argument. The utilitarian point of view (the end justifies the means) [13,14] is countered with the deontological (the end never justifies the means) [15]. Early complications described are wound infections, urinary tract infections, bleeding wounds that require surgical revision, thrombophlebitis, and pulmonary emboli occurring at a rate between 0.2 and 5.9% [16,17] (Table 1). The perioperative mortality lies between 0.06 and 0.03% [16,18–20]. Late complications are primarily scar problems, hypertension, and proteinuria. Late and mild incisional pain was reported in 10.5% and incisional hernia in 3.6% [17]. Hypertension occurs in 8.5–48% of living kidney donors (males often than females) but not more often than in a similar age group of the population and not more often then in siblings who are not nephrectomized and do not have a renal disease (hereditary component of hypertension in such families) [16,17,20–25] (Table 2). Thus, there is doubt as to the causality between kidney donation and later hypertension.

Hyperfiltration [26,27] and, after some years, proteinuria occurs in up to 39% of donors [16,20–25] (Table 3). The proteinuria is mostly in a range of 150–750 mg/day. However, the Brenner working group was not successful in documenting a progressive increase in proteinuria and a reduction in kidney function even late after kidney

Table 1. Intra-operative and immediate post-operative complications associated with kidney donor nephrectomy.

Acute complications	Weiland *et al.* [17]	Dunn *et al.* [16]
Total number of donors	628	314
Wound infections	2.2%	3.5%
Urinary tract infections	4.7%	2.9%
Urinary retention	n.m.	2.2%
Pulmonary atelectasis alone	5.9%	n.m.
Pulmonary atelectasis/fever	n.m.	34.7%
Pneumonia	3.0%	0.6%
Pneumothorax	4.0%	n.m.
Pulmonary oedema	1.8%	n.m.
Pulmonary embolus	0.5%	0.3%
Tracheostomy	0.3%	n.m.
Severe wound bleeding	0.6% (re-operation)	0.6% (retroperitoneal)
Thrombophlebitis (superfic.)	0.5%	1.9%
Adrenalectomy	0.3%	0.3%
Splenectomy	0.2%	0.9%
Acute depression	n.m.	0.6%
Transcient hypertension	n.m.	1.3%
Total	17.0% (107/628)	46.8% (147/314)

The overall frequency of acute complications (46.8%) in Nashville [11] includes the post-operative rise of temperature, which is not the case for Minneapolis and the analysis [16] (17.0%)
n.m. = not mentioned

donation [22]. Williams *et al.* in Philadelphia and Miller *et al.* in New York were equally unsuccessful [23,25] as we were in a study of living kidney donors up to 21 years after donation [28].

2. Criticism has been rightly directed at the lack of insurance coverage in case of a catastrophe following the kidney donation. If, for example, a young father were to die during a kidney donation due to an anaesthetic incident, there is at present no institutionalized donor life insurance available which would provide financial aid to the surviving dependents. The donor should also be automatically insured against a possible need for dialysis, so that she/he can obtain it without incurring any personal costs. In Germany, there is a case of a retired live donor who required dialysis years after donating his kidney but, lacking adequate insurance, had to pay partially out of his own pocket, thereby ruining himself financially. A mailed questionnaire to 70 life insurance companies in the United States revealed that all would be willing to insure healthy living kidney donors and only one company would have raised the premium for such an individual [14]. This inquiry asked, however, for the willingness to insure donors after donation while we would look for cover to include the operation.

3. How voluntary can a donation really be? If a partner asks for the donation of a kidney, is it possible to say no without a lack of love and solidarity being assumed? Is there not some hidden form of pressure for a donation?

4. On the other hand, does the result of this great gift later imply the obligation to eternal gratitude and fidelity? How can one ever leave a partner who has donated one a kidney?

5. There are also immunological doubts. The HLA match between spouses is usually poor. It is not unusual for a complete mismatch to occur. Can one risk such a transplantation at all? A woman who has borne the children of her spouse may be immunologically sensitized against him.

6. Anybody agreeing to a kidney life donation programme between non-blood relatives could, in the course of time, become more generous with the criteria for accepting donors. With the first non-related living donations begins the 'slippery slope' which may start slowly but could steadily lead to commercial living donations. At the EDTA Congress in Amsterdam in 1996, during a discussion of the pros and cons of non-related living kidney donation. several nephrologists from developing countries in the audience warned that the official acceptance of the non-relative living donation in Europe could lead to criminal misuse in their countries.

7. A strong objection is, finally, the fear that with the spread of both relative and non-relative living donations, efforts to promote cadaver organ donations would decrease further. On the other hand,

Table 2. Rate of hypertension in relation to the years after donation

Study	Incidence
Miller *et al.* (New York) [23] (≥ 2 to 15 years after donation) ≥ 160/90 mmHg	31% (9/29)
Weiland *et al.* (Minneapolis) [17] (≥ 3 years after donation) diastolic blood pressure ≥ 90 mmHg	8.5% (40/472)
Talseth *et al.* (Oslo) [24] (≥ 9.9 years after donation) diastolic blood pressure ≥ 90 mmHg	15% (10/68)
Anderson *et al.* (Rochester) [21] (≥ 10 years after donation) hypertension not defined	19% (19/100)
Dunn *et al.* (Minneapolis) [16] (≥ 10 years after donation) blood pressure ≥ 160/95 mmHg	22% (4/19)
Hakim *et al.* (Boston) [22] (≥ 10 years after donation) diastolic blood pressure ≥ 90 mmHg	48% (25/52)
Williams *et al.* (Philadelphia) [25] (≥ 10 years after donation) blood pressure ≥ 140 / ≥ 90 or on antihypertensive drugs	47% (18/38)
Najarian *et al.* (Minneapolis) [20] (≥ 20 years after donation) on antihypertensive drugs	32% (20/63)

Table 3. Incidence and degree of proteinuria late after donation

Study	Incidence
Dunn *et al.* (Nashville) [16] (≥ 6 months to 14.5 years after donation) proteinuria ≥ 150 mg/day (max. 300 mg/day)	5% (6/137)
Miller *et al.* (New York) [23] (≥ 2 to 15 years after donation) proteinuria > 150 mg/day	39% (14/36)
Talseth *et al.* (Oslo) [24] (≥ 9.9 years after donation) proteinuria > 185 mg/day proteinuria > 500 mg/day (688–5790 mg/day)	24% (16/67) 6% (4/67)
Anderson *et al.* (Rochester) [21] (≥ 10 years after donation) proteinuria > 95 mg/day	13% (13/100)
Hakim *et al.* (Boston) [22] (≥ 10 years after donation) proteinuria > 250 mg/day proteinuria > 500 mg/day	25% (13/51) 8% (4/51)
Williams *et al.* (Philadelphia) [25] (≥ 10 years after donation) proteinuria > 150 mg/day	10/38 (26%)
Najarian *et al.* (Minnesota) [20] (≥ 20 years after donation) proteinuria > 150 mg/day proteinuria > 500 mg/day (521–750 mg/day)	23% (12/52) 6% (3/52)

it should be noted that in Spain in 1995 it was possible to harvest enough cadaveric kidneys to shorten the waiting list without carrying out one single ERLKD. Living kidney donations would thus not be necessary if the cadaver kidney resources were fully utilized, as has happened in Spain and similarly in Austria. The inadequate number of transplantable cadaveric kidneys arises not from a lack of suitable donors, but rather the failure to make potential donors actual donors [29].

4. Discussion and outlook

Anyone wishing to start an ERLKD programme must be thoroughly familiar with the arguments for and against ERLKD and adapt his own programme accordingly. The early complications must be made clear to the potential donor in advance and measures must be taken to avoid them. Venous thrombosis and emboli, for example, can be largely prevented. Kidney donation by women does not lead to later pregnancy complications, so that younger females who plan to have children in the future need not be advised against donation [30]. In the current experiences of the prospective Swiss living donations register [31], it seems that microalbuminuria in the donor is often connected to insufficiently or untreated hypertension. The donation must therefore be linked with careful post-operative monitoring of the kidney donor. A systematic search must be made for the occurrence of a microalbuminuria and hypertension, and treatment must be started. The interest of an ERLKD centre in a donor must not end the moment the kidney has been donated.

The problem of the poor insurance coverage for kidney donors can no longer be accepted [34]. The rare occurrence of a catastrophe (this has not yet happened in Switzerland) should keep the insurance premium for an obligatory living donor risk insurance low. The premium payment should initially be borne by the institution, which profits most from the saving of dialysis costs.

An independent donor advocate, preferably from outside the transplantation team (in Basel, for example, it is the Department of Psychosomatics of the University), must be given the task of trying to identify any living donor candidate who feels forced into the donation but dares not speak freely about it. Such a person should be helped to word a refusal and give a plausible reason, if possible with a solid physical basis (positive cross-match, too great a bodily risk, etc.), which does not compromise the relationship with the recipient. It should be pointed out that donors who were questioned years later, in the few investigations available at present, have almost without exception expressed themselves as feeling positive about the donation [32,33].

Every transplantation team which has traditionally made efforts to find a proper HLA match, must first surmount its own psychological barriers if it wishes to transplant fully incompatible partner kidneys. Two multicentre statistics and several single centre analyses are proof of the success [2,4–11]. It is difficult to find an immunological reason for this. A possible mechanism is the avoidance of the ischaemic reperfusion damage which strengthens the immunogenicity of cadaver kidney transplants (ischaemia-induced expression of DR and adhesion molecules).

Although the 'slippery slope' argument is anti-innovative, it must not be totally ignored. Anyone who begins an ERLKD programme undertakes the responsibility strictly to avoid any commercial organ purchase in his programme and region. The only obvious weak points are profit-oriented private clinics, which lack neurosurgery and intensive care units and have no access to cadaver organs but who could start a commercial living donor programme under the label 'emotionally related'. Thus it is recommended that right from the start living kidney donor transplantation be permitted only in large public hospitals. The fears that European recommendations could be misused in developing countries can then be no grounds for delaying good, non-commercial programmes in Europe.

Finally, the argument that cadaver organ donations will suffer at the expense of an active living donor programme should be taken seriously, and at the same time the experience of Spain should be kept in mind. The success of the Spain cadaveric organ transplant programme is coupled to the activity of a large number of well trained transplant co-ordinators in all transplant centres (often more than one per centre), composed mostly of intensive care physicians. In contrast, for example in Switzerland, we have barely a single nurse working as transplant co-ordinator at transplant centres. Currently, there are also lively political and psychological streams in some of the German speaking regions that are aimed against brain death diagnosis and cadaver organ acquisition. The success of cadaveric organ harvesting in Austria is largely based on a traditional system of presumed consent, without a need to ask the relatives for their permission to perform an autopsy or to remove organs. The majority of families do not, therefore, know that organs have been removed from their brain-dead relatives. This, however, would not find a politically sustainable majority in Germany and Switzerland and would not be used by many intensive unit medical doctors and anaesthetists who are responsible for the care of the brain dead, even if it would be legally allowed by now. It therefore seems rather unlikely, on financial, political and psychological grounds, that the Spanish and Austrian recipe for success can be simply copied in Germany or Switzerland.

It is thus tempting to give preference to the living donor and to dispense with the diminishing cadaver organ donations (when comparing the first half-year of 1994 to that of 1996, a reduction of over 50% in Switzerland is noted). This would, however, be detrimental to all those who do not possess a motivated living donor and especially for all those who require an urgent heart, lung or liver transplant. Anyone who starts an ERLKD programme should also actively promote cadaveric organ donation within his centre and supply area. ERLKD is not a substitute for cadaveric organ donation, only a welcome addition.

There is a great probability that ERLKD will be a success, not at the expense of cadaver kidney transplants but rather at that of dialysis. Presently, too little use is made of the emotional motivation of donors from the social circle of the partner, close friends, relatives by marriage, etc. Greater quality of life and socio-economic advantages will help make a primary transplantation acceptable in place of dialysis. People suffering from progressive renal diseases will less frequently be refused the possibility of a primary living donor transplantation instead of dialysis. Moreover nephrologists will have to learn to look in time for emotionally related donors, when closely related kidney donors are not available. Nephrologists, transplantation clinicians and even family doctors should raise awareness in chronically ill renal disease patients of the possibility of ERLKD [34,35] and motivate them to prepare for this eventuality.

References

1. Ogden DA. Donor and recipient function 2 to 4 years after renal homotransplantation. Ann Intern Med 1967; 67: 998–1006.
2. Squifflet JP, Pirson Y. Poncelet A, Gianello P, Alexandre GPJ. Unrelated living kidney transplantation. Transplant Int 1990; 3: 32–5.
3. Land W, Dossetor JB (eds). Organ replacement therapy: ethics, justice and commerce. Springer Verlag, Berlin, 1991.
4. Alfani D, Pretagostini R, Rossi M et al. Living unrelated kidney transplantation: a 12 year single-center experience. Transplant Proc 1997; 29:191–4.
5. Berloco P, Alfani D, Bruzzone P et al. Is unrelated living donor a valid organ source in renal transplantation? Transplant Proc 1991; 23: 912–13.
6. Binet I, Bock AH.Vogelbach P et al. Outcome in emotionally related living kidney donor transplantation. Nephrol Dial Transplant 1997. In press.
7. Pirsch JD, Sollinger HW, Kalayoglu M et al. Living unrelated renal transplantation: results in 40 patients. Am J Kidney Dis 1988; 12: 499–503.
8. Sollinger HW, Kalayoglu M, Belzer FO. Use of the donor specific transfusion protocol in living unrelated donor-recipient combinations. Ann Surg 1986; 204: 315–19.
9. Abouna GM, Panjiwani D, Kumar MSA et al. The living unrelated donor – a viable alternative for renal transplantation. Transplant Proc 1988; 20: 802–4.
10. Smits JMA, Persijn CG, De Meester JMJ. Living unrelated transplantation: the new alternative? Transplant Int 1996; 9: 252.
11. Terasaki PI, Cecka JM, Gjerston DW, Takemoto S. High survival rates of kidneys from spousal and living unrelated donors. New Engl J Med 1995; 333: 333–6.
12. Jones JW, Gillingham KJ, Sutherland DER et al. Successful long-term outcome with 0-haplotype-matched living related kidney donors. Transplantation 1994; 57: 512–5.
13. Guttmann T. Living kidney transplantation: aspects of legal philosophy. Zeitschr Transplmed 1993; 5: 75–87.
14. Spital A, Spital M. Kidney donation: reflections. Am J Nephrol 1987; 7: 49–54.
15. Kant I. Die Metaphysik der Sitten (1797). Reclam (Ditzingen) 1996.
16. Dunn JF, Richie RR, MacDonell RC, Nylander WA, Johnson HK, Sawyers JL. Living related kidney donors – a 14 year experience. Ann Surg 1986; 203: 637–43.

17. Weiland D, Sutherland DER. Chavers B. Simmons RL. Ascher NL, Najarian JS. Information on 628 living-related kidney donors at a single institution with long-term follow-up in 472 cases. Transplant Proc 1984; 16: 5–7.
18. Bay WH, Hebert LA. The living donor in kidney transplantation. Ann Intern Med 1987; 106: 719–27.
19. Levey AS, Hou S, Bush HL. Kidney transplantation from unrelated living donors: time to reclaim a discarded opportunity. New Engl J Med 1986; 314: 914–16.
20. Najarian JS, Chavers BM, McHugh LE, Matas AJ. 20 years or more of follow-up of living kidney donors. Lancet 1992; 340: 807–10.
21. Anderson CF. Velosa JE, Frohnert PP et al. The risks of unilateral nephrectomy: status of kidney donors 10 to 20 years postoperative. Mayo Clin Proc 1985; 60: 367–74.
22. Hakim RM, Goldszer RC. Brenner BM. Hypertension and proteinuria: long-term sequelae of uninephrectomy in humans. Kidney Int 1984; 25: 930–6.
23. Miller J, Suthanthiran M, Riggio RR et al. Impact of renal donation: Long-term clinical and biochemical follow-up of living donors in a single centre. Am J Med 1985; 79: 201–8.
24. Talseth T, Fauchald P. Skrede S et al. Long-term blood pressure and renal function in kidney donors. Kidney Int 1986; 29: 1072–6.
25. Williams SL. Oler J, Jorkasky K. Long-term renal function in kidney donors: a comparison of donors and their siblings. Ann Intern Med 1986; 105: 1–8.
26. Bock, A, Gregor M, Huser B, Rist M, Landmann J, Thiel G. Glomeruläre Hyperfiltration nach unilateraler Nephrektomie bei Gesunden. Schweiz Med Wschr 1991; 121: 1833–5.
27. Terwee P, Tegzess AM, Donke Ab JM. Pair tested renal reserve filtration capacity in kidney recipients and donors. JASN 1994; 4: 1798–808.
28. Spartà G. Basler Lebend-Nierenspender. 1 bis 21 Jahre danach. Thesis, University of Basle. 1994.
29. Kreis H. Why living related donors should not be used whenever possible. Transplant Proc 1985; 17: 1510–14.
30. Buszta C, Steinmüller DR. Novick AC et al. Pregnancy after donor nephrectomy. Transplantation 1985; 40: 651–4.
31. Thiel G. The Swiss living kidney donor registry since 1993. Kidney Int. 1996; 50: 1436.
32. Sharma VK. Enoch MD. Psychological sequelae of kidney donation. A 5–10 year follow-up study. Acta Psychiat Scand 1987; 75: 264–67.
33. Spartà G, Thiel G. How living related kidney donors think about their organ donation 1 to 21 years later. Kidney Int 1993; 44: 262.
34. Daar AS. Living-organ donation: time for a donor charter. In: Terasaki PI. Cecka JM (eds). Clinical Transplants 1994. UCLA Tissue Typing Laboratory. Los Angeles 1995, pp. 376–80.
35. Spital A. Do US transplant centers encourage emotionally related kidney donation? Transplantation 1996; 61: 374–77.
36. Spital A. Life insurance for kidney donors – an update. Transplantation 1988; 45: 819–20.

Index

G.M. Collins, J.M. Dubernard, W. Land and G.G. Persijn (eds). Procurement, Preservation and Allocation of Vascularized Organs 375–381
© 1997 Kluwer Academic Publishers.